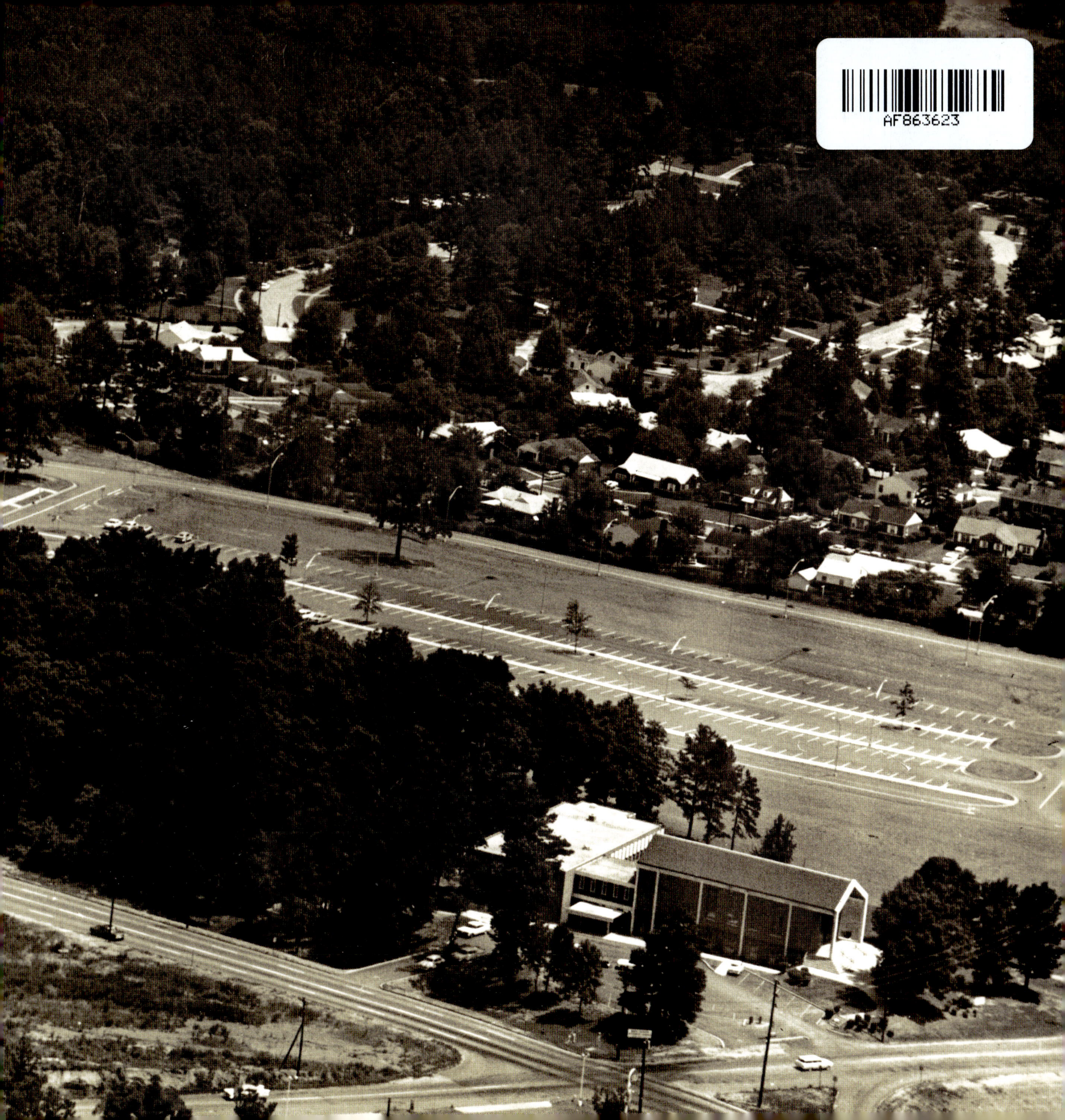

AF863623

The DeKalb Medical Story

Mytch Stubbs

Susan Parry

THE DEKALB MEDICAL STORY

FROM BERRY PATCH TO HEALTHCARE SYSTEM 1957–2007

Written by Wytch Stubbs, MD
& Susan Parry, RN

DeKalb Medical

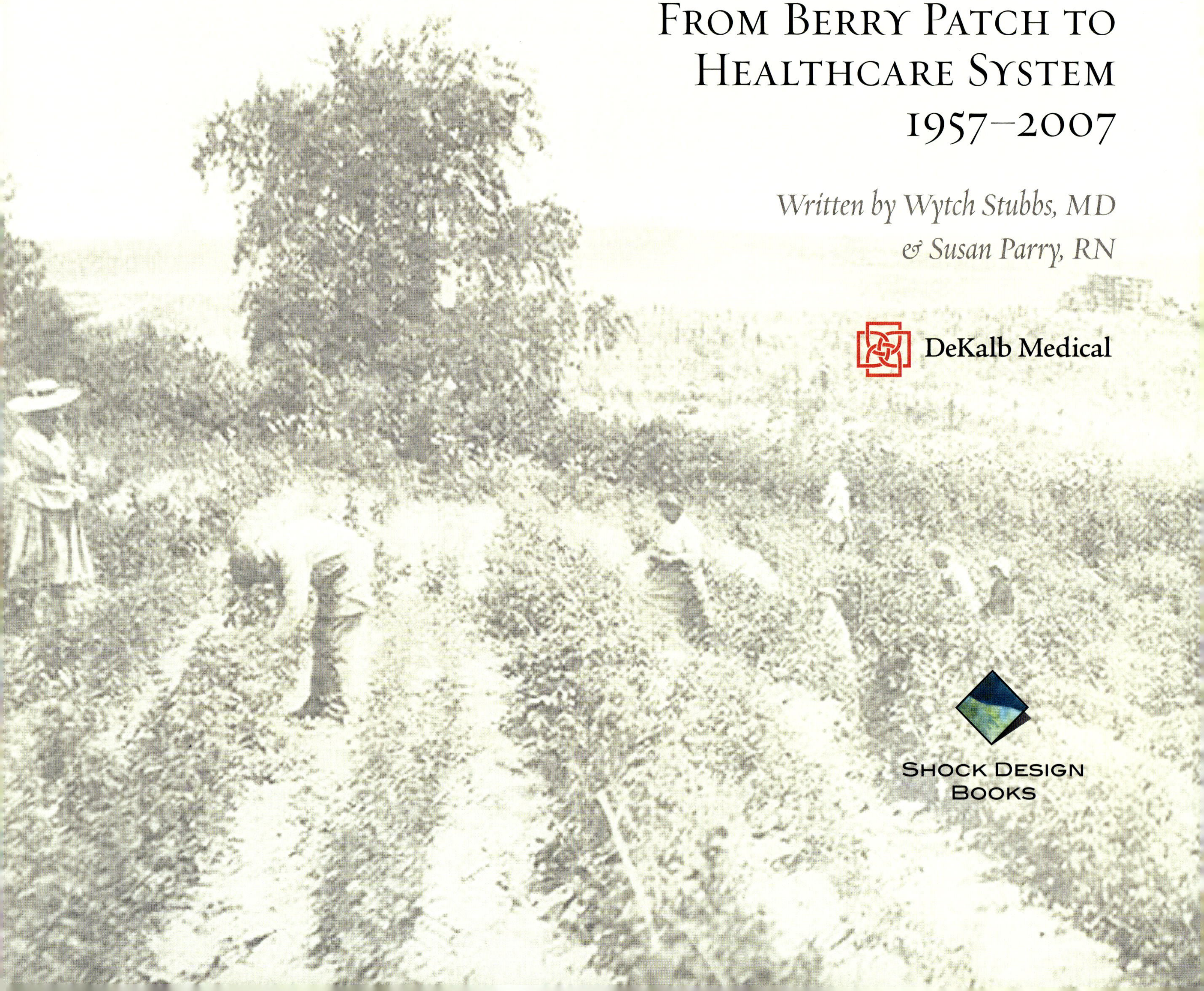

SHOCK DESIGN BOOKS

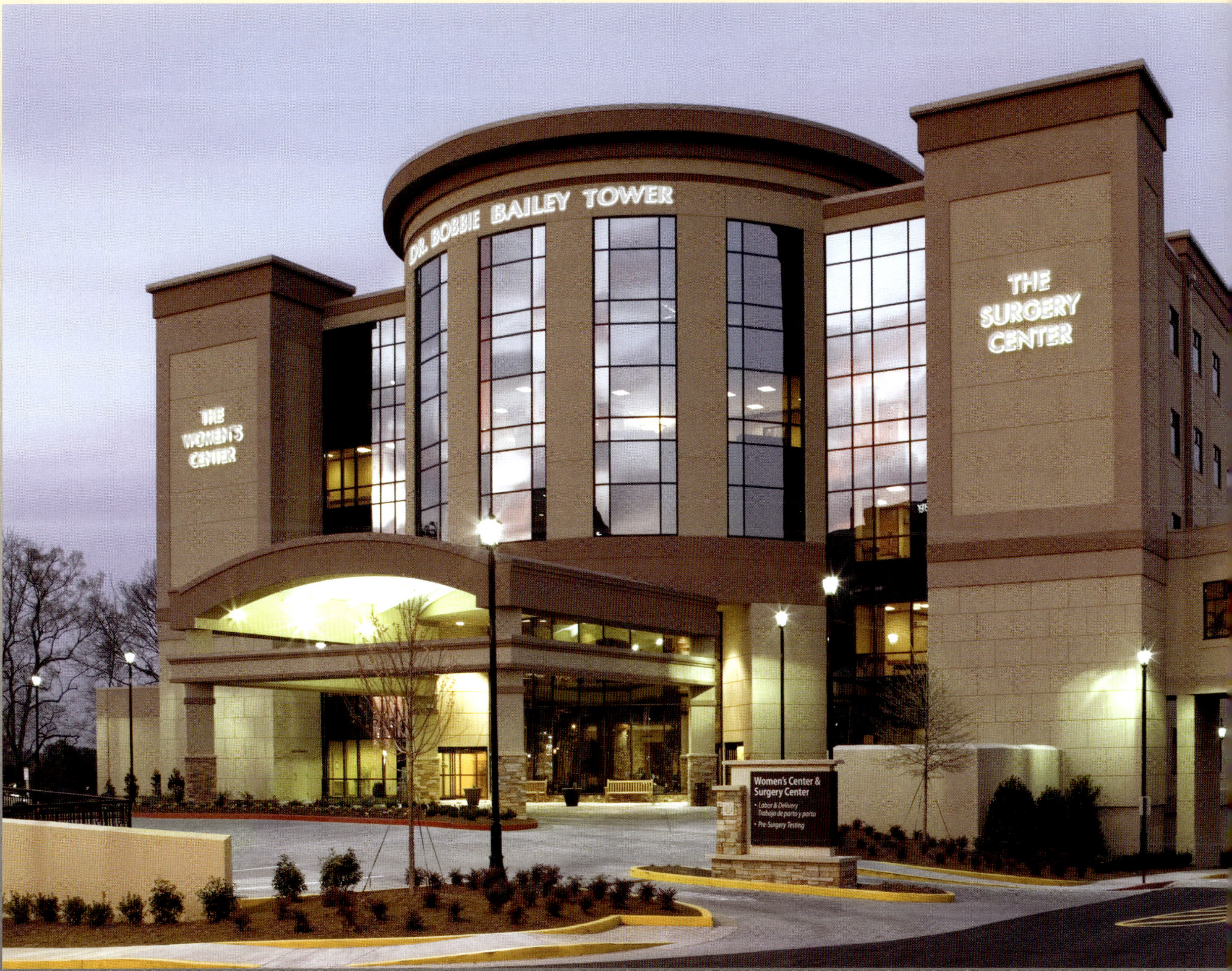
DR. BOBBIE BAILEY TOWER
THE WOMEN'S CENTER
THE SURGERY CENTER
Women's Center & Surgery Center
• Labor & Delivery
Trabajo de parto y parto
• Pre-Surgery Testing

Shock Design Books

A division of Shock Design & Associates, Inc.
984 Emerson Avenue, Studio A
Atlanta, GA 30316
www.shockdesign.com

Text copyright ©2009 Wytch Stubbs, MD, and Susan Parry, RN

All rights reserved. This book, or parts thereof, may not be reproduced in any form without written permission excepting brief excerpts for use in publicity and reviews..

Book development, design, and production: Laurie Shock
Picture research: Wytch Stubbs, MD, Susan Parry, RN, and Laurie Shock
Editor: Amy Bauman

Manufactured in Korea

First Edition

ISBN: 978-0-9824779-0-8

LC: 2009927767

Picture Credits

Jacket front, (background) Library of Congress, (top to bottom beginning top left) painting by Charles Wilson Peale, 1780; Courtesy of the Georgia Archives, Vanishing Georgia Collection dek084-85; Courtesy of the Georgia Archives, Vanishing Georgia Collection dek385-85; ©Bothwell-Jenkins, Slay and Brown; ©1969 Robin Johnstone; DeKalb Medical Archives; DeKalb Medical Archives; ©2009 Billy Howard Photography, Inc.; Jacket back flap, ©2009 Billy Howard Photography, Inc..

Unless otherwise noted, images are part of the DeKalb Medical Archives. Front endsheet, ©1962 Aero-Graphics, Inc.; p.ii–iii, (background) Library of Congress; p. iii, © Bras Field Gorrie, LLC; p. xvi, (1) painting by Charles Bird King, (2) painting by Charles Wilson Peale, 1780, (3) Courtesy of the Georgia Archives, Vanishing Georgia Collection ful0116, (4) Library of Congress, (5) Courtesy of the Georgia Archives, Vanishing Georgia Collection ful0313; p. xvii, (1) public domain, (2, above) Courtesy of Emory, Atlanta, (3) Courtesy of the Georgia Archives, Vanishing Georgia Collection dek035, (4) Courtesy of the DeKalb History Center, (5) ©Bothwell-Jenkins, Slay and Brown; xix, (top rt.) ©Chegwidden, Holmes & Dorsey; xx, (top left) Chegwidden, Holmes & Dorsey; xxiii; xxiv, painting by Charles Wilson Peale, 1780; p. 1, (top) Library of Congress, (inset) Courtesy of the Georgia Archives, Vanishing Georgia Collection dek385-85, (bottom) Courtesy of the Digital Library of Georgia, map by H. S. Tanner, 1823; p. 2, (left) Courtesy of Stone Mountain Park, GA; p. 3, (color inset) Courtesy of the U.S. Navy Art Collection, Washington DC, painting by V. Zveg, 1976, (b/w inset and rt.) Courtesy of the DeKalb History Center; p. 4, (left) Courtesy of the Georgia Archives, Vanishing Georgia Collection ful0116, (right) Courtesy of Georgia Archives, Vanishing Georgia Collection ful0119; p. 5, Courtesy of the DeKalb History Center; p. 6, (left) Courtesy of Emory, Atlanta, (rt.) Carl Vinson Institute of Gov't., the University of Georgia, drawing by Samuel Ireland, 1785, print by Ed Jackson; p. 7, (left) Courtesy of the Georgia Archives, Vanishing Georgia Collection 413-85, (top rt.) Courtesy of the DeKalb History Center, (bottom rt.) Courtesy of the Georgia Archives, Vanishing Georgia Collection dek439-85; p. 8, Courtesy of the Georgia Archives, Vanishing Georgia Collection ful0131; pp. 10, Courtesy of the Georgia Archives, Vanishing Georgia Collection dek035; p. 11, Courtesy of the Georgia Archives, Vanishing Georgia Collection dek042; p. 12, ©Bothwell-Jenkins, Slay and Brown; p. 13, (top) Library of Congress; p. 14, (bottom) Courtesy of the DeKalb History Center; p. 16, (top) Courtesy of the Georgia Archives, Vanishing Georgia Collection ful0028, (bottom) Courtesy of the Georgia Archives, Vanishing Georgia Collection dek084-85; pp. 19–21, ©Bothwell-Jenkins, Slay and Brown; p. 25, ©1960 Joseph T. Jackson; p. 29, Courtesy of the Bill Evans, Jr. Family Archives; p. 31, (top) Library of Congress; p. 43, ©Bothwell-Jenkins, Slay and Brown; pp. 44–45, ©1962 Aero-Graphics, Inc.; p. 46, ©1969 Robin Johnstone; p. 47, (top) Library of Congress; p. 49, ©1969 Robin Johnstone; p. 51, ©1969 Robin Johnstone; p. 54, Dwight Ross Jr. / *Atlanta Journal-Constitution*; p. 58, Dwight Ross Jr. / *Atlanta Journal-Constitution*; p. 60, ©1969 Robin Johnstone; p. 65, (top) Library of Congress; p. 73, (top) Library of Congress, (inset) ©Moreland Photography; p. 85, (top) Library of Congress; p. 92, ©Bill Mahan; p. 93, (top) Library of Congress; p. 107, Chegwidden, Holmes & Dorsey; p. 113, ©Bill Mahan; p. 114, ©1961 Lee Studio; p. 115, (top) Library of Congress; p. 124, (top rt.) ©Bill Mahan; p. 124, (bottom rt.) ©Bill Mahan; p. 125, ©Connie Lisenby; p. 126, (top rt.) ©Bill Mahan, (bottom left) ©Bill Mahan; p. 127, (top rt.) ©Ross DeLoach, Northlight Photography; p. 128, (top center) ©Richard T. Bryant, (top rt.) ©Richard T. Bryant; p. 129, (left) ©Bill Mahan; p. 130, (top left) Thrasher Family Archives; (top rt.) Eberhart Family Archives; p. 131, (top) Library of Congress, (bottom) Thrasher Family Archives; p. 132–133, Thrasher Family Archives; p. 135, Thrasher Family Archives; p. 138, Eberhart Family Archives; p. 139, (bottom) ©Chegwidden, Holmes & Dorsey; p. 144, Gerlach Family Archives; p. 145, (top) Gerlach Family Archives; p. 150, Norwood Family Archives; pp. 154–155, (background) Library of Congress; p. 170, ©Max20; p. 236, ©1969 Robin Johnstone; p. 245, ©Dick Ashe; p. 256, ©2009 Billy Howard Photography, Inc.; p. 274, ©Chegwidden, Holmes & Dorsey; p. 292, ©2009 Billy Howard Photography, Inc.; p. 299, (bottom rt.) ©Cheryl Norman; p. 300, (left) ©Chegwidden, Holmes & Dorsey; back endsheet, ©2009, Billy Howard Photography, Inc.

Although every effort has been made to ensure the accuracy and reliability of the information and credits in this book, mistakes due to human error are possible. Should a discrepancy or error be found, please notify us so that we may update our records and correct the information in future editions or publications.

This story is dedicated to

William P. Tatum

who said it deserved to be told and

who, for more than a quarter of a century,

was a vital contributor to it.

Contents

DeKalb Medical's Mission

The mission of DeKalb Medical
is to improve lives
through the delivery
of health and wellness services
in partnership with our physicians.

DeKalb Medical's Values

Diversity
Respect
Healing
Service

Preface

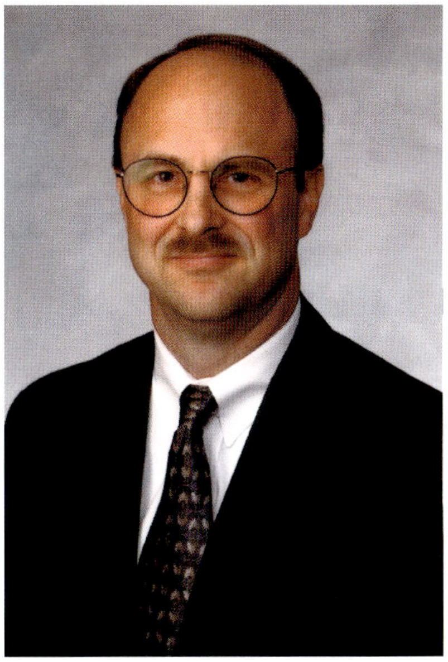

In 1957, one year after I was born, a group of community leaders put their hands and hearts together to create a new institution. This book is a work of love by many of the people who have invested their time, talent, and treasures into that institution.

It's very noteworthy that DeKalb Medical sprouted in a forty-acre berry patch, one that "was well-known to the community because of its abundant growth of strawberries and blackberries … The public was invited to help themselves to the delicious fruit free of charge." What a wonderful word picture of what DeKalb Medical has become over the last 50 years!

It is a place where the community can still help itself to produce good fruit, through the faithful investment of its time, talents, and treasure for the common good.

Its growth has been abundant indeed, producing a rainbow variety of services to a wonderfully vibrant and diverse community.

The reason people were able to pick berries free of charge in the 1950s was because of the generosity of a few with the means and the heart to bless many. That same ethic continues today, without which this institution could not prevail.

Bob Wilson, long-time chairman of the DeKalb Medical Foundation, and a loved and respected voice in our community, often speaks of the important role institutions play in any community. "Institutions, such as schools, churches, and hospitals, are an indispensable component of the foundation of any healthy community. They bring and hold people together for the common good and often do so amidst tensions and changing expectations in life."

From its humble beginnings in a berry patch, the people of DeKalb Medical have been privileged to serve people in need for 50 years. This book is a tribute to those people—past, present, and future—who joyfully give of themselves here to help others in need.

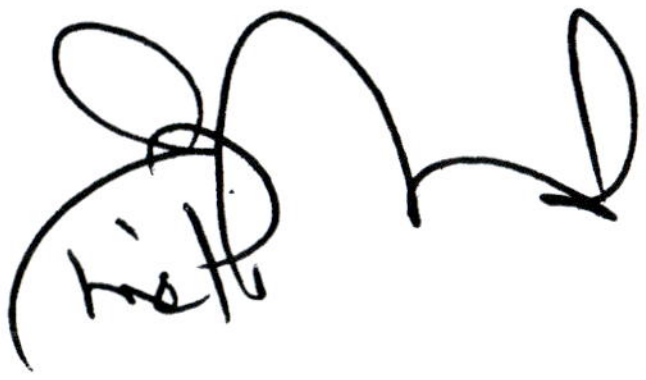

Eric P. Norwood, FACHE
President and CEO
May 2009

Introduction

DeKalb Medical's age often is identified in terms of when DeKalb General Hospital opened in May 1961. Its life, however, began long before then. It had its origins in the creation and growth of DeKalb County of which it has been a vital participant. It was officially conceived when the Board of Commissioners of Roads and Revenues of DeKalb County constituted and appointed the first DeKalb County Hospital Authority on September 19, 1957. The Authority's Constitution stated that "the general purpose of the Authority shall be to erect and operate one or more hospitals for the care of the sick in the county." *The DeKalb Medical Story* rightfully acknowledges the background out of which the need for the hospital emerged, the gestation period when the first trustees created the mission and managed the birth of the facility, and the ensuing years that witnessed the growth and services of the institution and the fruits of its labor.

When the DeKalb County Hospital Authority purchased forty acres of land facing North Decatur Road in 1958 from the Scott Estate, the property was well-known to the community because of its abundant strawberries and blackberries. The public had been invited to help themselves to the delicious fruit free of charge. Today that forty acres is the hub of a prominent health system that includes three hospitals, four professional office buildings, a Wellness Center, a Women's Center and Surgery Center, the Charles B. Eberhart Cancer Center, a Wellness on Wheels vehicle, a series of primary care centers, a charitable foundation, a community outreach program and many other facilities and services.

The Authority built and opened its first hospital on the forty-acre berry patch in 1961 and called it "DeKalb General Hospital." In 1988 the trustees changed the name of the hospital to "DeKalb Medical Center" to reflect the expanded services and expertise offered by the institution. In 1992, the governance of the hospital was restructured whereby the Authority retained ownership but leased its facilities and its assets to a private, nonprofit entity, DeKalb Medical Center, Inc., (DMC) and its parent company, DeKalb Regional Healthcare System, Inc., (DRHS). The new structure would take advantage of multiple opportunities for growth and development that were not possible under existing Georgia Hospital Authority law.

In 1976 the Hospital Authority acquired forty acres of land in South DeKalb County facing I-20 East expressway. DRHS opened a combined medical office building and outpatient diagnostic and treatment center in 1994, a second medical office building combined with an outpatient surgery and minor emergency center in 2001, and a 100-bed acute care hospital in 2005. In 1994 DRHS purchased the operating rights to the privately owned Decatur Hospital in downtown Decatur, and in1998 purchased the physical plant. Today the health system is known as DeKalb Medical, and the three hospitals are called DeKalb Medical at North Decatur, DeKalb Medical at Downtown Decatur, and DeKalb Medical at Hillandale.

In 2005 former Authority and board chairman William P. Tatum said the DeKalb Medical story deserved to be told. President and CEO Eric Norwood and the DRHS Board of Directors approved and endorsed its recording. The story told herein is divided into three sections. The first section consists of a timeline that identifies chronologically many of the significant events that have occurred in DeKalb Medical's history. The second section includes ten chapters that describe major developments in the history of the organization. The third section seeks to tell the story of many departments and services, and it contains a series of appendices.

The journey from berry patch to the current health system was made possible by a host of individuals who demonstrated an undying commitment to the well-being of the community, a vision of what should be done and what could be done, a tenacity to stay the course in the face of unrelenting challenges, and an integrity that rallied the trust, confidence and support of the community, physicians, and staff who joined them to make it all possible. It has been our privilege to relive and tell their amazing story.

—Wytch Stubbs, MD and Susan Parry, RN
May 2009

Acknowledgments

No research project could be accomplished without the contributions of many who give their support and encouragement and who provide essential information and insights. *The DeKalb Medical Story* is the result of such invaluable contributions.

The list of those who made this project possible is long and worthy of our attempted recognition and gratitude. William P. Tatum initiated the journey when he said the story deserved to be told. Eric Norwood, president and CEO, and the DeKalb Medical Board of Directors immediately endorsed and commissioned the project and made available the necessary documents, materials, and resources.

The Editorial Board that gave us direction and encouragement included Earnest Atkins, Duane Blair, John R. Gerlach, Wilma Hipps, Judy McMahan, Eric Norwood, Floyd Sanders, Bill Sublett, and William P. Tatum.

The Publications Board that identified the source of funds for publishing the book, chose its design, and determined the uses to which it would be devoted included Eric Norwood, Nancy Lawson, Leigh Minter and Cheryl Iverson.

Many individuals played enormously helpful roles along the way. Nancy Lawson secured all the official documents from their storage sites, kept us supplied with printer cartridges and paper, and arranged our many required meetings. Hospital attorney James Rawls volunteered to review the original draft to help us avoid legal and confidentiality potholes. Doris Jones and Dannie Bell assisted with the early research and editing. Diane Erdeljac reminded us of the importance of preserving our historical documents. Melissa Forgey, executive director, and Karen Kopanezos, archivist, of the DeKalb History Center placed the resources of the center at our disposal and provided copies of rare photographs. Joanne Thrasher Hauserman and her mother Helen Thrasher found and provided prized photographs and documents. Marilyn Barry and Tim Lammers of the Health Sciences Library located treasured resources. Mary Meek of Volunteer Services brought to our office and hauled away thirty-three years of Auxiliary scrapbooks for our review and use. Linda Tierney guided us toward many of the Public Relation's valuable resources; and Cheryl Iverson, Teresa Whitesel, and Tahira Carpenter were patient and enormously helpful in securing documents and photos and permission for their use.

Many shared their time, remembrances and stories through interviews and conversations that added information not to be found anywhere in written form. Those who made contributions included Jackie Anderson, Earnest Atkins, Marilyn Barry, Becky Beagle, Duane Blair, Emy Blair, Cathy Booker, Cathy Boyles, Dean Brown, Dan Callahan, Carol Campbell, Betty Castellani, Mary Chambers, Charles "Chip" Clifton, Jay Coffsky, Faye Cole, Nancy King Curdy, Helen Ebaugh, Paula Eissner, Grover Evans, Ann Fears, Mary Kay Flake, Carole Fortenberry, Opal Hopkins Fyffe, John

R. Gerlach, Robert Gibbs, Patrick Green, Ellen Hargett, Naomi Harman, Susan Bales Harris, Roslyn "Roz" Heath, Mary Hollis, Patricia Horton, Margie Hunter, Martin Isganitis, Norman Jacobs, Marti Jaynes, Della Johnson, Julia Hunter Jones, Martha "Cookie" Kalember, William Keeton, Barbara Kleynen, Carl Lallerstedt, Barbara Lewis, Mary Mallison, Frank Matthews, Scott McAuley, Ron McCranie, Kevin McMullen, Jo Ann Morgan, Gay Newton, Eric Norwood, Paul Olander, Patrick O'Neal, Mike Paul, Bonnie Phipps, Helen Scherer, George Sessions, Gail Shackleford, Beth Singleton, James Solomon, Bill Sublett, William P. Tatum, William "Bill" Townsend, Pat Vinton, Nancy Ward, Gertrude Weiser, Cathleen Wheatley, Sally Williams, and Mary Woody. Others generously offered to be interviewed, but a publication deadline prevented our taking advantage of their generosity.

Our special thanks to our publisher, Laurie Shock of Shock Design Books, who patiently and skillfully guided us through the publication process and who transformed our raw materials into a work of art; to Amy Bauman, our talented editor; and to Billy Howard, our gifted photographer.

Finally we offer our heartfelt thanks to our spouses, Jo Anne Stubbs and Richard Parry, for their support and patience in a project we promised to complete in six months but that evolved into four years.

—Wytch Stubbs, MD, and Susan Parry, RN
May 2009

The DeKalb Medical Story

Timeline

1821 1822 1836 1864 1892

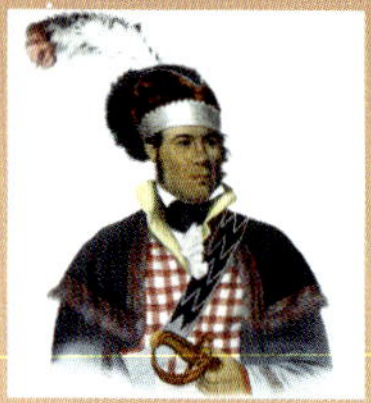
Creek Indian William Macintosh, "White Warrior"

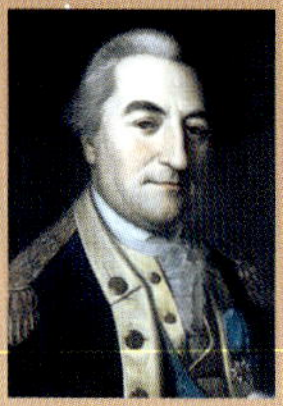
Johann DeKalb

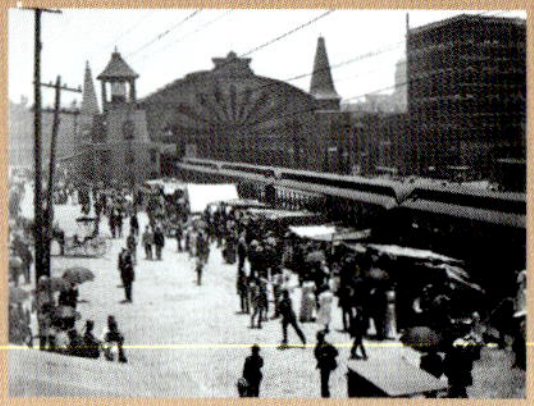
Early Atlanta

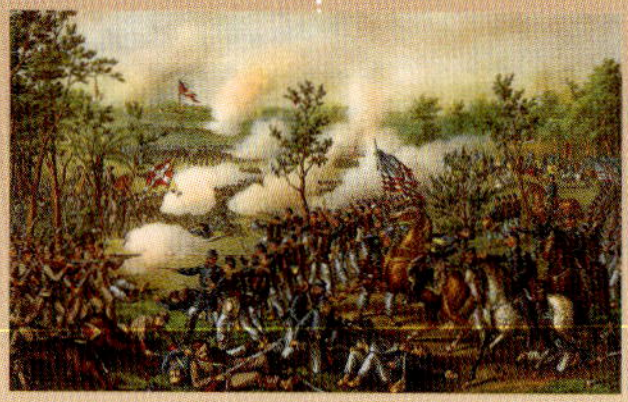
The Battle of Atlanta

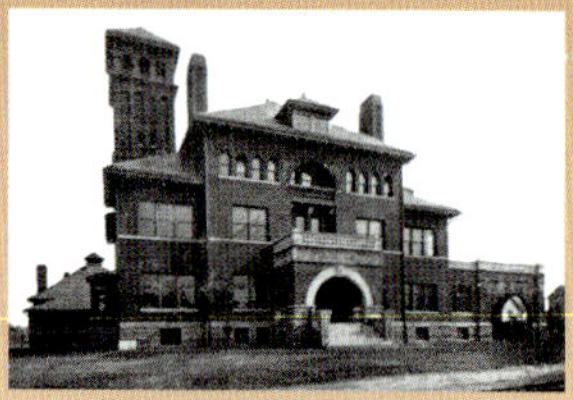
Grady Memorial Hospital

1821
- The Creek (Muskogee) Indians ceded the last of their Georgia land south of the Chattahoochee River to the United States government.

1822
- DeKalb County was created from a portion of Henry County and small portions of Gwinnett County and Fayette County to become Georgia's 56th county, named for General Baron Johann DeKalb.

1823
- The city of Decatur was incorporated and designated as the DeKalb County seat.

1834
- Emory University began as the Methodist Church's Georgia Manual Labor School at Oxford, Georgia, was chartered as Emory College in 1836, and opened as Emory University on the Atlanta campus in 1919 with land and money donated by Coca Cola founder Asa Griggs Candler.

1836
- Atlanta, originally called "Terminus" because it was the terminal site for several railroads, was re-named Marthasville in 1843 and Atlanta in 1845.

1838
- Oglethorpe University was established in Midway, Georgia, moved to downtown Atlanta in 1870, closed in bankruptcy in 1872, and reopened at its present location in 1915.

1853
- Fulton County was created from the northern and western portions of DeKalb County.

1864
- The Battle of Atlanta, much of it fought in DeKalb County, destroyed DeKalb County's segment of the Georgia Railroad.

1880
- St. Joseph's Hospital, begun as the Atlanta Hospital by four nuns of the Sisters of Mercy, a Roman Catholic religious order, was relocated to Courtland Street and renamed St. Joseph's Infirmary. It later moved to its present location in 1978 and renamed St. Joseph's Hospital.

1889
- Agnes Scott College, begun as Decatur Female Seminary in a home donated by a Presbyterian minister, was renamed and chartered as Agnes Scott College in 1906.

1892
- The original Grady Memorial Hospital opened, followed in 1912 by separate facilities for white and black patients, then after World War I by a third facility, and in 1958 by the present facility. The Fulton-DeKalb Hospital Authority was created in 1945, and the governance restructured to create the Grady Hospital Corporation, Inc., in 2007.

1897
- The City of Stone Mountain almost replaced Decatur as the DeKalb County seat.

1901
- Atlanta Medical Center, begun as the Tabernacle Baptist Infirmary on Courtland Street in downtown Atlanta, was relocated several times, sold to the Georgia Baptist Convention, renamed Georgia Baptist Hospital in 1913, and later sold to the for-profit Tenet Corporation and renamed Atlanta Medical Center.

1904
- Piedmont Hospital, begun as the Piedmont Sanatorium at the corner of Capitol Avenue and Crumley Street, was renamed Piedmont Hospital in 1925 and relocated to its present location in 1955.

1905
- Emory University Hospital, begun as Wesley Memorial Hospital, a Methodist hospital in a mansion at the corner of Auburn Avenue and Courtland Street, was relocated to a new facility on the Emory University campus in 1922, funded by Asa Griggs Candler, and renamed Emory University Hospital in the mid-1930s.

1908
- Emory Crawford Long Hospital, begun as the Davis-Fisher Sanatorium on Crew Street near the former Atlanta Stadium, was relocated to its present location in 1911, renamed the Crawford W. Long Memorial Hospital in 1931, donated to Emory University in 1940, and renamed Emory Crawford Long Hospital in 1955.

1915
- The Emory University School of Medicine was the name given to the Atlanta Medical College.
- The Scottish Rite Hospital for Crippled Children was established.

1924
- DeKalb Medical Society was created as a re-activation of the old DeKalb County Medical Protective Society that was formed after the Civil War.

1925
- J. Rufus Evans, MD, moved to DeKalb County from New Orleans to become the director of the DeKalb County Department of Public Health, a position he held for twenty-five years.

1927
- Columbia Theological Seminary relocated from Columbia, SC, to Decatur.

1928
- Henrietta Egleston Hospital for Children was established.

1938
- Elks Aidmore Hospital was established.

1939
- Scott Candler Sr. was elected sole DeKalb County Commissioner, a position he held until 1955.

1941
- The Georgia General Assembly passed the Hospital Authorities Law authorizing county governments to establish hospital authorities.

1946
- Congress passed the Hill-Burton Act authorizing federal and state funds to be used for hospital construction.
- DeKalb County was chosen as the site for the Centers for Disease Control and Prevention (CDC).

1948
- J. Rufus Evans, MD, began speaking to civic associations about the need for a new hospital in DeKalb County

1952
- DeKalb County passed a $1 million general obligation bond to build a new hospital in the county.
- Scott Candler Sr., Julius A. McCurdy, and J. Rufus Evans presented tentative architectural plans and the site for a hospital to the Georgia Department of Public Health. The plans were put on hold when no matching state and federal funds were available.

1953
- The Emory Clinic was established, making Emory Hospital less available to DeKalb County physicians.

1955
- Scott Candler Sr., retired as the sole DeKalb County Commissioner.

1957
- A five-man DeKalb Board of Commissioners replaced the sole commissioner practice.
- The General Assembly established the DeKalb County Bond Commission.
- State and federal Hill-Burton matching funds for hospital construction became available to DeKalb County.
- DeKalb County passed a second hospital bond in the amount of $1,405,000 for a hospital in the county.

1905 1915 1939 1948 1958 1960 1961 1970

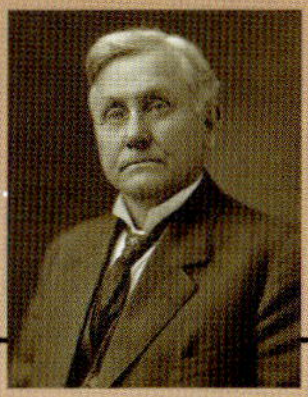
Asa Griggs Candler

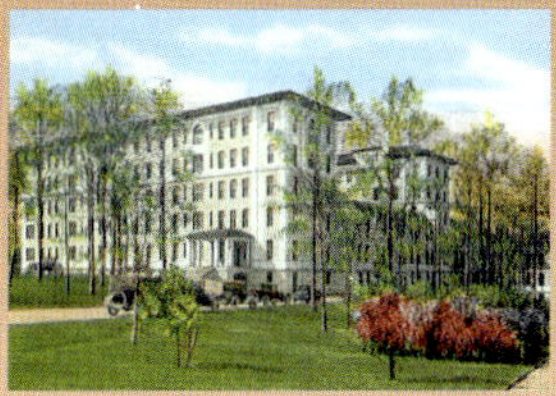
Wesley Memorial Hospital before it became Emory Hospital

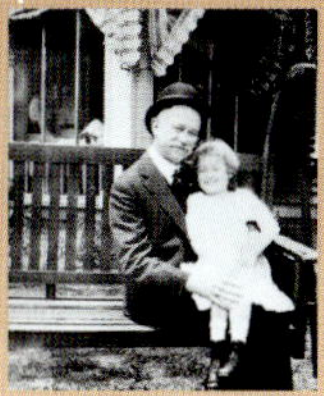
Scottish Rite Hospital

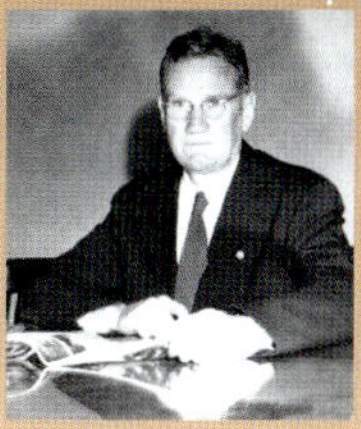
Scott Candler, Sr.

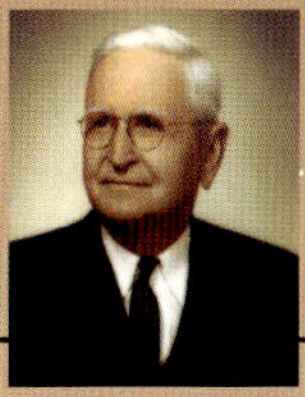
J. Rufus Evans, MD

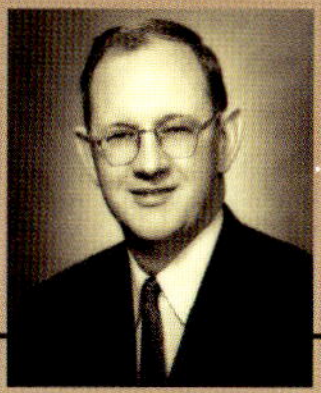
William H. Thrasher

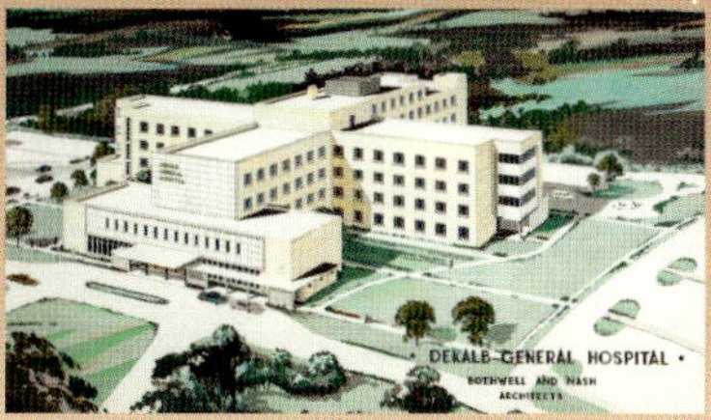

DeKalb General Hospital

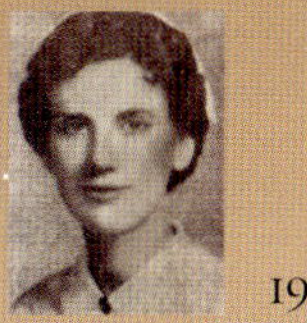
Opal Hopkins, RN

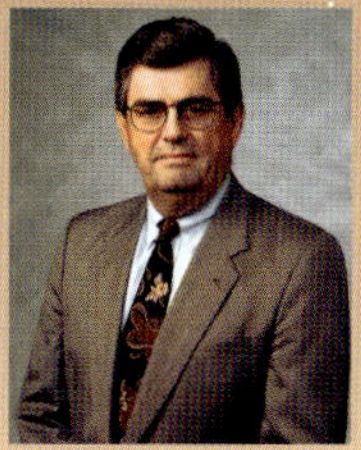
Charles Eberhart

- The DeKalb Board of Commissioners appointed a seven-man DeKalb County Hospital Authority: J. Rufus Evans, MD, J. Ross McCain, PhD, Julius A. McCurdy, JD, Wash W. Lively, M. E. Smith, R. L. Mathis Jr., and Hugh Rowland. The Authority elected Evans as its chairman.

1958
- The Hospital Authority purchased forty acres of land from the Booker Scott estate for $160,000, chose "DeKalb General Hospital" (DGH) as the hospital's name, retained George Dillard as hospital attorney, selected William H. Thrasher as the hospital administrator and Nash and Bothwell as the hospital architects.

1959
- T. C. Brittain Company was selected as the general contractor to build DeKalb General Hospital with a low bid of $3,518,628, which was $827 lower than the second-lowest bid.
- May 15—A groundbreaking ceremony was held for DeKalb General Hospital.

1960
- Opal Hopkins, RN, (later Fyffe) was named director of Nursing, Charles Anderson treasurer-controller, and Ted E. Barner assistant administrator.
- Frank Morgan, MD, was selected as radiologist and Frank Matthews, MD, as pathologist.
- July 17—A ceremony was held to lay the DeKalb General Hospital cornerstone.

1961
- George Sessions, MD, was chosen as anesthesiologist.
- January—The contractor turned keys to the hospital over to the Hospital Authority and administration.
- The Medical Advisory Committee of the DeKalb Medical Society provided DGH with its first medical staff bylaws and rules and regulations, and processed its initial applications for medical staff membership and privileges.
- March—L. C. Buchanan, MD, was named first chief of staff.
- April 21—A dedication ceremony was held.
- April 26—Three days of open house were attended by 20,000 visitors.
- May 1—DeKalb General Hospital (DGH) opened, and Stacy Stull, daughter of Mr. and Mrs. Thomas Stull, was the first baby born at DGH, delivered by John Fristoe, MD, six hours after the hospital opened.
- May 2—Martha Ivey, the first surgical patient, underwent thyroid surgery by L. C. Buchanan, MD, with Anibal Adan, MD, the anesthesiologist.
- Forty Red Cross (Gray Ladies) volunteers began serving DeKalb General Hospital.
- The DeKalb Junior Service League opened a gift shop.
- The Hospital Authority approved a budget of $93,450 per month for May – September, and for the first fiscal year beginning October, 1961.
- *The General InDecatur* was launched as the employee newsletter.

1962
- Ted Barner resigned as assistant to the administrator with no successor until John R. "Jack" Gerlach was hired in 1968.
- Oral surgeons became the first non-MD professionals admitted to the medical staff.

1963
- A Medical Library was established under the supervision of Frances Black, director of Medical Records.
- DeKalb General Hospital received its first three-year certification by the Joint Commission on the Accreditation of Healthcare Organizations (JCAHO).

1964
- Congress passed the Civil Rights Act prohibiting discrimination in public places.
- The new Veterans Administration Hospital opened on Clairmont Road.
- Richard Hackney, MD, the first African American physician, joined the medical staff in the General Practice Department.

1965
- Congress passed Title 18 of the Social Security Act (Medicare) and Title 19 of the Social Security Act (Medicaid).
- Following a civil rights complaint, the Hospital Authority passed a resolution stating that DGH would assign patients according to medical needs without distinction as to race, color, religion, or national origin.
- DGH contracted with DeKalb Emergency Group (Freeman Simmons, MD, Tom Lowry, MD, Thomas Cooper, MD and Ted Rheney, MD) to provide full-time medical coverage to the Emergency Department, the first such arrangement in the southeast. Luther Vinton, MD, later succeeded Thomas Cooper.
- The DGH School of X-ray Technology was established with Jo Ann Kilpatrick (later Morgan), director.
- Opal Hopkins Fyffe, RN, resigned as director of Nursing, to be succeeded by Margaret Ford, RN.

1966
- The Blue Alert system was inaugurated for patients with cardiac or respiratory arrest.
- DGH bought "a small computer for the business office" which did not perform as expected, and it was returned.
- The Hospital Authority deeded 4.5 acres of land to the DeKalb County Department of Public Health for its main county facility.

1967
- The DeKalb Board of Commissioners voted to finance $4 million in revenue anticipation certificates for the DGH renovation and expansion.
- The Authority's "Long Range Plan" called for a "satellite hospital and related hospital services in the South DeKalb area" and identified a portion of the Honor Farm in Panthersville as a possible site for the facility.
- Administrator Thrasher appointed an Advisory Committee that told him employee turnover was like a "mass exodus" due to inadequate salaries and benefits.

1968
- July—A groundbreaking ceremony was held for the expansion project to double the capacity of the hospital and add a mental health unit and a skilled nursing facility. Robert E. McKee of Dallas, Texas, was the general contractor. The project cost $10,904,229.
- John R. "Jack" Gerlach was named assistant to the administrator.
- The Georgia State Nurses Association (GSNA) activated the American Nurses' Association economic security program, and many DGH nurses assigned their collective bargaining rights to the GSNA as their agent to address their grievances about inadequate salaries, benefits, professional recognition and other issues. The Authority refused to recognize the GSNA as the nurses' bargaining agent.
- Nurses picket in protest over the Authority's refusal to recognize their bargaining agent.

1969
- January 16—Margaret Ford, RN, was dismissed as director of Nursing.
- January 17—Naomi Harman, RN, was named director of Nursing and Opal Hopkins Fyffe, RN, special assistant to the administrator.
- January 22—100 of the hospital's 130 nurses activated their resignations in mass.
- September—J. Rufus Evans resigned from the Authority, and Waldo Sowell was elected chairman.
- Psychiatry became the ninth medical staff department.
- The first separate Coronary Care Unit (CCU) was opened.
- DGH built a Child Care Center for children of employees.
- Rodney Sperry resigned as director of Building Services and was succeed by Daniel Goolsbee.

1970
- Charles Eberhart was named director of Administrative Services, John Gerlach director of Patient Care Services, Bill Sublett director of Personnel and Perry Stephens assistant director of Personnel.
- Attorney Ed Dorsey of the Powell Goldstein law firm succeeded George Dillard.
- DeKalb County voted a $1,950,000 bond for

Timeline

DE KALB GENERAL HOSPITAL

1971 · 1973 · 1974 · 1975 · 1976 · 1978

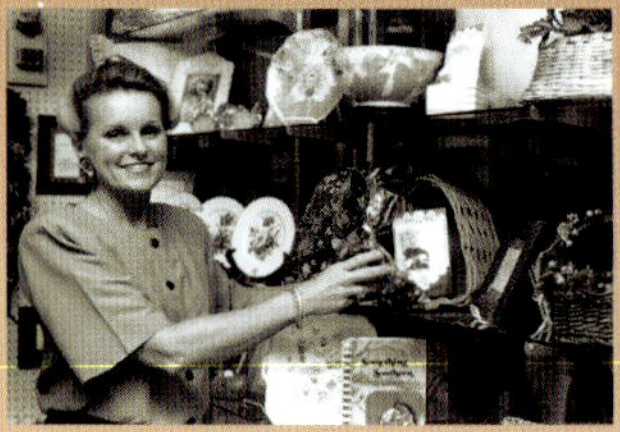
Paula Austin, The Dogwood Shop

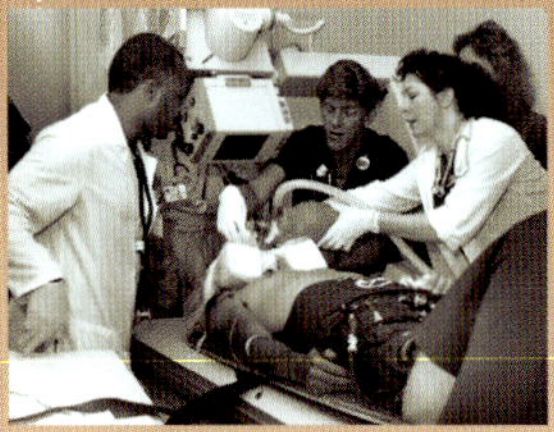
Emergency Department

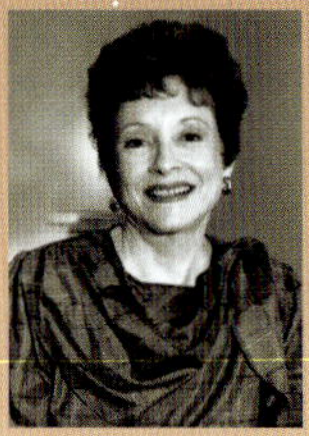
Naomi Harmon, RN

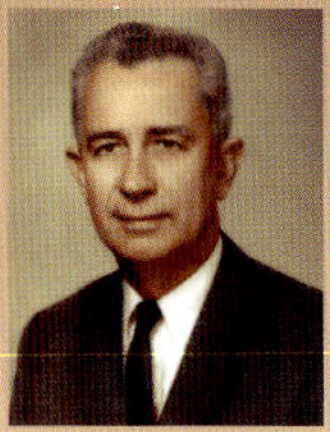
Waldo Sowell

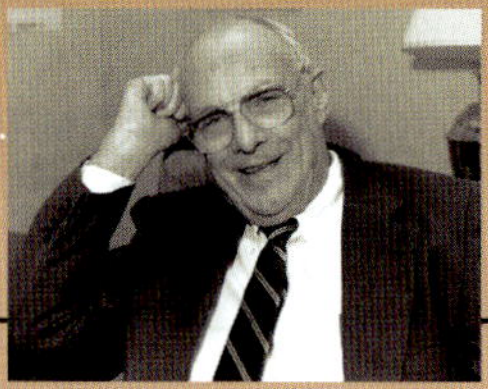
William P. Tatum

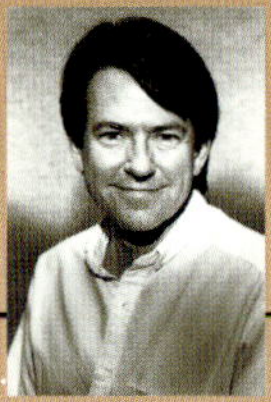
Michael Armand, MD

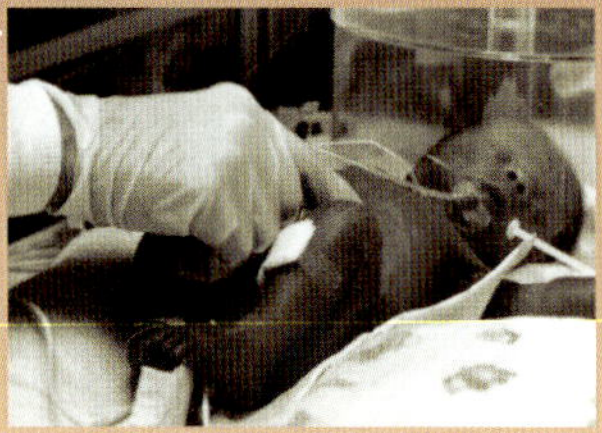

the Hospital Authority for land, a hospital and related medical facilities in South DeKalb County.
- The DeKalb Medical Employees' Federal Credit Union was established.
- The Junior League's Gift Shop was relocated to an area near the hospital entrance.
- The Radiology Department established a Nuclear Medicine service.

1971
- July—The expansion/renovation project was completed, doubling the size of the hospital to 640 beds (503 acute, 44 mental health, 93 long-term care/skilled nursing facility).
- The Mental Health Unit was opened.
- The federal government conveyed to the Authority a deed for 39.25 acres of the Honor Farm in Panthersville for a hospital, but the Metropolitan Atlanta Council survey reported an excessive number of hospital beds and no need for a hospital in South DeKalb.
- The DeKalb Junior League withdrew from operating the gift shop and formed a Hospital Guild to continue the service. The Guild renamed the gift shop The Dogwood Shop.
- DGH purchased a computer for the business office for $70,250.
- The Social Service Department was established with Esther Russell, MSW, director.
- The laboratory was expanded from 2,500 square feet to 10,000 square feet.

1972
- William Thrasher resigned as DGH administrator to become executive director of the DeKalb County Hospital Authority.
- DGH ceased selling cigarettes in its vending machines.
- Training and Education, an In-service Section of Nursing Service, became the Training and Continuing Education Section of the Personnel Department.
- The IV (Intravenous) Team was created.
- The DeKalb County Department of Public Health occupied a portion of the Mental Health Unit.
- The Physical Therapy Department opened with Dilys Jagger, RPT, director.
- J. Rufus Evans, MD, received the Georgia Hospital Association's Distinguished Service Award.

1973
- Charles Eberhart succeeded William Thrasher as administrator of DGH, and Douglas L. Buchner succeeded Eberhart as director of Administrative Services.
- Decatur Hospital opened as a private, for-profit, 6-story, 120-bed facility owned by Decatur Professional Investors, which included key members of the DGH medical staff.
- The Hospital Guild joined the Georgia Hospital Association's Council on Auxiliaries and became the DeKalb General Hospital Auxiliary.
- A Tumor Registry was established.
- A Cardiac Rehabilitation Program was established.
- Emergency Medicine became the hospital's tenth medical staff department.
- The General Practice Department was renamed the Family Practice Department.

1974
- John Manfredi, MD, joined the medical staff as DGH's first medical oncologist.
- John Harrel, MD, was named DGH's first director of Medical Affairs.
- Marilyn Gibbs (later Barry) was named medical librarian.
- William Thrasher was named director of Hospital Relations.
- DGH purchased a computer system from Avnet to handle admissions, discharge, and transfer functions, and it later sued Avnet for failure to perform.
- Doctors of Osteopathic Medicine became the second non-MD professionals admitted to the medical staff when the Authority overrode a negative vote of the medical staff.
- DGH displayed its first logo.
- The Authority approved a four-phase development concept for creating medical facilities in south DeKalb County.

1975
- John Harrel, DMA, established a Tuesday morning continuing medical education (CME) program.
- The first newsletter for the medical staff, *Communiqué*, was distributed.
- The 50-bed Skilled Nursing Facility on 2700, completed in 1971, opened after four years of negotiations with the state over a license requirement. Naomi Harman, RN, DGH's director of Nursing, was named its administrator.

1976
- Waldo Sowell died from injuries sustained in a fall, and William P. Tatum was elected chairman of the Hospital Authority.
- The Hospital Authority purchased 41.83 acres of land on Hillandale Road facing I-20 East in South DeKalb County for $327,000 for its South DeKalb medical campus.
- The DGH Auxiliary donated $20,000 to establish the first Pulmonary Function Lab with William Reichert, MD, medical director and Clare Hart, RPFT, as technologist.
- DGH purchased its first Computerized Tomography (CT) scanner.

1977
- The new Dimension 2000 Telephone System was installed for $20,000, converting rotary phones to touch tone.
- The Authority returned the Honor Farm property to the federal government.
- The DGH Auxiliary created a 5.5 acre Dogwood Memorial Park on the northwest corner of the campus for beauty, relaxation and meditation in honor of the Hospital Authority.
- The state denied a DGH CON application to purchase a 6 MEV linear accelerator for radiation therapy.

1978
- Attorney James C. Rawls of the Powell Goldstein law firm succeeded Ed Dorsey as hospital attorney.
- Bill Sublett succeeded Douglas Buchner as director of Administrative Services, and Perry Stephens succeeded Bill Sublett as director of Personnel.
- DGH shut down the Avnet computer system due to poor performance and successfully sued Avnet for reimbursement.
- Wayne E. Spangler, MDiv, became DGH's first chaplain.
- Michael Armand, MD, pediatrician and neonatologist, established DGH's Neonatal Intensive Care Unit (NICU).
- Kathy Hayes was named DGH's first director of Volunteer Services.
- March 6—J. Rufus Evans, MD, DGH champion and first Hospital Authority chairman, died.

1979
- DGH replaced the Avnet computer system with a Huff, Barrington and Owns (HBO) Medpro system for admissions, discharge, and transfer functions.

1980
- The Training and Continuing Education Section of the Personnel Department became the Training and Education Department.

1981
- A portion of the 4200 medical-surgical nursing unit was dedicated to oncology services.
- The Diagnostic and Treatment Center was opened with Carole Fortenberry, RN, manager.
- The Ambulatory Surgery Center opened adjacent to inpatient surgery at a cost of $7.3 million.
- The Physical Therapy, Occupational Therapy, and Speech Therapy departments were relocated into one central Rehabilitative Services Center.

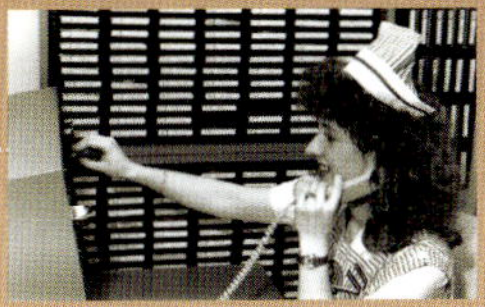

Tel-Med

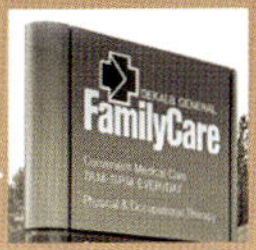

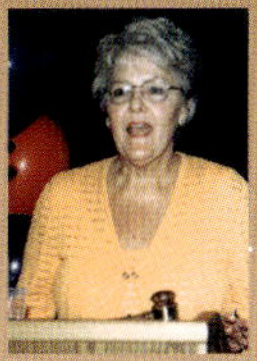

Judy McMahan

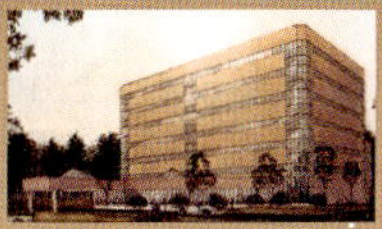

Professional Office Building

1982 1985 1986 1988 1989 1990 1991

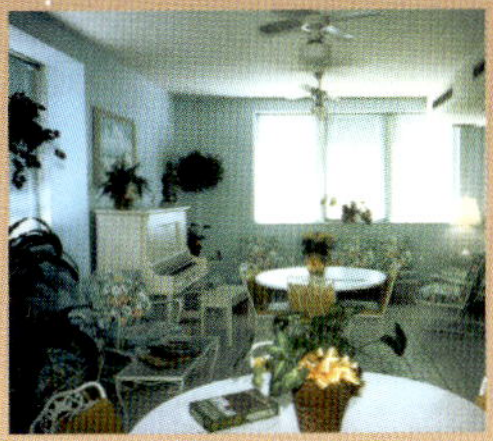

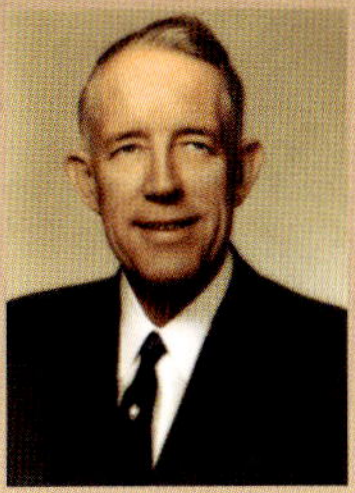

Wash Lively (right) funded The Lively Room (above).

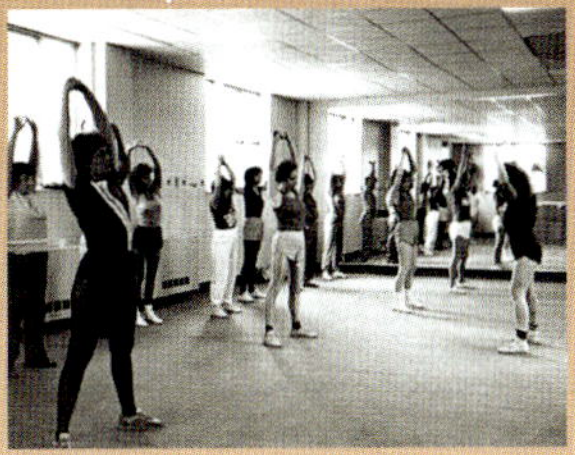

Women's Wellness Center

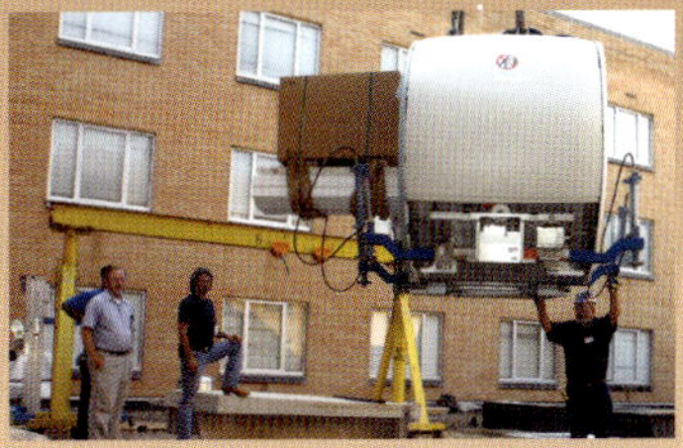

MRI for Diagnostic Imaging Center

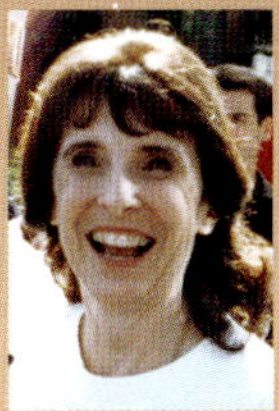

Betty Castellani

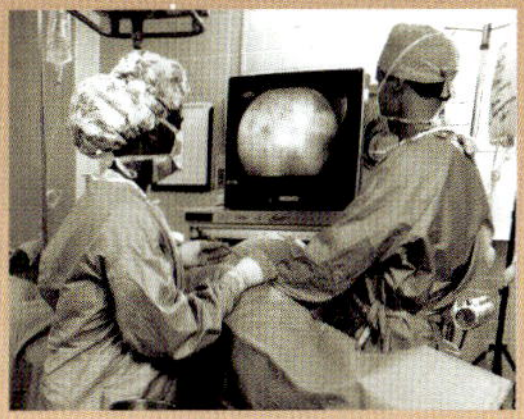

Laparoscopic Surgery

1982

- Tel-Med, manned by members of the DGH Auxiliary, was installed for public medical information on a variety of health-related topics.
- DeKalb County Department of Public Health relocated its community mental health program from the Mental Health Unit due to a lack of funds, and the Authority purchased full ownership of the facility from the federal government.
- The firm of Chegwidden, Holmes & Dorsey replaced Bothwell, Jenkins, Slay & Brown as hospital architects.
- The Lively Room, funded by trustee Wash Lively, was created in the 4200 solarium for the use of cancer patients and others.
- An 81,000-square-foot renovation and expansion project was completed for Ambulatory Surgery, the Diagnostic and Treatment Center, Rehabilitation Services, the nurseries, and the maternity unit

1983

- Medicare initiated the Prospective Payment System to pay hospitals a pre-determined payment according to a patient's diagnosis.
- November 12—William H. Thrasher, DGH's first administrator, died.
- Martha Nodal (Kalember) succeeded William Thrasher as director of Hospital Relations.

1984

- National Medical Enterprises, Inc. (NME), a for-profit corporation, filed a CON application with the state to build a hospital in South DeKalb County. DGH opposed the application, and the state rejected NME's application.
- Faye Sophy, RRA, succeeded Frances Black, RRA, as director of Medical Records.
- The Diagnostic Breast Center opened on the ground floor in space previously occupied by the Mental Health unit.

1985

- The Women's Wellness Center was opened on the ground floor of the Mental Health Unit, with Holly Wolfe, RN, manager and was renamed the Wellness Center in 1987 when it added services for men,.
- Anesthesiologists established the Pain Treatment Center, named in memory of Mark Coppage, MD, a former department member who was killed in an auto accident.
- A Congestive Heart Failure Program was established.
- "Tendercare" became the trade name for DGH's maternity services and other women's services.
- DGH initiated the WorksWell Program for the prevention and rehabilitation of on-the-job injuries.

1986

- DGH became a member of the Volunteer Hospital Association (VHA) of Georgia.
- Bonnie L. Phipps succeeded Charles Anderson as chief financial officer (CFO).
- The state denied DGH's CON application to build a 100-bed acute care general hospital in South DeKalb County.
- DGH opened the Diabetes Medical Center on the 1700 nursing unit with David Jacobson, MD, medical director and Peggy Jenkins, RN, department head.
- DGH opened the FamilyCare South DeKalb on Covington Highway in South DeKalb County and purchased the FamilyCare Tucker, both to provide for minor emergencies and illnesses.
- DGH replaced the HBO Medpro computer system with Shared Medical Systems' (SMS)INVISION.
- Hospital Corporation of America, Inc., (HCA) filed a CON application with the state to relocate Doctors Osteopathic Hospital from Tucker to a site on Lawrenceville Highway and rename it Northlake Regional Medical Center. The state approved the application.

1987

- Betty Castellani, DMin, was named associate chaplain.
- DGH leased the services of a mobile lithotripter unit to crush kidney stones.
- Wash Lively, original member of the Hospital Authority and long-time chairman of the Finance Committee, died.

1988

- DGH opened FamilyCare Decatur on the edge of the DGH campus.
- The Diagnostic Imaging Center (DIC) opened in front of the main hospital building and was connected to the hospital by a tunnel.
- A Magnetic Resonance Imaging (MRI) machine was purchased and installed in the DIC.
- The Emergency Department was expanded.
- Six VIP suites were opened on 3200 and 4200, and the corridor on the first floor was renovated.
- The College of St. Francis was brought on campus and offered bachelors degrees and masters degrees to members of the staff.
- Wytch Stubbs, MD, succeeded retiring John Harrel as director of Medical Affairs.
- Physicians held the first Medical Staff Leadership Retreat.
- The hospital name was changed from DeKalb General Hospital to DeKalb Medical Center (DMC) on the recommendation of the medical staff and approval of the Hospital Authority.

1989

- DMC became a Level 3 Trauma Center as part of the state's trauma network.
- Administrator Charles Eberhart established service line development teams for cancer, cardiology, surgery, mental health, and women and infants services.
- The DMC Cancer Center was established with Betty Castellani, director.
- DGH opened a Pediatric Rehabilitation Center on Winn Way and an Inpatient Rehabilitation Center on 3700.
- The cafeteria was expanded from a seating capacity of 175 to 275.
- The ArthritisCare Center was established in the FamilyCare Decatur Center.
- The first Nightingala fund-raising event was held at the suggestion of Robin Dretler, MD, and his wife Muffie Michaelson.
- A groundbreaking ceremony was held for the first Physician Office Building (POB).
- The New Day Substance Abuse program was established in the Mental Health Unit.

1990

- DMC contracted with four internists, the Medical Emergency Associates (MEAs), to be its first hospitalists.
- The Hospital Authority established the DeKalb Medical Center Foundation, suggested by Judy McMahan, with McMahan as the first board chairperson and Dana Jackson (later Rawls) the first director.
- The DeKalb Rape Crisis Center opened in the DMC Emergency Department.
- Smoking was banned in all Authority facilities, and smoking areas were provided outside.
- A Cardiac Catheterization Laboratory was opened.
- The construction of the Central Energy Plant and Incinerator was completed.
- Laparoscopic surgery was introduced at DMC.
- The medical library was renamed the Health Sciences Library.
- DMC offered Sleep Disorders assessment and management.
- Nurse midwives were approved to work in DMC's maternity services under the supervision of their obstetrician employers.
- The maternity unit was renovated, a high-risk antepartum unit opened, five labor-delivery-recovery rooms added, and the term nursery combined with the postpartum unit to form the Mother-Baby Unit.

1991

- The first Professional Office Building opened with eight stories and 150,000 square feet to provide physician office space, a pharmacy, a snack bar, a full-service bank and hospital services.
- Construction was completed on a 3-level parking deck.

Timeline

1992

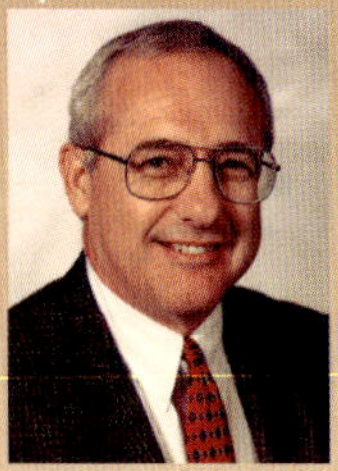

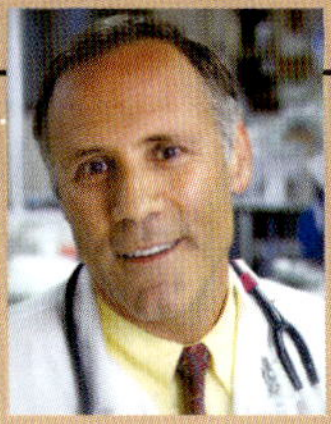

Pat L. Mathis (left) and Richard Leff, MD, (above).

1993

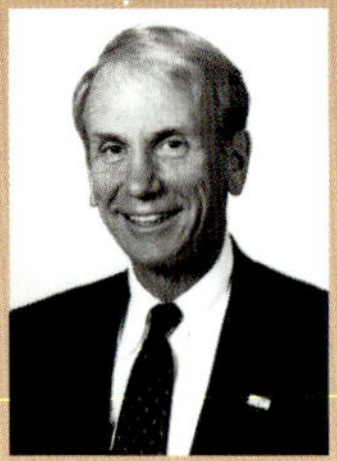

Charles Gindon

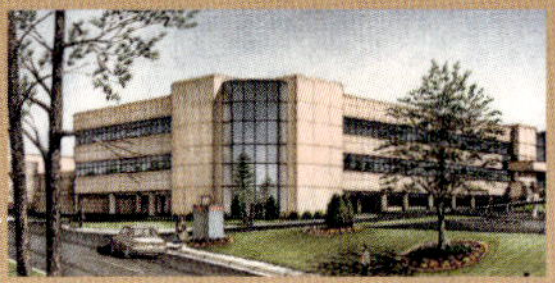

Maternity/Surgery Center

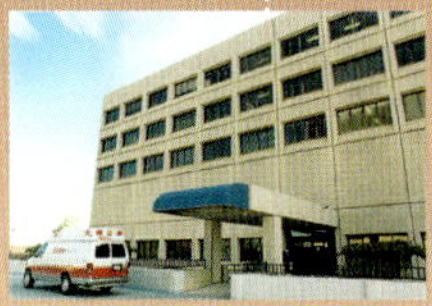

Decatur Hospital

1994

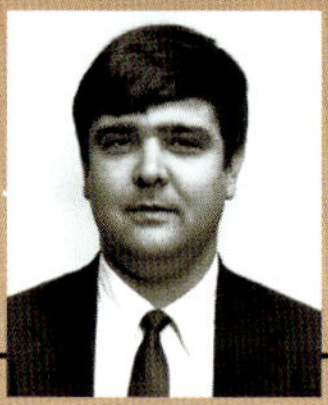

michael Kinstler, MD
DPHD Chairman

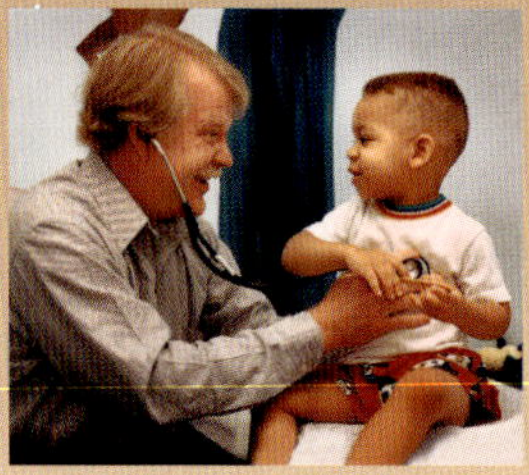

Primary Care Division

1995

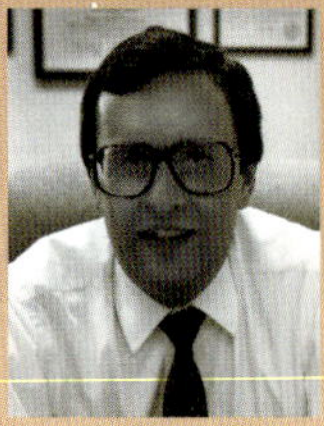

John R. "Jack" Gerlach

1996

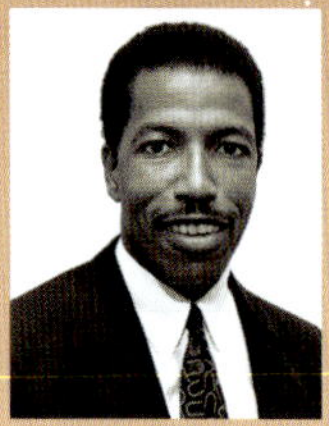

Oliver Lee

- DMC purchased the 300 Winn Way building from neurosurgeons and neurologists to house Information Technology services.
- A Chest Pain Emergency Center was opened in the Emergency Department.
- A third new hospital telephone system was installed.
- A new WorksWell rehabilitation facility was opened at the Snapfinger Woods Industrial Park in south DeKalb County.
- Paula Eissner, LMSW succeeded Esther Russell as director of the Social Services Department.
- Clayton Bailey succeeded Daniel Goolsbee as director of Building Services.
- The Breast Center was relocated to the ground floor in the first Professional Office Building.

1992

- March—The hospital governance was restructured and the Hospital Authority leased its assets to DeKalb Medical Center, Inc., (DMC) a private, nonprofit organization.
- December—The DeKalb Regional Healthcare System, Inc., (DRHS) was incorporated as a nonprofit parent company of DMC, Inc.
- Charles Eberhart was named CEO of DMC and DRHS, John Gerlach was named COO of DMC and DRHS, and Bonnie Phipps was named CFO of DMC and DRHS.
- Ninfa Saunders, RN, succeeded Naomi Harman, RN, director of Nursing with the title of administrator of Patient Care Services.
- Betty Castellani, DMin, succeeded Wayne Spangler, MDiv, as director of Pastoral Services.
- Pat L. Mathis succeeded William P. Tatum as chairman of the Hospital Authority when Tatum was elected chairman of the DMC and the DRHS boards.
- The DMC Cancer Center established Georgia's first Stem Cell Transplant program (an alternative to traditional bone marrow transplantation) for cancer patients needing high-dose chemotherapy with Richard Leff, MD, medical director.
- DMC opened a Medical-Psychiatric Unit.
- DMC contracted with Peachtree Hospice to provide an inpatient hospice unit on 3700, the first such arrangement in Georgia.
- The inpatient Diabetes Medical Center was replaced with the Outpatient Center for Diabetes Education.
- The DeKalb Medical Center employees created W.H.A.T., a voluntary giving program to support the Foundation and other charitable and service-related causes.
- Oliver Lee was named chairman of the DMC Committee on South DeKalb, and Julia Hunter (Jones) was named director of the South DeKalb Project.

1993

- Pat L. Mathis succeeded William P. Tatum as chairman of the DMC Board, and Charles Ginden succeeded Tatum as chairman of the DRHS Board.
- William P. Tatum, CEO, of Property Resources, Inc., contracted with DRHS to manage the system's physical properties.
- DRHS incorporated Decatur Health Resources, Inc., (DHR) to purchase the Decatur Hospital operation from OrNda Healthcorp.
- DRHS purchased its first primary care practice and established its Primary Care Division with Andy Morley, MD, director.
- Construction was completed on the Women's and Surgery Pavilion at a cost of $15,280,000 to include fourteen operating rooms and twelve maternity suites.
- Mary Kay Kiesling succeeded retiring Martha Nodal as director of Hospital Relations and Resource Services.
- The Health Sciences Library was expanded and relocated to the ground floor.
- The family of Mark Coppage, MD, anesthesiologist, established a nursing scholarship in his memory.
- A new Child Care Center was opened, and a management contract was signed with AmeriCare Company.
- Paul C. Browne, MD, obstetrician-perinatologist, established DMC's Maternal-Fetal Medicine service for high-risk expectant mothers.
- The state denied DMC's CON application to perform open heart surgery.
- DeKalb Medical Society established the volunteer Physicians' Care Clinic to provide medical care to uninsured and underinsured DeKalb County citizens.
- The hospital chapel was relocated to an area near the hospital entrance.
- DMC broke ground for a combined outpatient diagnostic and treatment center and a medical office building on Hillandale Drive in South DeKalb County.

1994

- DRHS/DHR purchased the operation and management rights for Decatur Hospital from OrNda Corporation for $6 million, and continued leasing the building from Decatur Professional Investors.
- Charles Eberhart was named chairman of the DHR Board of Directors and Carol Nikola was retained as CEO of Decatur Hospital.
- DRHS began alliance discussions with Rockdale, Emory, Northside, St. Joseph's and PROMINA health systems.
- DMC opened primary care centers at East Park near Stone Mountain, Virginia Highlands, Jimmy Carter Boulevard, Killian Hills and Five Forks Trickum Road.
- The DeKalb Physician Hospital Organization (DPHO) was incorporated to align physician and hospital incentives and to enhance the quality and efficiency of medical care provided. Michael Kinstler, MD, was elected chairman.
- The DRHS Board of Directors approved plans to construct the second Physician Office Building on campus.
- DMC established the South DeKalb Advisory Committee with Oliver Lee, chairperson.
- DMC opened its three-story medical office building/outpatient diagnostic center on the South DeKalb Hillandale property.
- The Herbert E. Kann Outpatient Cancer Treatment Center was opened in the first Professional Office Building.
- August—CEO Charles Eberhart was diagnosed as having a malignant brain tumor.
- Charles Eberhart was selected as the first non-physician to be awarded DeKalb Medical Society's Julius McCurdy Citizenship Award.
- The DMC and the Decatur Hospital mental health services were combined into a new Behavioral Health Services Department.
- The DMC Foundation successfully concluded a $1.5 million campaign for the surgery and maternity center and launched a 1994–1996, $1.6 million campaign to renovate and expand the Emergency Department.

1995

- March—The cancer center was named The Charles B. Eberhart Cancer Center.
- May 28—CEO Charles B. Eberhart died.
- John R. "Jack" Gerlach was named CEO of DMC and DRHS.
- Floyd Sanders, MD, succeeded Pat L. Mathis as chairman of the Hospital Authority.
- The Red Cross Volunteers program was disbanded nationwide, and the majority of DMC's members joined the DMC Auxiliary.
- Emergency Department physicians became employees of DMC rather than contract physicians.
- The credit union became the MedCom Federal Credit Union.
- DRHS entered into a partnership agreement with Strategic Decision Systems, Inc., and Behavioral Health Partners, Inc., developed by Gary Lang, to manage and market the DRHS mental health services.
- The Rehabilitation Services Department was renamed the Rehab Results Group.
- The outside contract for respiratory therapy services was terminated and brought in-house as the Respiratory Care

DeKalb Medical Center
PROMINA

1997 — 1997 — 1998 — 1999 — 2000

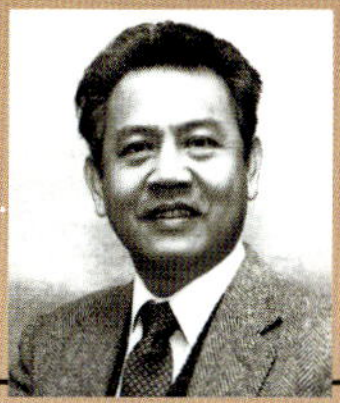

Tong Huynh, MD

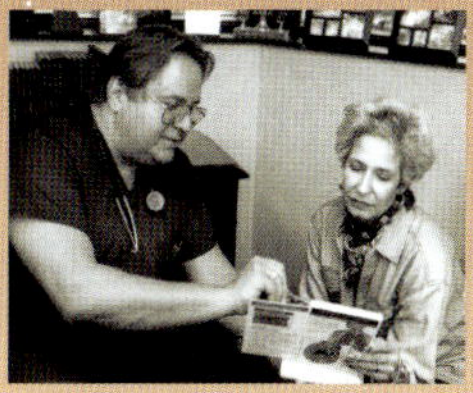

Thomas DeMarini, MD

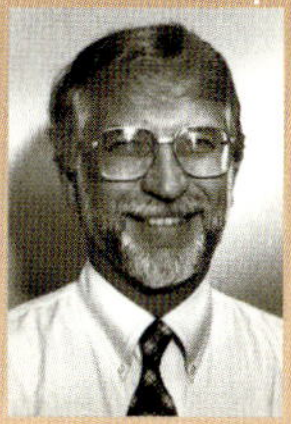

Alex Parkinson, MD

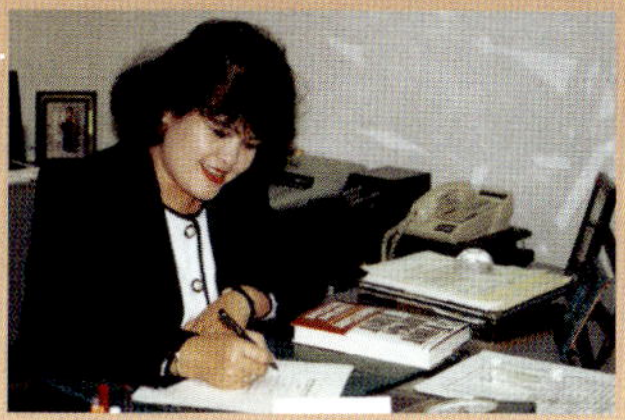

Ninfa Saunders, RN

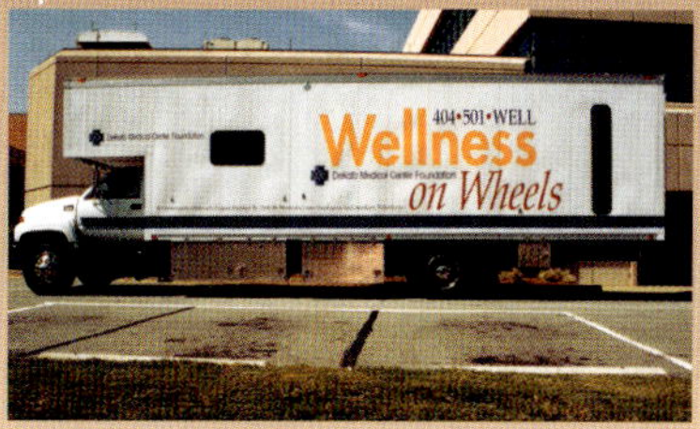

Wellness on Wheels

Department, to be responsible for respiratory services, the sleep lab and the pulmonary function lab.

- The Congestive Heart Failure program was established.
- The three-level parking deck was expanded, and a parking area was created adjacent to the second Professional Office Building under construction.

1996

- The second Professional Office Building opened on the central campus with seven stories, 156,400 square feet, physician offices, a new Wellness Center (18,000 sq. ft.), The Charles B. Eberhart Cancer Center, the Diagnostic Breast Center, the Herbert E. Kann Outpatient Cancer Treatment Center, and the DMC Outpatient Laboratory.
- DMC opened its new and expanded Emergency Department, Intensive Care/Coronary Care Unit and Diagnostic Treatment Center.
- DRHS discontinued alliance discussions with Rockdale, Emory, St. Joseph's, and Northside health systems and pursued negotiations with PROMINA.
- Kenneth Robinson succeeded Bonnie Phipps as CFO when Phipps became president of the PROMINA Health Plan.
- Richard Schmidt succeeded Carol Nikola as executive director of Decatur Hospital.
- Oliver Lee succeeded Floyd Sanders, MD, as chairman of the Hospital Authority.
- Maureen Vandiver succeeded Judy McMahan as the second Foundation Board chairperson.
- Paul Crank, MD, succeeded Wytch Stubbs, MD, as director of Medical Affairs.
- DMC negotiated an agreement with Mercer University to offer an on-campus master's degree in business administration for staff and physicians.
- McClellan Cox, MDiv, was named as associate chaplain.
- The DMC Foundation successfully completed its $1.6 million campaign for the new Emergency Department and launched a $5 million 1996–2001 Community Partnership 2000 campaign.
- DMC served as a member of the 1996 Olympic Games Hospital Network, providing staff, supplies, and equipment for the first aid stations located at the Stone Mountain Park venue. Betty Castellani, DMin, was nominated to be an Olympic torch bearer.
- IV Team nurses were transferred from the Pharmacy staff to Nursing Services, and staff nurses were trained to administer IV therapy.

1997

- June—DRHS became the 5th member of PROMINA along with Gwinnett, WellStar, Piedmont and Southern Regional health systems.
- The DeKalb Physician-Hospital Organization (DPHO) became the DRHS Local Integrated Delivery System (LIDS) for PROMINA.
- The Dogwood Shop was doubled in size.
- DRHS purchased land for the International Primary Care Medical Center on Buford Highway.
- DRHS' mental health partner, Behavioral Health Partners, Inc., contracted with PROMINA to market and manage its mental health services.
- DMC merged the Social Services Department, Utilization Review, Case Management, and Discharge Planning into one department, Medical Management Services (later named Care Management).
- The Charles B. Eberhart Cancer Center established an on-campus linear accelerator radiation therapy service.
- Decatur Hospital established a Long-Term Acute Care Unit (LTAC) with Thomas DeMarini, MD, medical director.
- Alex Parkinson, MD, succeeded Frank Matthews, MD, who retired after thirty-six years, as chief of Pathology and medical director of the Laboratory.
- The new and expanded Laboratory opened with 18,000 square feet of space.
- The Quality Council (later renamed Performance Improvement Council) was established by John Gerlach.
- Charles Eberhart was awarded posthumously the 1996 Georgia Hospital Association's Distinguished Service Award.

1998

- DMC purchased a home health service with Southern Regional Medical Center as a partner.
- Ninfa Saunders, RN was named chief operating officer (COO) of DMC.
- Duane Blair, MD, succeeded Pat L. Mathis as chairman of the DMC Board of Directors.
- The state denied DMC's request to build an "Alternative Healthcare Model" outpatient hospital in south DeKalb exempt from a CON application.
- The South DeKalb Advisory Committee recommended applying to the state to build an "outpatient hospital" with outpatient surgery, a recovery area, rehabilitation services, minor emergency center, and physician offices.
- DRHS/DHR negotiated the purchase of the Decatur Hospital facility and ground lease from Decatur Professional Investors for $6 million.
- DMC completed a pedestrian bridge linking the hospital and parking deck.
- The International Medical Center on Buford Highway opened with Tong Huynh, MD, medical director.
- DMC and DRHS Boards approved a Medical Staff Development Plan to limit physician additions to the medical staff according to need and ability to support them.
- The DMC Outpatient Surgery Center was expanded.
- Dan Callahan succeeded Clayton Bailey as director of Building Services.

1999

- Susan G. Sciullo succeeded Kenneth Robinson as CFO.
- Construction was begun in South DeKalb on Georgia's first "outpatient hospital" as recommended by the South DeKalb Advisory Committee and approved by the state.
- J. Randall Carroll succeeded Maureen Vandiver as the third Foundation Board chairperson.
- The Wellness on Wheels (W.O.W.) mobile health van was purchased to provide, in partnership with the DeKalb County Board of Health, community and health services to the county's underserved citizens.
- The DMC Foundation sponsored the staffing of a pilot children's health project in Decatur City Schools to ensure that all children have access to a primary care health provider.
- Doctors of Podiatric Medicine became the third non-MD professionals to be admitted to the DMC medical staff with James L. Bouchard, DPM as chief of the section.
- The Primary Care Division opened an outpatient Senior Health Center at Decatur Hospital and the inpatient Acute Care for the Elderly (ACE) unit at DMC.
- WellStar Health Systems withdrew from PROMINA.
- A robot system (aka "D'Spenser") was installed in the pharmacy to dispense commonly used drugs.
- The Diagnostic Imaging Center acquired open MRI technology.
- Ron McCranie, RRA, succeeded Faye Sophy, RRA, as director of Medical Records.

2000

- Judy McMahan succeeded Duane Blair, MD, as chairman of the DMC Board of Directors.
- Duane Blair, MD, succeeded Charles Ginden as chairman of the DRHS Board of Directors.
- Sarah Sloan succeeded Randall Carroll as the fourth Foundation Board chairperson.
- Jerilyn Bing succeeded Mary Kay Kiesling as director of Risk Management/Compliance.
- The Training and Education Department was renamed the Education Services

Timeline

2001 — 2002 — 2003 — 2004

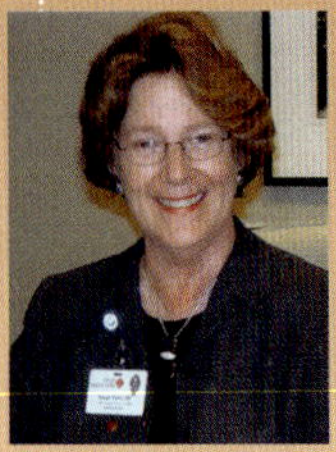
Susan Parry, RN

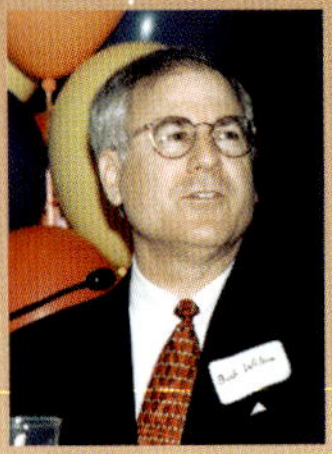
Robert "Bob" Wilson

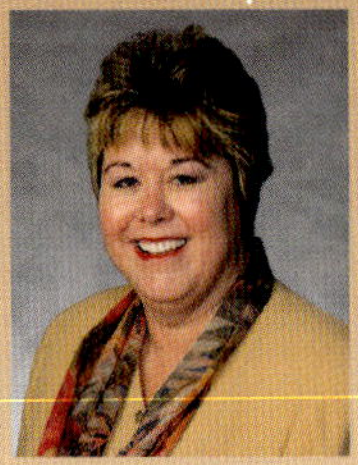
Cynthia Adgate (Davis)

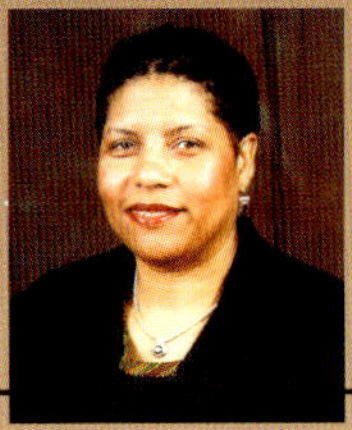
Delphyne Lomax

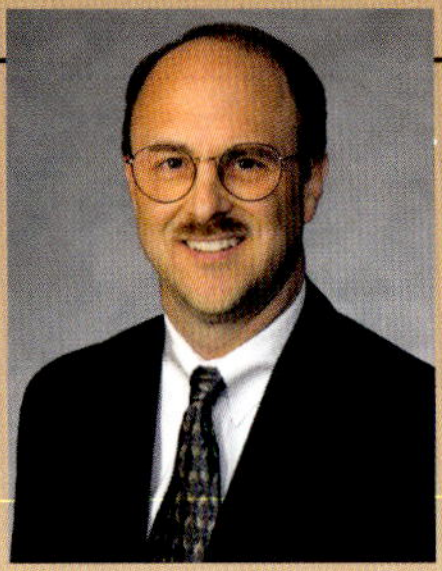
Eric Norwood

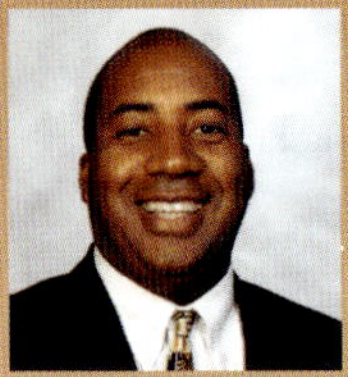
Albert Scott, MD

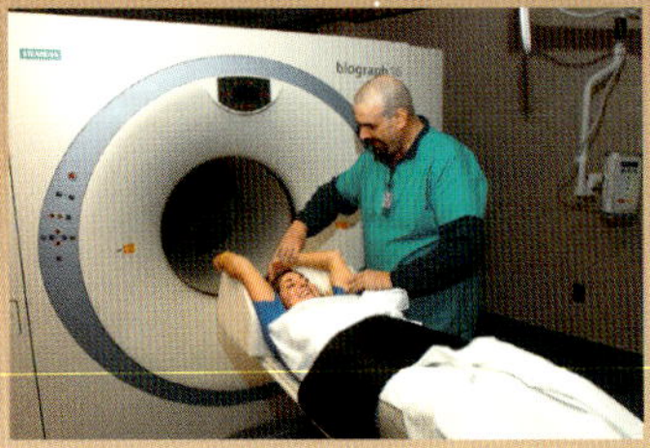
PET/CT Scanner

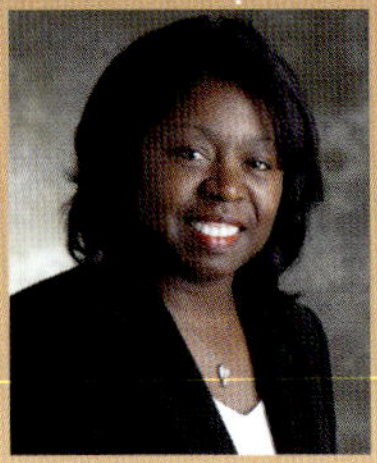
Julia Hunter Jones

Department.

- DRHS closed its acquired home health service due to poor financial performance and established an in-house Home Health Department.
- DRHS closed the Behavioral Health Partners mental health management operation due to mounting financial losses and continued its in-house Behavioral Health Department.
- South Fulton Hospital filed for bankruptcy.
- DMC opened a forensic toxicology laboratory.
- DMC expanded its osteoporosis program with state-of-the-art bone-density testing technology.
- The hospital earned a top CARE Quality Award for its treatment of patients with congestive heart failure.
- DMC was one of five hospitals in the nation to use H Works, a Health Care Advisory Board program, to find solutions for nursing recruiting and retention.

2001

- Susan Parry, RN, succeeded Ninfa Saunders, RN, as vice president of Patient Care Services and chief nursing officer.
- DMC opened the Outpatient Hospital at Hillandale with its physician offices, outpatient surgery, and minor emergency center; and FamilyCare South DeKalb on Covington Highway relocated to the Hillandale facility.
- DMC filed a new CON application with the state to build a full-service, acute-care 100-bed hospital on its Hillandale property; and two months later Tenet Healthcare Corporation filed a competing CON application to build a similar hospital at the Stonecrest Mall area.
- Robert E. Wilson succeeded Sarah Sloan as the fifth Foundation Board chairperson.
- DMC Foundation successfully met its $5 million goal for the 1996–2001 "Community Partnership 2000" campaign.
- The DeKalb Medical Auxiliary reached its 1 millionth hour of service to the medical center.
- DMC established the Coumadin® Clinic.
- The Radiation Oncology Center expanded and upgraded its capabilities.
- DMC purchased for $2 million American Management Systems' (AMS) SOVERA system to electronically scan and store medical records and patient financial information.
- A new DMC Chapel was completed and named in honor of donors Pete and Jerri Pike.
- Lynne Anderson succeeded Jerilyn Bing as director of Risk Management/Compliance.
- Bonnie Phipps succeeded Bernard Brown as CEO of PROMINA.
- Albert Wildstein, MD, succeeded Michael Kinstler, MD, as DPHO chairman.

2002

- Eric Norwood was named COO of DMC and DRHS.
- Bonnie Phipps resigned as CEO of PROMINA to become CEO of St. Joseph's Hospital.
- PROMINA faced severe financial difficulties.
- Skip Wright succeeded Richard Schmidt as executive director of Decatur Hospital.
- Cynthia Adgate (Davis) was named DRHS' first vice president for Information Technology and chief information officer (CIO).
- Judy McMahan was awarded the 2001 Georgia Hospital Association's Distinguished Service Award.
- The South DeKalb Advisory Committee was restructured as the South DeKalb Hospital Planning Board with Delphyne Lomax, chairperson.
- Nancy Rampell, MD, succeeded Paul Crank, MD, as director of Medical Affairs.

2003

- Eric Norwood succeeded John Gerlach as president and CEO of DMC and DRHS.
- Piedmont Hospital withdrew from PROMINA leaving DeKalb, Gwinnett and Southern Regional health systems as the three remaining members.
- PROMINA ceased providing managed care contracting for its members, returning that responsibility to local member organizations.
- DRHS allocated $8.5 million to convert its old SMS INVISION computer system to a browser-based version of INVISION, making it compatible with other computer program installations underway.
- The fifty-bed Skilled Nursing Facility on 2700 was closed due to financial losses.
- DMC sold the FamilyCare South DeKalb building and its property on Covington Highway to a private developer.
- Gail Winston, RN, succeeded Holly Wolfe, RN, as director of the Wellness Center and Health Promotions.
- The DMC and DRHS Boards rescinded the 1998 Medical Staff Development Plan and initiated a physician recruitment program to meet the new demand for physicians.
- The DeKalb Medical Society's Physicians' Care Clinic received the Georgia Hospital Association's Community Leadership Award.
- The DMC Foundation launched a 2003–2005 $5 million "Diagnosing the Future" campaign.
- Bill Sublett retired as director of Administrative Services with thirty-three years of service with perfect attendance.
- Cheryl Iverson was named vice president of DRHS Marketing and Business Development.
- The state gave final approval for DMC to build a 100-bed acute-care hospital in south DeKalb County, and construction began.

2004

- John Shelton was named executive vice president and COO of DMC and DRHS.
- Brent Robinson, RN, succeeded Susan Parry, RN, as vice president of Patient Care Services and chief nursing officer.
- DRHS reorganized its governance structure to make the DRHS Board the true parent board with Duane Blair, MD, chairman of the DMC, DHR, and DRHS boards.
- DeKalb Regional Healthcare System was renamed the DeKalb Regional Health System.
- Community Committees were established for DeKalb Medical at Hillandale, DeKalb Medical at Downtown Decatur and DeKalb Medical at North Decatur.
- Gordon Church resigned as PROMINA CEO.
- PROMINA downsized and reorganized with only six remaining shared services, including a purchasing group. The PROMINA name was dropped by the remaining members.
- The Diagnostic Imaging Center acquired a PET/CT scanner.
- The McKesson "Meds Manager" computer system was installed in the Pharmacy.
- The new DMC front entrance façade was completed.
- The credit union became the MembersFirst Federal Credit Union.
- Nancy Rampell, MD, resigned as director of Medical Affairs and the position was discontinued.
- Julia Hunter Jones was named vice president and administrator of DeKalb Medical at Hillandale.
- Albert Scott, MD, became the first African American chief of staff at North Decatur, and Cornelius Flowers, MD, became the first chief of staff at Hillandale.
- DMC was one of forty nonprofit hospitals nationwide named in a class action suit as not meeting its charitable obligation, all claims being dismissed by the courts in 2006.
- April—The Health Insurance Portability and Accountability Act (HIPPA) went into effect aimed at protecting health insurance coverage for workers and their families and protecting patient privacy, but creating heavy compliance demands on all providers.
- April—Healthvision's physician Internet Portal System was installed to permit authorized users remote access to the hospitals' websites for lab results, EKG tracings and reports, radiology images and

2005

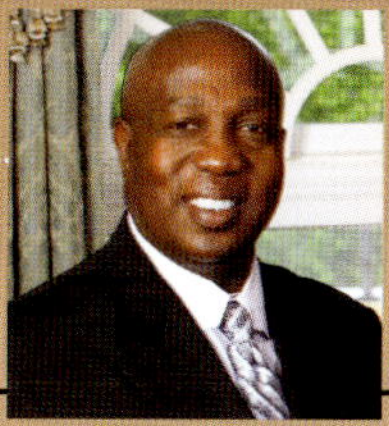

Gregory Levett Sr.

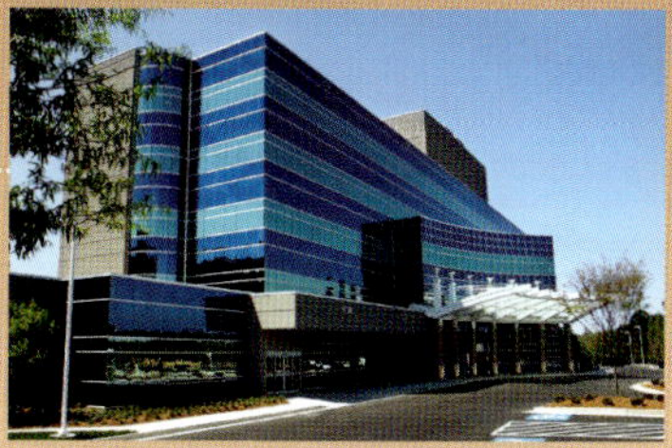

DeKalb Medical at Hillandale

2006

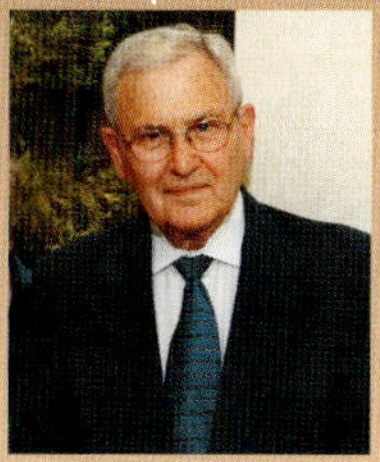

H. Duane Blair, MD

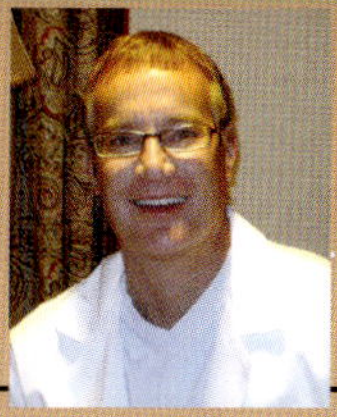

David Holladay, MD

DeKalb Medical

2007

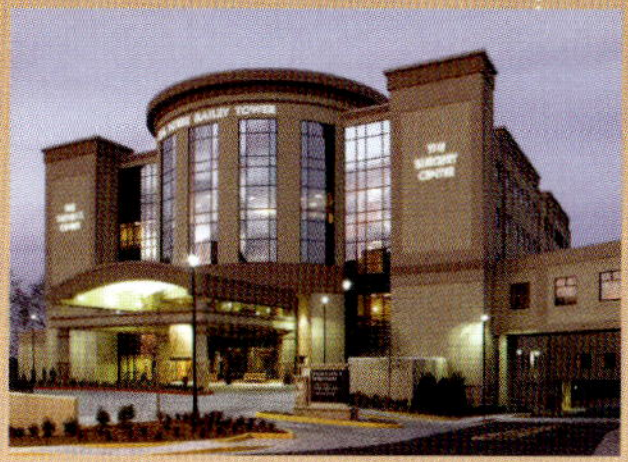

Women's Center and Surgery Center

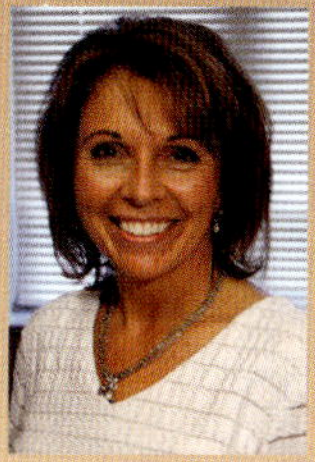

Cathleen Wheatley, RN

2008

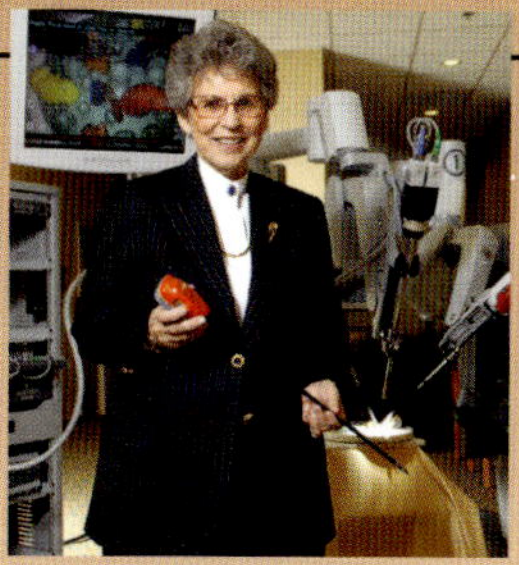

Bobbie Bailey with da Vinci robot

reports, and other information pertaining to their patients.

- July—DRHS "went-live" with the Sunrise Clinical Manager System as the foundation for the Computerized Physician Order Entry (CPOE) system and computerized clinical documentation by nurses and doctors.
- DRHS and the DPHO developed the concept of hospital-physician clinical integration and established the DeKalb Quality Institute to provide the data and leadership with Steve Meurer, PhD, as executive director.
- W. P. Tatum sold Property Resources, Inc., DeKalb Medical's property management company, to Meadows and Ohly Company.
- The state approved the CON application for the Women's Center and Surgery Center on the North Decatur campus.

2005

- Diane Harden succeeded Susan Sciullo as CFO.
- July—The DMC Hillandale $66.6 million, six-story, 191,000-square-foot, hospital opened as Georgia's first all-digital hospital, including the use of CPOE and computerized clinical documentation.
- FamilyCare Tucker was sold.
- Gregory B. Levett, Sr. succeeded Oliver Lee as Chairman of the Hospital Authority.
- *Dateline DeKalb* replaced *InDecatur* as the DRHS employee newsletter.
- A new telephone system was installed linking the three hospitals and the professional office buildings.
- DMC Foundation exceeded its 2003-2005 $5 million goal for the "Diagnosing the Future" campaign and launched a $6 million 2006–2009 campaign, "Building a Healthier Tomorrow."
- The Georgia Department of Community Health denied DMC's application to be one of the ten hospitals in the state to participate in a Johns Hopkins clinical trial to determine the efficacy and safety of performing angioplasty procedures for heart-attack patients in community hospitals without on-site open heart services.
- DRHS contracted with the California Emergency Physicians Medical Group to provide physician coverage for the North Decatur and Hillandale Emergency Departments in place of employed physicians.
- Scott W. McAuley, RPh, succeeded Lee Underwood, RPh, who retired after thirty-four years of service, as director of Pharmaceutical Services.
- Kevin McMullen, PT, was named director of DeKalb Rehabilitation Services.

2006

- DRHS initiated a joint management venture with surgeons for its Ambulatory Surgery Center.
- H. Duane Blair, MD, received the 2005 Georgia Hospital Association's Distinguished Service Award.
- DeKalb Medical Foundation launched its 2006–2009 campaign, "Building A Healthier Tomorrow."
- Alex Parkinson, MD, retired as chief pathologist to be succeeded by Hilary Hargreaves, MD, and William McNeill, MD.
- Behavioral Health Services closed its outpatient service.

2007

- The new $55 million Women's Center and Surgery Center opened with an underground parking deck.
- DRHS faced severe financial challenges.
- The positions of vice president and administrator of Downtown Decatur and vice president for Information Technology/ chief information officer were discontinued.
- DMC discontinued its designation as a state's Level 3 Trauma Center.
- DeKalb Medical contracted with Sodexho, Inc., to provide nutrition services to the three campuses.
- Occupation Health and Infection Control were divided into two departments.
- The IV Team service was downsized to a core of nurses to support floor nurses needing assistance.
- David Holladay, MD, was named medical director of DeKalb Medical's Radiation Oncology Department.
- HCA closed Northlake Regional Medical Center which Emory University purchased and reopened.
- Facing the possibility of Grady Memorial Hospital's bankruptcy and closure, the Fulton-DeKalb Hospital Authority agreed to lease its operation to a private, nonprofit governing body, the Grady Hospital Corporation, with the promise of grants from foundations, the business community and the state.
- Clay Fowler succeeded Julia Hunter Jones as vice president and administrator of DeKalb Medical at Hillandale hospital.
- Oliver Lee succeeded Duane Blair, MD, as chairman of the DRHS Board, the DMC Board and the DHR Board.
- Cathleen Wheatley, RN, succeeded Steve Meurer, PhD, as senior vice president and executive director of Quality, Care Management, Information Technology and Infection Control.
- Brent Robinson resigned as VP, Patient Care Services and CNO, a national search for his successor was launched.
- Betty Castellani was selected as the third non-physician to be awarded DeKalb Medical Society's Julius McCurdy Citizenship Award.
- The name "DeKalb Medical" was chosen to signify the health system, and the hospitals were designated as DeKalb Medical at North Decatur, DeKalb Medical at Downtown Decatur, and DeKalb Medical at Hillandale.
- A new DRHS logo was created.
- Radiation oncologist, Dale McCord, MD, and medical oncologist, Bruce Feinberg, DO, initiated plans for a Radiation Treatment Center at Hillandale.
- CPOE and computerized clinical documentation went live hospital-wide at the North Decatur campus.
- DeKalb Medical negotiated a contract with Visiting Nurse/Hospice Atlanta to be its preferred provider for home health services.
- A History Preservation Center Committee was established to preserve and manage documents pertaining to DeKalb Medical's history.
- The new chapel at DeKalb Medical at Hillandale was completed and named in honor of donors Pete and Jerri Pike.

2008

- Bobbie Bailey's gift of $3.3 million completed the 2006–2009 Foundation campaign and launched the next campaign that included acquiring the da Vinci robot for Surgical Services.
- Jan Gannon, RN, is named Vice President of Patient Care Services and chief nursing officer.

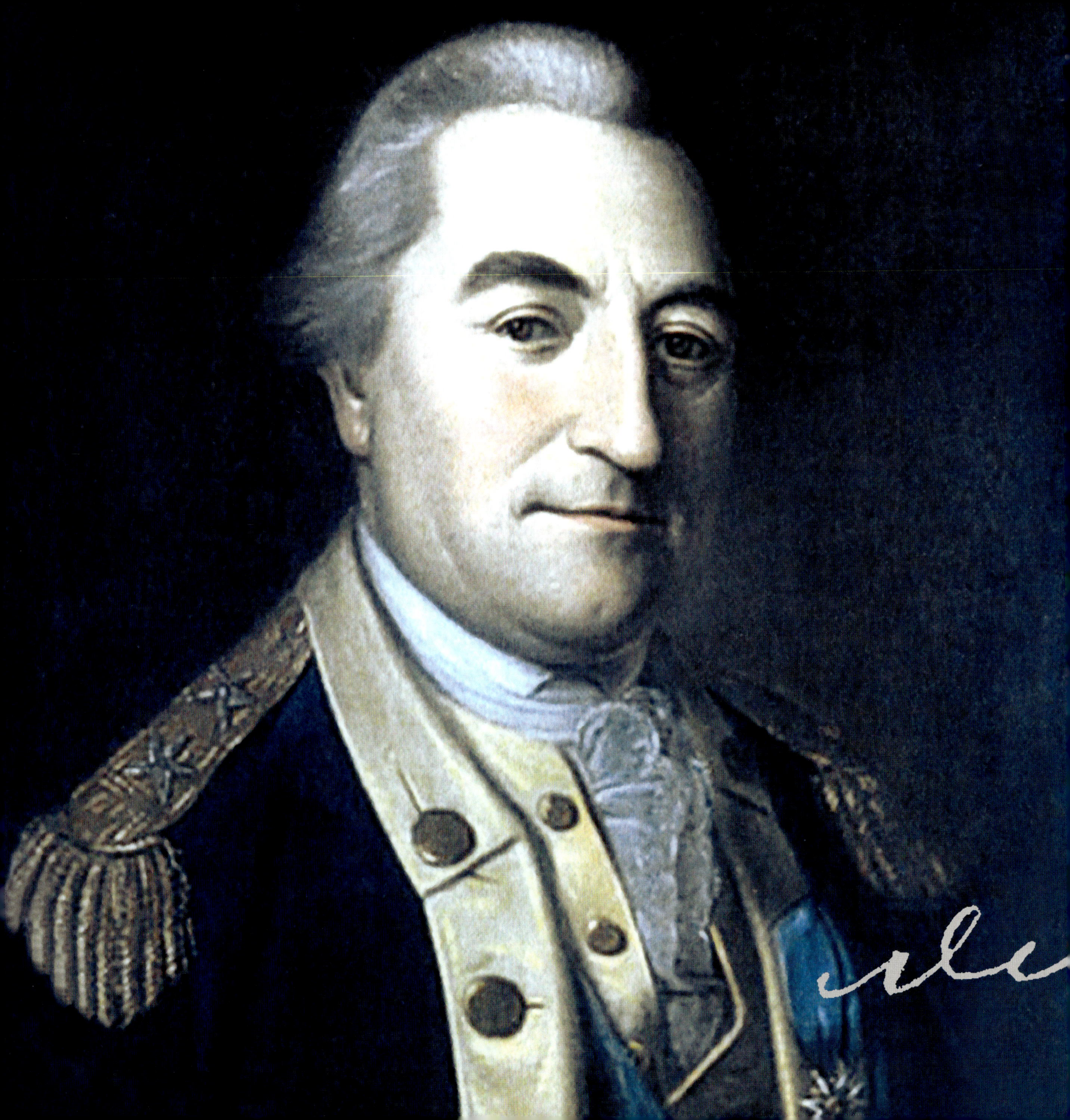

CHAPTER ONE

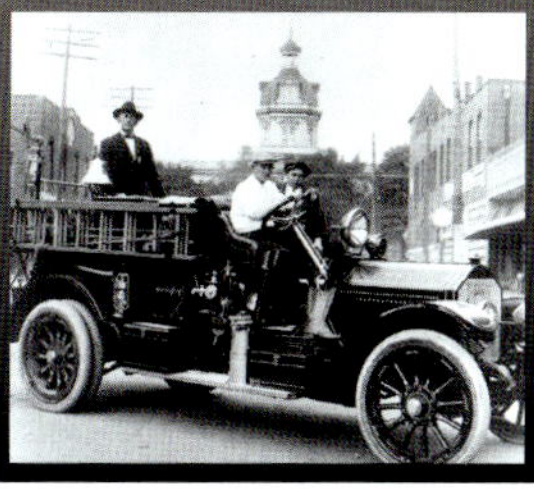

DeKalb County Comes of Age

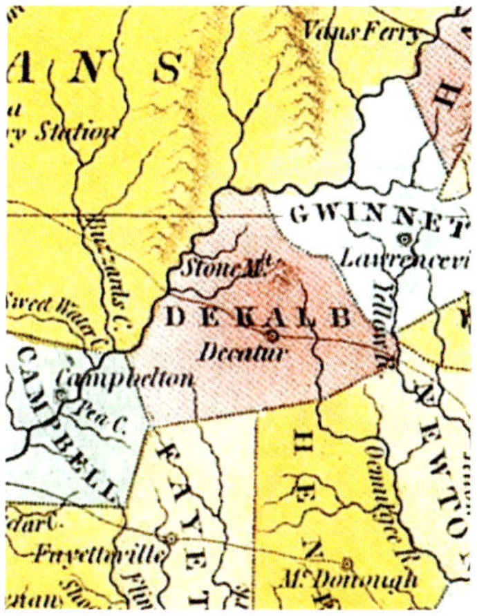

Opposite: French soldier, Baron Johann DeKalb, was the only general in the American Revolution who died on the battlefield fighting next to the average foot soldier. DeKalb County was named in honor of him. His signature appears below. **Above:** Map of DeKalb County, Georgia, 1830.

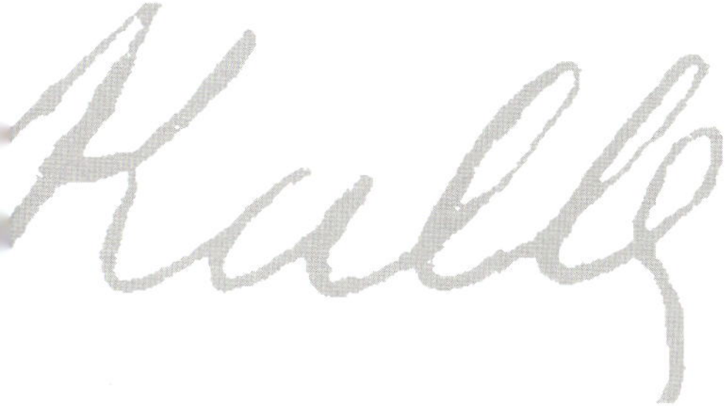

On April 21, 1961, DeKalb General Hospital was dedicated "to the glory of God and to the improved health of mankind." DeKalb County officials, the DeKalb County Hospital Authority, community physicians, the hospital's leadership and staff, and approximately four hundred interested citizens gathered in front of the hospital to join in the celebration. That event was the culmination of vision, commitment, sweat, and toil on the part of many community heroes who labored tirelessly for more than a decade to make DeKalb General Hospital a reality. It also was the culmination of a historical evolution that saw DeKalb County come of age.

At the Treaty of Paris that officially ended the American Revolution in 1783, the defeated British transferred most of their land holdings in America to the thirteen colonies. As a result, Georgia's western border extended to the Mississippi River. In 1802, when Thomas Jefferson was president, Georgia ceded title to all of its territory lying west of the current Georgia-Alabama line to the federal government in return for $1.25 million and the government's promise to remove all American Indians from Georgia soil.[1]

Among the American Indians in Georgia, the Cherokee people occupied most of north Georgia, and the Creeks occupied the southern part of the state that lay below the Chattahoochee River.[2] In keeping with its promise, the federal government extracted a series of treaties from the Georgia native people so that by 1827 the Creeks held claim to no Georgia land, and by 1835 the Cherokees had given up north Georgia.[3] The government made good on its promise.

Georgia immediately divided the land acquired through these treaties into counties. In 1822, DeKalb became the state's fifty-sixth county.[4] It, along with counties in several other states, was named for Baron Johann DeKalb, the French army officer who fought and died on the side of the Americans in the Revolutionary War.[5] Of course, he wasn't always French, he wasn't always a baron, he wasn't always "Johann," and he wasn't always "DeKalb." He had been born Hans Kalb, the son of a German peasant. Hans left home at the age of sixteen to become a French soldier of fortune. When he learned that only noblemen could become officers, he gave himself the title of "baron."[6] He later assumed the name of a French acquaintance, Jean DeKalb, and finally altered his name to the more Germanic, Johann DeKalb. He was one of several French soldiers who came to America with Marquis de Lafayette in 1777,[7] offered his services, was appointed major general in the Continental army, and fought gallantly in the Battle of Camden, South Carolina, where he died in 1780 after being wounded eleven times. He has the distinction of being the only general in the American Revolution to die on the battlefield fighting next to the average foot soldier. He is alleged to have uttered as his last words, "I thank you for your generous sympathy; but I die the death I always prayed for—the death of a soldier fighting for the rights of man."[8]

Transportation was limited in the early days of the county. A weekly stage from Milledgeville to Stone Mountain and Decatur was one of the few forms of public transportation. There were few passable roads, and early settlers frequently used old Indian trails. Three that were used most heavily were the Hightower Trail, the Sandtown Trail, and the Peachtree Trail. Eventually the Hightower Trail became the boundary line between DeKalb County and Gwinnett County.[9] The Sandtown Trail ran westward from DeKalb County along the present DeKalb Avenue from Decatur to what is now Five Points in downtown Atlanta.[10] The Peachtree Trail ran along the top of the Chattahoochee Ridge from near Toccoa to what now is Buckhead and Five Points.[11]

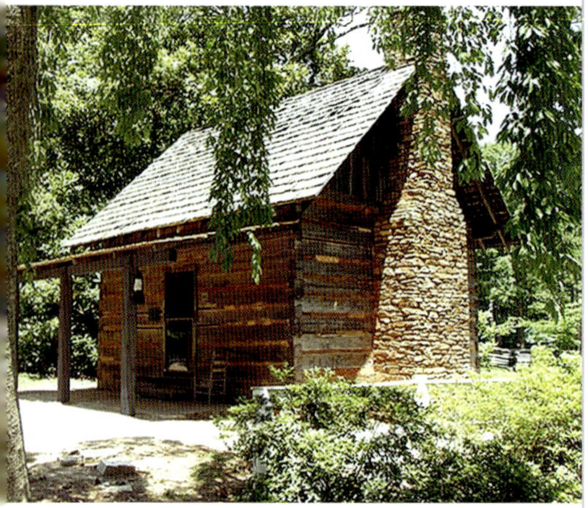

Chapman Powell, MD built the "Medicine House" near the corner of Clairmont and North Decatur Road in the early 1800s. He treated Cherokee Indians and whites with his own herbal medicines.

Physicians came to DeKalb County shortly after it was established. Jeanne O. Gibbs[12] and Calvin Weaver, MD,[13] each wrote of the history of medicine in DeKalb County. Chapman Powell, MD, and Ezekiel N. Calhoun, MD, arrived in 1827. Powell lived near the present intersection of Clairmont Road and North Decatur Road and built a log cabin that the Cherokees called "Medicine House," where he treated the whites and the native people alike with his own compounded herbal preparations. A plaque commemorating the Medicine House remains at the site today. The original house is now located in Stone Mountain Park. But Calhoun and Powell each held claims to fame in addition to being physicians. Powell became sheriff of DeKalb County in 1833, and Calhoun was commander of the eighty-four-man Volunteer Light Infantry that took part in putting down a renegade Creek uprising in southwest Georgia.

Thomas Holley Chivers, MD, came to Decatur in 1856 and became one of the county's most famous physicians. His fame, however, did not come from his being a physician, for he never practiced medicine in the county. Instead he was best known for his eleven volumes of poetry, for his music, and for his inventions that included a machine for unwinding silk cocoons. A long-time friend and correspondent of Edgar Allen Poe, Chivers claimed that Poe plagiarized one of his poems when Poe wrote his famous "The Raven."[14]

Many DeKalb physicians served in the Confederate army, and after the war several played key roles in rebuilding their devastated community. They also formed the DeKalb County Medical Protective Society, the forerunner of the present-day DeKalb Medical Society. The society became inactive in the early 1900s, but was reactivated and received its charter from the Medical Association of Georgia in 1924 with Wiley S. Ansley, MD, as president.[15]

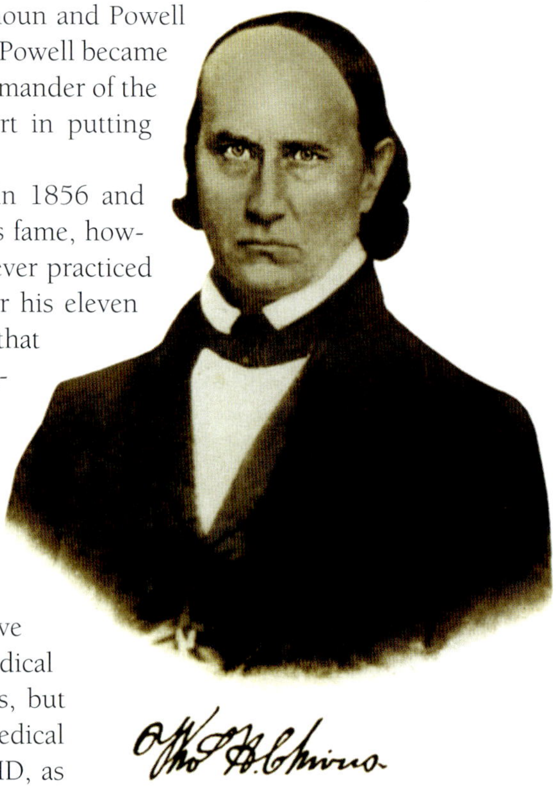

Thomas Holley Chivers, MD

The city of Decatur was named for Commodore Stephen Decatur, a naval hero in the War of 1812. It was incorporated and designated as the county seat in 1823. In 1824 the citizens constructed a log cabin courthouse on the northwest corner of the original town square over a dungeonlike basement that was used for the county jail.[16] In 1829 they built a second courthouse, also wooden,[17] that was destroyed by fire in 1842 along with practically all of the county's records. The county built a brick courthouse in 1847, with a portico, steps, and two granite columns on the east side.[18] The building was later replaced in 1898 with the granite structure that still stands on the old courthouse square, though the interior was reconstructed after being gutted by fire in 1916.[19]

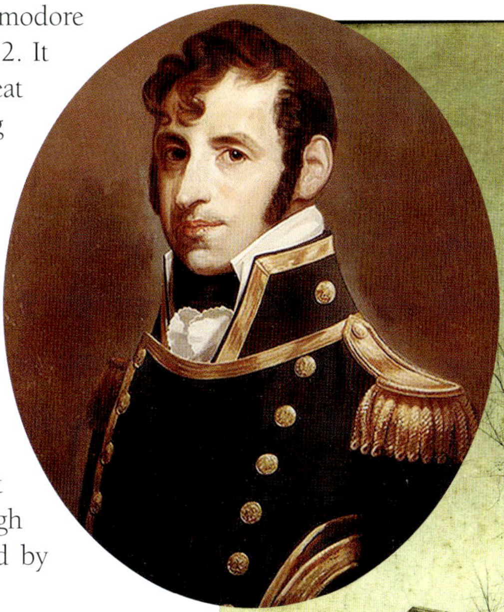

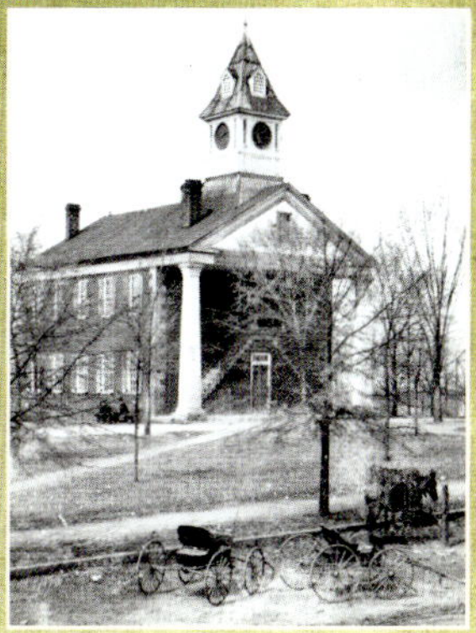

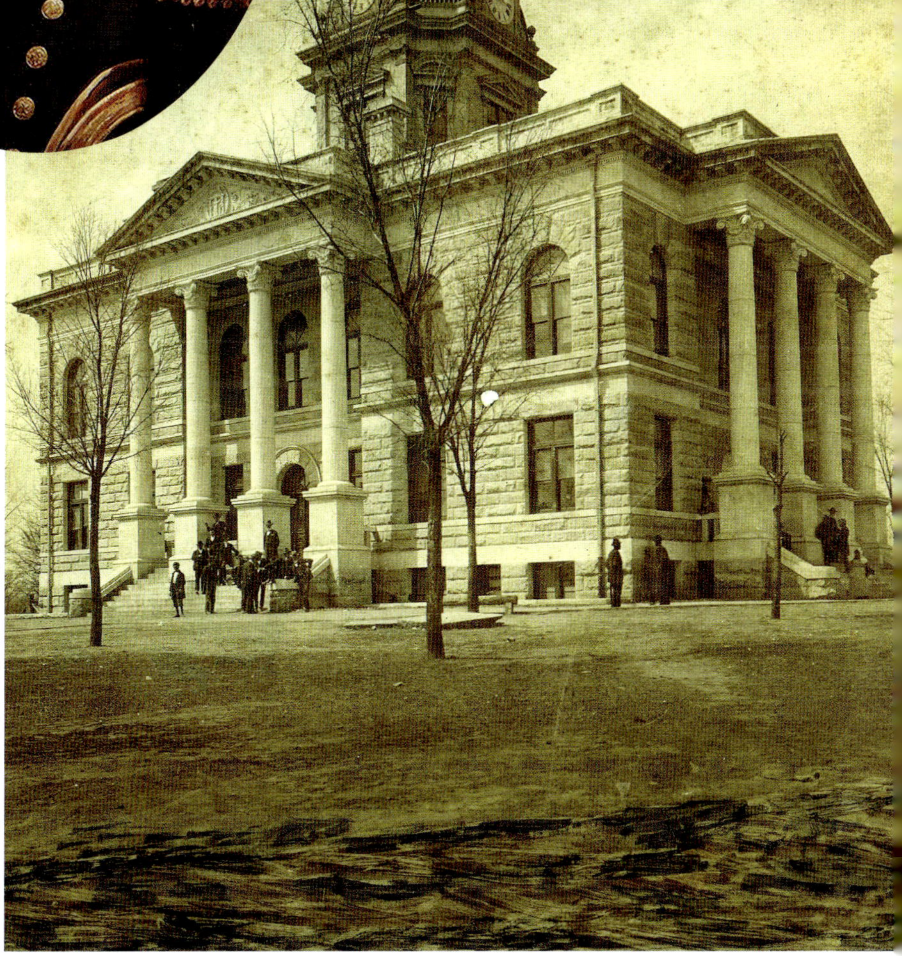

In the 1890s Decatur almost lost its designation as the county seat when the citizens of Stone Mountain petitioned to have it relocated to their thriving community. The issue was put to a county referendum, and a majority chose Stone Mountain over Decatur by a vote of 814 to160. The Georgia Supreme Court declared that election to be valid. When the issue went to the Georgia General Assembly for its approval in November 1897, a majority of the legislators voted eighty-five to sixty in favor of Stone Mountain. That vote, however, was twelve less than the two-thirds majority required by the state constitution to make a change.[20] So Decatur remained the county seat.

The coming of the railroad was a major boost to DeKalb's economy. Decatur, however, missed a golden opportunity when it turned down the chance to be the end of the line for the Georgia Railroad that originated in Augusta.[21] Decatur's citizens said they did not want the noise, smoke, and confusion that might be associated with a train terminal.[22] So, instead, Atlanta agreed to be the terminating point for the Georgia Railroad and other lines. Because of that designation, Atlanta was originally known as Terminus but was renamed Marthasville in 1843 after the daughter of Wilson Lumpkin, the town mayor and former governor.[23] In 1845 the city was given the name Atlanta, allegedly suggested by John Edgar Thomson, chief engineer of the Georgia Railroad. He said Atlanta was the feminine form of the masculine Atlantic in the Western and Atlantic line that ran from Chattanooga to Atlanta.[24]

Top left: Commodore Stephen Decatur was a naval hero in the War of 1812. The city of Decatur, Georgia, was named for him. **Above inset:** A DeKalb County courthouse was built in 1847 to replace the previous wooden structures. **Above:** A new granite courthouse was built in 1898 and still stands today in the Decatur city square.

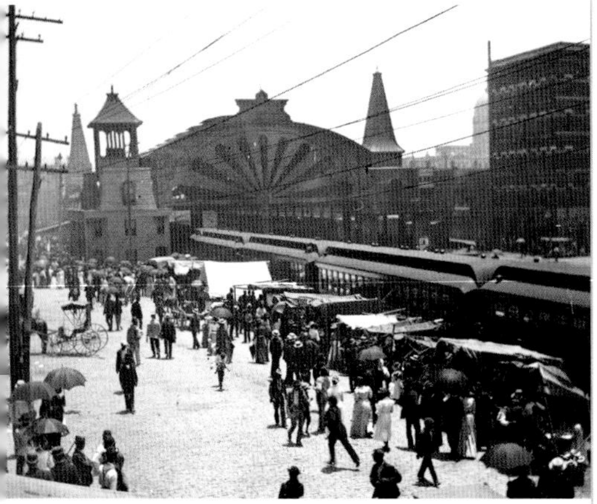

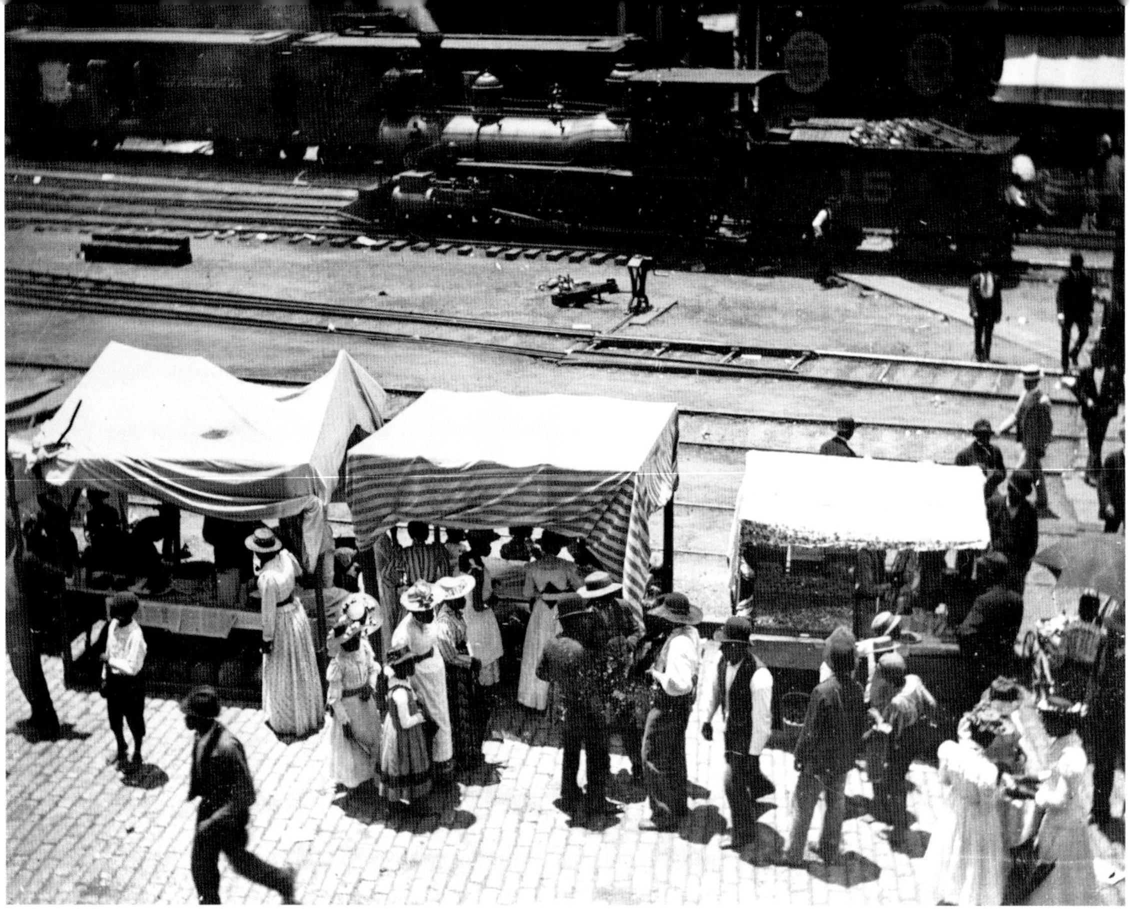

Above and right: Atlanta was a bustling and rapidly growing city in the mid-to-late 1800s. In 1868, it became the state capital of Georgia.

As a transportation hub, Atlanta experienced an explosive growth and vitality that eluded Decatur. In 1853 the legislature created Fulton County, which included the city of Atlanta, out of the western half of DeKalb County. And the city's growth resumed after the Civil War, when, in 1868, Atlanta succeeded Milledgeville as the state capital. The new capitol was constructed at a cost of just under $1 million and dedicated on July 4, 1889.[25]

By this time, the economy of DeKalb County also began to flourish. Important industries included quarrying for granite that was in great demand as building stones, growing and ginning cotton, truck farming, dairy farming, and grain milling (hence such roads as Browns Mill, Tilly Mill, and Henderson Mill).[26] Scottish immigrant John Keay Davidson Sr. owned one of the major quarry sites in and around Lithonia.[27] Richard F. Sams, a Georgia Institute of Technology graduate, was one of the best known truck farmers in the county. He developed techniques such as irrigation, refrigerated storage, and the use of hothouses—concepts that eventually were incorporated into the agricultural program at the University of Georgia.[28]

Towns emerged rapidly. There were only three incorporated cities in the county before the Civil War: Decatur incorporated in 1823, Stone Mountain (originally known as New Gibraltar) in 1825, and Lithonia in 1856. After the war, Doraville was incorporated in 1871, Clarkston in 1882, Chamblee in 1908, Avondale Estates in 1927, and Pine Lake in 1935. Tucker, though thriving, was never incorporated as a city. Avondale Estates was originally known as Ingleside. George Willis purchased the town in 1924 to develop it as a model suburban city and gave it its present name.[29]

The earliest schools in the county were small, private institutions such as the Donald Fraser School on Clairmont Road in Decatur and the Lithonia Academy in Lithonia. In 1825 DeKalb County

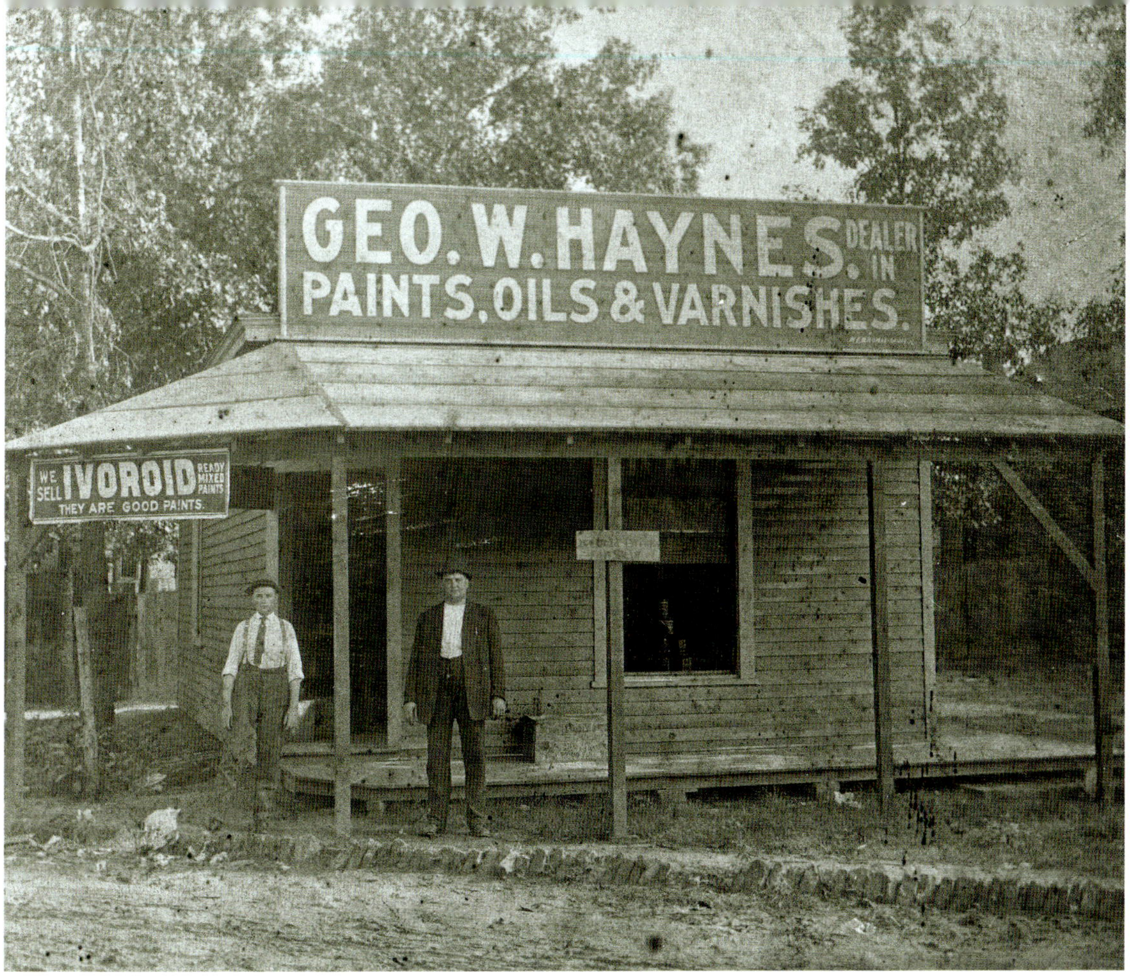

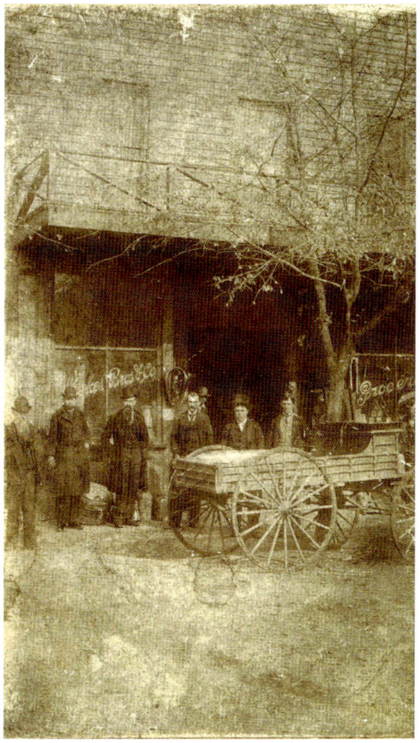

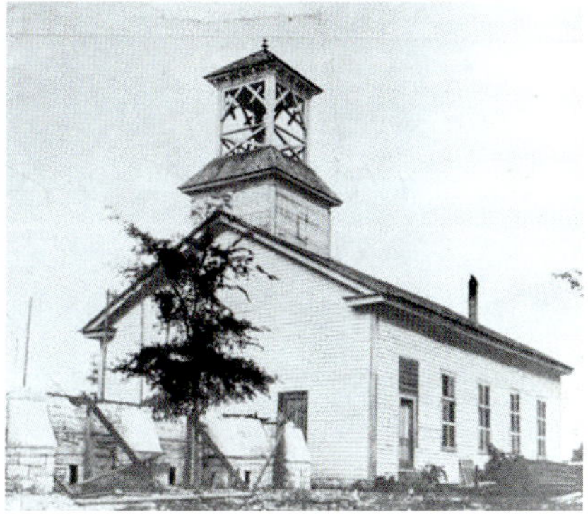

Above left: George W. Haynes store in Decatur. **Top:** Thomas Ramspeck's store in Decatur. **Above:** The Methodist Church in Decatur in the mid-1800s.

opened its first semipublic school, the DeKalb Academy in Decatur. Tuition was two cents a day for the lower grades and three cents a day for students in higher grades. The state supplemented the academy with three cents a day per pupil. Early in the 1900s, both the city of Decatur and DeKalb County created the present-day public school system.[30]

The state of Georgia and DeKalb County were at the forefront of establishing institutions of higher education. Georgia was the first state in the nation to establish a state-chartered institution of higher education when it created the University of Georgia in 1785.[31] DeKalb County would have its own outstanding institutions of higher learning in Emory University, Oglethorpe University, Agnes Scott College, and Columbia Theological Seminary.

Emory originated in 1834 when the Methodist Church established a preparatory school at Oxford in Newton County known as the Manual Labor School. This school was designed to provide Georgia youth with a place where they could receive an education while working on a farm to learn farming skills and to earn money to pay for their education and keep. In 1836 the Georgia legislature granted the Methodist Church a charter to expand the school into a college. It was named Emory after Methodist Bishop John Emory and opened in 1838 with four faculty members and fifteen students. Emory was closed for five years during the Civil War when its buildings were used as a temporary hospital and its library and equipment were destroyed. Even when the college reopened, it struggled financially because of the difficult financial times associated with the Reconstruction.

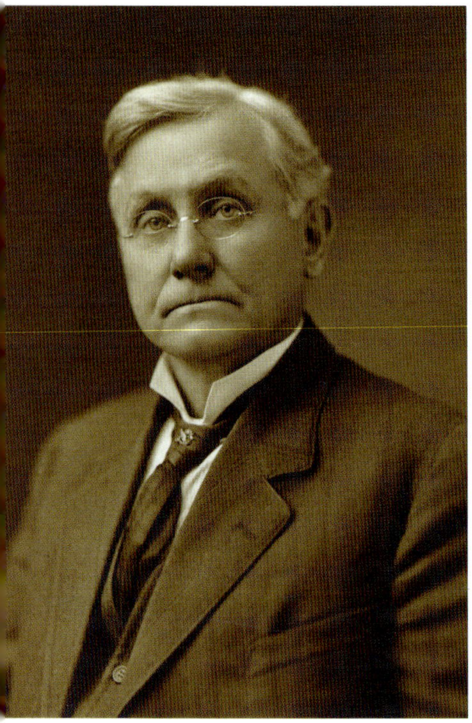

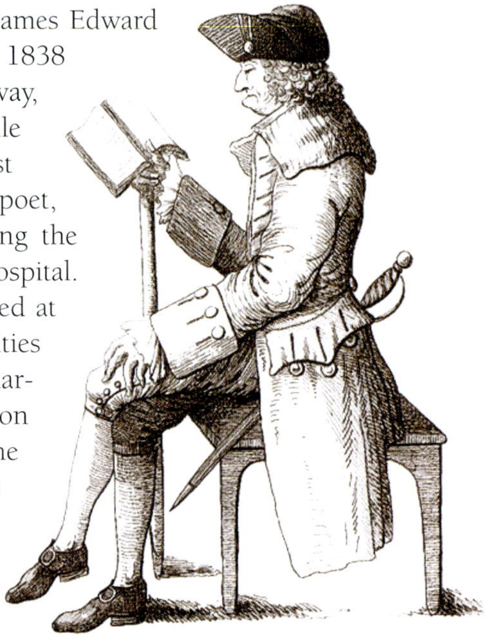

Above: Asa Griggs Candler, Atlanta druggist, founder of The Coca-Cola Company, and mayor of Atlanta 1916–1919. **Right:** James Edward Oglethorpe, the founder of Georgia and for whom Oglethorpe University was named.

In 1914 Asa Griggs Candler, who owned the Coca-Cola Company, offered Emory $1 million and seventy-two acres of land in the Druid Hills community to move to Atlanta. His younger brother, Warren Candler, was a bishop in the Methodist Church and past president of Emory College at Oxford. The Methodist Church accepted his offer, maintained a two-year undergraduate program at Oxford, and moved the four-year college to Atlanta where it would be the core of the university that was chartered in 1915. Construction of the new Emory University campus began in 1915 and was completed in 1919 to accommodate the college, the School of Theology, the Business School, the Law School, and the Graduate School.[32]

Oglethorpe University, named for Georgia's founder James Edward Oglethorpe, was chartered and commenced operations in 1838 with four faculty members and twenty-five students in Midway, a small community near Milledgeville, Georgia. Milledgeville was still the capital of Georgia. One of Oglethorpe's most prominent graduates in the class of 1860 was Sidney Lanier, poet, critic, and musician. Like Emory, Oglethorpe closed during the Civil War when its buildings were used for barracks and a hospital. Once reopened, it moved to Atlanta in 1870 and was located at the site of the present-day Atlanta City Hall. Financial difficulties forced it to close again in 1872. It remained closed until rechartered in 1913 and reopened in 1915 at its present location on Peachtree Road. It "arose from the ashes" largely due to the heroic fund-raising efforts of Thornwell Jacobs who became the school's president for nearly three decades.[33]

Agnes Scott College was established in 1889 when Rev. Frank Gaines, pastor of the Decatur Presbyterian Church, donated a home in Decatur for the Decatur Female Seminary, an all-girls school. It opened with four faculty members and sixty-three students. Col. George Washington Scott, grandfather of Scott Candler Sr. who later would play a pivotal role in the development of DeKalb County, helped the school become a college. He donated $40,000 to provide a permanent home for the school on the condition that it be named after his mother, Agnes Irvine Scott. The school was chartered as Agnes Scott College in 1906 and became the first institution of higher education in Georgia to receive accreditation from the Southern Association of Colleges and Schools.[34]

Columbia Theological Seminary was founded in 1828 in Lexington, Georgia, by several Presbyterian ministers. It moved to Columbia, South Carolina, in 1830 where it got its name before relocating to Decatur in 1927.[35]

DeKalb County experienced an exploding population growth in the twentieth century. The 1900 census recorded 21,112 residents. By 1930 the number rose to 70,278, and by 1950 the census figure was 136,395. Between 1950 and 1960, DeKalb County was one of the fastest growing counties in the nation, and by the end of the decade it had 256,782 residents, a growth of more than 88 percent.[36]

While the rapid population growth gave the county something to celebrate, it also presented a challenge to provide the necessary services and infrastructure. Roads were in poor condition.

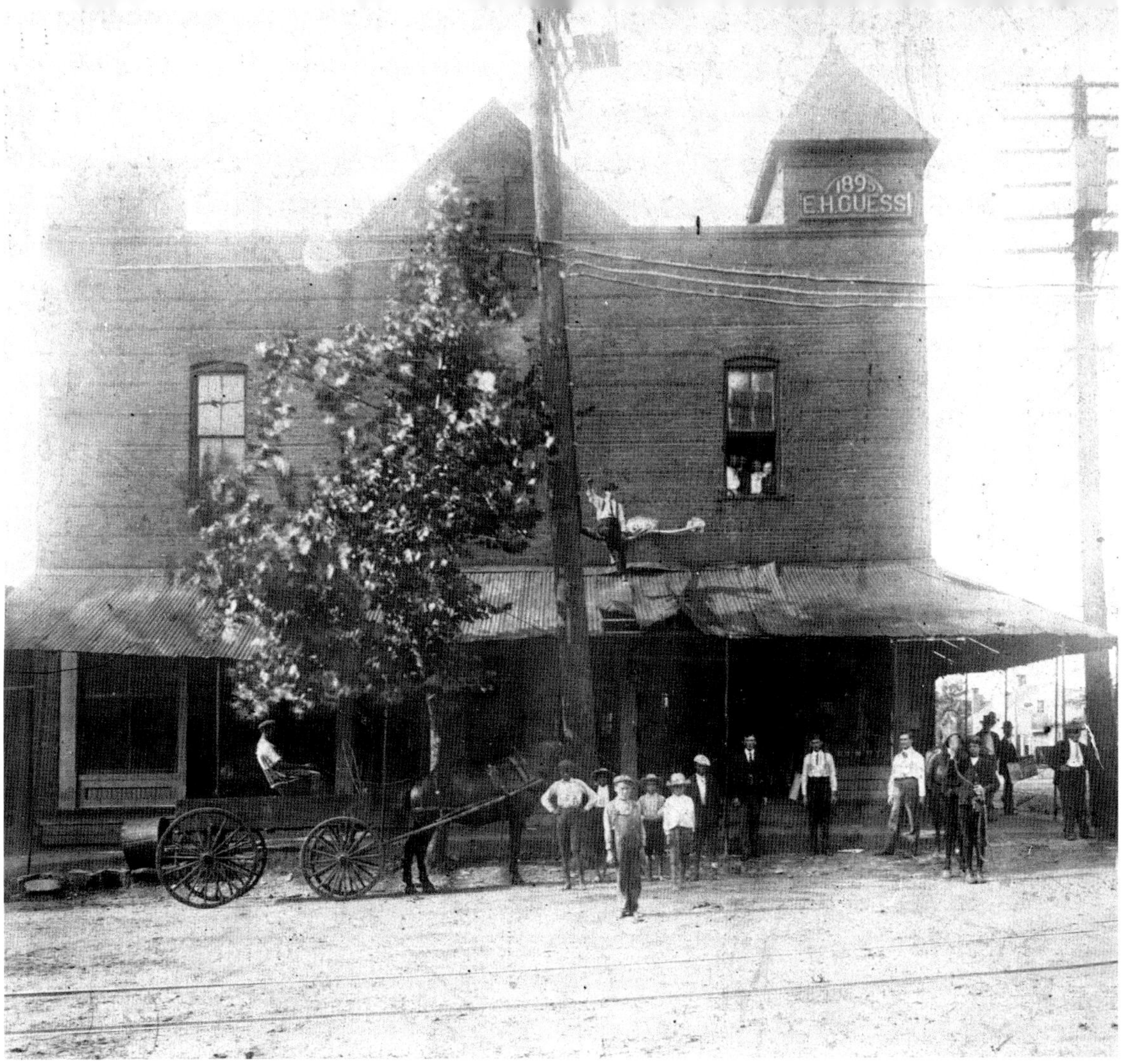

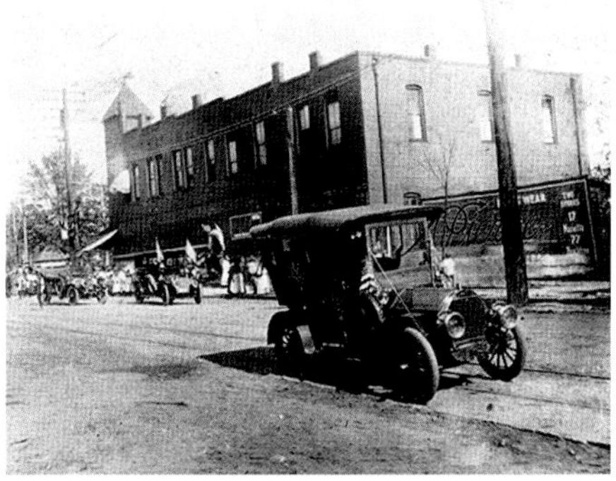

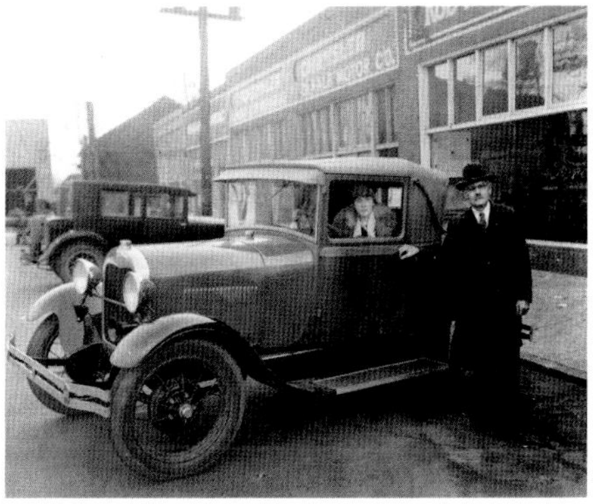

Left: Henry Simeon Rogers' general store in downtown Decatur, 1910. **Top:** A parade of the first cars in Decatur ca. 1912–1916. **Above:** A Model A Ford on the square in Decatur.

The portion of Ponce de Leon Avenue that ran through Decatur was not paved until 1914. Public transportation was in short supply. A streetcar line constructed in 1915 ran from Stone Mountain through Decatur to Atlanta. The county needed a water system, sanitation services, and police and fire protection. In 1934 Druid Hills residents subscribed to a private fire protection service out of Nashville, Tennessee. The county faced many urgent needs.[37]

Scott Candler Sr., known to many as "Mr. DeKalb," would help the county meet many of those needs. Candler was born in 1887, attended Davidson College, and received a law degree from Atlanta Law School. He served as mayor of Decatur for seventeen years and was elected the sole DeKalb County Commissioner of Roads and Revenues in 1939, a position he held until 1955. During those sixteen years, he exercised sole control over the county's financial operations, and he helped the county realize an unprecedented period of growth, new industries, new services, and new facilities.

Under his leadership, the county paved four hundred miles of road, opened the Decatur-DeKalb Library, constructed a large water system for the entire county from the Chattahoochee River, persuaded General Motors (GM) to locate its assembly plant in Doraville, recruited nearly seventy other industrial companies to the county, opened DeKalb-Peachtree Airport on a portion of the old Camp Gordon built in 1917 for use in World War I, located the Internal Revenue Service on the remaining portion of the that land, helped establish the Fulton-DeKalb Hospital Authority that allowed Grady Memorial Hospital to serve Fulton and DeKalb's indigent residents, established residential sewer service and garbage collection, enhanced the DeKalb Police Department, and helped bring the Stone Mountain Memorial Park and its Confederate Memorial carving to completion as a nationally acclaimed tourist attraction.[38]

One of the legendary stories about Candler says that when he met with officials of General Motors in an effort to encourage them to build a multimillion dollar automobile assembly plant in Doraville, the GM automotive officials finally agreed to the terms he offered. They asked when the county commission would meet to confirm the concessions Candler proposed. Candler allegedly replied, "We just met, and I voted 'yes.'"[39]

One of the most urgent unmet needs facing the county in the 1950s was a hospital to serve the exploding population and the area's growing number of physicians. Atlanta had several hospitals, but there was a void in DeKalb County.

Saint Joseph's Hospital was established in 1880 when four nuns of the Sisters of Mercy, a Roman Catholic religious order, arrived in Atlanta and opened the Atlanta Hospital in a small house on Baker Street. This hospital, which was the first medical facility in the city following the Civil War, later moved to a three-story building on Courtland Street (now the site of the Marriott Marquis Hotel) where it was known as the Saint Joseph's Infirmary. In 1978 it was relocated to its present location in North Atlanta where it became Saint Joseph's Hospital of Atlanta.[40]

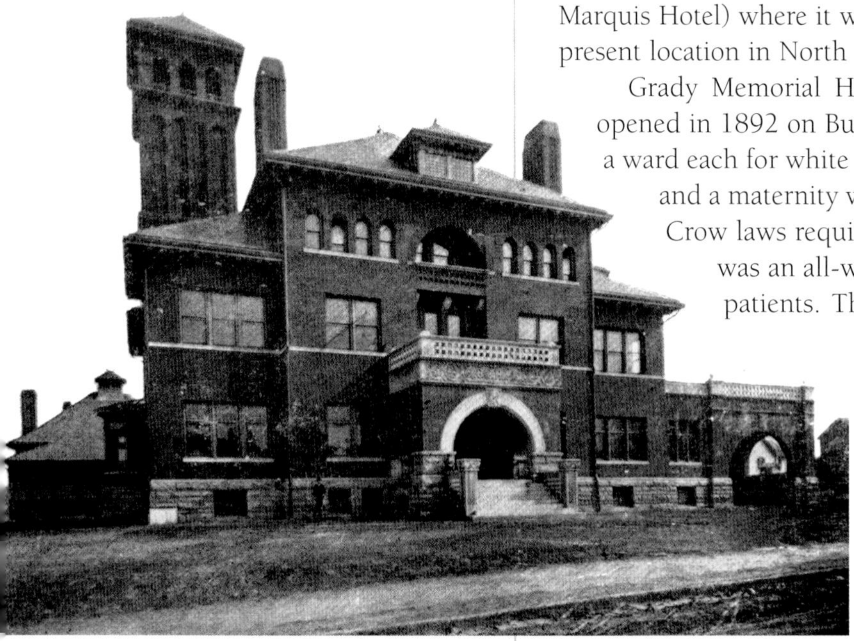

Grady Memorial Hospital on Butler Street in Atlanta.

Grady Memorial Hospital, named for the Atlanta Constitution editor Henry W. Grady, opened in 1892 on Butler Street. It contained one hundred beds and ten rooms that included a ward each for white males, white females, black males, and black females, a children's ward, and a maternity ward. When a second Grady was constructed in 1912 the state's new Jim Crow laws required segregation of the races and the construction of two hospitals. One was an all-white facility, and the other at Armstrong and Butler Street was for black patients. Those separate facilities were often referred to as "the Gradies," a name that many people continue to use today. A third Grady Hospital was constructed following World War I, and the present structure opened in 1958.

The city owned, financed, and operated Grady Hospital until the Fulton-DeKalb Hospital Authority was established in 1945 and assumed responsibility for its operation. Fulton County and DeKalb County each contributed tax revenue to support the Authority with the requirement that Grady provide health services for the indigent citizens of the two counties.[41]

Georgia Baptist Hospital became Atlanta's third hospital. In 1901 Leonard Broughton, MD, a physician and the pastor of the Tabernacle Baptist Church in downtown Atlanta rented a "dilapidated" five-room house on Courtland Street for $25 a month and opened the Tabernacle Baptist Infirmary for "down and out" people who had nowhere else to go for their medical care. He later moved the infirmary to Spring Street, then to Luckie Street, and finally bought land at the corner of Bartow and Luckie Street where he built a fifty-room facility. Broughton installed a telephone system that connected his pulpit at the Tabernacle Church with each patient's bed in the infirmary so that each could listen to his Sunday evening prayers, songs, and sermons. One of the infirmary physicians said it was a wonderful idea because those who had trouble sleeping were in dreamland after five

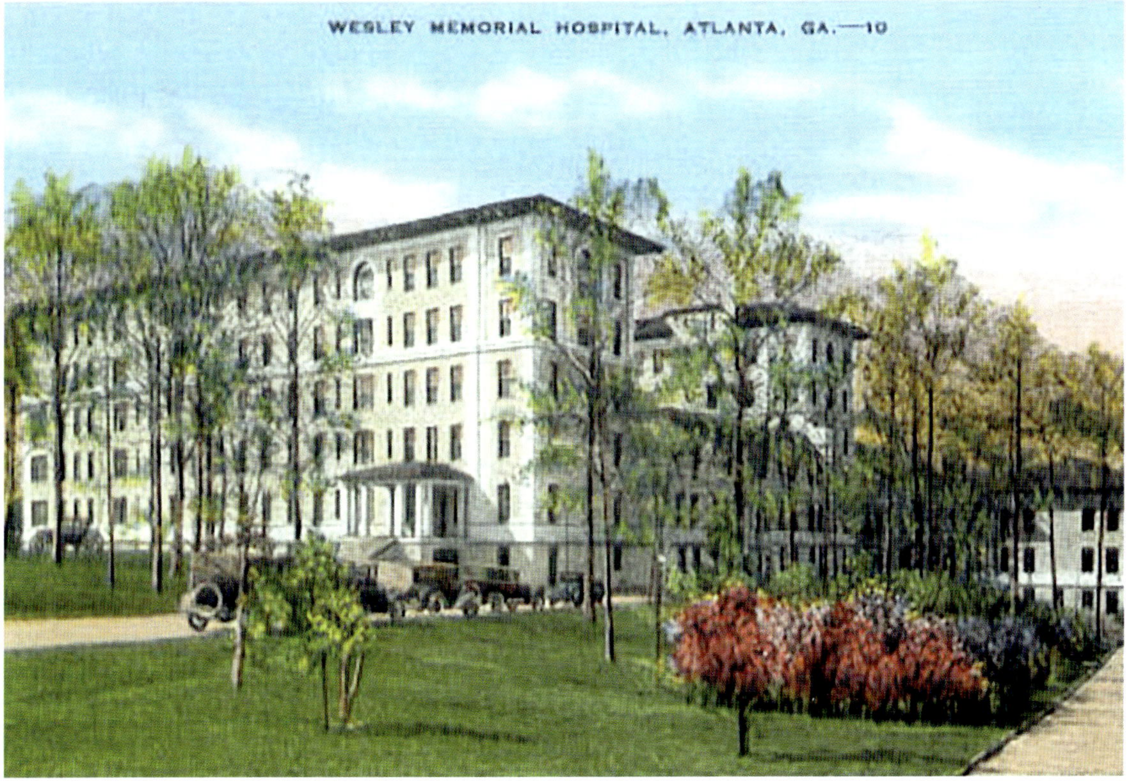

Left: Wesley Memorial Hospital in Atlanta before it became Emory University Hospital.

minutes of listening to Broughton's sermons. The Georgia Baptist Convention purchased the Infirmary in 1913 for $75,000, most of which was used to pay off the infirmary's debt. It was rechartered as Georgia Baptist Hospital in 1915 and moved to its present location on Boulevard in 1926. Currently, under the ownership of Tenet, a for-profit hospital corporation, the hospital now is known as Atlanta Medical Center.[42]

Emory University Hospital had its origin as Wesley Memorial Hospital in downtown Atlanta. In 1903 members of the Atlanta First Methodist Church said there was the need for a Methodist hospital in Atlanta. Asa Candler (who in 1914 would make it possible for Emory University to move to Atlanta) and his brother Warren offered $50,000 for a hospital if the Atlanta congregation would raise $150,000. The congregation met that challenge. The state granted a charter in March 1904, and the church purchased a sixteen-room mansion on the corner of Auburn Avenue and Courtland Street that Sherman's army had spared when it torched Atlanta. Wesley Memorial Hospital opened as a fifty-bed facility in August 1905. By 1922 patient volume had outgrown the space. Asa Candler offered to build a new, 275-bed hospital on the new Emory University campus. It continued to bear the Wesley Memorial name until the mid-1930s when it was renamed the Emory University Hospital.[43]

Piedmont Hospital originated in 1904 when Ludwig Amster, MD, a Jewish immigrant from Austria-Hungary, leased the Smith House at the corner of Capitol Avenue and Crumley Street (at about the position of the infield in the old Fulton County Stadium) as a medical and surgical clinic. He called it the Piedmont Sanatorium, a name it retained until 1925 when it became Piedmont

Hospital. It was a private institution governed entirely by physicians until its first lay board member was elected in 1940. In 1944 the trustees purchased eleven acres on Peachtree Road and in 1953 bought additional, adjacent acreage from Atlanta attorney Hughes Spalding Sr. In 1954 the hospital broke ground for a its present $5 million, 217-bed facility.[44]

Crawford Long Hospital, named for the Georgia physician considered the first to use ether as a surgical anesthetic, was established in 1908 as the private Davis-Fischer Sanatorium. Luther Fischer, MD, and his former medical school instructor, Edward Campbell Davis, MD, leased a small twenty-six-bed hospital on Crew Street (near the present-day Turner Stadium) formerly used as a private hospital for railroad workers. They soon needed a larger facility. They purchased property at 35 Linden Avenue against the advice of friends who said it was "too far out of town" and opened a new brick 85-bed facility in 1911. In 1921 they expanded it to 225 beds. Before Davis died in 1931, he and Fischer rechartered the hospital as a nonprofit organization and gave it the Crawford W. Long Memorial Hospital name.[45]

In 1940 Fischer and the board of trustees gave the hospital to Emory University with two conditions. First the hospital would continue to be operated by the trustees as a distinct unit "without interference from the university" during Fischer's lifetime. Second Fischer and his wife could continue living in their apartment atop the newly constructed wing of the hospital as long as they both should live. In the early 1950s, Fischer turned over most of his administrative responsibilities to Wadley Glenn, MD. By 1953 both Dr. and Mrs. Fischer had died, and the hospital became the Emory Crawford Long Hospital.[46]

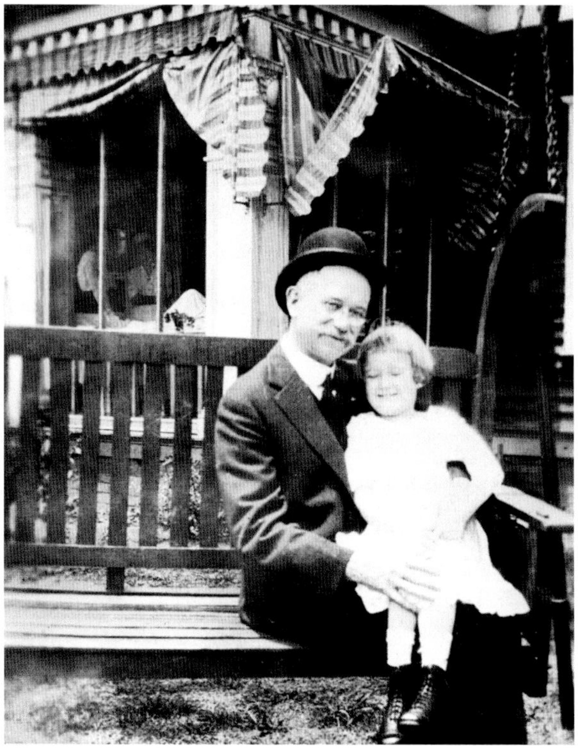

Right: Forrest Adair with a young child at Scottish Rite Hospital for Crippled Children. He, along with Mrs. William C. "Bertie" Wardlaw Sr., founded the hospital in 1915.

Metropolitan Atlanta also was the home of the old Veterans Administration Hospital on Peachtree Road, the Scottish Rite Hospital for Crippled Children that was established in 1915,[47] the Henrietta Egleston Hospital for Children that was started in 1928,[48] the Elks Aidmore Hospital (built in 1938) originally for crippled and handicapped children and later expanded to offer services to handicapped adults,[49] and the Hughes Spalding Children's Hospital opened in 1952 for black patients.[50] DeKalb County was the site chosen for the Centers for Disease Control and Prevention (CDC) that opened in 1946.[51]

Atlanta also had a prominent medical school. The Emory University School of Medicine had its origins in the Atlanta Medical College, founded in 1854, and the Southern Medical College, founded in 1878. The two colleges merged in 1898 to become the Atlanta College of Physicians and Surgeons. In 1913 the Atlanta College of Physicians and Surgeons merged with the Atlanta School of Medicine (founded in 1905) to become the Atlanta

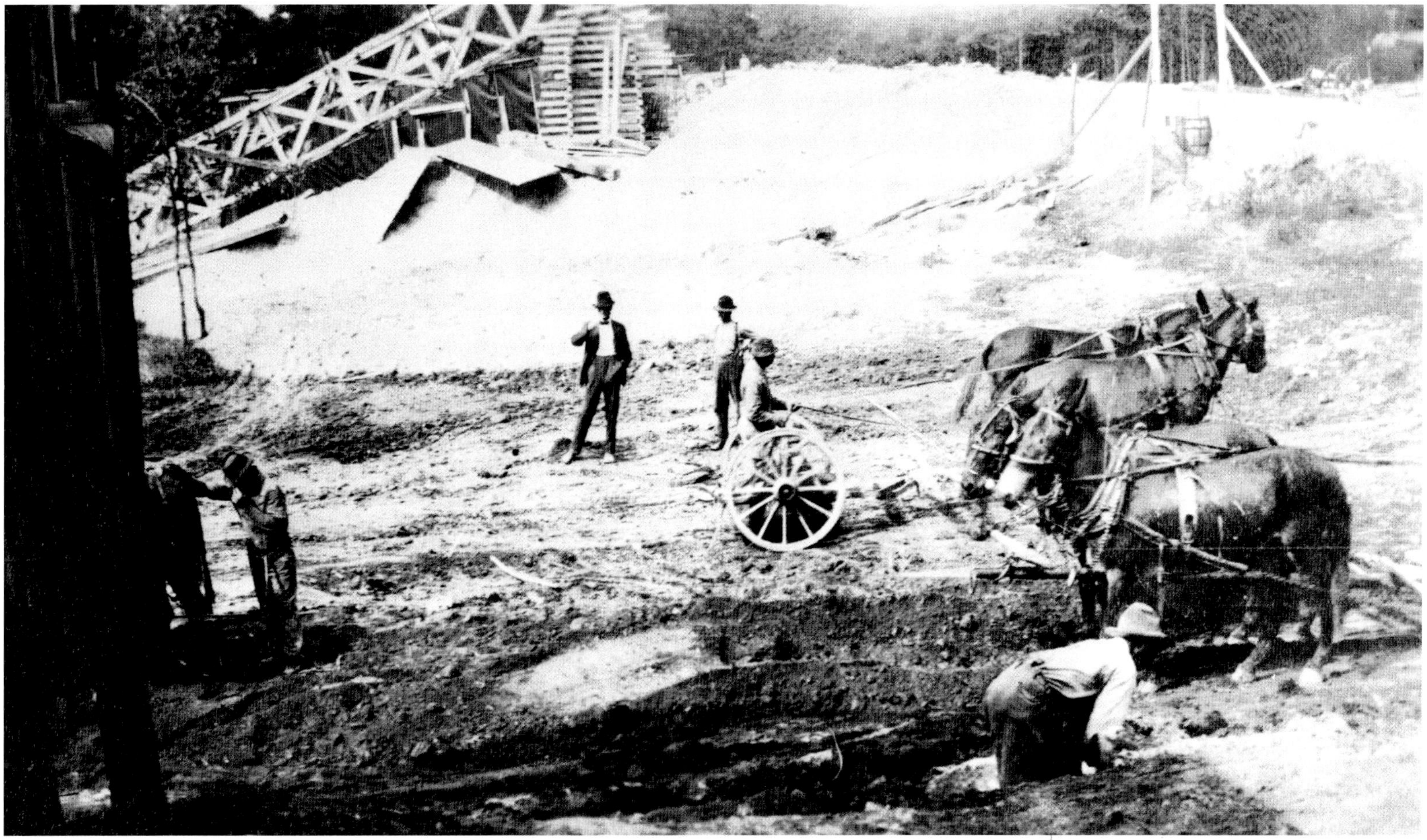

Medical College. In 1915 the Atlanta Medical College was renamed the Emory University School of Medicine.[52]

Excavation of land for the Emory Medical School in DeKalb County.

Despite all these facilities and resources, DeKalb County needed another hospital. Emory Hospital was, of course, located in the county. Many of the county's physicians were graduates of the Emory School of Medicine, had trained in its internship and residency programs, were on the staff of the hospital and held teaching positions in the School of Medicine. Emory Hospital, however, became increasingly unavailable to the community physicians and their patients. First the Emory School of Medicine was becoming identified as a specialty institution that focused on teaching and research. In addition the number of physicians on the School of Medicine faculty who used the hospital grew rapidly when the Emory Clinic was formed in 1953. The clinic was a partnership of faculty physicians that gave the physicians a way to have a private practice of medicine to generate additional income for themselves and the School of Medicine.[53] For both these reasons, there were fewer Emory Hospital beds available for use by community doctors.

In light of the county's exploding population, the growing physician base, and the shrinking number of available hospital beds, something needed to be done to provide a community hospital in DeKalb County. The citizens, physicians, and leaders of the county began looking for how this could be accomplished.

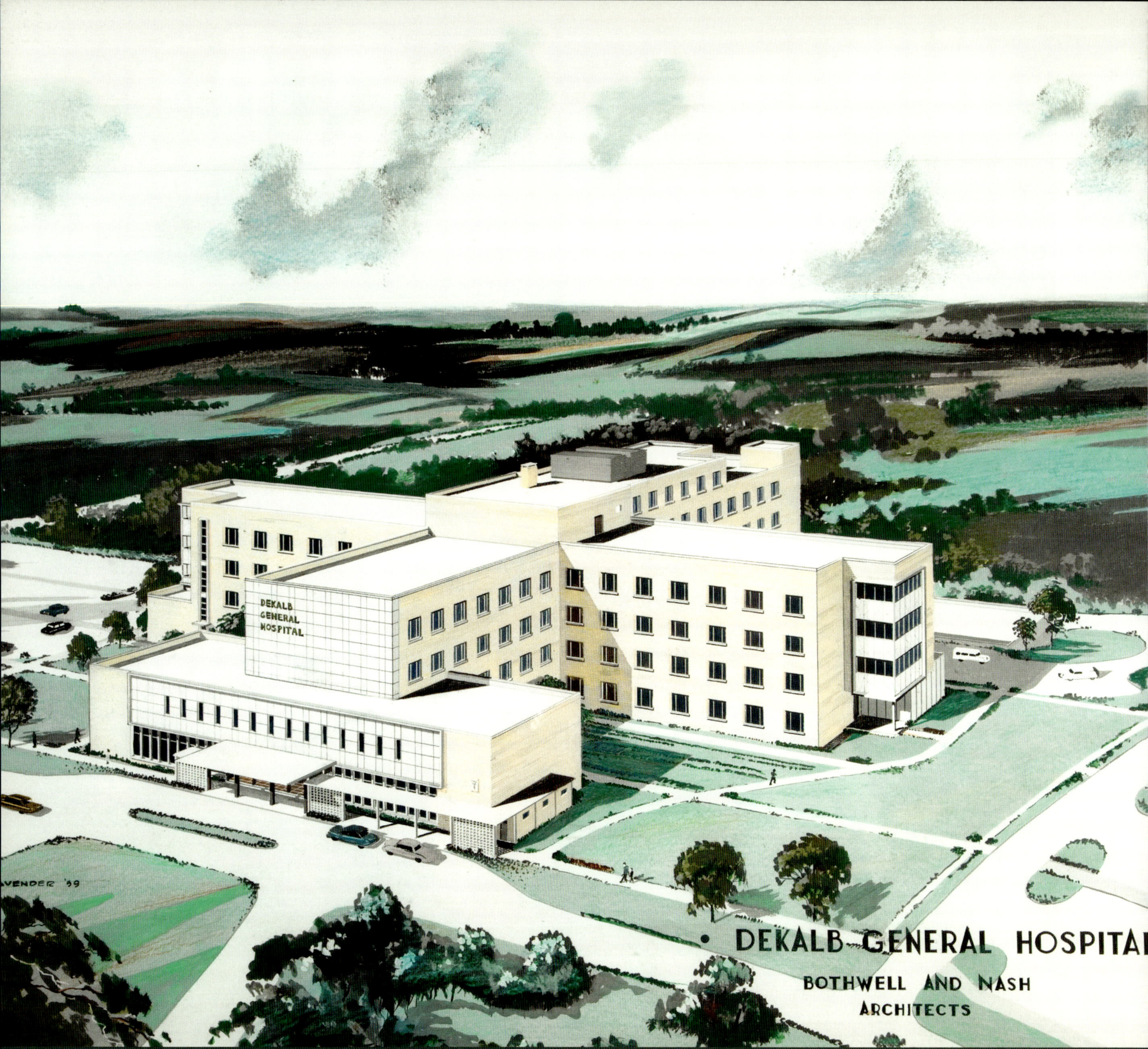
DEKALB
GENERAL
HOSPITAL
DEKALB GENERAL HOSPITAL
BOTHWELL AND NASH
ARCHITECTS

CHAPTER TWO

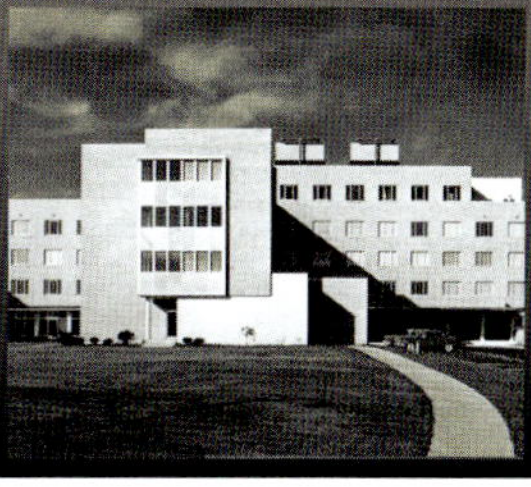

DeKalb General Hospital Becomes a Reality

"I just made a decision and did it and didn't worry about it."

—J. Rufus Evans, MD
on his leading a crusade for building a hospital

While DeKalb County had had a contract with Grady Memorial Hospital since 1945 to provide medical services for its indigent patients, the county's physicians needed a facility where they could care for their patients, and the nonindigent citizens needed a local hospital where they could receive care. Prominent organizations supported the idea of a new hospital in DeKalb County. The Georgia Department of Public Health surveyed metropolitan Atlanta and confirmed the need. The DeKalb County Medical Society petitioned for a hospital, the Decatur Lions Club voiced its support, and Decatur newspapers gave their endorsements. Of course there were dissenters. One Atlanta newspaper declared that building a hospital with local, state, and federal funds was illegal.[1] Some Atlanta physicians opposed it because they feared the loss of referrals from DeKalb County. A few politicians voiced opposition, and some homeowners objected to the increased traffic and congestion that a hospital might bring.

Among those involved in the discussion, however, three men emerged who not only saw the need for a new hospital but who had the will and the skill to make it happen. Those three were J. Rufus Evans, MD, who was the medical director of the DeKalb County Department of Public Health; Scott Candler Sr., the sole DeKalb County commissioner; and Julius A. McCurdy, former state legislator, the attorney for DeKalb County, a founding partner of the McCurdy and Candler Law Firm, and a founding director of the Decatur Federal Savings and Loan Association.[2] These three men became a formidable team committed to building a hospital for the physicians and citizens of DeKalb County. Candler was once quoted as saying that Evans would tell them what to do, Candler would get it done, and McCurdy would tell them how they could pay for it and make it legal.

Evans led the crusade for a hospital. Despite the dissenting voices, he said, "I just made a decision and did it and didn't worry about it."[3] At the ceremony to lay the hospital cornerstone in 1960, Scott Candler said the hospital was "a memorial to Dr. Rufus Evans."[4]

Evans was born in Walton County in 1898 and received his medical education at Tulane University. He married the former Sarah McCurdy and was in practice in New Orleans when, in 1925, he was invited to become the medical director of the DeKalb County Department of Public Health, a position that he held for twenty-five years. The department was housed in a small building on Ponce de Leon Avenue, and the entire staff consisted of Evans, two nurses, a secretary, and a sanitation engineer.[5] Evans was instrumental in forming

The three men who were a formidable team committed to building a hospital for DeKalb County were: *right*, Julius A. McCurdy; *far right*, J. Rufus Evans; and *bottom*, Scott Candler.

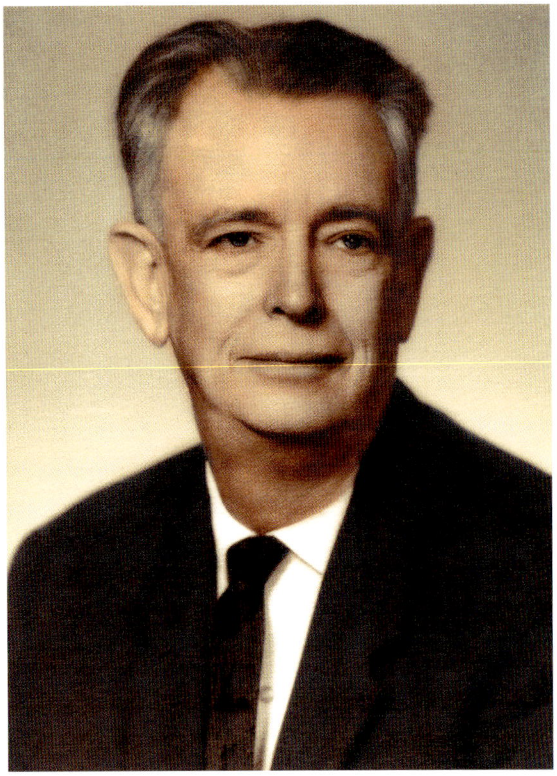

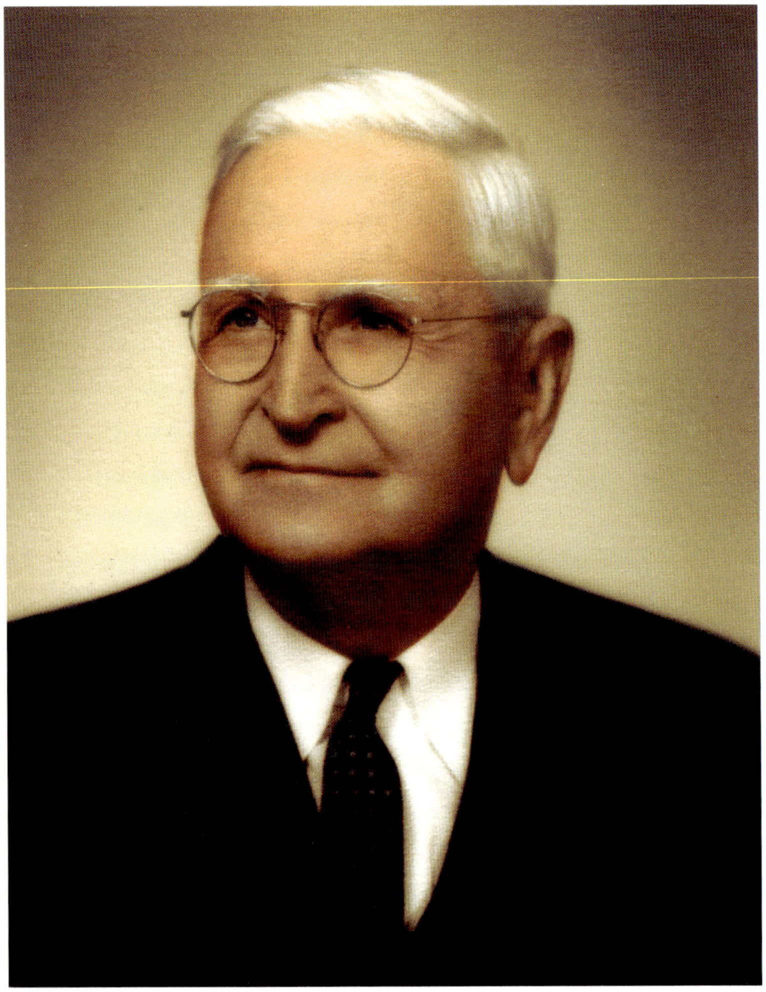

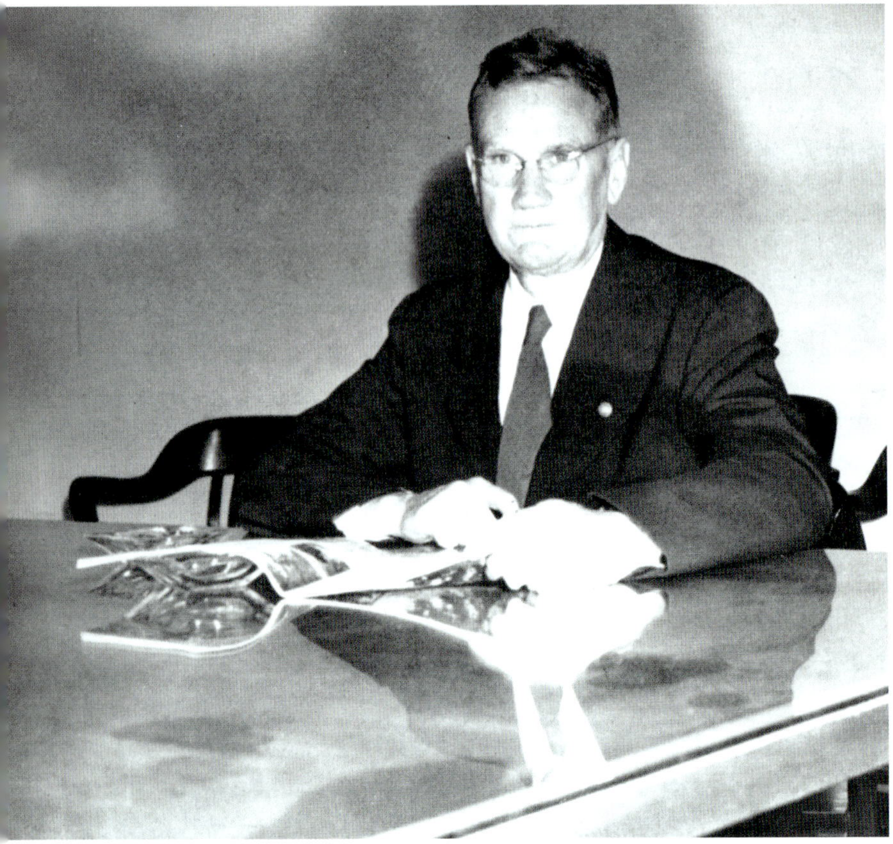

the DeKalb Medical Society and was its president from 1935 to 1942.[6] While still medical director of the health department, he also joined his brother-in-law in his Stone Mountain medical practice part-time.

Having advocated the need for another hospital in the county for several years, in 1952 Evans enlisted the support of Scott Candler and Julius McCurdy in the cause to build one.[7] That year Candler, as sole commissioner, approved the election of a $1,000,000 general obligation bond for a hospital, and the citizens voted for it. The three leaders anticipated that state and federal Hill-Burton funds would be available to match the bond money. The Hill-Burton Act, which had been enacted in 1946, authorized federal grants to states to survey for the need of additional hospitals, to plan for their construction, and to assist in financing their construction.

Confident of those matching funds, Candler hired the architectural firm of Bothwell and Nash to develop plans for a hospital. He chose a site facing North Decatur Road that eventually would become the hospital's location. When the trio presented their plans to the Georgia Department of Public Health, however, the state said Hill-Burton funds were not available.[8] So the plans for a new hospital in DeKalb County had to be put on hold for another five years.

Candler stepped down as sole commissioner in 1955, but he remained a powerful voice in the county's affairs, and he continued campaigning for a hospital. A five-man board of commissioners replaced the one-man commissioner system, and the Georgia General Assembly created the ten-member DeKalb County Bond Commission to advise the county commissioners concerning bonds. J. Rufus Evan was one of those bond commission members.[9]

In 1957 Candler, Evans, and McCurdy learned that state and federal Hill-Burton funds were now available for a hospital. They petitioned the county commissioners, the bond commission recommended a second bond election in the amount of $1,405,000 bond, and the citizens once again approved it.[10] DeKalb's hospital was a step closer to reality, and it would be the first hospital in greater Atlanta built with the aid of Hill-Burton funds.

The county commissioners' next task was to create an organization with the legal authority to build and operate a hospital. In 1941 the Georgia General Assembly had passed the Hospital Authorities Law that authorized county commissioners to create "hospital authorities" to build, operate, and maintain hospitals in their counties.[11] The law specified that each authority would consist of a board of trustees of not less than five nor more than nine members with staggered terms, all of whom must reside in the county. Based on that law, the commissioners passed a resolution on September 19, 1957, establishing the DeKalb County Hospital Authority.

The commissioners appointed seven trustees to the Authority: J. Rufus Evans a leader in the effort to build the hospital; J. Ross McCain, Presbyterian minister and retired president of Agnes Scott College; Julius A. McCurdy; Wash W. Lively, dairy owner and owner of the Brownlee and Lively Realty Company; M. E. Smith, retired principal of Chamblee High School in DeKalb County; R. L. Mathis Jr. manager of the prominent Mathis Dairy farm in the county; and Hugh Rowland, executive vice president of the East Atlanta Branch of the Trust Company of Georgia.[12]

The Authority held its first meeting at the East Lake Club on September 25, 1957. McCain called the meeting to order and presided until officers were elected. The meeting's first and only order of business was to elect the following officers: J. Rufus Evans was elected chairman; J. Ross McCain became vice chairman; and Julius A. McCurdy was elected secretary-treasurer.[13]

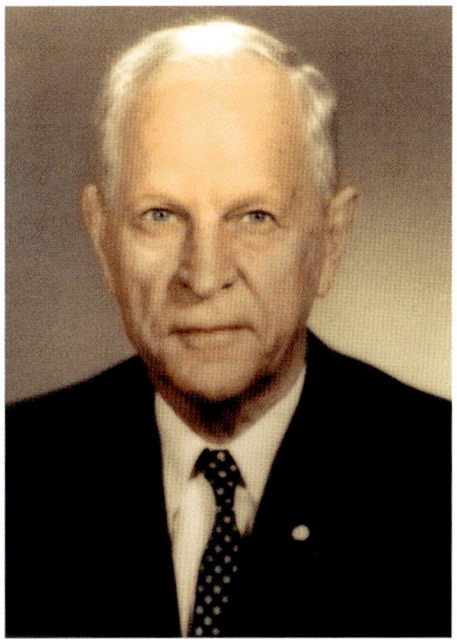

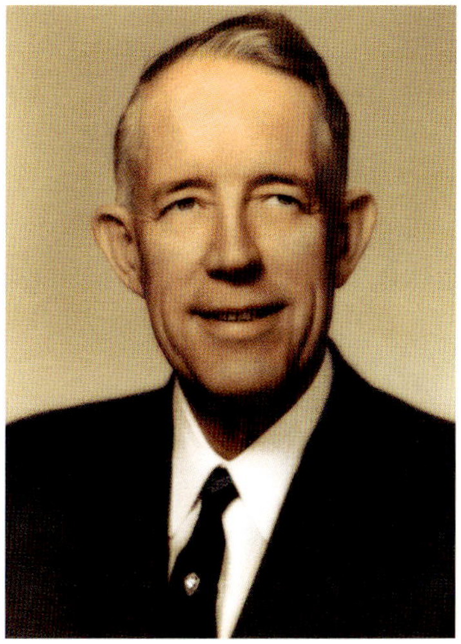

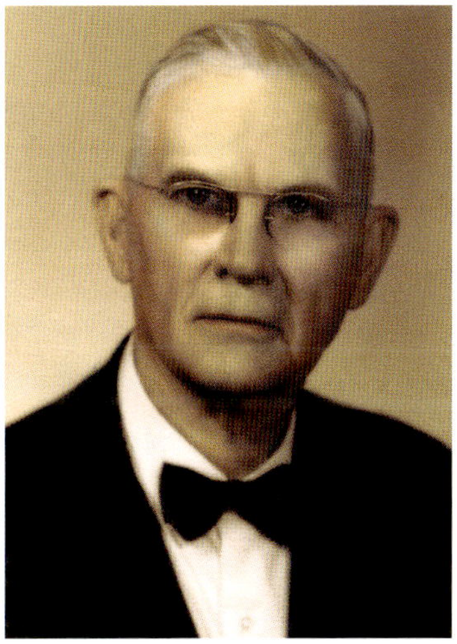

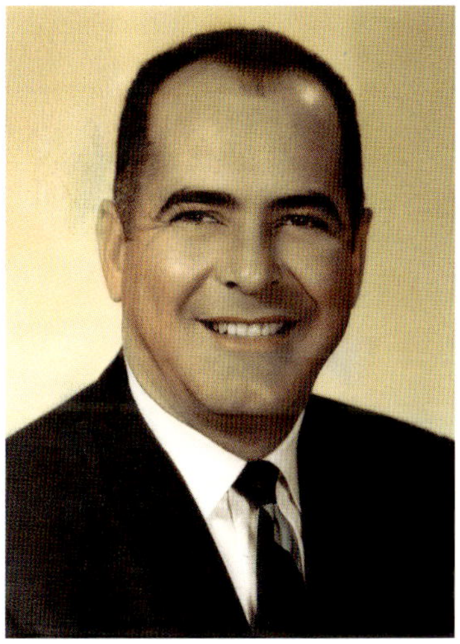

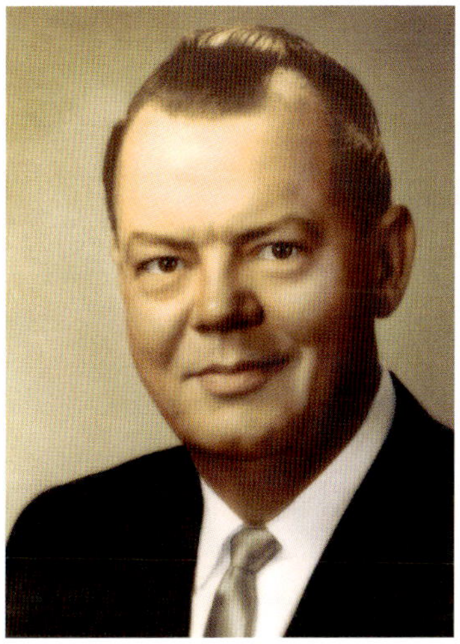

Seven trustees were appointed to the newly formed DeKalb County Hospital Authority in 1957: opposite, J. Rufus Evans and Julius A. McCurdy; top left, J. Ross McCain; top right, Wash W. Lively; center left, M. E. Smith; center right, R. L. Mathis Jr.; and left, Hugh Rowland.

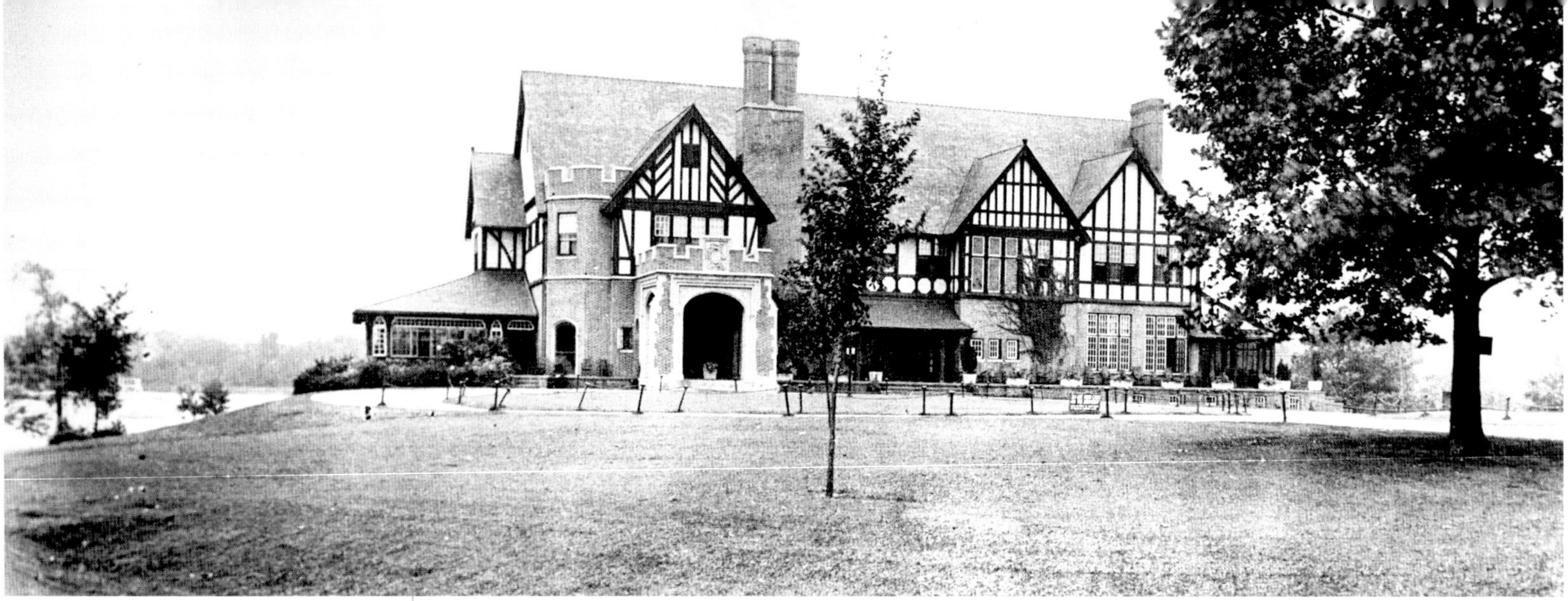

Above: It was at the East Lake Club on September 25, 1957, that the DeKalb County Hospital Authority had its first meeting. **Below:** A forty-acre property on North Decatur Road, known for its strawberry and blackberry plants, was chosen as the desired site for the new hospital. **Opposite background:** Plat of the property where the Authority chose to build the new hospital.

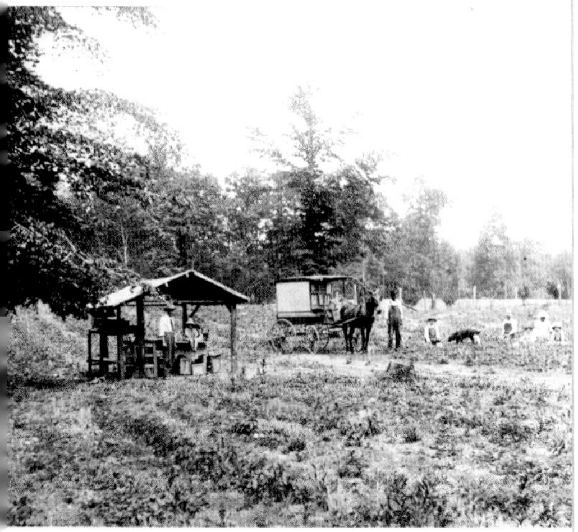

At the Authority's second meeting, Evans appointed Lively chairman of a committee to find a site for the hospital and McCain chairman of a committee to recommend an architect. McCain's committee not surprisingly recommended Bothwell and Nash, the same architectural firm that Scott Candler had engaged to prepare preliminary hospital drawings in 1952. It was a respected firm, and the architects already understood the project that the trustees envisioned. They would be responsible for producing architectural drawings and for assisting in preparing the many detailed applications for state and federal funding.

Lively's site committee considered several locations and finally recommended four potential properties for the Authority's consideration: (1) the former Booker Scott farm, then owned by the Scott Estate, that faced the then unpaved North Decatur Road Extension (the site tentatively selected by Candler in 1952);[14] (2) the County Work Camp in South DeKalb County; (3) the House property on LaVista Road; and (4) a site on Clairmont Road that Emory University officials said might become available.[15]

The trustees chose the Scott Estate property and determined that they would need forty acres. The site was a hilltop wooded tract just east of Church Street and a short distance south of Scott Boulevard. It was in the geographic center of DeKalb County. The property was well known to the community because it contained many strawberry and blackberry plants, and the public traditionally was invited to pick as many berries as they wanted at no charge. Members of the community still recall the delicate fragrance that emanated from the field when the strawberries were in season. North Decatur Road that fronted the property was, at the time, an unpaved extension from Scott Boulevard. It was not officially opened to Memorial Drive until December 1961, seven months after the hospital opened.[16]

The trustees engaged three real estate appraisers to recommend a price they should offer for the property. Two out of the three said the property was worth $4,000 an acre, or $160,000 for the entire forty acres. Evans and McCurdy approached Milton C. Scott who represented the Scott Estate and offered to purchase forty acres at $4,000 an acre. Scott said he would prefer selling only twenty-seven acres, or thirty acres if absolutely necessary. He asked for $5,000 an acre but said he would consider $4,500 an acre.

McCurdy wrote to Scott in response.[17] His letter reflects the tenacity, the skill, the sense of stewardship, and the vision of those early trustees:

February 28, 1958

Dear Milton:

Your letter of February 20 was submitted to the Hospital Authority and was given long and serious consideration. I was requested to write to you and to give you the consensus of opinion developed at this meeting.

First, let me explain why the members feel that forty acres should be obtained at the present time. We realize that it will not be needed immediately for the hospital contemplated, but we are confident that DeKalb's growth will make additions to the hospital necessary within the next few years. We are sure that living quarters for interns, nurses, and hospital personnel will need to be provided. Of course, parking must be available for all these facilities.

A convalescent wing, where the chronically ill can be treated, and a rehabilitation center is also a possibility. It may be that in the future it would be advantageous to move the clinic and health department to some building close to the hospital.

Of course, all of these, except the present two-hundred-bed hospital, are the subject of future planning; but since there would be no other adjoining property in the future, except the property which we acquire now, a majority of the members of the Authority believe that we should obtain at least forty acres.

Regarding the price, we all realize that people are likely to differ on property valuations, and we are satisfied that the price which you quoted, in your opinion, was a fair price. All of the members of the Authority feel the heavy responsibility which falls upon them as members of the Authority. For this reason, we have not tried to fix our own valuation.

As Dr. Evans and I explained to you, the Authority selected three real estate men who have experience in property of this kind, and requested them to give us an appraisal. Two of these men fixed a value of $4,000 per acre, and one fixed a value of slightly less than that. None of the members of the Authority feel that they would be justified in offering more than the highest appraisal received by us.

I have tried to state the views of the members of the Authority. I have been further authorized to submit to you and your associates an offer of $4,000 per acre for forty acres of land, including that shown in the plat which you furnished us, dated November 1957, and adjoining property to be mutually agreed upon.

I hope that you will give this offer favorable consideration.

Yours truly,
Julius A. McCurdy
Secretary-Treasurer

A week later Scott agreed to sell the Authority forty acres at $4,000 an acre. He requested the right to claim the trees cleared from the property[18] but later decided he did not want the timber. The sale of the forty acres for $160,000 was closed on May 1, 1958.

The Authority next had to decide on the size of the hospital and the scope of services it would provide. As they would do time and again, the trustees turned to the community physicians for guidance. McCain surveyed the doctors for their estimate of the number of beds and services that would be needed. When he tabulated the results of his survey, he found the doctors recommended building a 938-bed facility. Fortunately McCain and the other trustees realized that the bed count recommended by the physicians was "a bit confusing"[19] and proceeded with plans for a 200 bed hospital rather than one with 938 beds.

At its September 1958 meeting, the Authority conducted a lengthy discussion concerning the name of the hospital. They approved a motion to name it "DeKalb General Hospital" and submitted the name to the Georgia Department of Public Health, which gave its approval.[20]

The next agenda item was the selection of a hospital administrator. Chairman Evans asked McCain to bring a recommendation to the Authority. There were eight candidates, all of whom had at one time or another served on the staff of the state health department.[21] Among these, William H. Thrasher was the one who most caught the attention of the trustees. He was administrator of Athens General Hospital in Athens, Georgia.

In February 1958 McCain wrote to Thrasher and requested that he send the Authority his written ideas regarding:

> *What the Authority should do and when. . . . What employees we should have and in what order secured and at what cost . . . up to the day of opening . . . and then into the first year or two of operation? . . . What we may expect to spend for equipment, supplies, and all such items, with some guess perhaps as to landscaping. . . . Will all of this be paid for before the hospital opens? . . . What charges we should make when operations begin and what chances there may be to avoid deficits? . . . What kind of cushioning against red ink ought to be provided? . . . What extent of services to be offered, whether to buy some of them from nearby hospitals or provide them all ourselves? . . . Do we need to run our own cafeteria and laundry? . . . How we should proceed in competition with some of the best hospitals in the country to secure good nurses, interns, trained orderlies and other servants. . . . How may we enlist enough of the [doctors] to provide plenty of patients? How may we best set up a medical staff so as to serve the county well and yet have very high standards? How may we provide for a strong Christian influence at the hospital?*[22]

To this McCain added,

> *Our Personnel Committee knows that each prospective officer would like at once to come and look over the site and plans first of all, before making any [of these requested] suggestions. However, we have too many people on our list to arrange this. Also, we feel that we have too many to begin any personal interviews or [to make] visits to the hospitals being run by our applicants.*[23]

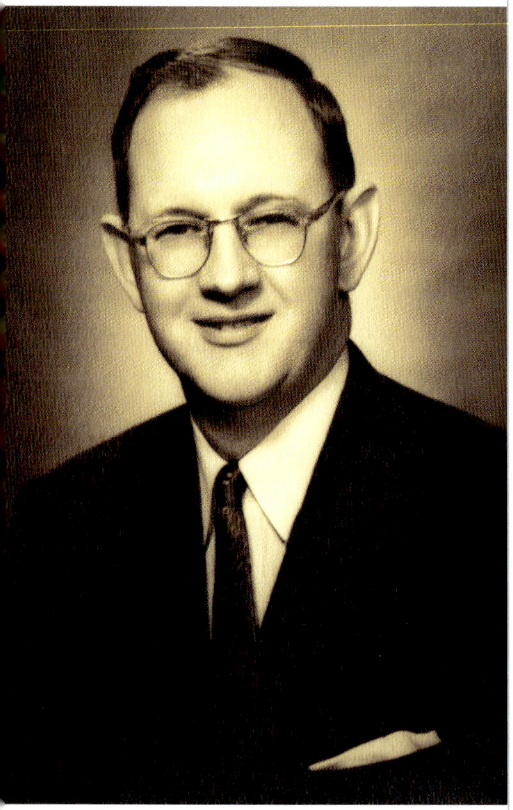

William H. Thrasher was hired as hospital administrator of DeKalb General Hospital and began work on August 1, 1958, even though no hospital existed yet. He held multiple important roles until the hospital opened its doors on May 1. 1961.

Thrasher was left to produce a document that provided all that the Authority wanted to know without seeing the plans or the site, without meeting with the trustees, and without having more information than McCain provided in his letter.

He did just that. In the same month that he received this enormous request, he submitted to the Authority a twenty-page document outlining his ideas about everything that had been requested of him and more.[24] The Authority was sufficiently impressed that it gave Thrasher an interview in March, and the trustees offered him the job of being the hospital's first administrator with an annual salary of $10,000 plus $100-a-month car allowance. Thrasher accepted the offer.

He began work on August 1, 1958. Since there was no hospital at that time, he found office space first in the county health department offices and later moved to a building on Atlanta Avenue in downtown Decatur. He served multiple roles. He was the hospital's public relations agent and, in that role, shared plans for the hospital with organizations and the media throughout metropolitan Atlanta, elicited interest in and support for the hospital, and prepared for special events such as the ground-breaking and dedication services. In another facet of his work, he collaborated with the architects in finalizing the hospital plans and worked alongside the contractor in its construction. He assisted in preparing the documents required for local, state, and federal funds. He recruited a corps of managers to plan for and obtain the equipment, the supplies, the personnel, and establish the business organization needed to open and operate the hospital. He oversaw the training of the personnel in the various departments and services. He worked with the DeKalb Medical Society to recruit, credential, and organize physicians for the medical staff. And when the hospital opened on May 1, 1961, he was there to manage the facility and its services.

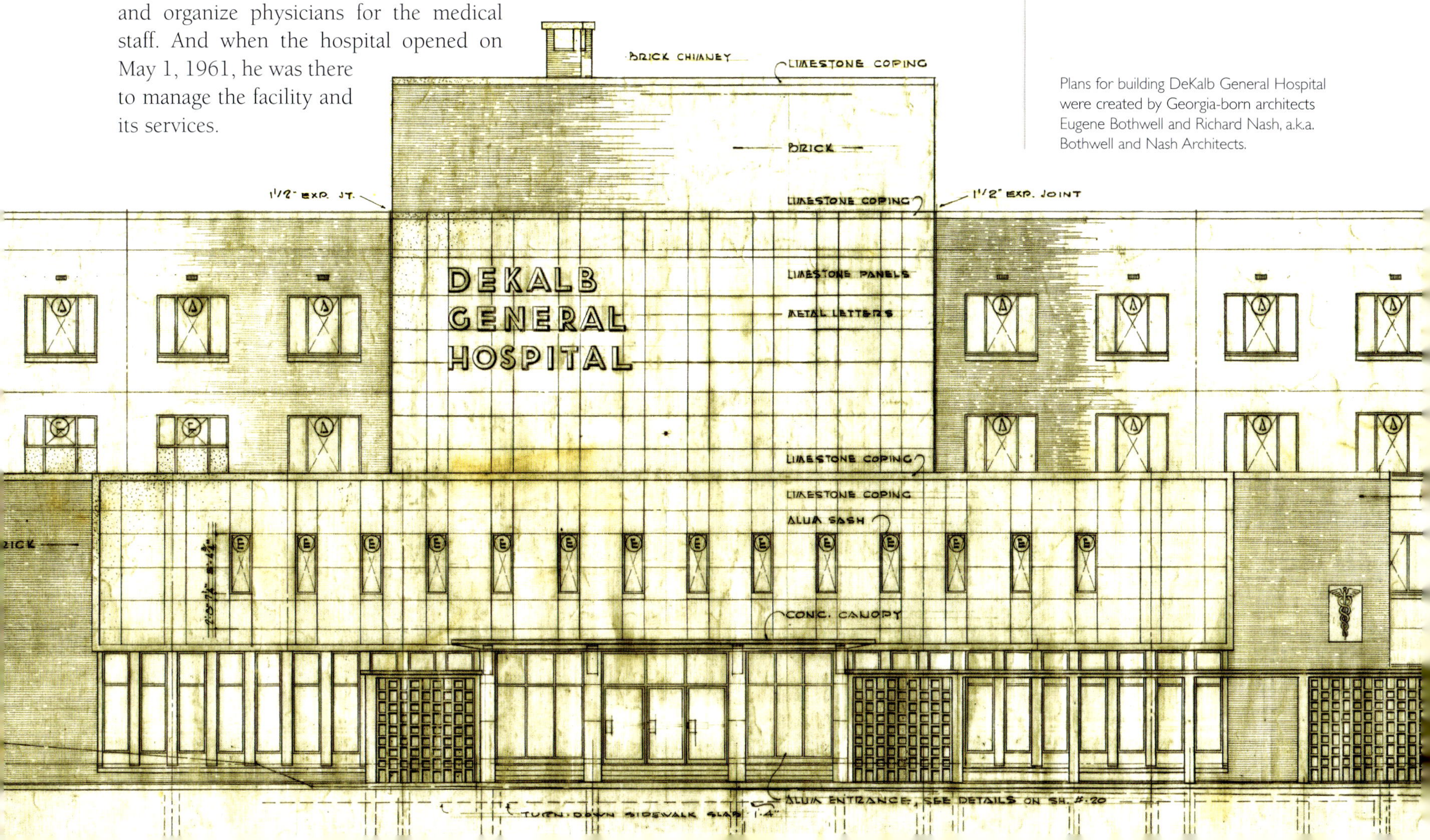

Plans for building DeKalb General Hospital were created by Georgia-born architects Eugene Bothwell and Richard Nash, a.k.a. Bothwell and Nash Architects.

While the trustees had the assurance of the county's two bonds for the hospital—the first for $1,000,000 in 1952 and the second for $1,405,000 in 1957—as well as the promise of matching state and federal Hill-Burton funds, they still faced the daunting task of getting their hands on the promised money.

First they had to get official approval of all their plans from the state and federal agencies. That involved a host of steps that included approvals of a narrative description of their plans, the architectural drawings, a list of equipment and its budget, and acceptable soil testing. Each phase of the application had to be approved first by the Georgia Department of Public Health and then by federal agencies. Getting approval was not easy. Multiple revisions of the architectural plans were required. Major pieces of equipment that the hospital considered essential for good patient care were described as "gold plating" by the state and rejected outright.

Finally the trustees had to commit to two long-term obligations. First they had to promise to provide a certain amount of "uncompensated care" as free or discounted services. In addition to this, they had to make a "community service" pledge to provide all of their services to anyone living within the facility's service area who had some ability to pay, and they were to make available their emergency services to everyone regardless of ability to pay.[25]

"...we want everything about the hospital to be characterized by heart interest in each patient, whether rich or poor."

— J. Ross McCain

After satisfying those conditions, the state and federal agencies still refused to distribute funds until the Authority demonstrated that it had stayed within budget, had used its local funds in an appropriate manner, and had paid all its bills in a timely manner. Even then the state and federal agencies spread out their disbursements in as many as seven installments.[26] On one occasion the Authority had to borrow $110,000 from a local bank to pay the balance due on equipment so that it could document that it paid its bills in a timely manner to qualify for state and federal payments.[27] The Authority received its first payment of state and federal funds in February 1960, eight months after hospital construction got underway.[28]

The Authority also had to meet certain conditions before it could receive the local bond funds, but those conditions were less difficult than the ones imposed by the state and federal agencies. First the bonds had to be sold. The sale was completed in April 1959.[29] Next the Bond Commission had to approve the architectural plans and all contracts.[30] Finally the Authority had to complete all phases of its Hill-Burton application before the bond money could be transferred.[31] The last of those conditions finally were met in April 1959, and the county transferred approximately $2,500,000, including accumulated interest, to the Authority. The Authority opened a construction account at the Trust Company of Georgia[32] and engaged the Trust Company to handle the investment of their funds.[33]

With the bond money in hand, the Authority was able to accept construction bids. Sixteen contractors submitted bids ranging from $3,518,628 to $3,846,000. The low bid came from the T. C. Brittain Company of Decatur, and it was awarded the general construction contract. Brittain's bid came in only $827 lower than the one from Batson-Cook Company. Separate contracts were issued for laundry and kitchen equipment.

The trustees held a groundbreaking ceremony at the building site on Friday, May 15, 1959. Evans, as chairman of the Authority, and Claude H. Blount, chairman of the DeKalb Board of Commissioners, wielded shovels that symbolically initiated DeKalb General Hospital's construction.

McCain was the principal speaker and explained the hospital's plans for a tiered patient-care system known as "Progressive Patient Care." The seriously ill would receive "the same intensive

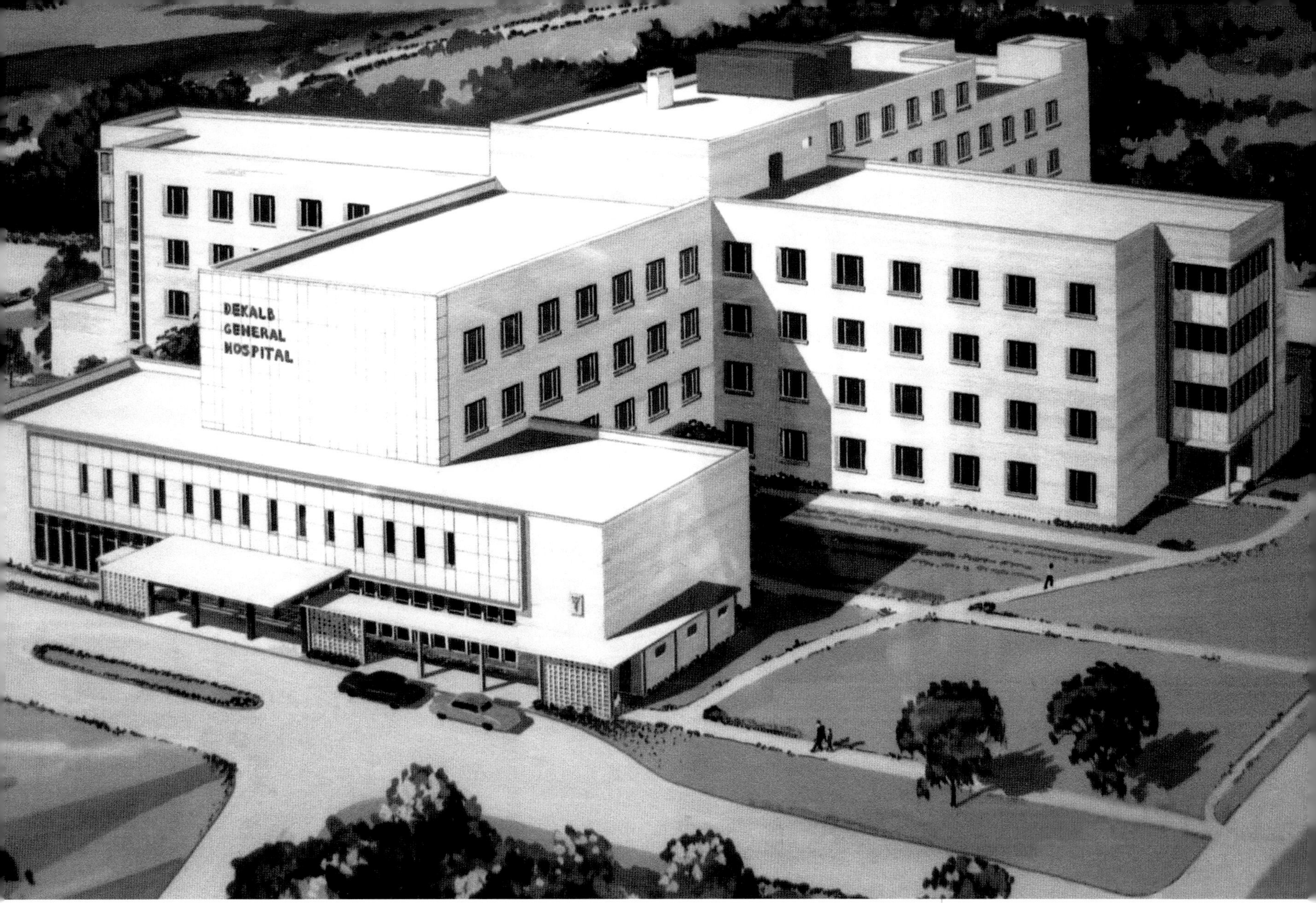

Three-dimensional rendering of the proposed hospital design by Bothwell and Nash Architects.

care they might expect from a private nurse." Those less ill would receive an "intermediate" type care. The third level of care was reserved for those who are recovered sufficiently to allow "self-service." They would be expected to do most of their own housekeeping, and they would be at liberty to walk around and visit with other patients.[34] The three-level concept of patient care, especially the plan for an Intensive Care Unit, was unique among hospitals in the southeast. McCain described the purpose of the institution as envisioned by the trustees:

> *The sole end and purpose of all our efforts is to take the best care possible of the sick people, primarily of this county. We wish to prevent illness as well as to cure it. We expect to have the best facilities in the state and some of the best skill which doctors need, but we want everything about the hospital to be characterized by heart interest in each patient, whether rich or poor.*[35]

"We have other dreams . . . one hundred beds for old folks who simply need a home . . . a first class clinic . . . a school of nursing . . . quarters for the families of patients to stay without the expense of hotels and taxicabs"

— J. Ross McCain

Then McCain spoke of the future vision of the hospital:

> *We have other dreams for our forty acres and for the fastest growing county in the state. We hope before long to add stories and to provide for four hundred rooms. We count on a wing for convalescents who need to be near to the hospital but do not need its high prices. We wish also one hundred beds for old folks who simply need a home and are not yet sick. We hope to have the county public health services on our land and to cooperate with many of their projects. Possibly a first class clinic will be possible for outpatients. We envision a school of nursing and a home for nurses. Perhaps a doctors' building may be needed. We wish to have quarters for the families of patients to stay without the expense of hotels and taxicabs. We want unlimited parking without charges.*[36]

The Brittain Company commenced work in early June 1959 and promised to complete the hospital in twenty months.[37] With hospital construction underway, Thrasher went to the Authority to request more administrative help. He outlined a minimum of forty-six tasks for which he was responsible, including hiring 250 to 300 people to fill 125 jobs, developing policies and procedures, purchasing and installing approximately ten thousand pieces of equipment at a cost of nearly $500,000, and overseeing the construction process. He asked permission to hire an assistant administrator and a secretary. The trustees discussed his request at length but concluded that "although an assistant administrator might be justified at this particular time, from a public opinion standpoint it would be better to wait a little longer. A motion was carried that the administrator be authorized to employ only a secretary at a monthly salary not to exceed $300."[38] Despite the forty-six daunting tasks, Thrasher would have to wait another full year before the Authority felt the time was right to let him hire an assistant administrator.

In the fall of 1958, the Authority turned to the task of selecting a hospital-based radiologist, pathologist, and anesthesiologist to assist in planning for their service areas and to be in place when the hospital opened. The trustees asked the DeKalb Medical Society to recommend physicians for those positions. The society appointed a Medical Advisory Committee that included Homer Allen, MD, as chairman, L. C. Buchanan, MD, George Mitchell, MD, and Freeman Simmons, MD.

Five physicians applied to be the hospital radiologist: Frank E. Morgan, MD, David Tanner, MD, Walter Sale, MD, Robert Quattlebaum, MD, and Henry Johnson, MD. The advisory committee met with all the candidates and recommended Morgan as its first choice. It also recommended that, if the Authority could not work out a satisfactory contract with Morgan, Tanner of Augusta would be its next choice.[39] The Authority was able to work out a suitable contract with Morgan, and he became DeKalb General Hospital's radiologist.

Three physicians applied for the position of hospital pathologist: Robert J. Peace, MD, Hugh V. Bell, MD, and Frank Matthews, MD. The Medical Advisory Committee met with each candidate and recommended Bell as their first choice with Matthews as runner-up.[40] But when Bell and the Authority could not come to terms over financial arrangements, Bell withdrew his application. The trustees then turned to Matthews and arrived at an agreement. Some members of the committee later confided that, given Frank Matthews' outstanding record of success as the hospital's pathologist, they were glad that their first choice had not worked out.

In March 1961 the Authority approved George Sessions, MD, as its anesthesiologist. Sessions, like Morgan and Matthews, would be a contract physician rather than a hospital employee. Unlike the radiologist and pathologist, however, Sessions would work on a fee-for-service basis with no guarantee from the hospital. He would be responsible for his own billing and collections as well as the salaries of his staff. The Authority advanced him a loan of $500 a month for the first six months to help with hiring an associate and a nurse anesthetist.[41] He recruited Anibal Adan, MD, as anesthesiologist and Sarah Brockman, CNA, as nurse anesthetist to join him before the hospital opened in May.

With those three hospital-based physicians in place, Thrasher turned his attention to recruiting individuals for three key administrative positions: a director of Nursing, a chief financial officer (at the time referred to as treasurer-controller), and an assistant administrator (Thrasher would finally get his year-old wish). He chose Opal Hopkins, RN, as director of Nursing, Charles Anderson as treasurer-controller, and Ted E. Barner as assistant administrator.

Hopkins was a member of the nursing school faculty and staff at Georgia Baptist Hospital.[42] She received a diploma in nursing from the Georgia Baptist School of Nursing in 1952 and a bachelor of science degree in nursing education from the University of Georgia in 1956. When recruited, she was an instructor in the Nursing Education Department at Georgia Baptist Hospital.[43]

Most of Hopkins's experience was in nursing education. Her only administrative experience had been, for a brief time, as head nurse of a sixteen-bed medical-surgical unit at Georgia Baptist Hospital. Because of her limited administrative experience, Thrasher asked her to write out how she would proceed at DeKalb General if she were chosen for the job. Looking back she said she relied on some simple mathematics and a lot of common sense to come up with her recommendations. She substituted the number of beds that DeKalb General planned to have—two hundred—for the sixteen she was accustomed to dealing with, and used that as a basis to plan for staff, supplies, and equipment. She also identified the areas where she would need expert advice and described how she would go about obtaining and utilizing that advice. She planned to hire specialty head nurses, seek input from physicians, visit other community hospitals, and solicit advice from drug companies and vendors.[44]

Thrasher liked her practical plan, and he also appreciated her background in nursing education. Since DeKalb General would not initially have a school of nursing, he recognized the need for leadership in education to orient and train the new staff of nurses, affiliating students from neighboring nursing schools, nurses' aides, orderlies, and ward clerks. Before the hospital opened, Thrasher negotiated with the dean of the Emory School of Nursing to have its students rotate through DeKalb General for their clinical practice. He also anticipated having a number of licensed practical nurses (LPNs) on the staff along with registered nurses (RNs). In his mind, Hopkins's training and experience in education would be a significant asset to the hospital.[45]

To Opal Hopkins's surprise, especially when she later learned of the outstanding qualifications of some of the other candidates, Thrasher offered her the position of director of Nursing. When he made the offer, he told her that he liked her and that he thought they would work well together.[46] The trust that he had in her would be key not only to his hiring her but also to the role she would play in the crisis in Nursing Services nearly a decade later. She accepted his offer in February 1960,[47] served as a consultant for the next few months, and officially began her duties as director of Nursing in September 1960.[48] She remained in that position until the summer of 1965.

In early 1960 when looking for a treasurer-controller, the name of Charles Anderson, a certified public accountant in Albany, Georgia, was suggested to the trustees.[49] Evans asked Wash W. Lively to chair a committee to look into Anderson's qualifications and to bring a recommendation to the Authority. Lively later reported that his committee had met with Anderson and had found him to be

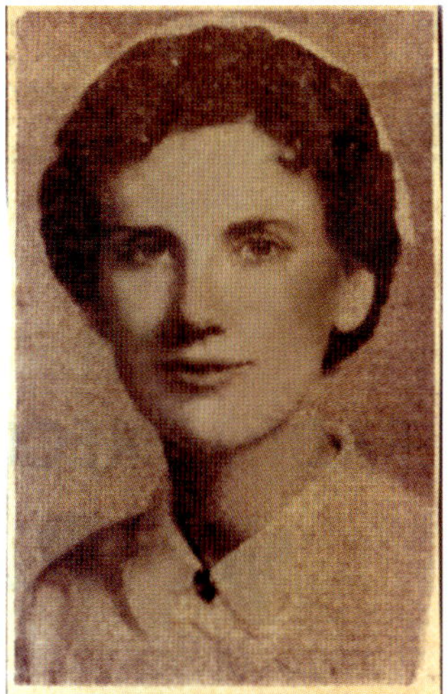

MRS. HOPKINS

Native Georgian To Head Nurses At New Hospital

Mrs. Opal Hopkins has been selected as director of the nursing department of the new DeKalb General Hospital, now under construction at North Decatur Rd. and the Lawrenceville Highway.

Mrs. Hopkins, a native of Carroll county, graduated from Mt. Zion High School near Carrollton in 1949. She was graduated from Georgia Baptist Hospital School of Nursing in 1952, and from the University of Georgia in 1956 with a Bachelor of Science degree in Nursing Education.

She has been on the staff at Georgia Baptist Hospital since 1952, and a member of its School of Nursing faculty since 1955. Mrs. Hopkins is a member of the National League for Nursing and the American Nurses' Association.

Applications for other positions in the Nursing Department, as well as in all other departments, are still being accepted, according to William H. Thrasher, administrator of the new hospital. Mr. Thrasher stressed that most of the personnel will be employed around the first of next year, since the hospital will be completed and opened in the early spring. Applications may be obtained by calling DR 7-2678 or by visiting the temporary administrative offices at 215 Atlanta Avenue in Decatur.

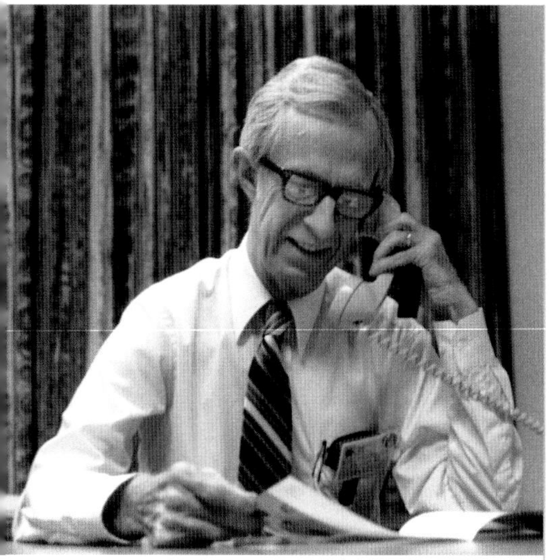

Charles Anderson became DeKalb General's first chief financial officer (treasurer-controller). He held that position for twenty-six years.

"of good character and thoroughly qualified to do the work." The committee said, however, that the hospital needed only a part-time person in that position for the time being. The Authority authorized the committee to offer a part-time position to Anderson "to be paid on a per diem schedule rate rather than a fixed salary" until such time as a full-time treasurer-controller was needed.[50] Anderson accepted the offer and became DeKalb General's first chief financial officer in May 1960, a position he held until his retirement twenty-six years later when he was succeeded by Bonnie Phipps.

In April of 1960, the Georgia Department of Public Health wrote to Thrasher that he had an enormous task in front of him in selecting and installing the equipment that had to be in place before the hospital opened:

> *This is to advise you that someone should be appointed with as little delay as possible to start compiling the list of all your equipment needs. . . . Since this is an extremely tedious and time-consuming task, it will require the undivided attention of the person to whom this responsibility is assigned.*[51]

Thrasher probably took considerable delight in sharing that letter with the Authority, for it gave reinforcement to his year-old request for an assistant administrator. He went to the April meeting with the state's letter and the recommendation that Ted E. Barner be approved for the position. Barner, who held a master's degree in personnel administration and a master's degree in hospital administration, was the former director of Personnel at Athens General Hospital. He and Thrasher had worked together there.[52] The Authority authorized Thrasher to hire Barner at a salary of $7,200 per year. Barner remained in that position for two years until he resigned to become administrator of a hospital in Bainbridge, Georgia.[53] To Thrasher's disappointment, when Barner resigned, the Authority discontinued the position,[54] and it would be six years before it approved the appointment of the next assistant to the administrator, John R. Gerlach.

Hospital construction went smoothly. The Brittain Company stayed on schedule despite occasional bad weather. The Building Committee that included Chairman McCain, Evans, and Lively performed a heroic task. They worked closely with the administrator, the architect, and the contractor and gave monthly progress reports to the Authority. In addition to overseeing the construction of the building, they approved the equipment and furnishings to go into the hospital and selected bids from competing companies. Although the trustees usually went with the lowest bidder, occasions arose when they determined the lowest bidder did not offer the quality or specifications they considered essential. On those occasions even the conservative trustees selected companies that met their requirements but that were not the lowest bidders.

Some of their choices created challenges. In the fall of 1960, the state informed the Authority that its revised equipment costs exceeded those proposed in its application.[55] It said the Authority would have to reduce cost or solicit donations to make up the difference before the state and federal agencies could approve the equipment budget.[56] The federal agency increased slightly what it was willing to contribute, the Building Committee trimmed all of the costs that it could, the Authority raised a few thousand dollars in donations, and the county agreed to allow the Authority to use some of $200,000 it had budgeted for the opening of the hospital. Few, if any, of the tasks the trustees faced were simple or easy.

The Authority held a ceremony to lay the hospital's cornerstone in July 1960 when the project

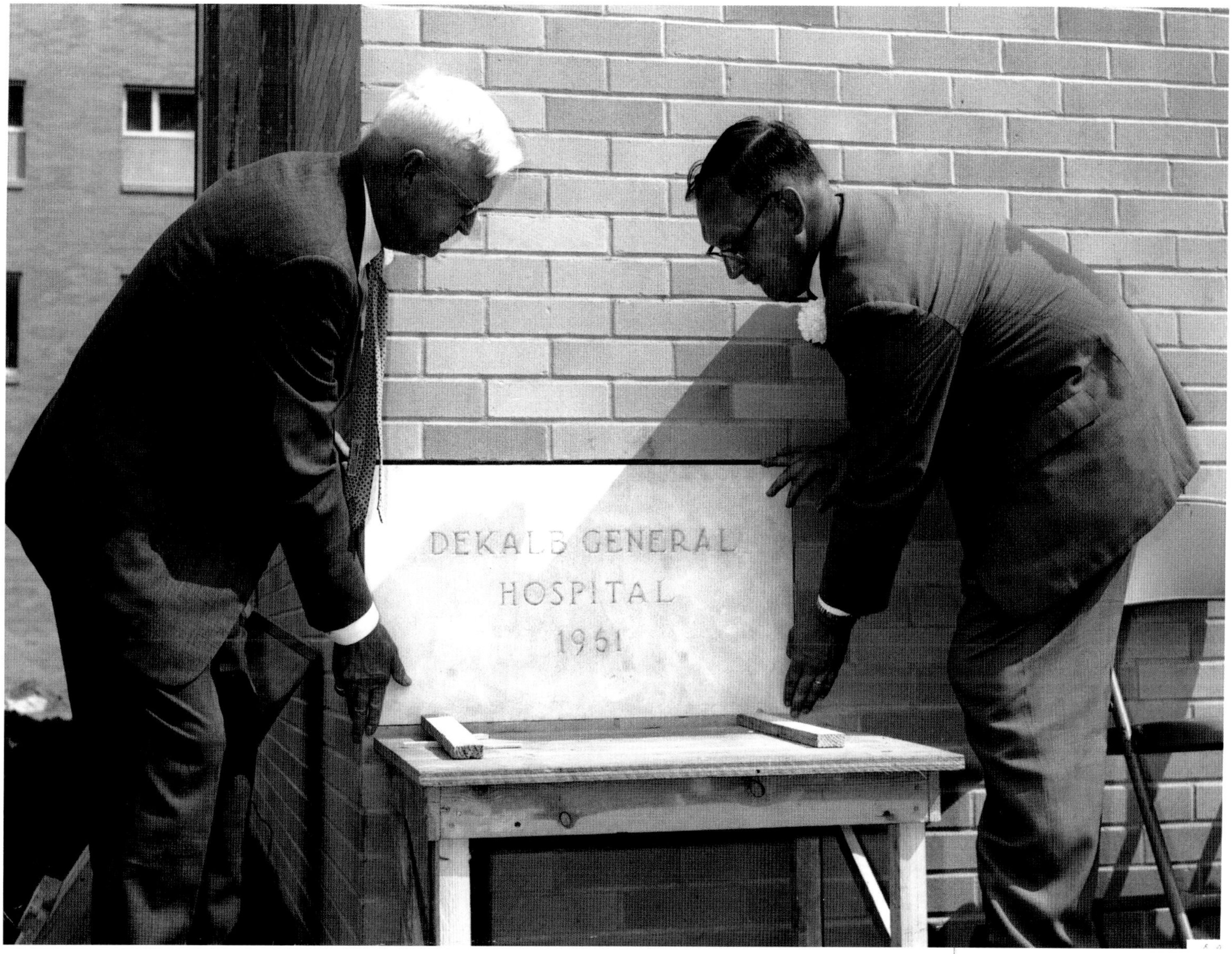

Authority Chairman J. Rufus Evans, MD, (left) and Administrator William Thrasher (right) lay the DeKalb General Hospital cornerstone during a ceremony in July of 1960.

was about 80 percent complete. Scott Candler was the principal speaker. A sealed box placed in the stone contained records of the DeKalb General Hospital development, a roster of the officials and citizens who participated over the years in its development, a statement of the hospital's philosophy, drawings and photographs of the building, and copies of newspaper articles announcing the cornerstone ceremony. The Authority insisted that the cornerstone be a simple stone with only the name, "DeKalb General Hospital," the date of its erection, and no names.[57]

The T. C. Brittain Company had promised to complete the hospital in twenty months. In January 1961, nineteen months after beginning construction, despite delays from bad weather, the contractor turned the hospital keys over to the trustees for their inspection. The staff that Thrasher had assembled moved from its temporary quarters into the hospital the first week in February on a "do-it-your-

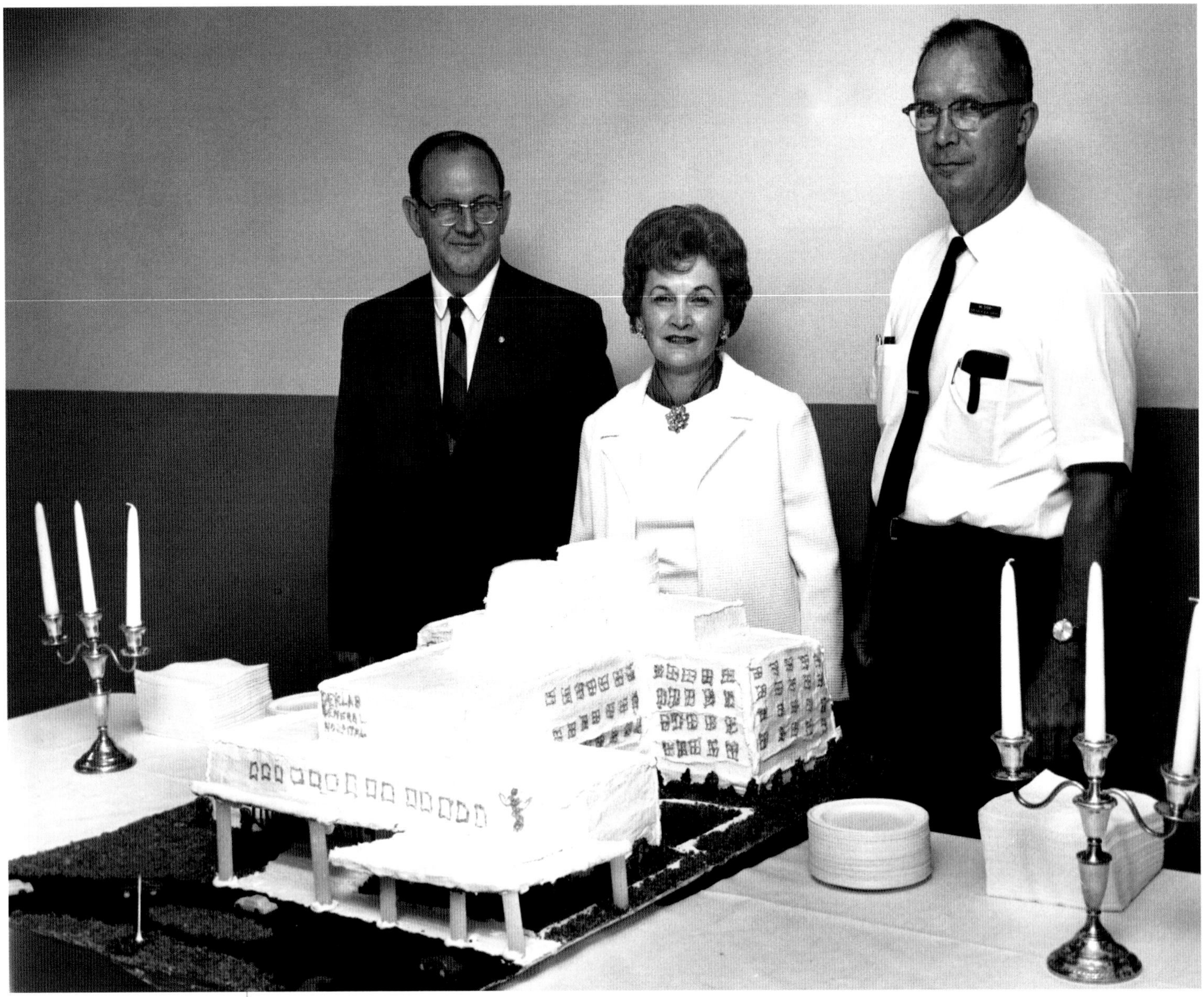

Administrator William Thrasher (left) with Mary Lou Hurt, director of Personnel (center), and Rodney Sperry, the hospital's first director of Building Services.

self" moving-in day. This was exciting, but there were many tasks yet to be completed before DeKalb General Hospital could open for business.

The Authority approved a budget for the first few months of operation, projecting a monthly operating expense of $93,450 from May 1 through September 30, 1961.[58] The Building Committee selected furniture manufactured by the Hill-Rom Company for patient rooms.[59] It also chose office furnishings and equipment as well as equipment for the operating rooms, Maternity, the Nursery, the Emergency Department, the Laboratory, and the Radiology Department.

In addition to Thrasher, Barner, Anderson, and Hopkins, the hospital's leadership staff included Frances Black, director of Medical Records; Arthur Woody, director of Pharmacy Services; Rodney Sperry, director of Building Services; Mattie Lou Meadows, director of Dietary Services;

Floyd Mitchell, director of Purchasing; Mary Lou Hurt, director of Personnel; Mary Lou Bothwell, director of Admissions; and Gee Aldridge, chief medical technologist for the Laboratory.[60]

Beyond this, Thrasher anticipated hiring, orienting, and training 250–300 staff members in as many as 125 job categories. There were approximately two thousand job applications on file for the available positions, most of which had come from DeKalb County residents.[61] Management had to develop policies and procedures for the defined work week, vacation time, holidays, sick leave, salary adjustments, pay periods, probation, pre-employment physicals, and other issues. The Business Office installed an IBM electronic accounting system, DeKalb General reportedly being only the second hospital in the nation to use the system.[62]

Despite a critical nursing shortage across the nation, Hopkins was successful in hiring 120 nurses. There were a number of factors in her favor. First of all she had a strong connection with the nurses at Georgia Baptist Hospital. She knew them, they knew her, and they thought well of her. She filled all the head nursing positions except one with nurses from Georgia Baptist. It also did not hurt that DeKalb General Hospital was new and was outfitted with state-of-the-art equipment; this and the fact that the Intensive Care Unit was a new and exciting concept in healthcare delivery were enticements for some nurses. And then there was the fact that many of the recruits lived in DeKalb County, and the commute to the new hospital with its ease of available parking was an attraction. Finally, DeKalb's nursing salaries were superior to those offered at other Atlanta hospitals at the time, although this would not hold true for long.[63]

On the hospital's opening day, Hopkins had a waiting list of nursing applicants. The majority of nurses she had hired were graduates of hospital diploma programs. All were female. Some were African-Americans, assigned to work on the first floor east wing where an all-black staff cared for black patients. Orderlies and Housekeeping personnel were the only African-American members of the staff who worked in both the black and the white areas of the hospital. Margaret Ford, RN, the director of Health and Training was a member of the staff and would become Hopkins' successor as director of Nursing in 1965. Naomi Harman, RN, the first night supervisor, also was a member of the nursing staff and would succeed Ford in 1969.[64]

Finally the trustees approved the physicians applying for the medical staff. They called on the Medical Society's Medical Advisory Committee again to develop a set of bylaws, to screen the medical staff applicants, and to serve as a temporary organizational committee until the hospital had enough physicians on staff to take over their own organization.

L. C. Buchanan, a member of the advisory committee, recommended that membership and privileges be based on the individual's medical qualifications rather than on privileges held in other hospitals. The trustees also agreed that members of the medical staff must be members of the DeKalb Medical Society since those doctors logically would be closer to the hospital and more available to take care of the emergencies.[65]

The Medical Advisory Committee developed medical staff bylaws; an application form for physician applicants to the medical staff; rules and regulations for the medical staff; and a procedure (only one page long!) for organizing the medical staff. The committee processed applications and made membership and privilege recommendations to the Authority until there were enough approved physicians on the medical staff to assume those responsibilities.

The initial medical staff departments included Anesthesia, General Practice, Medicine, Obstetrics and Gynecology, Pathology, Pediatrics, Radiology and Surgery.[66] The Department of

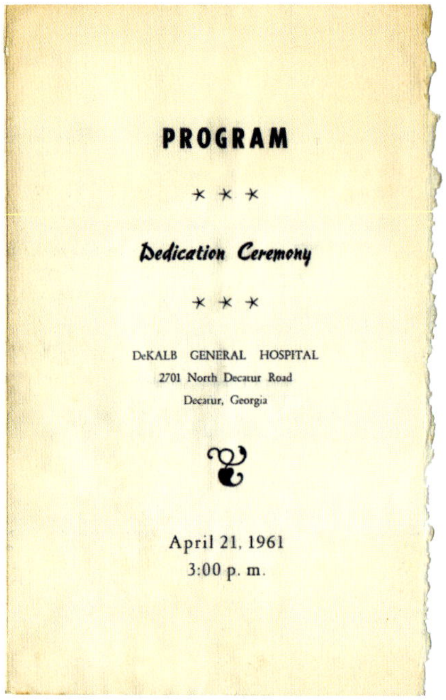

Above: The program for the hospital dedication ceremony on April 21, 1961. **Opposite:** J. Rufus Evans, MD, speaks at the dedication ceremony with William H. Thrasher seated behind Evans and Scott Candler Sr. seated to Thrasher's left.

Psychiatry would be added in 1971 and the Department of Emergency Medicine in 1973.

The Authority approved sixty-six physicians for membership and privileges on the medical staff prior to the opening of the hospital (see Appendix G) and named L. C. Buchanan as the first chief of staff.

DeKalb General Hospital was finally ready to open. It was built and equipped at a cost of $4,500,000. It covered 115,000 square feet, included a basement, and four stories, and had a two-hundred-bed capacity. The beds were spread over 128 private rooms, 26 semiprivate rooms, and a twenty-bed Intensive Care Unit.

The hospital was air conditioned throughout, and each patient room had an electric bed, its own thermostat, connection to a master antenna for television rental, a four-channel radio with pillow speaker, one channel being used for hospital broadcasting (including services from the chapel), and an intercommunication connection with the room's nursing station. Hot meals were delivered on aluminum carts that contained automatic toasters to serve fresh toast at the bedside.

A small chapel, open at all times, was located adjacent to the lobby. There were facilities for in-service training of employees. The X-ray equipment was considered the latest and best on the market with an automatic film processor that produced readable film in six minutes rather than the traditional one hour. The Radiology Department also had a cobalt therapy machine for treating cancer patients. Physicians had a lighted in-and-out register at their entrance and a selective paging system. The telephone system permitted conference calls. There were six hundred free parking spaces, one hundred of which were reserved for doctors.[67]

The trustees held a dedication ceremony on April 21, 1961, at which the facility was dedicated "to the glory of God and the improved health of mankind." Approximately four hundred people attended the ceremony, and as many as twenty thousand toured the hospital during three days of open house prior to its official opening to patients on May 1.

At the dedication ceremony, Thrasher said that the hospital would have a different atmosphere from the typical hospital in that the personnel were "trained to have a continuous interest in the patients, their families and friends," and would "look at their duties and their relationship with the patient as if they, themselves were the patient."[68] He pledged to "give the best care at the least cost to the patient. . . . We'll have a clean hospital, serving good food, with friendly personnel.[69]

In concluding his remarks, Thrasher summed up in three brief sentences the driving motivation behind the vision and the commitment of time and effort on the part of those who had worked for more than a decade to make DeKalb General Hospital a reality. He said, "The medical staff and personnel of DeKalb General Hospital are here to comfort you and to help you until you can help yourself, because you are not just another case to us. You are a human being in trouble—sick, frightened, and lonely—and taking care of you comes first. You are our reason for being here."[70]

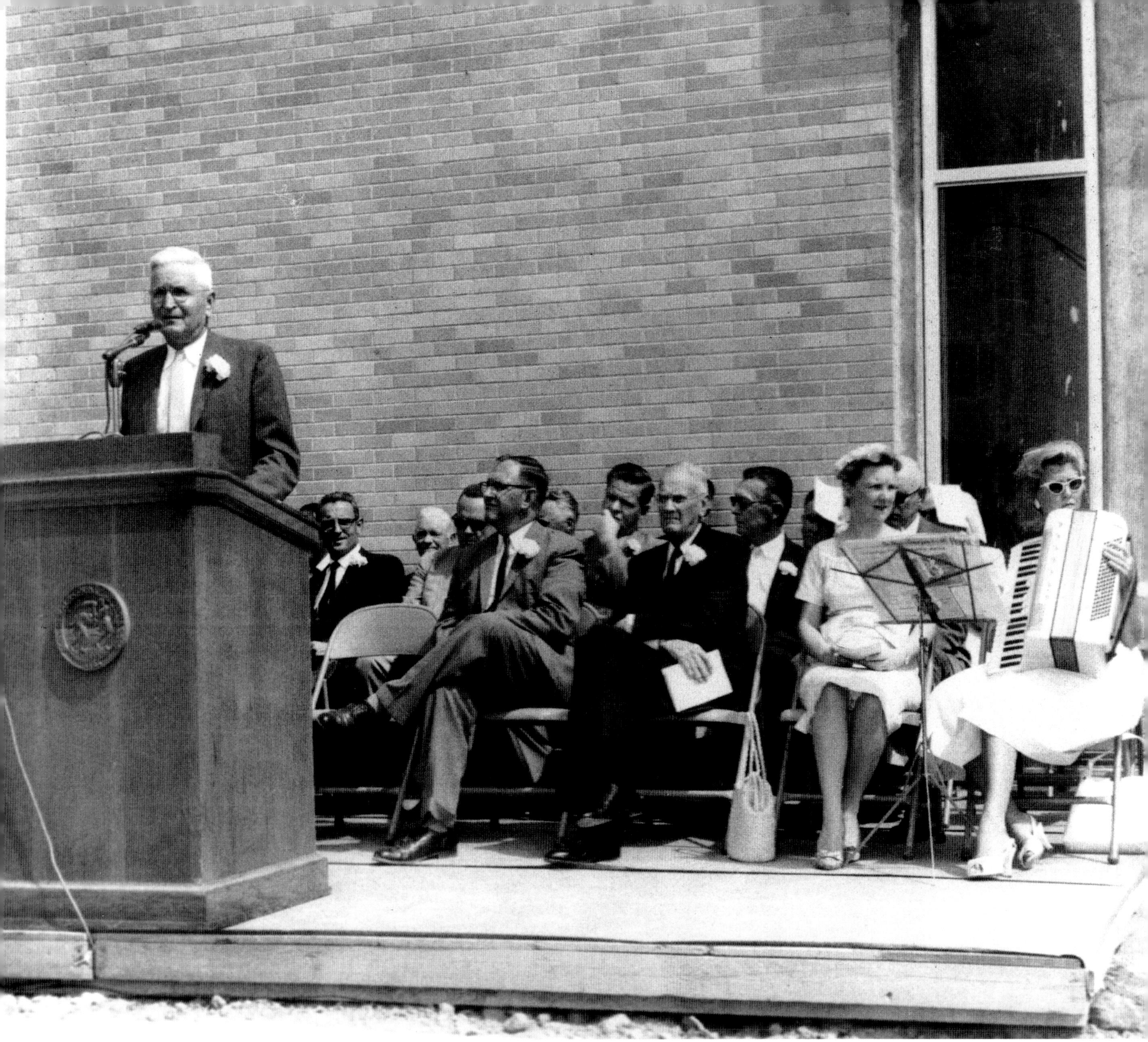

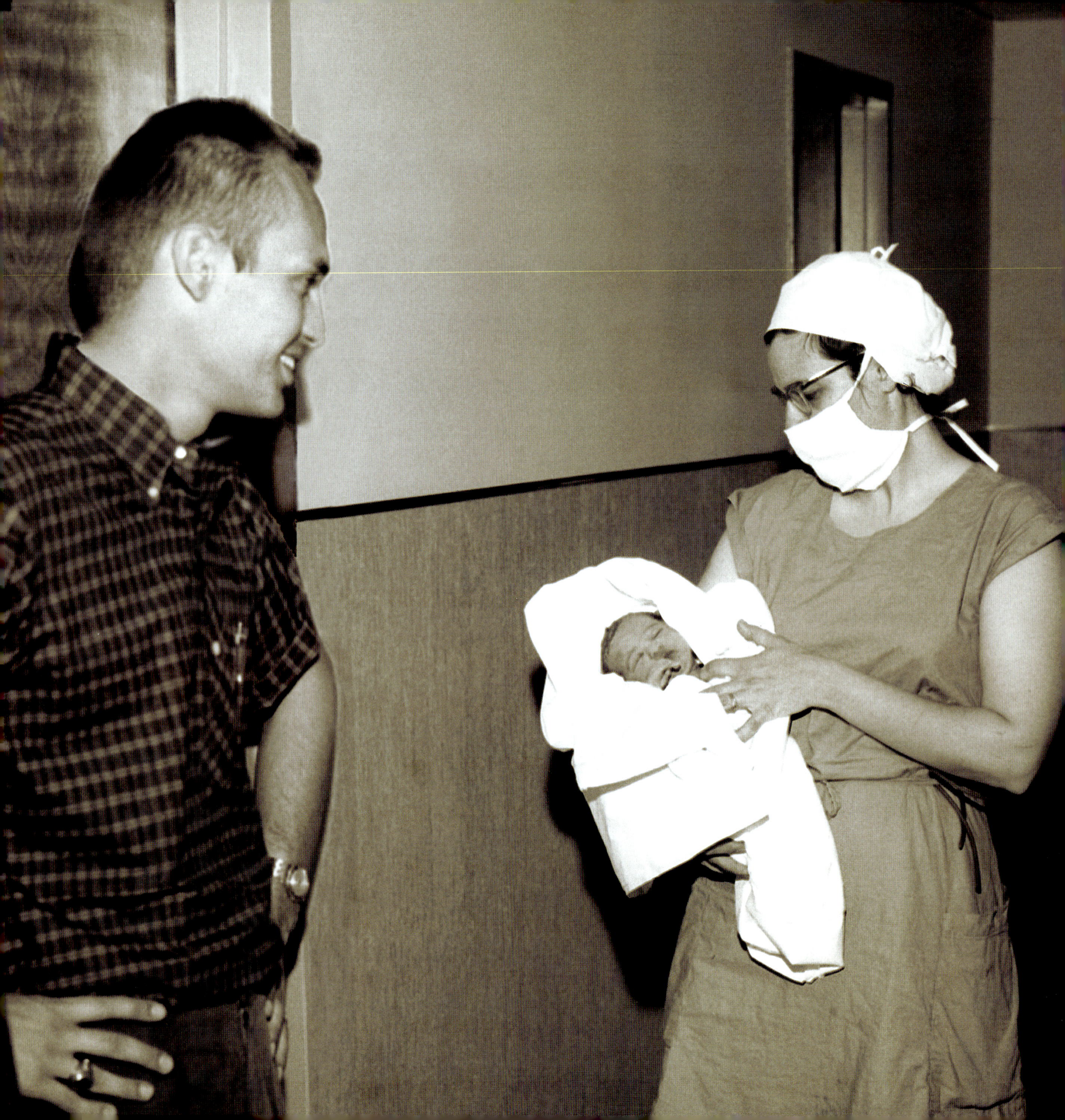

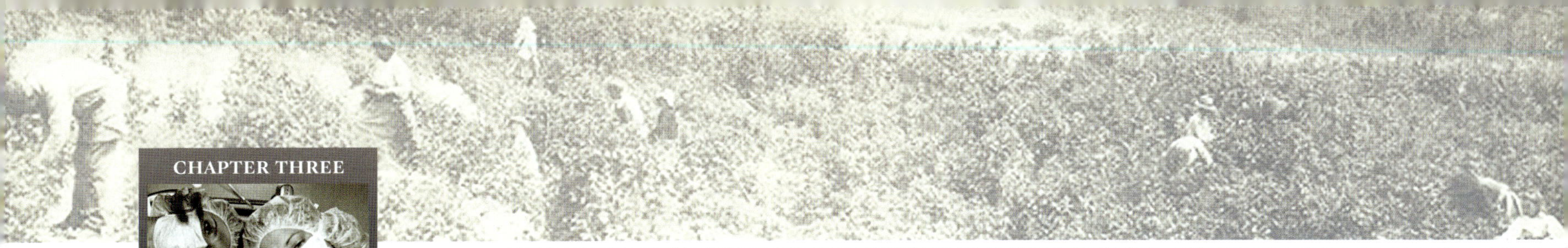

CHAPTER THREE

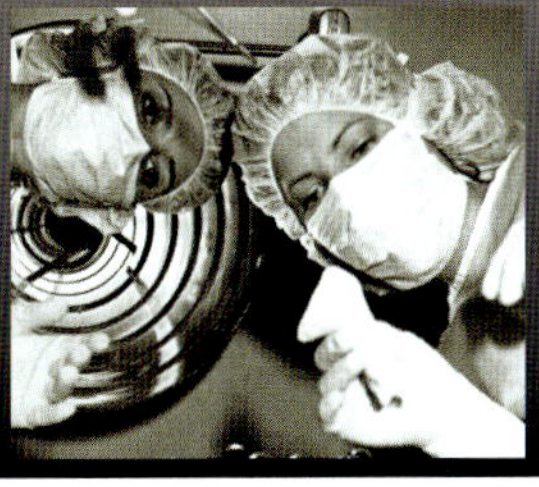

A Decade of Growth and Challenges

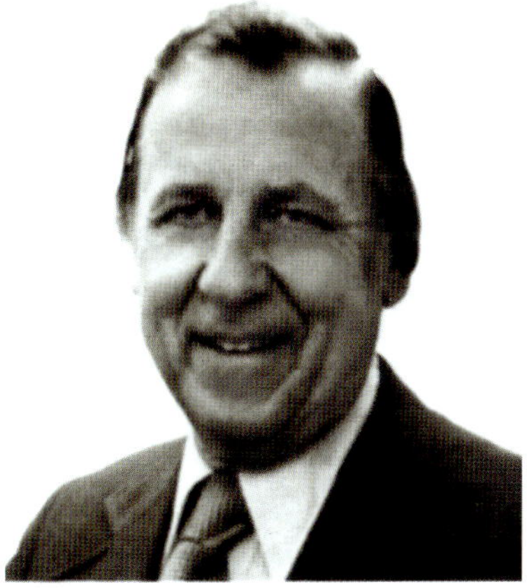

Above: L. C. Buchanan, MD, performed the first surgical procedure upon the opening of DeKalb General Hospital. **Opposite:** A nurse presents six-pound, eleven-ounce Stacy Elizabeth Stull to her father Thomas Stull. Stacy was the first baby born at the new hospital on the very day it opened its doors.

DeKalb General Hospital opened its doors at 9:00 am on May 1, 1961, amid a flurry of activity. John W. Fristoe, MD, admitted Mrs. Thomas E. Stull to the maternity service around noon, and at 3:04 pm delivered six-pound, eleven-ounce Stacy Elizabeth Stull, the hospital's first baby.[1] Stacy's father was a coach at Chamblee High School. As the first baby born at the hospital, Stacy and her parents received nearly forty gifts from members of the Decatur Merchants Association.[2] Twenty-five babies were delivered during the hospital's first week of operation.

On May 2, L. C. Buchanan, MD, performed thyroid surgery, the hospital's first surgical procedure, on Martha Ivey, mother-in-law of DeKalb General nurse, Peggy Ivey, LPN. Anibal Adan, MD, administered the anesthesia. On the same day, Richard Smoot, MD, performed a hernia repair, Lawrence Matthews, MD, a hysterectomy, and Catherine Foster, MD, a dilation and curettage (D & C).[3] During the first three weeks, thirty-seven doctors admitted 192 adults and delivered fifty-eight babies. The average daily inpatient census was forty-two. The Laboratory and Radiology Departments performed studies on 138 outpatients.[4] By July the average daily inpatient hospital census grew to sixty-nine.[5]

As with most new hospitals, DeKalb General faced challenges. During its first decade, it struggled with deficit finances, the issue of diversity, medical coverage for its Emergency Department, fraud on the part of one of its managers, changes in the governing body membership, the need to recruit replacements for two administrative leaders, inadequate space, external pressure from regulatory agencies, and a major crisis in Nursing.

Finances

At the May 1959 groundbreaking ceremony, trustee J. Ross McCain said the hospital would be "characterized by heart interest in each patient, whether rich or poor."[6] To qualify for state and federal Hill-Burton funds, the trustees were committed to providing a certain amount of uncompensated care and to provide emergency care regardless of ability to pay. The DeKalb County Hospital Authority, however, intended to operate the hospital without a deficit. When McCain wrote to William Thrasher as a candidate for the position of administrator, he said:

> *We would like to be told what charges we should make when operations begin and what chances there are to avoid deficits. What kind of cushioning against red ink ought to be provided?*[7]

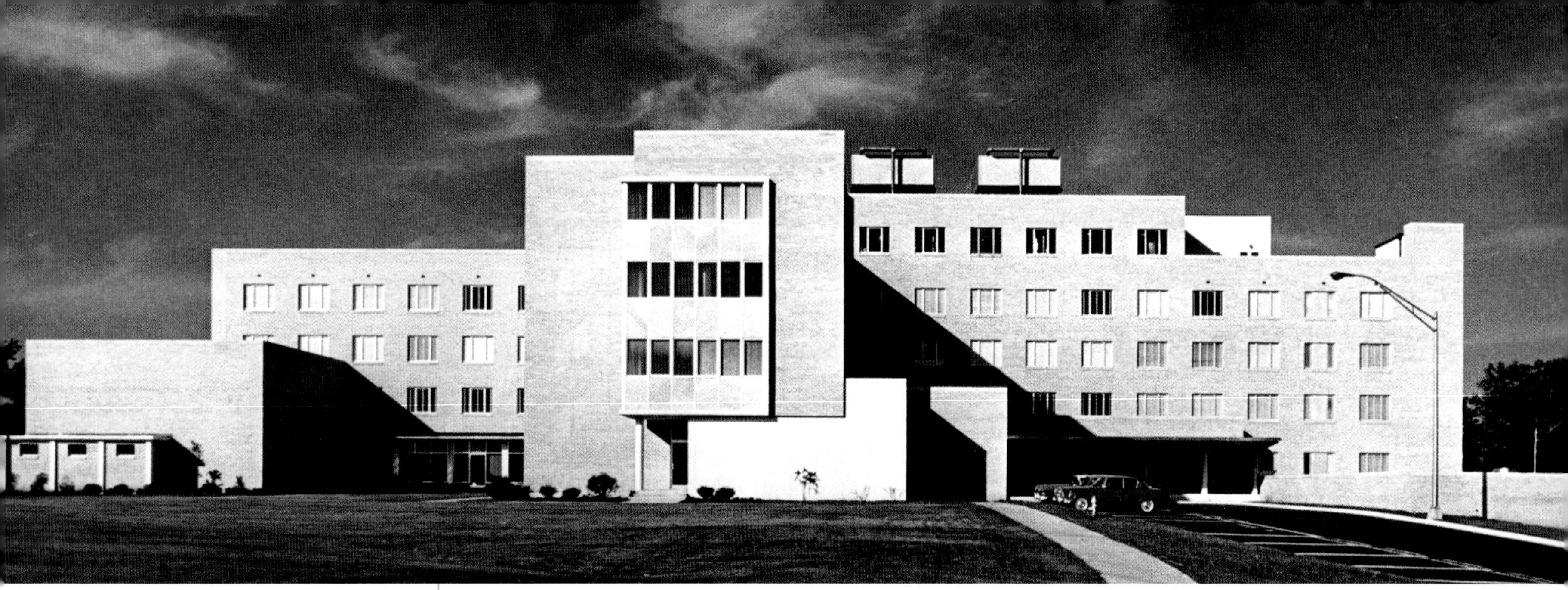

With its opening, DeKalb General Hospital would finally be able to provide the much needed health care to the surrounding community. Over time it would also become the flagship of the entire DeKalb Regional Healthcare System. This view is from the emergency parking area looking at the right side of the hospital.

The trustees wanted to keep expenses to a minimum and charge patients as little as possible, but avoid red ink.

Despite its commitment and Hill-Burton requirements to provide care regardless of one's ability to pay, the hospital unapologetically proclaimed that it was built for paying patients, not charity patients. The press quoted Thrasher as saying, "DeKalb General Hospital [wants] the 'right of patient selection' and therefore does not take charity cases." He added that DeKalb County taxpayers support Grady Memorial Hospital, and the county is required by its contract with the Fulton-DeKalb Authority to transfer its charity cases to Grady.[8] The DeKalb trustees did not mention charity patients in their preadmission brochure,[9] and they urged physicians to send their indigent patients to Grady.

The Authority also went to great lengths to ensure that its paying patients paid for the services they received. Patients scheduled for elective admission were required to submit a preadmission form to establish their financial status. The form asked for the patient's permission to review his or her credit rating, and the business office reviewed each elective patient's credit report. It contacted credit references listed on the preadmission form. If there was any question about a patient's ability (or willingness) to pay in full for the services received, the business office called the patient. If the patient did not satisfy the hospital that it would be paid for services provided, that patient's elective admission reservation was canceled.[10]

Patients who qualified financially for admission were asked to pay all charges not covered by insurance at the time of discharge. If they stayed in the hospital for a prolonged period, a representative from the business office presented them with their current bill at the bedside at the end of each week.[11]

Realizing that the hospital would have to take care of indigent patients despite efforts to discourage them, the trustees did two things to recover some of those costs. First they negotiated a contract with Grady Memorial Hospital in which Grady agreed to pay DeKalb General $22.50 a day, for up to twelve patients a month, for any DeKalb County indigent patient hospitalized at DeKalb General.[12] They also asked neighboring counties to pay for the services their indigent patients received at DeKalb General. For the most part, that was a futile effort. Commissioners for Rockdale County agreed to pay up to $250 for its patients, but they were alone in this.[13] Most other counties turned a deaf ear to that

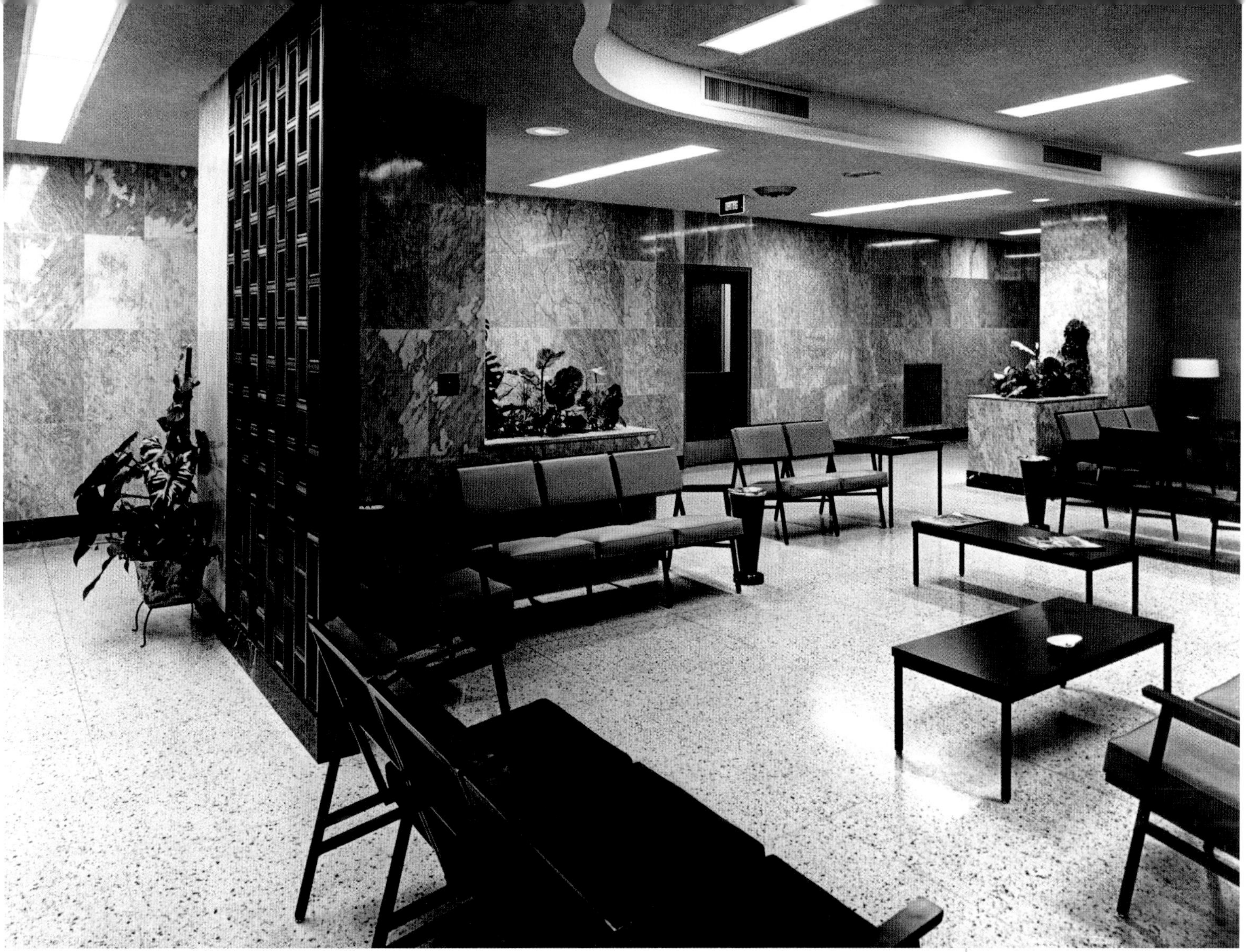

request, and the trustees found no legal basis to force them to pay.[14]

Despite its best efforts, bad debts and an increasing amount of indigent care caused the hospital's accounts receivable to grow. Dealing with accounts receivable became a regular agenda item at Authority meetings. The trustees considered asking physicians to indicate their patients' ability to pay but decided the doctors would not have that information or would not choose to provide it if they had it. The trustees also hired collection agents to collect debts due the hospital, but most of these agents had little if any success. One agent returned to the hospital the list of overdue accounts given to him a year earlier without having collected a dime.[15] Within three months of opening, 3 percent of the hospital's gross charges were deemed either uncollectible or charity cases.[16]

In addition to maximizing income, the Authority was adamant about containing costs. The trustees reviewed the operating budget at every meeting to compare expenses and income. They assumed direct and close control over how the hospital spent its money. They reviewed and approved all requests for equipment, travel, salary increases, and personnel acquisition. In 1964 Thrasher asked the Authority for a vote of confidence by authorizing him to employ additional personnel as he deemed necessary, make adjustments in beginning salaries as he deemed appropriate, establish a fair

The beautiful, spacious lobby at DeKalb General Hospital.

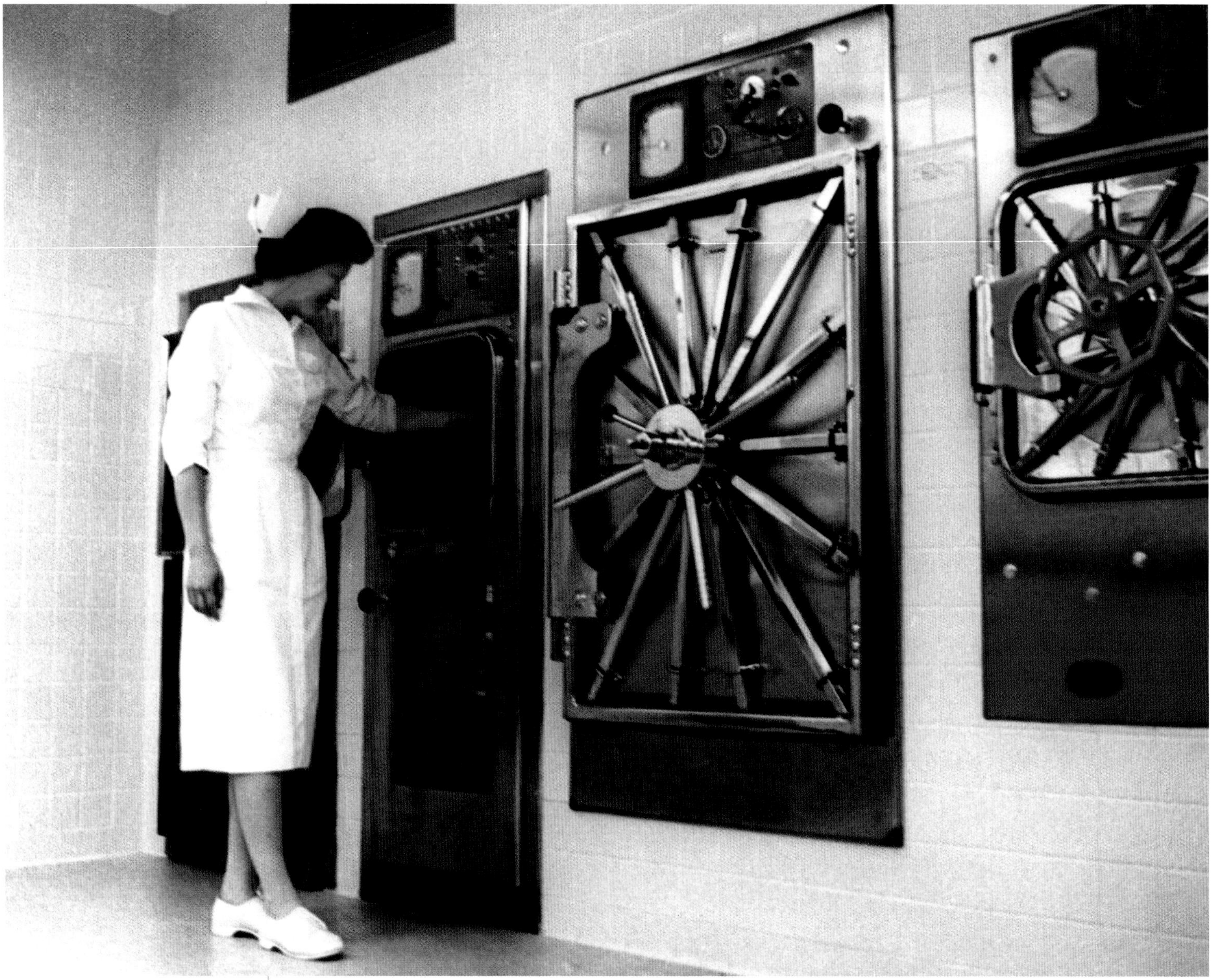

A nurse in the central supply area of the new hospital.

merit increase program, and make adjustments in hospital rates as needed. The trustees declined and said these matters should remain in their hands.[17]

No expense was too small to be evaluated, and no savings was too small to be celebrated. The Authority had to approve the kitchen's spending $398 to buy a blender.[18] One trustee objected strongly to the hospital's paying $50 for a Medical Records librarian to attend a meeting in Macon.[19] When the hospital physicians asked that a gate be installed for their parking lot, the Authority agreed on the condition that the doctors raise the $300 needed to pay for the gate.[20] The Authority was very pleased when it learned that the Christmas Open House for employees had, with many items donated, cost only $25.04.[21] It was important enough to note in the minutes that a change in one staff position saved the hospital $40 a month.[22]

The Authority deferred even desirable and needed expenditures if it deemed them unaffordable. It delayed the salary raises promised to those who had been on the staff for six months or more.[23] It deferred for three years establishing a depreciation account. It discussed having a hospital chaplain,[24] a retirement plan,[25] a credit union[26] and group insurance,[27] but determined that the hospital, at the time, could not afford those worthwhile initiatives. When certain positions became vacant, it often elected not to appoint replacements, or to combine positions, or to replace a position with a less expensive position. When Ted Barner, the hospital's first assistant administrator, resigned in 1962, neither he nor his secretary was replaced until John R. Gerlach was named assistant to the administrator six years later. When the director of Purchasing resigned, his responsibilities were decentralized and assigned to the director of Pharmacy and other department heads. When Margaret Ford, RN, resigned as director of Training and Health Services, her position was replaced by a supervisor of Training and Health at a lower salary.[28]

The Authority approved a monthly budget of $93,450 for each of the first five months of operation and $1,121,400 for the first fiscal year that began in October 1961. Despite its best efforts to maximize income and minimize cost, the hospital had a net loss of $152,000 in its first year of operation.[29] Its cash flow was so limited that accounts payable often were carried over from month to month, and honored bills were frequently paid after forty-five days rather than within the standard thirty days.[30]

Because of its deficit, the Authority did two things. It raised the hospital's room rates, and it called on the county for help. The room rate increases were minuscule compared to present-day charges. The Emergency Room fee was increased from $3 to $4, but only after the increase was approved by the Medical Staff Executive Committee.[31] In 1962 the Intensive Care Unit (ICU) rate was increased from $22 a day to $30.[32] As late as 1966 private-room rates were raised reluctantly from $25 to $27.50 a day, semiprivate rooms went from $20 to $22, and ICU rates went from $50 to $60.[33]

The hospital's major source of supplementary cash came from the county. It has been said that the hospital never used county tax dollars for its operational expenses. That is true for the last forty years. During the first six years, however, county support was a critical factor in keeping the hospital fiscally viable. The county contributed $200,000 to the hospital's operating budget in the calendar year 1961, $150,000 in 1962,[34] $100,000 in 1963,[35] $50,000 in 1964,[36] $30,000 in 1965,[37] and $30,000 in 1966.[38]

Federal legislation added more financial burdens to DeKalb General. In the federal year 1965–1966, Congress passed more social legislation affecting the healthcare industry than in all of the previous 190 years.[39] Most notable were two amendments to the Social Security Act (Public Law 89–97). President Lyndon B. Johnson proclaimed the concept of "The Great Society," and Congress passed Title 18, known as Medicare, to provide healthcare to the elderly, and Title 19, known as Medicaid, to provide health care services to the poor.[40] Medicare initially paid only 87 percent of hospital charges, and Medicaid paid even less.[41] Over time both programs paid less and less of hospital charges, and Medicaid eventually paid less than actual hospital costs.

Despite the challenges, by the mid-1960s the hospital gained sound financial footing. The Authority no longer turned to the county to supplement its operating budget. It funded its depreciation account retroactive to 1961, paid its bills on time, purchased new and expensive equipment, and established a savings account. Grave financial concerns, however, would return three decades later.

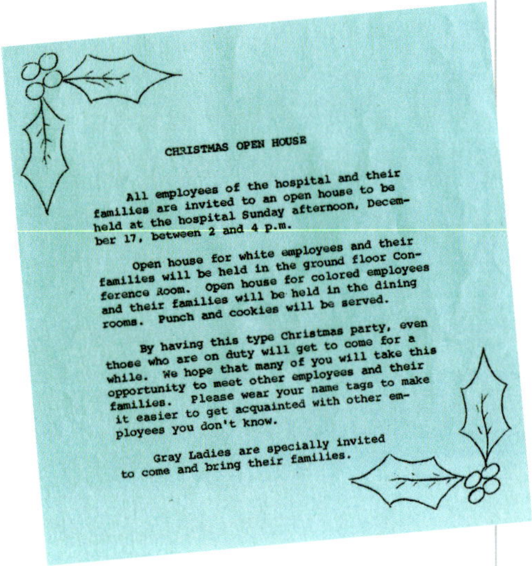

CHRISTMAS OPEN HOUSE

All employees of the hospital and their families are invited to an open house to be held at the hospital Sunday afternoon, December 17, between 2 and 4 p.m.

Open house for white employees and their families will be held in the ground floor Conference Room. Open house for colored employees and their families will be held in the dining rooms. Punch and cookies will be served.

By having this type Christmas party, even those who are on duty will get to come for a while. We hope that many of you will take this opportunity to meet other employees and their families. Please wear your name tags to make it easier to get acquainted with other employees you don't know.

Gray Ladies are specially invited to come and bring their families.

In its first year of operation, the hospital began to publish an employee newsletter. In the December issue, it notified employees of the segregated holiday open houses.

Diversity

In 1961 DeKalb General Hospital was one of the few hospitals in Atlanta to admit and treat African American patients, but it was segregated. The primary diversity issue was how to respect and treat African American patients and employees fairly and appropriately. Segregation generally was still an accepted condition at DeKalb General as elsewhere in the South. The east wing of the first floor and one of the four isolation rooms on the upper floors were designated for African American patients. Orderlies and housekeeping personnel were the only blacks to work in all-white areas. The hospital gave the DeKalb Junior League a special rate for the medical and surgical services it provided the league's sponsored black children.[42] It hosted its first Christmas Open House for employees and their families in December 1961, but the employee newsletter specified that the "open house for white employees and their families will be held in the ground-floor conference room. Open house for colored employees and their families will be held in the dining rooms. Punch and cookies will be served."[43]

There were no black physicians on the original medical staff, and available documents are silent on the number or names of African American nurses or physicians on the hospital staff in the early years. The application form for the medical staff asked for the physician's race, and there was at least one black physician. In February 1968, Thrasher reported to the Authority that "the [last] remaining negro on the staff, Dr. Richard Hackney, died on February 7, 1968."[44] Hackney had been admitted to the General Practice Department in February 1964 with no mention of his race at that time.[45]

In 1964 Congress passed Title VI of the Civil Rights Act that prohibited discrimination by any governmental agency that received federal funding (such as the Hill-Burton funds that DeKalb General had received) and required affected hospitals to show no "separation, discrimination or any other distinction on the basis of race, color, or national origin in any activity carried on in, by, or for the institution affecting the care and treatment of patients."[46]

A year later a committee of white and black DeKalb County citizens presented a petition to the Department of Health, Education, and Welfare (HEW) and to DeKalb General Hospital claiming job and patient discrimination. The petition accused the hospital of segregating patients by race, refusing to process African American job applications in the same manner as whites, assigning black employees to unskilled and low-paying jobs, and refusing to respond to specific complaints of racial discrimination.[47]

Representatives from HEW came to DeKalb General and investigated. They deemed the hospital to be in compliance with Title VI, with "no problems in terms of racial discrimination."[48] However, as a result of the complaint, the Authority declared in March 1965, "DeKalb General Hospital will comply with the law;" and in September 1965 it approved the following resolution: "Patients will be assigned to hospital facilities according to their medical needs with no distinction to be made on grounds of race, color, religion, or national origin."[49] The east wing for blacks became a pediatric wing, and the isolation room formerly designated for African American patients thereafter was designated as a general patient isolation room. Patients and staff were assigned to areas according to need.

William Page, regional director of HEW, wrote to the Authority, "If this policy is followed, it would not be beyond the realm of probability to have biracial occupancy of multibed rooms."[50] The Authority publicized its resolution in the press, and there is no record of further civil rights complaints at that time. Eight months later an HEW publication stated that DeKalb General Hospital "presents essentially no problems in terms of racial discrimination." The issue of diversity, however, would arise again in later years.

Changes in Governance

Five of the original seven members of the Authority either died or resigned before the end of the first decade. In September 1964 Julius McCurdy resigned and Hugh Rowland died.[51] Ross McCain died in 1965, M. E. Smith resigned in January 1969, and J. Rufus Evans resigned the following September. That left only R. L. Mathis, who would die in 1974, and Wash W. Lively who would remain on the Authority for thirty years.

Waldo Sowell replaced McCurdy; W. P. Tatum replaced Rowland; Floyd Sanders, MD, replaced McCain; Rufus Camp replaced Smith; and William Lewis replaced Evans.

When Evans resigned in 1969, the trustees elected Waldo Sowell as chairman and W. P. Tatum vice chairman, retaining W. W. Lively as secretary-treasurer.[52]

Evans' resignation from the Authority marked a major change in the organization. He experienced a heart attack in April 1969 and missed the April and May Authority meetings. In August he announced that, on the advice of family and physician, he was stepping down as chairman. At the September meeting, he added that he was resigning as an Authority member. When the other trustees asked him to reconsider, he said "it would be very difficult for [me] to sit on the board and not act like a chairman."[53] At his last meeting, he "asked only that the Hospital Authority continue to set money aside to cover emergencies and not hesitate to make a profit."[54]

His exodus from the Authority ended two decades of remarkable leadership and achievement. He had championed the need for DeKalb General Hospital, and he had been a key force in its creation. Once established, he was the acknowledged leader in charge. Evans never made a decision that the other trustees did not approve; and the trustees made no decisions without his approval. Throughout his tenure, he maintained a close relationship with county and state officials which enabled him to call on their support and resources on behalf of the hospital. When initiatives he championed were confronted with roadblocks, he found effective alternate routes. When the county commissioners said they could not get another bond passed to fund the hospital's needed expansion, Evans persuaded them to underwrite $4,000,000 in revenue anticipation certificates. When the state said they would not provide matching funds for the hospital's expansion, Evans said the hospital would pay for it with its own funds.

Thrasher once informed Evans that revised federal regulations for Hill-Burton hospitals required that DeKalb General convert its prized private rooms into semiprivate rooms because of their large size. Evans reportedly replied, "Hell, Thrasher, we'll make the rooms smaller." And he then ordered cabinets to be built in the private rooms making them just large enough to reduce the open square footage of the rooms to satisfy Hill-Burton requirements.[55]

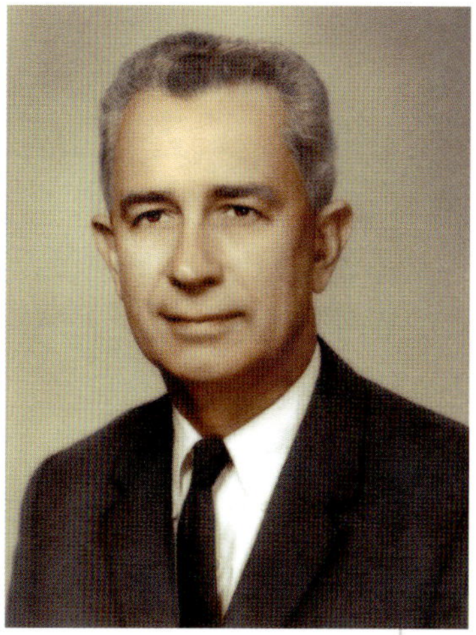

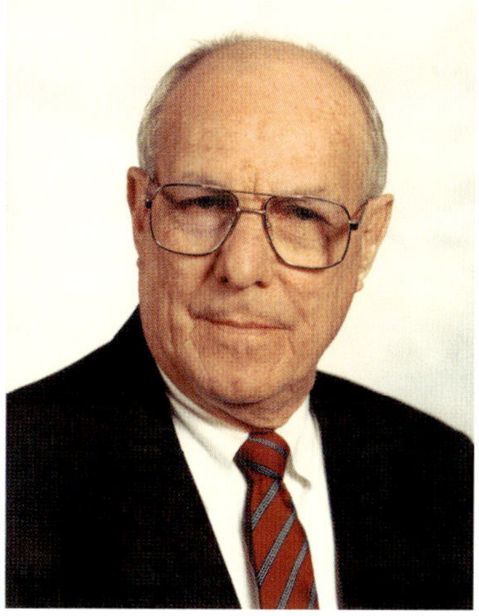

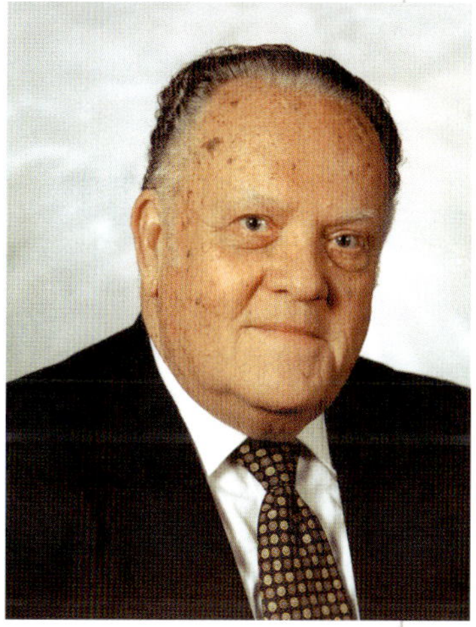

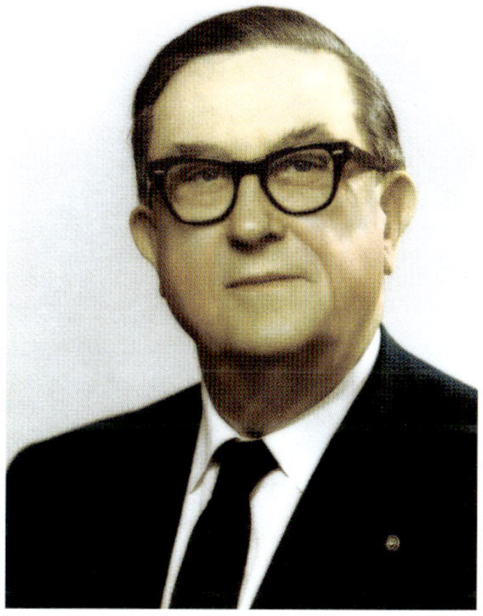

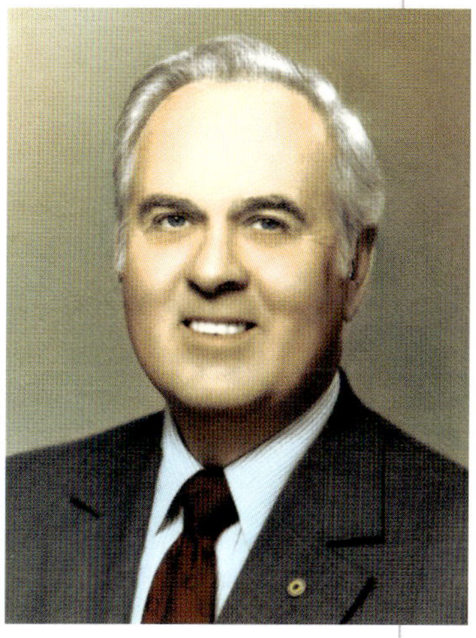

Clockwise beginning bottom left: William. E. Lewis, Floyd Sanders, MD, Waldo Sowell, W. P. Tatum, and Rufus Camp.

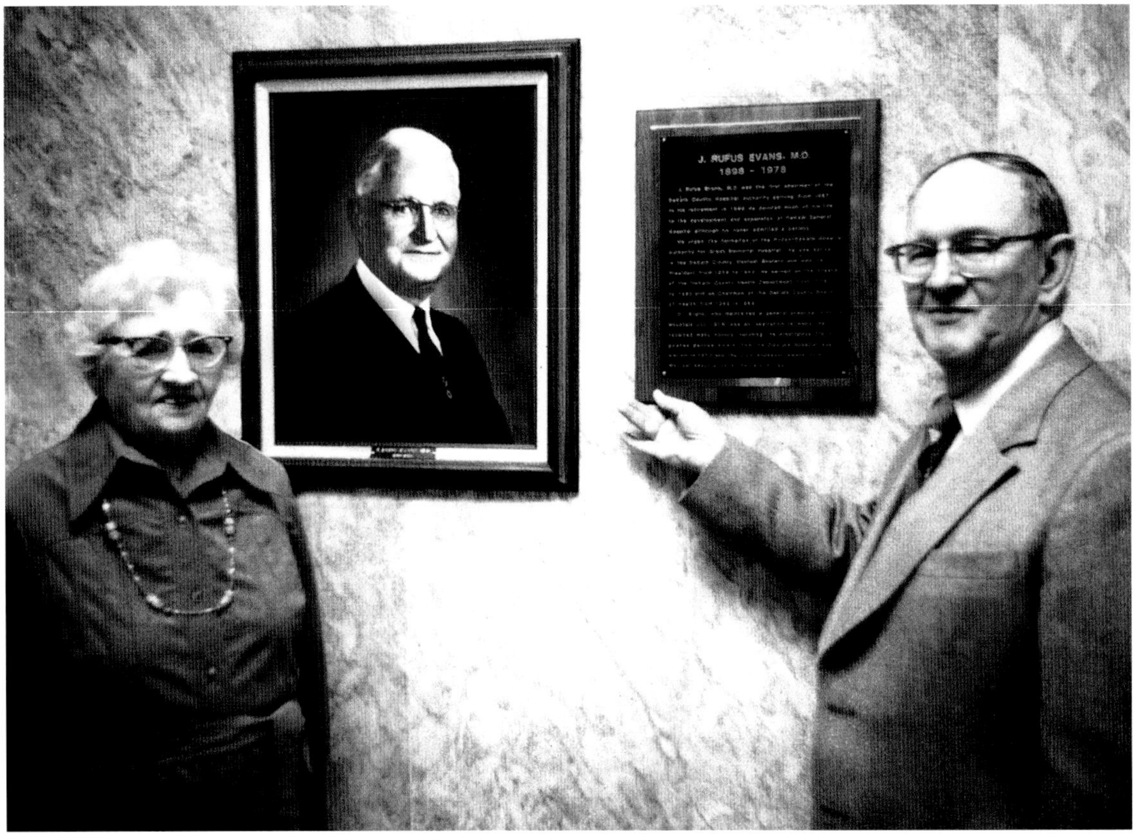

Mrs. Rufus McCurdy Evans and William H. Thrasher, director of Hospital Relations and former administrator, display a portrait in memory of J. Rufus Evans.

Thrasher once said that if he ever wrote a book about the hospital, one chapter would be entitled, "Hell, Thrasher" because that was how Evans introduced most topics when speaking to him. Earnest Atkins, MD, an early chief of staff who frequently attended the regular Evans-Thrasher morning meetings said that for a while he thought Thrasher's first name must be "Dammit," because he always heard Evans refer to him as "Dammit, Thrasher."

Chester Morse, MD, one of DeKalb General's original physicians and one of Evans's many admirers, referred to Evans as a "despot" but added that he was a "benevolent despot" who got good things done on behalf of the hospital that he loved and nurtured.

The leadership of the governing body continued to be enormously effective, but it was never the same once Evans stepped aside. Evans's leadership and accomplishments were legendary, and many organizations acknowledged his contributions. The Georgia Nurses Association named him the Doctor of the Year, and the Decatur Lions Club designated him the Senior Citizen of the year. He received the Leon Thomas Award from the DeKalb Chamber of Commerce, the Golden Deed Award from the Decatur Exchange Club,[56] and the Distinguished Service Award from the Georgia Hospital Association.[57]

Evans continued practicing medicine in Stone Mountain for six years after retiring from the Authority. He retired from his medical practice in 1975 at the age of 78 and died on March 6, 1978.[58] Despite the time, talent, and energy that he devoted to DeKalb General Hospital, Evans never admitted a patient to the hospital.[59]

Staffing the Emergency Department

The Emergency Department (originally known as the Emergency Room, or ER) proved to be one of the hospital's big surprises. In the planning stages, no one thought it would care for a large volume of patients or be a major player in the hospital's services. When being considered for the position of administrator, Thrasher wrote that the ER would likely play only a minor role since the hospital was planned for private, paying patients; and Grady Memorial Hospital, Georgia Baptist Hospital, and Emory Hospital each had busy, well-established emergency departments that took care of the community's emergency needs.

Based on those assumptions, the original Emergency Department consisted of a small area with only a few examining and treatment rooms, and the medical staff was expected to volunteer the medical coverage needed. An "ER Call List" designated the days when each physician was to be available to see ER patients. If a patient presented with problems outside the expertise of the on-call physician, there was a "Backup Call List" of specialists who could be summoned for assistance.

Within a year, however, the Emergency Department faced problems of space, staffing, patient volume, technology, and finances. As an interim measure, the hospital contracted with "house physicians," mostly residents, interns, and physicians in the process of establishing their practices to assume some of the ER responsibilities of the volunteer medical staff. The hospital paid the house physicians $500 to $700 a month.

Within two years, however, it became clear that changes were needed. The volume of patients rose rapidly. By 1963 as many as 2,000 patients a month presented for care. The volunteer medical staff was incapable of managing that volume while attending to their own growing medical practices. The house physician concept was inadequate. They were difficult to recruit and retain, and vacancies were common. They also varied in competence and in the quality of care they provided. They were not members of the medical staff and thus did not come under the jurisdiction and supervision of medical staff rules and regulations. Some were not licensed to practice medicine in Georgia, but the Authority hired whomever they could get.[60]

In 1963 the medical staff asked the Authority to consider other options for staffing the ER.[61] The trustees commissioned Thrasher, L. C. Buchanan, and Robert Gibbs, MD, to investigate what other hospitals were doing. They visited and studied models in operation in Pontiac, Michigan, and in Alexandria, Virginia. The Alexandria hospital contracted with a group of physicians for total emergency room care. In February 1965 Gibbs described that model in detail to the Authority. Freeman Simmons, MD, chairman of the Medical Staff Emergency Committee, said his committee endorsed the concept, and Evans said the plan sounded good to him. He asked the medical staff to review it and present the Authority with a specific proposal.[62]

The medical staff recommended what they called "the Alexandria Plan with modifications," and the Authority approved their recommendation. In June 1965 administration signed a contract with four well-known and respected community physicians: Freeman Simmons, Ted Rheney, MD, Tom Lowry, MD, and Thomas Cooper, MD. These four physicians closed their medical practices in the community and agreed to provide full-time medical coverage of the ER as contract physicians.[63] They were known as the DeKalb Emergency Group. When Cooper left the group in 1968, Luther Vinton, MD, another respected community physician, took his place and remained with the group for many years.

The DeKalb Emergency Group began work in July 1965, and they were an immediate success. The public praised their care as quicker and better than the previous arrangement, and the medical

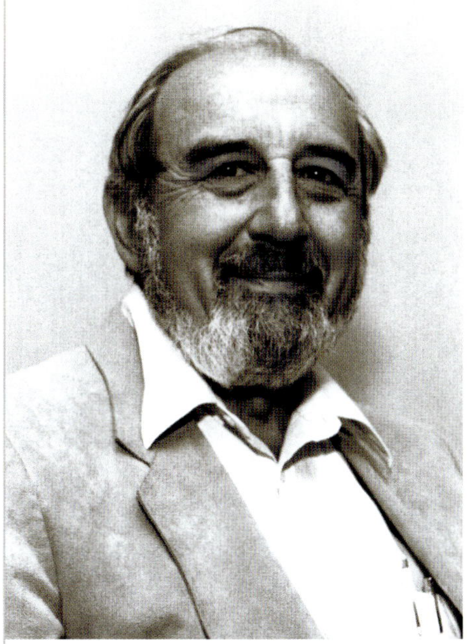

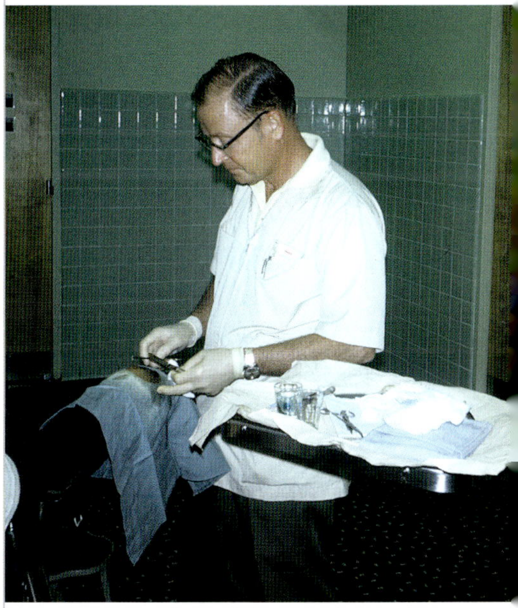

Top: Joseph Arnold, MD, a family physician still in practice, was an early house physician while waiting to open his own office. **Above:** Freeman Simmons, MD, was the first chief of the DeKalb Emergency Group and medical director of Emergency Services.

staff appreciated the consistent high quality of care the physicians provided. It was the first such arrangement among hospitals in the southeast, and it became a model that many other hospitals emulated. It also became a contributing factor in the emergence of Emergency Medicine as a specialty.

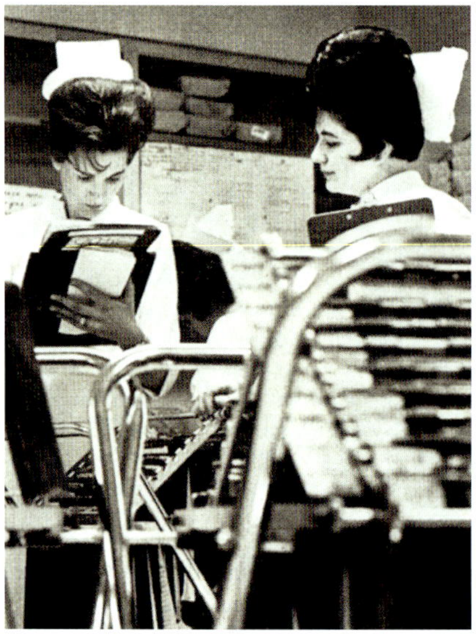

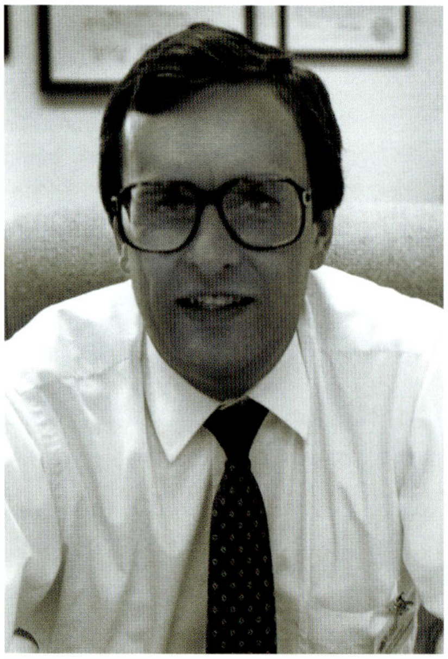

Top: Opal (Hopkins) Fyffe, left, with Naomi Harman, right. Fyffe was hoping that Harman would be her successor. **Above:** John R. "Jack" Gerlach, former part-time pharmacist at the hospital, was named assistant to the administrator in 1968 to assist with a planned major expansion of the hospital.

Replacing Two Key Administrative Positions

In its first decade, DeKalb General had to find a new director of Nursing and a new assistant to the administrator.

In 1963 Opal Hopkins reduced her responsibilities as the director of Nursing in order to care for her husband, Troy, who had developed acute leukemia. She called on her night supervisor and friend, Naomi Harman, RN, to serve as assistant director. She returned to her full-time position following Troy's death in 1963, but in March 1965 married David Fyffe, a Georgia Tech professor, and asked Thrasher to accept her resignation so that she might become a full-time homemaker. In July she wrote the following to Thrasher:

> *I would like for you to make arrangements for my position by September 30, 1965. My primary reason is due to a home situation. I have to take [my son] Larry out of the nursery the end of August and beginning September 1, I have to leave the office at 2:30 to pick him up at school. I do not feel, due to this problem, I can be responsible for the Nursing Department and all its countless problems. I will do whatever I can to assist you in securing a replacement for the position.*[64]

Now known as Opal Fyffe, she wanted Naomi Harman to be her successor. Thrasher, however, told her that while Harman was a competent diploma graduate from a hospital nursing program, the trustees wanted an academic degree nurse in that position. Fyffe then recommended Margaret Ford, RN, who had been the hospital's director of Training and Health Services in 1961 until she accepted the position of director of Nursing at Elks Aidmore Hospital in 1962. Ford had received a bachelor's degree in nursing education from the University of Georgia and a master's degree in nursing from Emory University. She had served as a first lieutenant in the Army Nurse Reserve Corps, as director of Nursing Education at Crawford W. Long Hospital and as a member and as president of the State Board of Nursing Examiners.[65] On August 4 Thrasher wrote to Fyffe, "Yesterday I employed Margaret Ford as director of Nursing to come with us on November 1, 1965."[66] As will be seen in chapter 4, Ford and Fyffe would each play pivotal roles in the crisis in Nursing Services that was to come.

The second change occurred when the hospital's first assistant administrator, Ted Barner, resigned in 1962 to become the administrator of another hospital. The Authority deferred replacing him for six years. In the summer of 1968, however, plans for a major hospital expansion project were underway and administrative responsibilities were expanding exponentially. The trustees authorized Thrasher to hire another assistant administrator, and he turned to former pharmacy employee, John R. "Jack" Gerlach. Gerlach had worked part time at DeKalb General as a registered pharmacist while pursuing a master's degree in hospital administration at Georgia State University. Having completed his graduate degree, he accepted the position of assistant to the administrator in October 1968. He joined the hospital staff in time to become involved in its major expansion project, to assist with the evolving crisis in Nursing Services, and to serve as acting administrator during Thrasher's illness in the spring of 1969.

A Major Expansion

At the groundbreaking ceremony for DeKalb General Hospital in May 1959 trustee J. Ross McCain described a vision of what the hospital's forty-acre site would eventually contain. He said, "We hope before long to add stories and to provide for four hundred rooms. We count on a wing for convalescents who need to be near to the hospital but do not need its high prices."[67]

Within three weeks after opening, the hospital was running out of bed space. The average daily census of patients quickly reached 85 to 90 percent, which meant essentially that all beds were full all of the time.[68] In 1965 the hospital admitted 12,000 patients.[69] Physicians could admit only those patients who had urgent or emergency conditions. And even with that stipulation in place, surgeons faced long waiting lists to get their patients on the surgery schedule and long delays in getting into the operating room on days when their patients were on the schedule. The hospital had to turn down qualified physician applicants to the medical staff "for lack of bed space or operating room time for their patients."[70]

Within three weeks after opening, the hospital was running out of bed space.... The hospital had to turn down qualified physician applicants...for lack of bed space or operating room time for their patients.

The concept of "Self Care," the third phase of the Progressive Patient Care program that the Authority envisioned, was "temporarily" suspended immediately after the hospital opened.[71] It never reappeared. When patients reached the third phase of being "able to care for themselves," they were discharged to make room for others. The hospital converted some private rooms into semiprivate rooms to provide additional beds.[72] In November, six months after opening, the trustees instructed the architects to prepare a plan for expansion and also a site plan to show all the facilities that eventually might be built on the hospital's forty acres.[73]

The trustees took the architectural plans to the DeKalb County commissioners to inquire about available local funds and to state and federal agencies to explore the availability of matching funds for the hospital's expansion.[74] All three bodies gave the trustees encouraging responses. DeKalb County officials agreed that expansion was needed and that the time was right. The state encouraged the Authority to move ahead with its planning and outlined the steps the trustees should take to get final approval.[75] The federal agency recommended that the hospital apply for a planning grant of at least $20,000[76] and said there was a good chance that Hill-Burton matching funds would be available as early as July 1965.[77]

Then the tide turned. The county and the state suddenly identified other priorities that they considered more important than the expansion of the hospital. The county commissioners said there was a need for "a facility for the chronically ill and infirm . . . a facility to care for the aged [that should be] placed on DeKalb General Hospital property" and run by the Authority.[78] The county even voted on a bond of $200,000 in 1963 for a one-hundred-bed facility and asked the Authority for eight acres of land facing Winn Way for the facility.

The trustees told the county that $200,000 was not enough money to build and operate what the commissioners wanted.[79] That amount of money would provide only for a forty-bed facility that would be too small to operate efficiently and profitably.[80] They advised the commissioners to wait until another bond issue could be passed for sufficient funds to build a one-hundred-bed facility that could be operated profitably.[81] The Authority also said it was reluctant to give up eight of its forty valuable acres for the facility.

Following that exchange, DeKalb County Commission Chairman Brince Manning told the Authority that DeKalb General could not count on the voters supporting a bond election to fund the hospital's expansion.[82]

Then the county commissioners made another request of the Authority. They asked for 4.5 acres on which the county would build the main office of the DeKalb County Department of Public Health. They first requested a plot adjacent to the North Decatur Methodist Church,[83] but the church objected to the facility's being located close by. Finally, in December 1966, the Authority deeded to the county 4.5 acres on the southwest corner facing Winn Way.[84] Once the trustees made that concession, the county commissioners voted in March 1967 to finance $4,000,000 in revenue anticipation certificates for the hospital's expansion.[85]

While local funds were now assured, state and federal matching funds remained uncertain. Despite the state's earlier encouragement, in 1965 it now cast doubts on the likelihood that state or federal Hill-Burton funds would be available.[86] The promised $20,000 federal planning grant also was canceled.[87] It eventually became clear that the state wanted the DeKalb County Hospital Authority and the county commissioners to solve one of its problems as a condition for getting matching federal and state funds.

In 1965 the Veterans Administration Hospital (VA) was moved from its old site on Peachtree Road in Brookhaven to a new facility on Clairmont Road in Decatur. The state was left with an abandoned hospital and twenty-two acres of land and no means of doing anything with it. It wanted the county to renovate the old hospital or build a new one, build a nursing home, and have the Hospital Authority operate both facilities.[88] The state insisted that DeKalb County and the Hospital Authority would have to attend to this project before state and federal funds would be available for DeKalb General Hospital's expansion.[89]

Brince Manning took a firm stand and told the state that DeKalb General's expansion was an urgent matter and that the county would not support a bond election for the VA Hospital project.[90] Rufus Evans made the Authority's position clear. He told the state that the Authority must attend first to the hospital expansion. After that the trustees would consider the VA Hospital project but would make no commitment to it.[91] He said that the Authority had a duty to take care of the hospital's urgently needed expansion even if it meant doing without state and federal matching funds.[92]

In that "battle of wills," the state blinked first. After the county commissioners voted in March 1967 to finance $4,000,000 in revenue anticipation certificates for the hospital expansion, John Venable, MD, director of the Georgia Department of Public Health, wrote that his department as well as the Community Council of the Atlanta Area would support DeKalb General Hospital's expansion with state and federal matching funds.[93] They would support not only the addition of hospital beds but also the construction of a mental health unit and a long-term care (nursing home) facility.[94]

With that assurance, the Authority instructed Bothwell and Nash Architects to prepare plans for a 93-bed long-term care unit and a 44-bed mental health unit, as well as plans for expanding the hospital beds from 216 to 403 beds.[95] The plans were completed and approved in November 1967.

Robinson Humphrey Company served as broker for the $4,000,000 in revenue anticipation certificates,[96] and Rufus Evans traveled to New York on January 15, 1968, to accept a check from their sale.[97] Since the plans included the construction of a long-term care facility, the county also released to the Authority the $200,000 from the 1963 bond election for a facility for the "chronically ill, infirm . . . and aged."[98]

Five general contractors bid on the project, and the contract went to the Robert E. McKee Company of Dallas, Texas, with a low bid of $7,937,000 for the basic construction, excluding

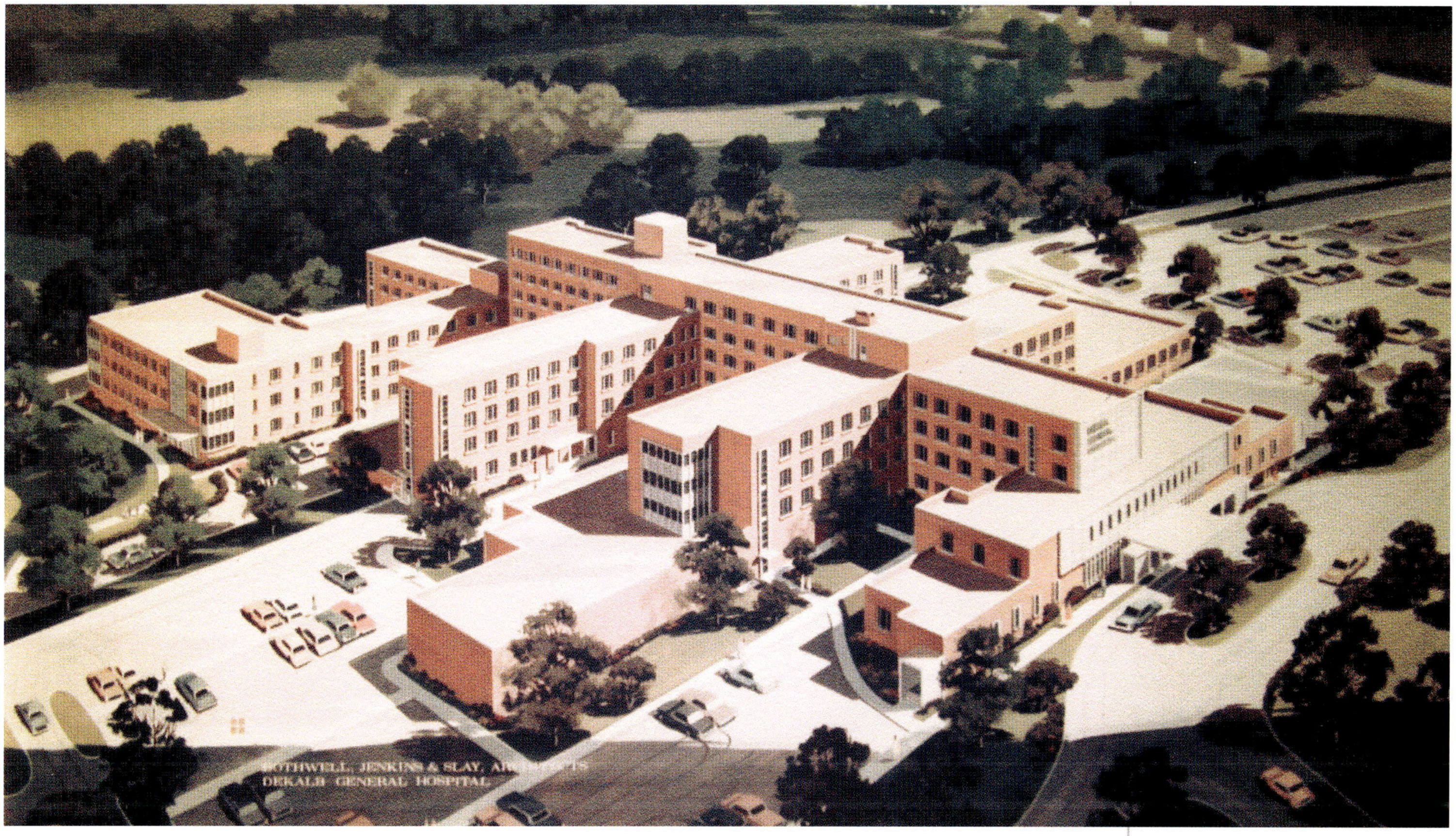

Architectural drawings by Bothwell and Nash for the hospital expansion project.

equipment and furnishings.[99] The Authority held a groundbreaking ceremony on July 1, 1968, which was also Evans's birthday.[100]

Everyone seemed content—everyone, that is, except Rufus Evans. He was still thinking. He reported at the July meeting of the Authority that he wanted to add two additional floors over the planned long-term care facility to give the hospital another one hundred beds. McKee Company estimated the addition would cost $1,018,687.[101] The trustees voted to add the two floors with hospital funds and a bank loan if necessary.[102] Now everyone, including Evans, was content.

The contractor anticipated that the expansion project would be completed by early December 1970. A three-month construction labor strike that began in July 1970, along with other delays, moved the completion date up to the fall of 1971.[103] The trustees held a dedication service in October 1971.[104]

The total cost of the project came to $10,904,229. Of this amount, federal dollars paid $4,139,249, the state gave $500,000, the county paid $4,200,000, and the hospital came up with $2,064,980 out of reserves.[105]

The end result of the project met many critical needs. Getting to the end result, however, was not easy. Six months after breaking ground for the expansion, the hospital faced a major crisis in Nursing Services. As a result of the ensuing labor strike and other delays, the project took nearly a year longer to complete than anticipated. The equipment ran $350,000 over the budget that had

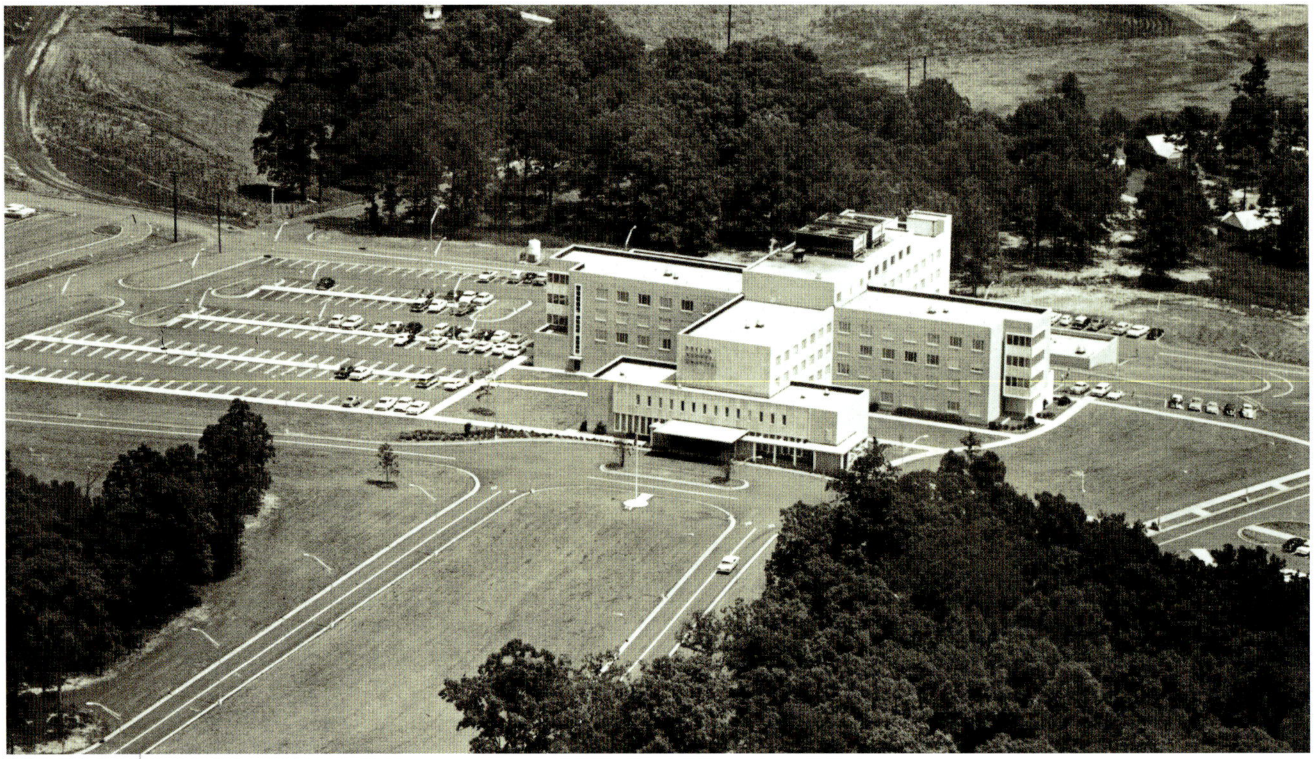

The aerial photograph, top, shows DeKalb General Hospital when it was first built in 1961. The aerial photograph, below, was taken in 1975.

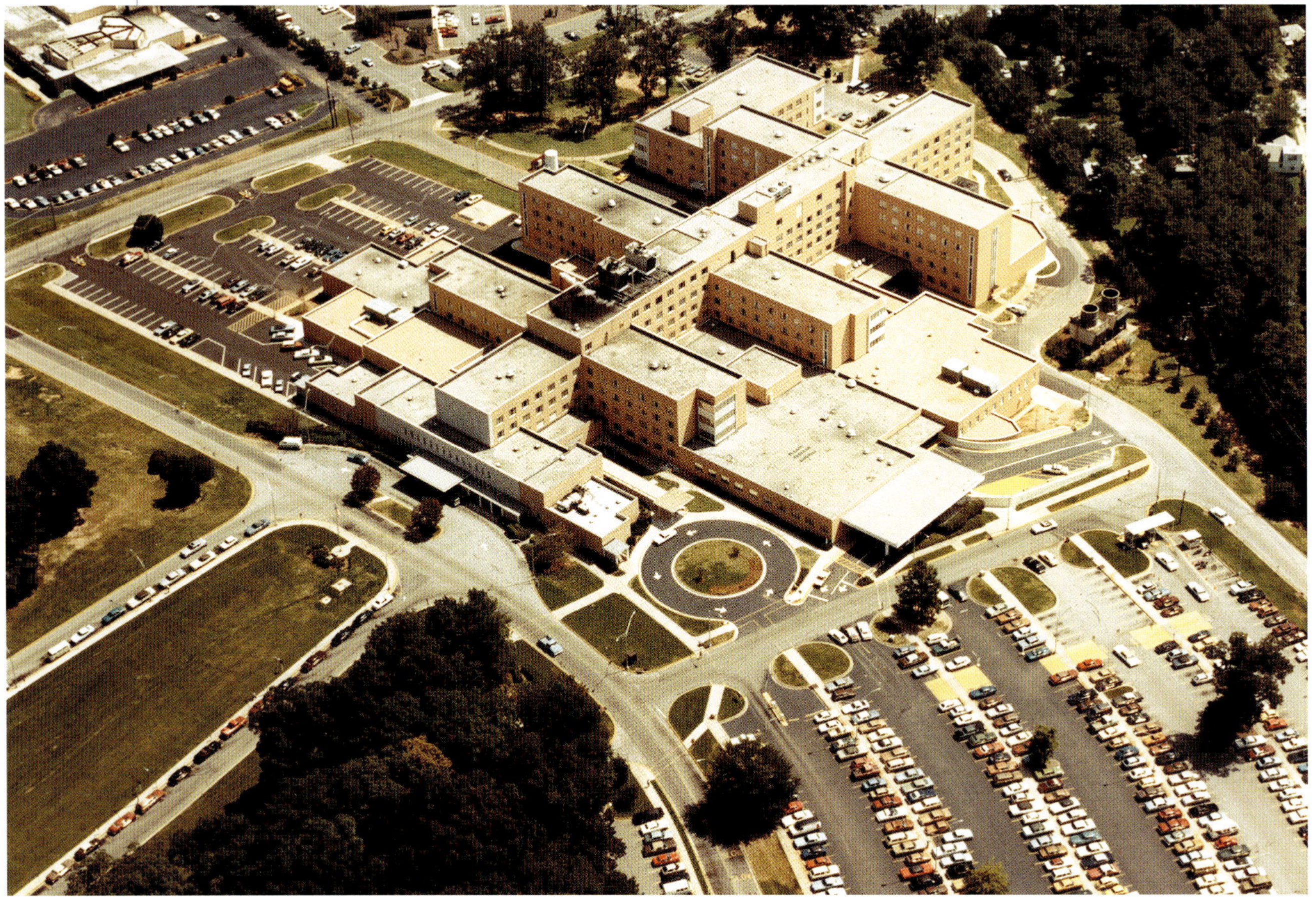

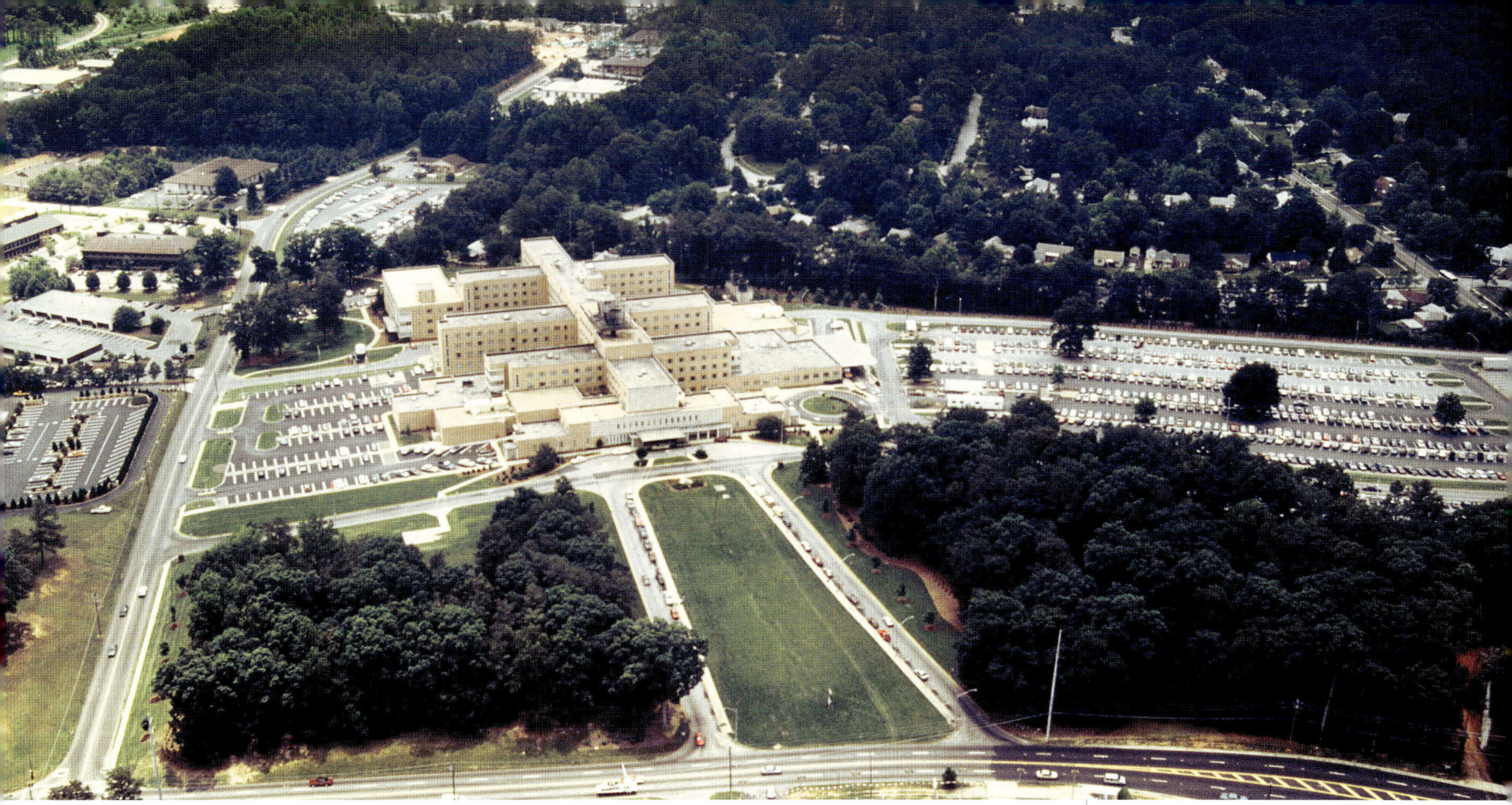

been submitted for federal and state funds, and the Authority had to find the additional money. Construction required closing sections of the hospital, making the bed shortage even more critical. The medical library was occupied by the EKG Department.[106] The cafeteria was closed during construction, the kitchen was relocated to the conference room and theater, and patient meals required the use of hot plates and microwave ovens.[107]

Once completed, however, the expansion project made DeKalb General the second largest hospital in the Atlanta area and one of the ten largest hospitals in the state.[108] It now had 503 acute beds, 44 mental health beds, and 93 long-term care beds for a total of 640 beds.[109] It had a 225-seat theater; new classrooms for in-service training; a new Coronary Care Unit and Intensive Care Unit, new Radiology Department and Laboratory space; a Pediatric Unit; a doubling of Surgery's operating rooms and recovery room; a quadrupling of the size of the Emergency Department with its own X-ray capabilities; two additional delivery rooms; two caesarean-section rooms; a new kitchen and dining area capable of seating two hundred people; a new room for vending machines; new administration and enlarged business offices; and an expansion of the Medical Records Department, the Laundry, and Central Supply.[110] DeKalb General Hospital now was ready for the expanded growth and needs of the community.

A Crisis in Nursing Services

As the end of the hospital's first decade approached, one of the most severe crisis in its history was evolving. The hospital would experience the sudden loss of 100 of its 130 nurses.

The photograph above shows the hospital in 1987.

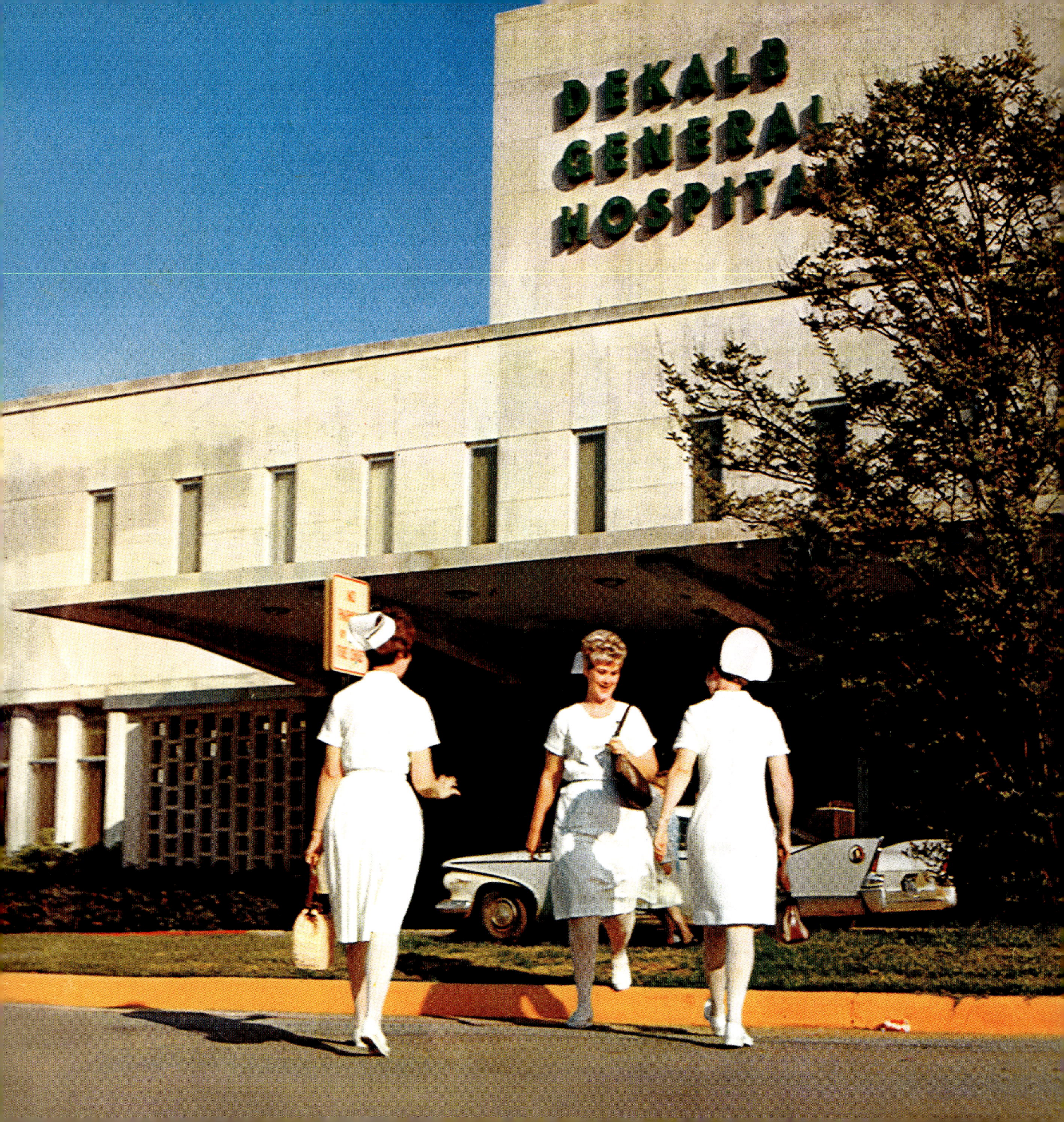
DEKALB
GENERAL
HOSPITAL

CHAPTER FOUR

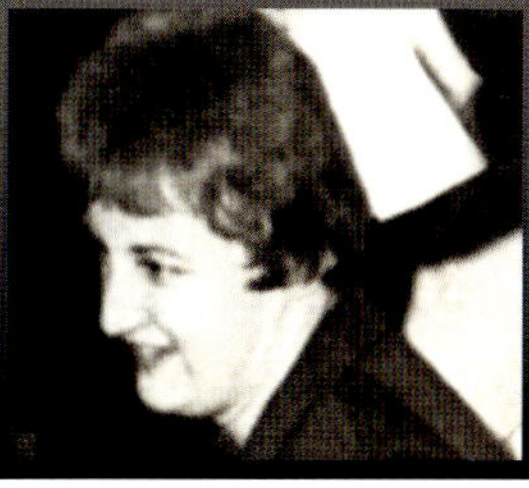

A Crisis in Nursing at DeKalb General Hospital

Opposite: Nurses outside the entrance to DeKalb General Hospital in 1969.

As director of Nursing, Opal Hopkins, RN, was very successful in recruiting nurses to DeKalb General Hospital prior to its opening. There was an element of excitement at the idea of working in a new hospital with good salaries and state-of-the-art equipment. The luster, however, faded as DeKalb General's nurses got down to work.

Within three weeks after the hospital opened, the census was so large that nurses had to care for more patients than anticipated. Patient room assignments and nursing assignments changed frequently. Nurses had to become acquainted with new models of nursing care and new policies and procedures.[1] They had to grapple with inconveniences in the design of their units. The bedpan "hoppers," for example, that were located at the end of the halls left nurses shaking their heads. "Did anyone even consult with nurses when they designed this place?"[2] they often asked.

On top of this, they had to deal with physician concerns and the concept of physician authority. At the August 1961 DeKalb County Hospital Authority meeting, L. C. Buchanan, MD, the hospital's first chief of staff, said physicians had concerns with the quality of patient care.[3] The Authority held a special meeting to consider nine physician recommendations, five of which made Nursing accountable to the medical staff. These five read:[4]

1. In all matters of patient care, nursing procedures, treatments, etc., the director of Nursing shall be responsible to the medical staff.
2. In instances where a physician desires to point out a specific deficiency in nursing treatment or patient care, the physician shall discuss the problem in a courteous manner with the nurse involved and/or the nurse in charge of the appropriate unit. If a satisfactory solution is not promptly obtained, the matter should immediately be reported to the director of Nursing and to a Nursing Committee of the medical staff.
3. The Nursing Committee shall meet regularly and shall keep accurately recorded all such complaints submitted to it together with the action taken in each instance, reporting same to the [Medical Staff] Executive Committee.
4. Professional problems suggesting a change in any nursing procedure or policy shall be reviewed by the Nursing Committee with the director of Nursing and a recommendation made to the [Medical Staff] Executive Committee. The action

taken by the Executive Committee, when approved by the Hospital Authority, shall be decisive in all matters.

5. The present program of in-service training for nursing personnel shall be reviewed by the Nursing Committee with the director of Nursing. This program of instruction should be expanded and regular instruction sessions should be conducted. . . .[5]

...the hospital's nurses did not receive the pay increase expected at the end of the first six months of employment. Nurses also were dissatisfied with the hospital's benefits—or lack thereof.

Nursing clearly was expected to answer to the medical staff as well as to administration.

To make the situation worse, the hospital's nurses did not receive the pay increase expected at the end of the first six months of employment. The Authority had promised all employees a raise "if funds are available."[6] But because of an operating deficit, the trustees did not authorize the salary increase until six months later in June 1962.[7] Furthermore other hospitals quickly caught up with and surpassed DeKalb General's salary scale.[8]

Nurses also were dissatisfied with the hospital's benefits—or lack thereof. They considered the policies on vacations, sick leave, and death leaves to be inadequate. The Authority asked its Finance Committee to make recommendations regarding these policies,[9] but when the committee met and recommended no changes, the Authority approved that recommendation.[10] Nurses asked for a retirement plan, but the Finance Committee said, as late as 1967, that "the hospital was not in a position at this time to recommend a retirement plan."[11]

In 1963 the nurses asked that the hospital provide a child care facility for its employees.[12] A year later administration said it still could not find a child care facility in the community willing to provide that service.[13] Even six years later, the hospital still did not have a child care center for its employees.

In the spring of 1963, Thrasher said the hospital was faced with an acute shortage of nurses.[14] The trustees authorized him to arrange for Licensed Practical Nurse (LPN) students at DeKalb Area Vocational School to train at DeKalb General.[15] The shortage, however, persisted. In May 1964 Opal Hopkins, Floyd Sanders, MD, chairman of the Nursing Committee, and Fincher Powell, MD, chief of staff, jointly sent a letter to the Authority alerting it to the critical nursing shortage and urging it to act promptly to deal with salaries and benefits.[16] When there appeared to be little or no response to their plea, Hopkins placed a letter of resignation on Thrasher's desk in protest over the apparent unwillingness of administration and the Authority to deal with the problem. Thrasher asked her to go with him to meet with Authority Chairman Rufus Evans. After hearing her case, Hopkins recalls Evans saying, "Thrasher, give this girl whatever she wants."[17] She rescinded her resignation, but the nurses saw the salary increases as minimal and felt little was being done to meet their expectations.

The nurses became even more concerned when, in 1968, they learned that the Authority planned to double the capacity of the hospital. The nurses appreciated the problem of inadequate beds, but they were convinced there would be an even greater nursing shortage if the hospital expanded and did not address the issue of salaries and benefits.

Coupled with dissatisfaction over salaries, benefits, and working conditions, there was a change in nursing leadership. As described in chapter 3, Opal Hopkins Fyffe resigned in 1965 following the death of her husband, Troy Hopkins,[18] and her subsequent marriage to David Fyffe.[19] Thrasher selected Margaret Ford, RN, as her successor.[20] Naomi Harman, RN, assistant director of Nursing, resigned to assist her husband in his new furniture business, later to take a position as night supervisor at Emory Hospital, and subsequently to become director of the Fountainview Convalescent Center.[21]

Opal Fyffe said that Ford's leadership style was different from hers. Fyffe described her own style as "open and friendly." She frequently surprised the nurses by working with them at the bedside. Margaret Ford, on the other hand, had a "private side" and approached her work with a professional demeanor. The nursing staff trusted her, but some of them thought of her as "cold."[22]

As soon as Ford assumed office, she was faced with the "countless problems in the nursing department" to which Fyffe referred in her resignation letter to Thrasher.[23] Ford alerted Thrasher to the critical difficulty of retaining nurses and urged him to address the inadequate salaries and benefits, including the lack of a retirement plan.[24] Thrasher presented recommendations to the Finance Committee,[25] and the Authority approved salary increases to $4,884 to compete with those offered by the new VA Hospital. While still significantly below what the American Nurses Association (ANA) recommended,[26] the trustees' action elicited a positive response. Approximately 325 employees signed a letter of appreciation addressed to the Authority.[27]

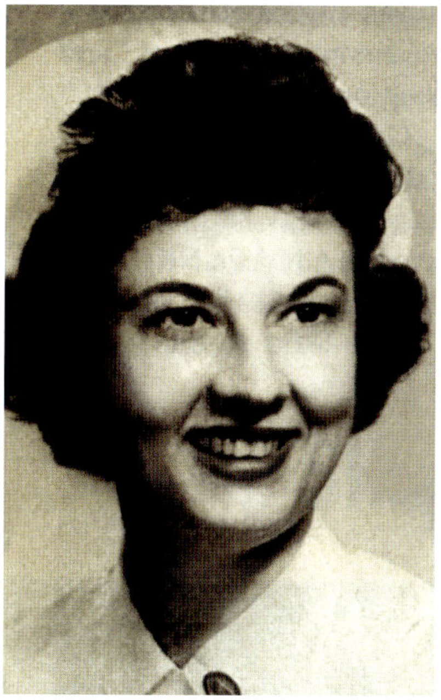

In 1965 William Thrasher hired Margaret Ford, RN, as the second director of nursing to replace Opal (Hopkins) Fyffe.

In the short term, those increases helped recruiting and retention. In June 1966 Thrasher reported that the turnover rate was the lowest it had been in three years. All but two vacancies were filled.[28] That relief, however, was short-lived. Ten months later, the hospital faced another acute nursing shortage[29] with "considerable unrest in the hospital regarding salaries," vacation time, the sick leave policy, health insurance, and other employee policies.[30]

In September 1967 Thrasher created an advisory committee made up of department heads from Nursing and other departments to give him feedback on how things were going in the hospital. At its very first meeting the members of the advisory committee told him they were gravely concerned about morale in the hospital. The committee characterized the turnover of employees as a "mass exodus."[31]

Finance Committee minutes reflect that Thrasher reported to the committee what he heard from his advisory committee and proposed "several changes in benefits related to vacations, sick leave, and holidays . . . . [But] after some discussion the committee recommended no change in the present policies. . . . He also recommended a retirement plan for employees, but it was agreed that the hospital was not in a position at [that] time to recommend a retirement plan. . . ."[32]

The Authority approved the decisions of the Finance Committee[33] but asked the committee to continue investigating a retirement proposal "because it was the feeling of many of the Authority members that a retirement system was necessary at DeKalb General."[34] Thrasher was unable to report any encouraging news to his advisory committee, and Ford continued losing disheartened nurses.

In the meantime, developments were taking place in the ANA and the Georgia State Nurses Association (GSNA) that would have a significant impact on DeKalb General Hospital.

In 1946 the ANA adopted an Economic Security Program and designated state nurses associations to serve as the exclusive agents for nurses to negotiate improved salaries, working conditions, and professional recognition. The State associations were encouraged to use lobbying, public relations, education, and collective bargaining.[35]

At its 1967 state convention, the GSNA adopted a resolution supporting nurses' rights to have a voice in determining employment conditions, to organize, to choose a bargaining representative, and to participate in planning and administering its nursing service. The GSNA affirmed its support of collective bargaining as "the most effective means of assuring nurses the right to participation in the implementation of high standards of employment and nursing practice."[36]

In February 1968 the ANA adopted a "New Approach" to its Economic Security Program that included direct financial support and staff assistance to state organizations. Alda Ditchfield, president of GSNA, and Leilee Ault, chairman of GSNA's Economic and General Welfare Committee, submitted a proposal to the ANA for GSNA that said Georgia was a key to collective bargaining for nurses throughout the southeast.[37] The ANA approved GSNA's proposal, committed $20,000 to the Georgia project, and sent New Jersey attorney Stanley Kravit to Atlanta to support GSNA's initiative.[38]

Some Georgia nurses opposed this aggressive way of dealing with nursing issues. Dana Hudson, director of Nursing at Georgia Baptist Hospital and a close friend and mentor to Opal Hopkins Fyffe,[39] resigned as executive secretary of GSNA in protest to its endorsement of collective bargaining.[40]

Hudson, while a friend and mentor to Opal Fyffe, on the other hand had several adversarial encounters with Margaret Ford. When Ford was president of the Georgia State Board of Nurse Examiners, she successfully opposed proposals that Hudson made to the board of examiners on behalf of the Georgia Baptist Hospital diploma nursing program.[41] Hudson's friendship with Fyffe and her unhappy encounters with Ford would play a role in future events at DeKalb General.

Over the three months following Stanley Kravit's arrival in Atlanta, the GSNA sponsored a series of informational conferences. Several nurses from DeKalb General attended those meetings with Thrasher's approval and financial support.[42] At the meetings, Kravit described the structure and functions of the New Approach Economic Security Program. Each institution would elect its own local unit from among participating nurses. The local unit would serve as GSNA's local collective bargaining agent. The local unit would elect a Negotiating Committee to handle grievances and a Professional Practice Committee to meet regularly with management to discuss patient care concerns and to serve as the liaison with administration and physicians. Members of the medical staff and the Professional Practice Committee would form a Joint Practice Committee to deal with problems arising out of the nurse-physician relationship.[43]

Several Atlanta institutions formed local units, including the Fulton County Department of Public Health, the DeKalb County Department of Public Health, the Cobb County Department of Public Health, and the Visiting Nurses Association of Atlanta. Kravit considered Grady Memorial Hospital a key to the success of GSNA's initiative in Georgia. There was indeed activity at Grady, but a local unit never materialized, in part due to the resistance of Grady's new director of Nursing, Mary Woody, RN, who opposed the GSNA approach.[44] The GSNA would then turn its attention to DeKalb General.

In October 1968 Margaret Ford surveyed nursing salaries in Atlanta area hospitals and found that DeKalb General's salary scale was below that of other hospitals. She sent the results of her survey with specific recommendations to Thrasher. Convinced that administration and the Authority were not going to act on Ford's recommendations, even before administration and the Authority responded, Frances Lubin, RN, an ICU nurse, and others decided to explore the possibility of participating in GSNA's program. Lubin called Stanley Kravit and arranged a meeting for November 7. At that meeting the nurses decided to form a local unit. Frances Purtymun, RN, ICU head nurse, was elected chairman, Carolyn Waters, RN, vice chairman, and Mary Beiser, RN, secretary.

Kravit said directors of Nursing should take a neutral position if unable to support the nurses' attempt at organization.[45] That said, the DeKalb local unit declared they would leave Margaret Ford "out of their business."[46]

The local unit conducted a survey from which it identified eight issues to be addressed with the hospital: (1) starting salaries and a standardized scale of increases, (2) a retirement plan, (3) changes in vacation and sick time, (4) maternity leave, (5) child care for employees, (6) more freedom from clerical and housekeeping duties to provide more time for bedside patient care, (7)

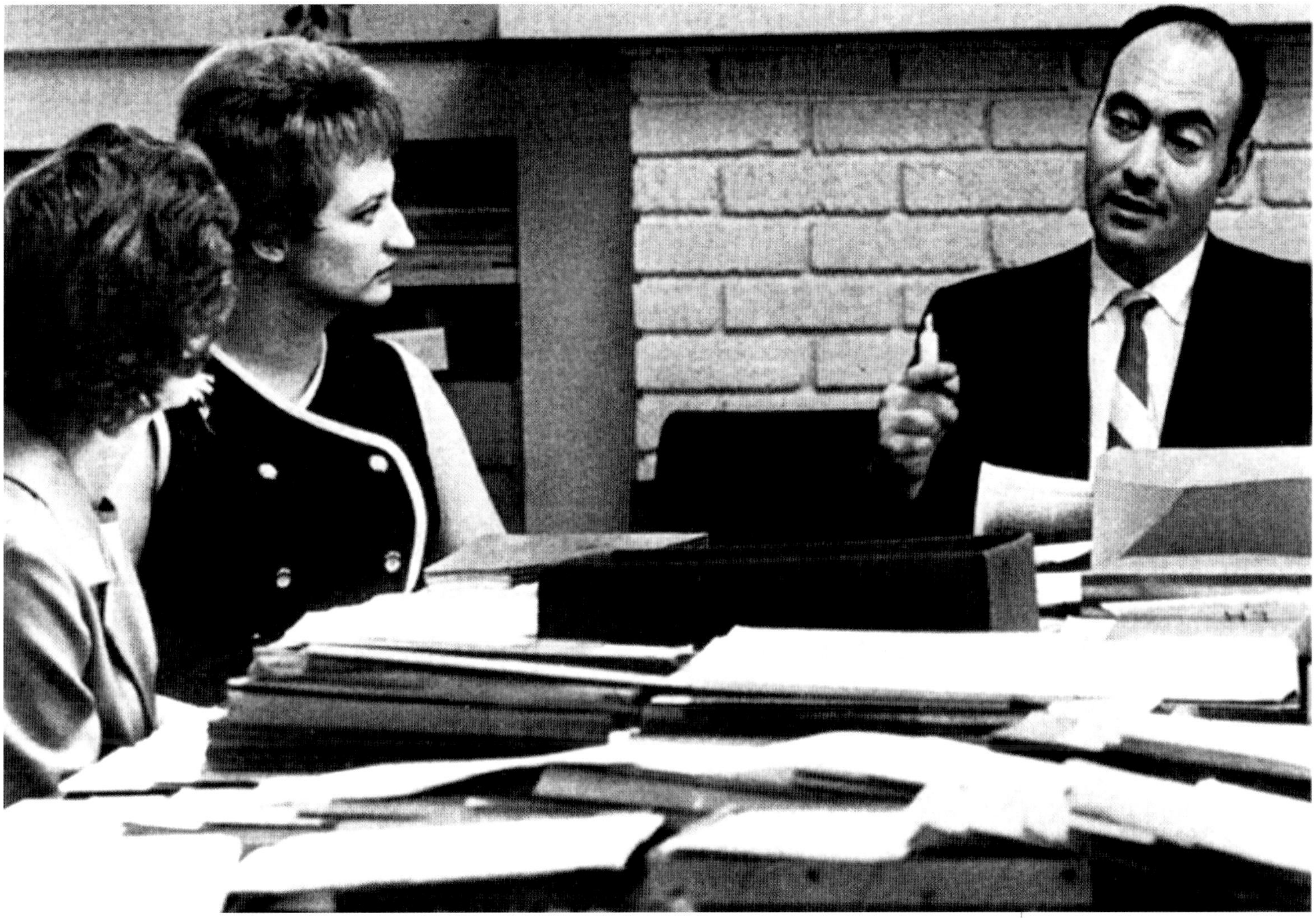

Attorney Stanley Kravit, director for GSNA's campaign to become the bargaining agent for Georgia nurses, meets with DGH nurses Lois Hudson and Bette Ann Brama.

improved orientation, and (8) improved continuing education and in-service education.

In mid-November, four days after the DeKalb nurses formed a local unit, Thrasher presented Ford's proposed recommendations to the Finance Committee. Those recommendations included two salary increases, one in February 1969 and one the following October. The Finance Committee reported to the Authority that they had "received this information, taken it under advisement, and [would] continue to study it and to work on it."[47] The Authority accepted their report.

Kravit tried to convince the nurses that collective bargaining by professionals for better nursing care was different from union activities that sought primarily to obtain better salaries.[48] The nurses would find, however, that DeKalb General's leadership would not accept that distinction.

Once the nurses formed a local unit, the trustees authorized Thrasher to retain the services of an attorney "to work with the hospital on their labor problems."[49] He hired Homer Deakins of Thompson, Ogletree and Haynsworth law firm. Deakins had a background in labor union issues.

By the end of November, 111 of DeKalb's 130 nurses had signed their bargaining rights over to the GSNA.[50] On December 2, 1968, Kravit sent the following letter to Thrasher:

I am writing on behalf of the Georgia State Nurses Association and the Registered Professional Nurses of DeKalb General Hospital to advise you and the DeKalb General Hospital Authority that the nurses employed by the DeKalb General Hospital have formed a Local Unit under the GSNA Economic Security Program. The purpose of the Local Unit is to negotiate a contract with the Hospital covering terms and conditions of employment and standards of professional practice.

GSNA has received an Assignment of Bargaining Rights from 111 nurses. Under our policies, when a Local Unit is certified, GSNA acts as bargaining agent. . . .

The Economic Security Program is authorized and supported by the American Nurses' Association. It is an integral part of the Association's goal of professional recognition for registered nurses. Whenever a group of nurses adopts this Program and desires to bargain professionally and collectively with the employer, we believe there is a tremendous potential for improving and maintaining quality nursing care.

The request to bargain is a gesture of respect toward the management of any health organization and, I trust, will be reciprocated by recognition of the professional nurses' right to participate in setting the terms and conditions of their employment. Through this participation, the Local Unit, the Association, and the Hospital can work together toward maximum commitment to quality health care for those we serve.

Looking forward to hearing from you, I am

Stanley Kravit, Director
Economic Security Project

Thrasher shared Kravit's letter with the Authority at its December 9 meeting. The Authority invited Ford to attend that meeting, and she and Thrasher gave the trustees the background on how DeKalb's local unit came into being.[51] That apparently was the only Authority meeting to which Ford was invited.

Attorney Deakins attended the December 9 meeting and advised Thrasher to respond to Kravit's letter by saying that "DeKalb General Hospital would not recognize the Georgia State Nurses Association as a bargaining agent, but. . . would be glad to receive any suggestions from the Georgia State Nurses Association president and director of the economic security project."[52] He advised the Authority to follow through with the salary and benefits adjustments recommended to the Finance Committee in November and said he would make recommendations at its next meeting. The trustees approved a motion "that the Finance Committee work toward improved salaries and fringe benefits for the personnel, and if necessary . . . meet in special session to take whatever action that is necessary."[53]

Prior to the next meeting of the Finance Committee, Deakins met with Margaret Ford, Mary Lou

Hurt, director of Personnel, Charles Anderson, treasurer-controller, and Thrasher to formulate proposals that he would take to the committee.[54] He took the following recommendations to the Finance Committee on December 16:

1. A general salary increase for all employees starting February 1969
2. An additional holiday for those employees with six months or more of continuous service
3. Beginning May 1969, an additional week of vacation for all employees with five years or more of service
4. After May 1969, vacation time to accumulate each pay period
5. After May 1969, vacation time may be used after six months of employment
6. As of January 1969, employees may accumulate up to sixty days of sick leave [rather than the current twenty days]
7. As of January 1969, all employees will be eligible for sick leave after six months of employment
8. The Finance Committee should continue to work toward the implementation of a retirement plan.[55]

The Finance Committee approved all eight recommendations.

Margaret Ford urged Thrasher, in the spirit of the holiday season, to inform the staff in a personalized Christmas letter of the approved package of salary and benefits, wishing them a happy holiday, and thanking them for their service to the hospital. Attorney Deakins, however, advised against Ford's suggestion, and the staff was only informed of the anticipated changes in the form of a memorandum attached to their next pay check.[56] The memorandum came late in the conflict and lacked an acknowledgement of the Christmas season or the personal words of appreciation that Ford recommended.

"If the object was to bring J. Rufus Evans to his knees, they should have realized that he only did that when he prayed."

— Opal Hopkins Fyffe

In the meantime, members of the local unit were discouraged, angry, and frustrated by Thrasher's response to Kravit that refused to recognize the local unit as GSNA's bargaining agent. They decided to take their case to the media, and for the first time discussed the possibility of mass resignation. They also made plans to engage in "informational" picketing and pamphlet distribution on Saturday and Sunday, December 28 and 29.

Thirty-four nurses picketed around the flagpole in front of the hospital on those two days and distributed a leaflet explaining their request for professional recognition. They picketed again on North Decatur Road in front of the hospital on the very cold morning of January 6.[57] They were careful not to obstruct access to the hospital.[58] But Thrasher, Ford, and Evans watched the picketing from the hospital window, and Evans allegedly said "I'll close the doors before I'll recognize the local unit."[59] Opal Hopkins Fyffe later reflected, "If the object was to bring J. Rufus Evans to his knees, they should have realized that he only did that when he prayed."[60]

The public and non-picketing nurses reacted negatively to the sight of picketing in front of the hospital and to seeing a picture of it on the front page of the newspaper. Administration called it unprofessional, the Medical Staff Executive Committee said the Authority was right to oppose third party negotiations, and the local press referred to it as a professional organization resorting to labor union tactics.

The local unit nurses, however, stayed their course. They met on January 2, 1969, and set January 13 as a deadline for the hospital to recognize the unit. If not recognized by then, they would submit letters of resignation effective February 24, the standard six-weeks' notice. At that

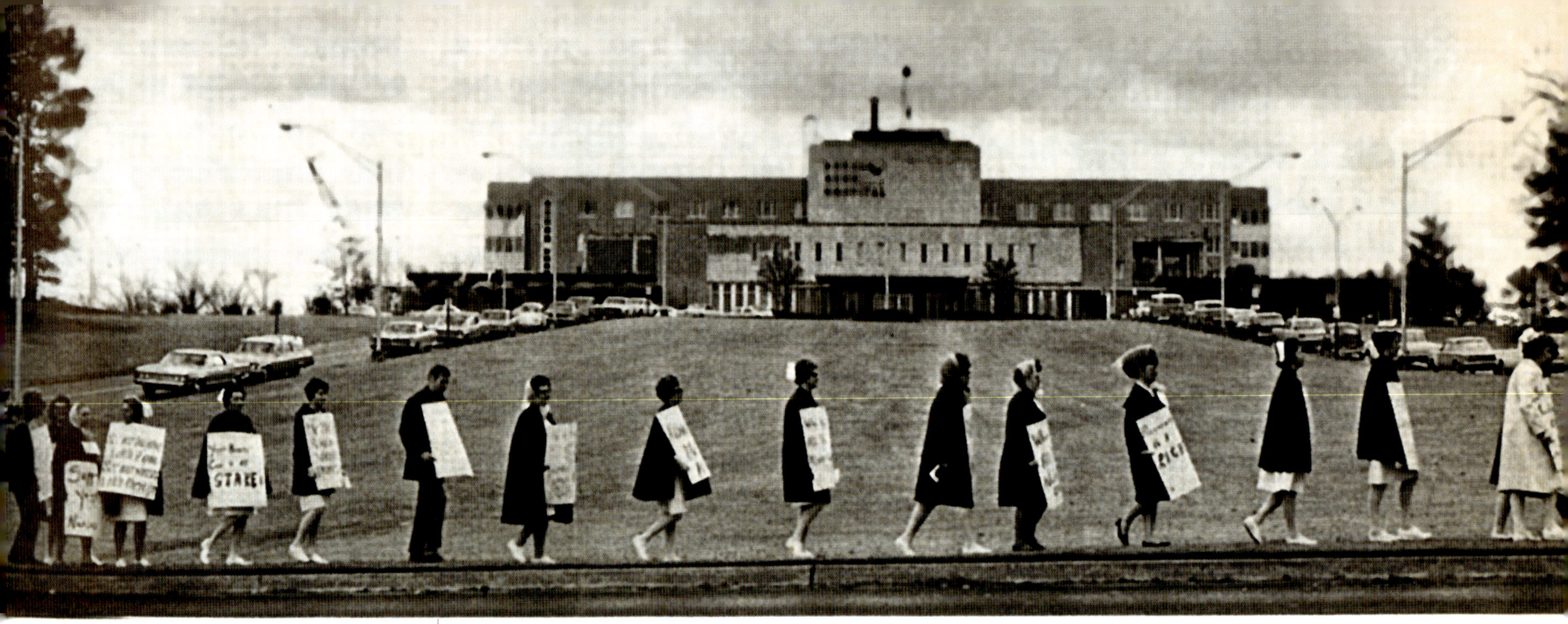

On a cold morning on January 6, 1969, DGH nurses picketed in front of the hospital on North Decatur Road hoping for recognition as a negotiating agent of the Georgia State Nurses' Association for better working conditions.

same meeting, they rejected Margaret Ford's plea for the nurses to negotiate apart from the local unit. They were not willing to relinquish their connection with the GSNA Economic Security Program.[61]

Thrasher met with members of the local unit's Negotiating Committee on January 3, and they advised him of their decision to submit letters of resignation. He stood firm in refusing to recognize the local unit as GSNA's bargaining agent and told the nurses he was shocked they would threaten to strike. After the meeting, he released a statement that declared resigning employees would not be reemployed.[62] Deep lines were being drawn in the sand.

Margaret Ford warned the nurses that administration would not recognize the local unit as the bargaining agent of the GSNA and would accept any resignation offered. On January 8 she wrote to Thrasher urging him to intervene for an immediate resolution of the standoff. In the note, she said, "In the event additional nurses resign, I cannot accept legal responsibility to care for patients unless we have minimal RN coverage." Then she added, "Our nurses' effort to achieve recognition and the right to discuss their problems with administration and the Authority cannot be considered wrong in terms of legal, moral, or professional standards."[63] Despite the neutral position she had attempted to take, Thrasher and the trustees interpreted those last words as Ford's tacit support of the local unit's actions.

On January 8 Kravit wrote to Thrasher requesting mediation either by the Federal Mediation and Conciliation Service or the Georgia Commission on Labor. The trustees, however, considered mediation appropriate only when an employer already agreed to recognition and a collective bargaining arrangement.[64] Since the Authority refused such recognition, Thrasher replied to Kravit, "Our Hospital Board has considered this request. We feel that no worthwhile purpose could be served in contacting these agencies and therefore decline your request."[65]

The nurses were true to their word. On Monday morning, January 13, 100 of the 130 nurses on staff presented their letters of resignations to Ford. She took them to Thrasher and said, "The nurses feel you have not heard me, you have not heard them, and they feel they have no alternative except to submit their resignations . . . ."[66] Thrasher reported having received the letters to the Authority at a called noon meeting of the Authority.

At that meeting the trustees conferred with Deakins as to how they might counter the threat of a mass resignation. They discussed the advisability of dismissing certain nurse leaders. In particular, they discussed Ford's stand on non-recognition. Thrasher and the trustees questioned her loyalty. Her January 8 letter to Thrasher advocating the nurses' "right to discuss their problems with administration and the Authority" raised the level of their doubts about her.[67]

Following that Authority meeting on January 13, Thrasher issued the following press release:

This morning we received resignations from a substantial number of nurses. Naturally, this comes as no surprise. Upon being advised of this development at its regular meeting today, the DeKalb County Hospital Authority has determined to stand by its original position not to extend recognition. We consider this threatened strike to be completely out of place in a hospital and directly contrary to the best interest of the community. The Authority has no intention of being coerced by such tactics. If these nurses carry out their threatened strike, the hospital will remain open, and we expect to continue to provide a high level of medical care for the community. In fact, plans are already underway to insure that the hospital will be adequately staffed in the event of any contingency.

We call upon these nurses to reconsider their position in the interest of the people in this community whose health and welfare they are pledged to serve. We repeat our continued willingness to work with the nurses at DeKalb General Hospital for the purpose of identifying and solving any and all problems which exist.[68]

"...he had a million dollar secret and an ace up his sleeve that he would play in the next few days."

— The Atlanta Journal, Jan. 16, 1969 referring to William Thrasher

On Thursday, January 16, *The Atlanta Journal* quoted Thrasher as saying "he had a 'million dollar secret and an ace up his sleeve' that he would play in the next few days."[69] The million dollar secret and the ace up his sleeve involved his former director of nursing, Opal Hopkins Fyffe, Naomi Harman, and a plan to dismiss Margaret Ford.

While the local unit was seeking recognition, Fyffe had occasion to visit her sister who had undergone surgery at DeKalb General. Fyffe said that, despite the coverage given to DeKalb's nursing situation by the media, she had paid it little attention and had had no contact with the nurses. She was unaware of the pending crisis until the day of her visit. When walking the halls to see her sister, however, she was "struck by the weird atmosphere."[70] She knew "in her gut" that "something bad was going on." After leaving her sister's bedside, she went to Margaret Ford's office and met with her for ten to fifteen minutes. She asked Ford what was going on. Ford replied, "We've run into a big problem with the RNs. The nurses are threatening to walk out." When Fyffe asked her what she was going to do about it, she said Ford replied, "There's nothing I can do. But there'll never be a walk-out. They're not going anywhere."[71]

Fyffe left Ford's office and went directly to see Thrasher. She told his secretary, "I've got to see him now." Thrasher acknowledged that the hospital had a problem with the nurses, but he felt things were going to be all right because "Margaret [Ford] is taking care of it." When Fyffe asked Thrasher what Ford was doing about the situation, he said, "The nurses are threatening, but she won't let it happen." Fyffe said she was convinced Ford had sold Thrasher "a bill of goods." She told him, "Margaret Ford is not going to help you. She'll let the nurses walk. She's not on your side. This would not have gotten to this point without help from the top. At best, she has been encouraging it by not doing anything about it. One hundred nurses don't walk out and the director of Nursing be blasé about it."[72]

Fyffe also had phone conversations with her old Georgia Baptist Hospital friend and mentor, Dana Hudson, who had openly opposed the GSNA Economic Security Program and who previously had adversarial encounters with Margaret Ford.[73] While the specific nature of those calls is unknown, Fyffe acknowledged that Hudson may have helped confirm her conclusions about the developments at DeKalb General and Ford's role in them.

"You are relieved of all authority, duties, and responsibilities as director of Nursing at DeKalb General Hospital."

— William Thrasher to Margaret Ford via telegram January 17, 1969

Thrasher called Fyffe at home the same afternoon of her visit to his office and asked her if she would be willing to come back to work at the hospital.[74] She told him she would if he and the board would agree to certain conditions: (1) she would work only part time and stay for a limited period to assist Thrasher, using a title of his choosing, (2) Margaret Ford had to go, (3) Naomi Harman would be the new director of Nursing, and (4) Thrasher and the board would agree to other recommendations she would have to deal with the situation.[75] Thrasher and Deakins called on Harman at home, and she agreed to accept the position of director of Nursing.[76] Thrasher and the trustees agreed to Fyffe's conditions.

On Thursday evening, January 16, a friend called Margaret Ford and told her of plans to terminate her publicly the following day. Ford called in sick the following morning and went to the GSNA headquarters to explore any available legal recourse she might have to prevent her pending termination. She found that she had none since she did not have a written employment contract with the hospital.[77] In the meantime, because he was unable to reach her by phone, Thrasher sent her a telegram informing her of her termination: "You are relieved of all authority, duties, and responsibilities as director of Nursing at DeKalb General Hospital. At your convenience, please contact me to discuss your future status."[78]

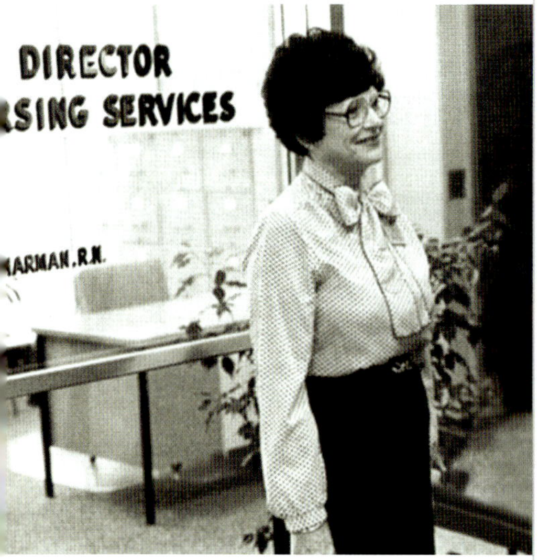

Naomi Harman became the new director of Nursing at DeKalb General Hospital.

At 1:00 PM on Friday, January 17, Fannie Mae Walker, assistant director of Nursing, also was terminated and ushered off the hospital grounds to her car. Ford had not forewarned Walker because she understood from the Thursday night call that only she would be terminated.[79]

Thrasher called a group of nurses together and informed them of the changes in leadership. Fyffe and Harman were present in uniform. Thrasher distributed a memorandum that said, "Effective immediately, Opal Fyffe, former director of Nursing, has been appointed special assistant to the administrator, and Naomi Harman, former assistant director of Nursing, has been appointed director of Nursing."[80]

Thrasher's first order to Fyffe and Harman said, "Please assure all nursing personnel that there will be no retaliation against anyone who has participated in the recent activity of the Georgia State Nurses Association. We sincerely hope that all nurses will remain on the job to fulfill their responsibilities to the patients. The hospital board has authorized me to make this assurance and will support my position in this regard."[81]

Thrasher and the trustees hoped that their swift, precipitous action would deflate the nurses' momentum and cause them to rethink their pending mass resignation. It had the opposite effect. Ford's termination only enhanced the emotions, energy, and determination of the nurses. The local unit held an emergency meeting on that Friday, January 17, which forty-seven nurses attended. Some urged an immediate walkout. Kravit instead advised the nurses to give at least a five-day notice in the hope that the hospital might change its position on recognition. At that meeting the nurses moved the effective date of their resignation up from February 24 to Wednesday, January 22.[82]

On Saturday, January 18, the Medical Staff Executive Committee convened in an emergency session to discuss the crisis and to explore any intervention it might offer. The physicians reaffirmed their support of the Authority's refusal to recognize the local unit for the purposes of collective bargaining, and they agreed that the very threat of a mass resignation by the nurses was deplorable and unprofessional. They acknowledged, however, that the nurses' grievances were legitimate and appropriate. Fincher Powell, chief of staff, appointed a committee to identify the nurses' specific grievances and to formulate a proposal to present to the Authority for their "sympathetic action."[83]

The physicians' committee met that evening and prepared a list of recommendations based on concerns shared by the nurses. The Medical Staff Executive Committee approved the recommendations and met with the Authority at 4:00 PM the next day, Sunday, January 19. L. C. Buchanan presented the committee's ten recommendations:

1. Establish a Professional Relations Committee consisting of five or six working nurses, four active physicians, two administrators, and two trustees
2. Revamp the nurses' workloads so that they have more time to attend to patient care and professional duties
3. Activate and maintain an enhanced in-service training program
4. Hire a full-time medical director responsible only to the Authority
5. Establish a retirement plan
6. Assure returning employees that there will be no reprisals
7. Improve the relationship of the Personnel Department with employees and clarify personnel policies
8. Establish a nursery for children of hospital employees
9. Establish and maintain convenient lounges for nurses
10. Allow nurses to arrange work schedules to pursue available programs of continuing education[84]

The DeKalb Medical Society issued an open letter to the Authority that endorsed similar recommendations.[85]

Authority Chairman Evans responded that a number of those recommendations already were under consideration and that all of them would be taken under advisement. He appointed two members of the Authority to serve with two members of the Medical Staff Executive Committee to form the recommended Professional Relations Committee, and he asked those four individuals to meet with "the loyal nurses" the following Monday morning to explain the actions of the Authority.[86] The Authority also voted to permit the attorneys to prepare the necessary papers for an injunction against the nurses' mass resignation and "at their discretion" request such an injunction.[87] There is no available documentation to indicate such papers were ever prepared or that an injunction was ever requested of the courts.

There also is no available record of a Monday morning meeting with "the loyal nurses" that Chairman Evans requested or a response by the nurses to the idea of a Professional Relations Committee as a negotiating vehicle. The nurses may have been receptive to it. The GSNA leadership, however, discouraged it. Stanley Kravit was quoted in *The Atlanta Journal* on Wednesday, January 22, as saying that the Professional Relations Committee proposal was inappropriate because the GSNA and its local unit still required recognition of the local unit as the nurses' collective bargaining agent. The opportunity to get both parties to an alternative bargaining table was thus aborted.[88]

A total of approximately one hundred nurses walked off the job at the end of their shifts on

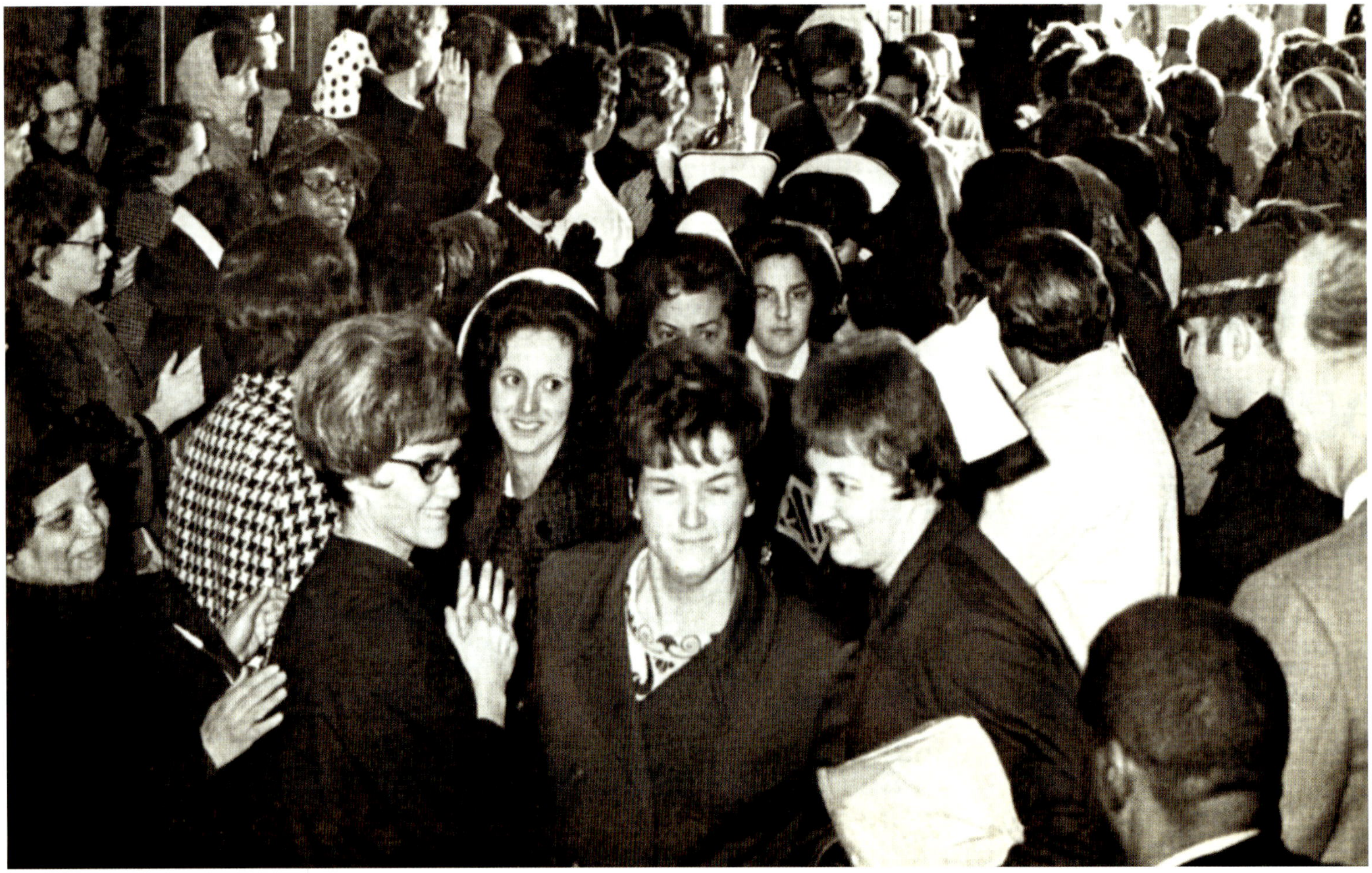

Approximately 100 DGH nurses resigned en masse on the evening of January 22, 1969.

January 22, leaving thirty employed nurses. "At 11 PM hundreds of people moved restlessly about the entrance steps and pressed around the plate glass doors. Some people were crying, some laughing nervously, some looking grim. Television cameras moved in on the scene, radio microphones were everywhere, photographers' flashbulbs popped. . . . Some nurses sobbed and went away quietly, some laughed, one shouted, 'Happiest day of my life'."[89]

One more opportunity emerged for reconciliation. On Friday, January 24, hospital attorney George Dillard stated publicly that "the nurses could form any kind of committee they want, . . . but could not bring in an outside agency . . . or come up with any type of compulsory collective bargaining agreement." Carolyn Waters, vice chairman of the local unit, responded for the unit, saying, "The nurses and their representatives will agree to meet with the Authority . . . on any neutral ground . . . [and never] claim in any form that the meeting amounts to recognition."[90] However, there is no record that such a meeting occurred.

On January 27 *The Atlanta Constitution* quoted Thrasher as saying the hospital remained unwilling to recognize the local unit, that there was "no hint of a settlement and the board does not intend to pursue one."

The *Decatur-DeKalb News* on February 5 quoted him as saying, "The nurses who have resigned can reapply for their jobs, and their applications will be considered on an individual basis." The hospital thus considered the issue closed and had a screening process to prevent the reentry of any known, disgruntled nurses who might create more problems.[91] The Medical Staff Executive Committee submitted to administration a list of nurses it recommended for accepting their resignation and not being welcomed back, but there is no indication that administration ever acted on that list.[92] Those resigning nurses who returned to DeKalb General were required to have the recommendation of a member of the medical staff.[93]

The mass resignation left approximately thirty nurses on the staff. Some of those thirty remaining nurses had been members of the local unit but decided their obligation to patients prevented them from affecting their letter of resignation. Mary Chambers and her nurses in Labor and Delivery, Elizabeth Powell, supervisor of the Emergency Department and Central Supply, Mary Mercer, head nurse in the Recovery Room, and Kay Watson, a staff nurse in Surgery, were among the members of the local unit who shared the concerns of the resigning nurses but who decided not to go through with leaving.[94]

Prior to the resignations on January 22, Opal Fyffe and Naomi Harman had recruited forty nurses and volunteers.[95] Two floors were closed, reducing the number of beds from 220 to 160; ambulances were instructed to take their patients elsewhere whenever possible; elective surgery was canceled; and only emergency patients were admitted.[96] Members of the medical staff and their spouses who held current nursing licenses volunteered to take duty assignments in the units that were kept open. The expansion and renovation project underway had already closed some beds, reducing the number of nursing replacements needed and minimizing to a slight degree the impact of the resignations.

DeKalb General remained in operation, though the ensuing months were not easy. The hospital had to rebuild the nursing staff, cope with a shortage of beds and operating time, and continue the construction project. Within a month of the resignations, Harman reported to the Medical Staff Executive Committee that she had sixty-three full-time nurses on staff in addition to temporary nurses and volunteering physicians' wives.[97] By October, Thrasher reported to the Authority that there were only three vacancies among the six hundred total hospital employees, and the physicians attending that meeting "agreed that the nursing care at this time was back to the level it was in January and as good or better as any hospital in the Atlanta area."[98] Most of the remaining inconveniences such as noise, closed beds, and restricted services were associated with the construction project. The Joint Commission on Accreditation of Healthcare Organizations conducted its regularly scheduled inspection in March 1970 and granted the hospital another three-year accreditation.[99]

Whether incidental or related to the stressful times, Evans sustained a heart attack in March 1969, and Thrasher suffered a heart attack the following May. Both recovered, though Evans resigned from the Authority the following September on the advice of his family and physician.[100]

The Hospital Authority's refusal to recognize the local unit as the negotiating agent for the nurses and the subsequent resignations essentially sealed the fate of the GSNA's efforts to achieve collective bargaining in any Atlanta or other Georgia hospitals. The GSNA did not renew Stanley Kravit's contract at the end of 1969, renamed the New Approach Program, and abandoned the concept of strikes, mass resignations, or any form of work stoppage.[101]

Despite the difficulties, the hospital became a better employer and assumed a new attitude in dealing with its employee relations. Authority member W. P. Tatum laid down the challenge

Administrator William Thrasher looking over the DGH expansion project with Naomi Harman, RN, new director of Nursing, and Opal Hopkins Fyffe, RN, the first director of Nursing.

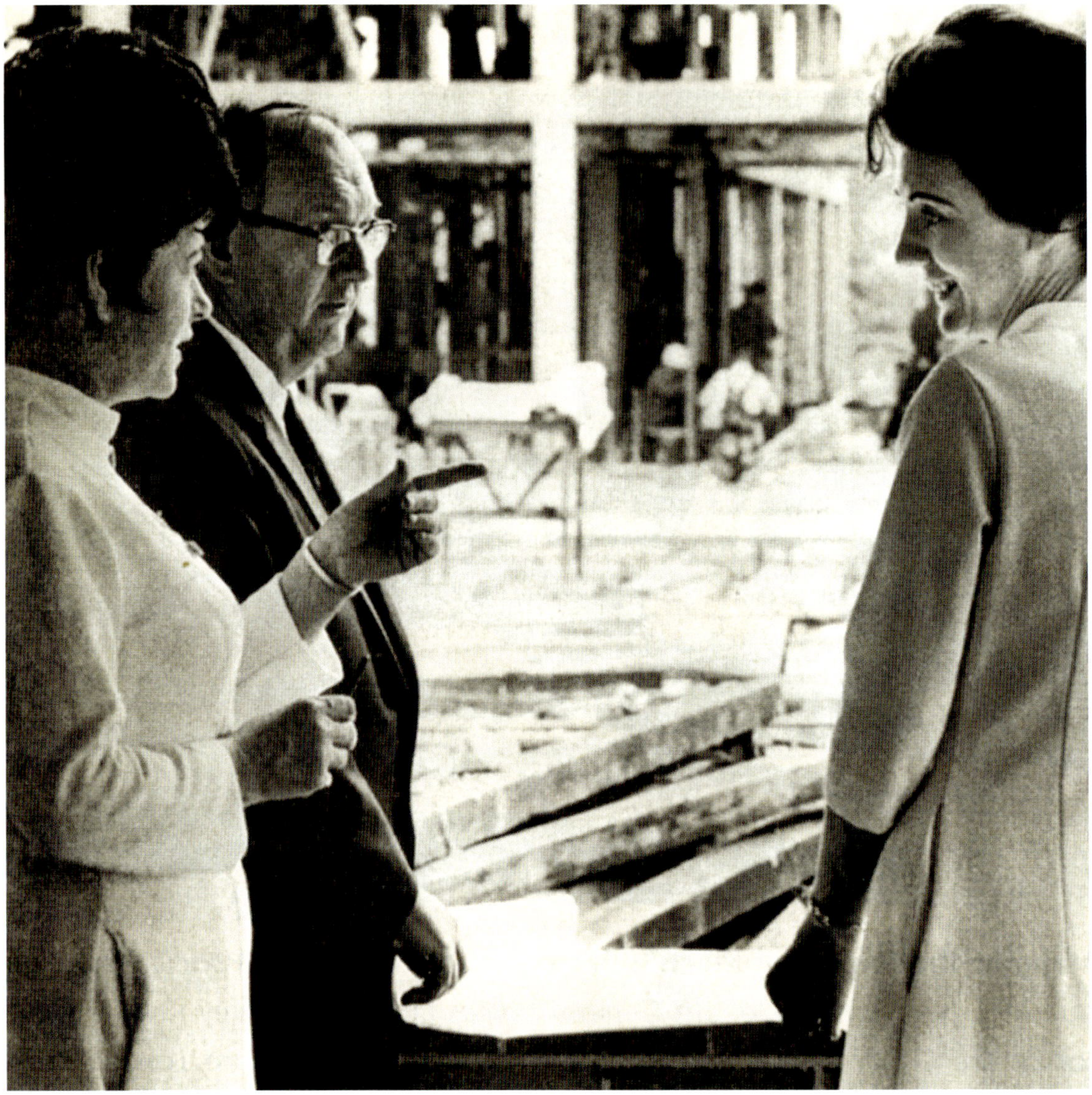

when he said to the trustees that "the Authority was going to have to decide if we were going to be the leader or the follower in personnel relations. . . . We have to attract good people to DeKalb General Hospital, and we can no longer play catch-up with the other hospitals and local employers."[102]

Within a short period of time, the hospital met nearly all of the requests of the resigning nurses except recognition of the local unit as GSNA's bargaining agent. Within two weeks of the resignations, assistant to the administrator John Gerlach announced that a temporary nursery was in operation in one wing of the hospital,[103] and the Authority subsequently approved the construction of a permanent facility.[104] In addition to the salary increases made in February, others were scheduled for October and again for six months later.[105] Team nursing was initiated, additional ward clerks were hired, and housekeeping personnel were assigned to each floor to free up nurses for more direct patient care.[106]

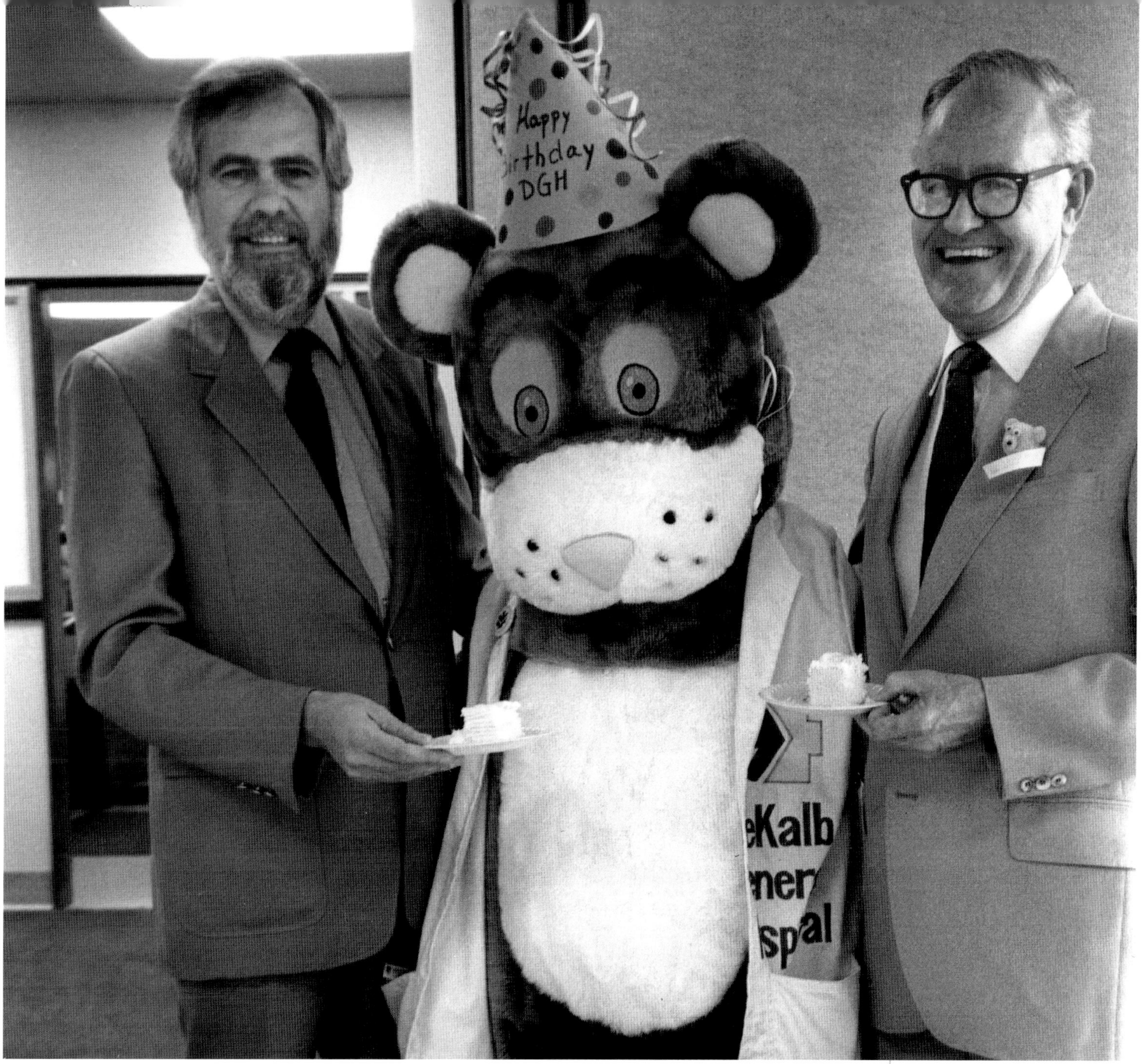

Bill Sublett, left, was named director of Personnel in 1970, and Perry Stephens, right, was named assistant director.

After exploring the establishment of a Professional Relations Committee as recommended by the Medical Staff Executive Committee, the Authority approved instead the formation of an Employee Council. The council was chaired by a member of the Authority and co-chaired by a member of the senior administrative staff, was composed of members from most hospital departments, met monthly, and reported directly to the Authority.[107]

Bill Sublett was named director of Personnel in 1970, and Perry Stephens became assistant director of Personnel. Employment policies were standardized, and salary adjustments were based on a merit system. Orientation and in-service training programs were enhanced, vacation and sick leave changes recommended by employees were approved, a life insurance policy was created, and a credit union was established. A consultant was hired with instructions to develop a retirement plan by October 1970, a check-cashing privilege for employees was approved, and the pharmacy was authorized to fill prescriptions for employees.[108] Nurse managers were given additional authority to run their units.

The walkout, however, took its toll. The resigning nurses paid dearly. Some of them reapplied and were rehired by DeKalb General Hospital. Many took nursing positions in other Atlanta hospitals and in physician offices. A few left the nursing profession to pursue other careers. Margaret Ford became the director of Nursing at the new Georgia Retardation Center.[109]

Despite the ability of most nurses to obtain other positions, most experienced a significant sense of loss. Many grieved over losing a place in the hospital in which they had been happy despite the grievances.[110] They were disillusioned, feeling that they had been set up and abandoned by the GSNA and the ANA.[111] They felt misunderstood and abandoned by administration, the Authority, the physicians, the public, and even some nursing colleagues. Many were confused and discouraged about the status and the future of their profession.

Despite the hospital's surviving and thriving, it, too, paid a price. It lost many excellent, dedicated, and highly competent nurses who were devoted to the hospital and who were committed to quality patient care. It suffered a reputation in the community for not caring about its employees or being able to deal with their grievances in a constructive way. Some doctors and patients from the community chose to use other hospitals. Qualified nurses were reluctant to apply to DeKalb General, unsure of whether it was a good place to work. The loss of trained and experienced nurses put the hospital's quality of care at risk. The discord that prevailed and the ultimate loss of one hundred nurses diminished the collegial, caring, comfortable, and safe environment that once was a tangible part of the hospital's "personality" and ambiance.

It was a crisis and a loss that many believe did not have to happen and should not have happened.[112] Many things might have been done differently to prevent it.

Margaret Ford, as director of Nursing, might have taken a more assertive role both in dissuading the nurses from their alliance with the GSNA and their fidelity to the course of collective bargaining to correct their grievances. She might have been more assertive and effective in making the case for her nurses with the medical staff, Thrasher, and the trustees. Opal Fyffe, it will be recalled, had been willing to resign in protest because of the resistance she faced in meeting the needs of her nurses.

Thrasher might have been more assertive in persuading the trustees to deal urgently and decisively with his employees' low morale and the "massive exodus" caused by inadequate salaries and benefits. He was the nurses' point of contact and the one on whom they depended to make their case to the governing body. Even though, on more than one occasion, the trustees had made it clear that they, not he, were in charge of day-to-day operational decisions, Thrasher might have chosen this occasion to take a stronger stand before the trustees.

Thrasher and the Authority might have been more cautious in accepting Opal Fyffe's on-the-spot conclusion that Margaret Ford was behind the nurses' agitation, that "she had to go," and that firing Ford would defuse the momentum of the resigning nurses and make them rethink their decision to resign. Ford had attempted to be neutral, had been excluded from the activities of the local unit, and had urged her nurses to negotiate apart from the local unit; and her precipitous firing only inflamed and entrenched the nurses in their decision to resign.

The physicians, who traditionally had the ear of administration and the Authority and a close relationship with the nurses, might have become involved much earlier and been more definitive in their efforts to intervene. Their emergency meeting to formulate a set of recommendations on behalf of the nurses occurred only three days before the walkout—only after the die was cast, emotions were dominant, and time had run out.

When planning for the expansion of the hospital that would double its bed capacity, administration and the Authority might have involved nurses more in the planning process, heard their concerns about the challenge of staffing the new facility with qualified personnel, and worked with them on a strategy to deal with their legitimate concerns. As it was, groundbreaking took place six months before their walkout without any apparent meaningful consultation with them.

The GSNA might have selected an attorney to work with the nurses other than "a Yankee from New Jersey" with a labor union background who, despite the rhetoric of "professionalism," presented the nurses' case in union terms. As well, the trustees might not have chosen an attorney that came from a labor union background to advise them on how to deal with the crisis.

The GSNA might have been less determined to have the DeKalb General nurses, regardless of the cost to them, establish its reputation as a powerful negotiating agent capable of bringing a hospital's leadership to its knees. Instead of holding to its rigid, entrenched position, it might have released the nurses from their commitment and advised them to consider other alternatives for addressing their concerns at DeKalb General.

The DeKalb General nurses might have been less trusting regarding several issues: (1) accepting GSNA's insistence that the administration, the Authority, the public, and even other nurses would "buy" the distinction between unionization and collective bargaining by an outside agent for professional recognition, (2) believing that administration and Authority would back down from its refusal to recognize the GSNA as the nurses' bargaining agent, (3) failing to anticipate the emotionally negative effect their picketing would have on the Authority and administration, physicians, the public, and other nurses, and (4) failing to appreciate the legal equivalence of a concerted mass resignation and work stoppage with a strike.

Both the nurses and the hospital leadership might have endeavored to engage more in creative negotiations to achieve "win-win" outcomes rather than in the inflexible posturing that prevailed.

The administration and trustees might have been more proactive than reactive and might have made a more concerted effort to create meaningful dialog and communication. The trustees repeatedly announced that they would be willing to meet with the nurses to discuss their issues, but there is no evidence that they undertook any concrete initiatives to bring the nurses to the bargaining table.

Administration and Authority might have appreciated more fully the concept of professionalism that had developed historically in the nursing profession. Repeatedly looking to the LPNs and associate degree nurses to "fill the gap" and provide for the hospital's nursing needs raised questions about that awareness and appreciation. Thrasher's confidence in Fyffe and Harman as representatives of "the old school" reinforced management's orientation toward the nursing profession.

The nurses who left got on with their lives, some back at DeKalb General, and the hospital continued on its path of growth and service. The hospital survived and moved on to be a better employer. One can only speculate what would have been the rest of the story if some of the things that might have been done had been done, and if the resignations that didn't have to happen had not happened.

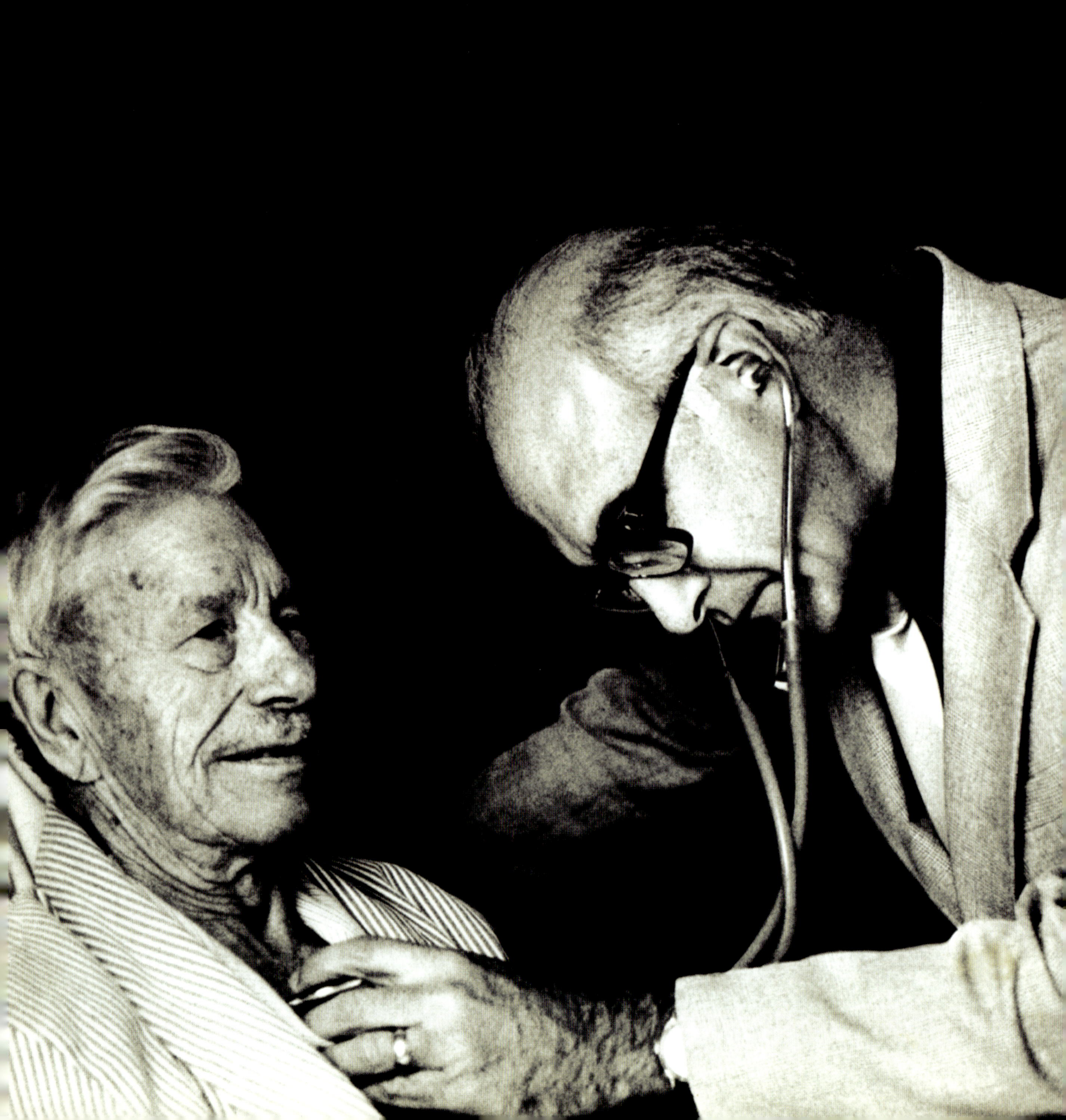

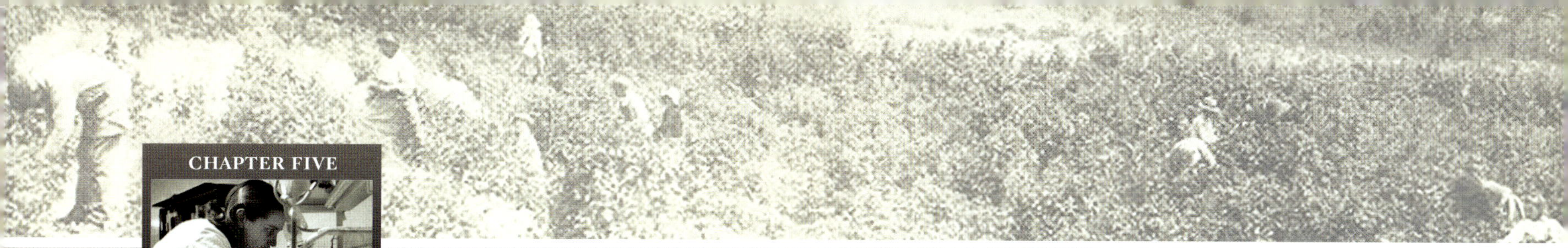

CHAPTER FIVE

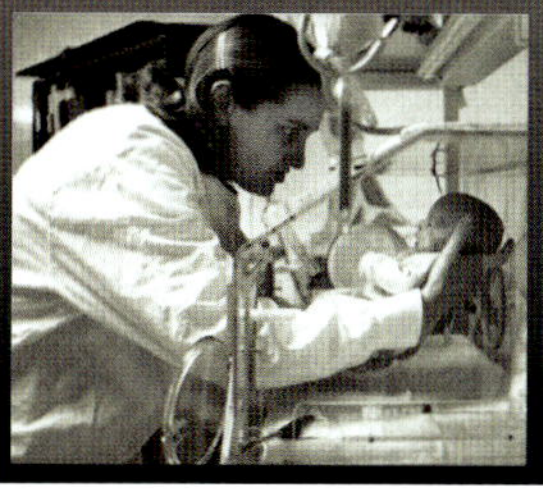

Two Decades of Prosperity and Expansion Leading to Restructuring

DeKalb General Hospital's second and third decade, the 1970s and 1980s, were among its most prosperous years, the years with the least challenges and difficulties, and the years filled with growth and the expansion of new facilities and services. The mass resignation of nurses was behind the hospital, its 1971 major expansion and renovation project was complete, its medical staff was growing in number and expertise, its management and governing leadership was competent and stable, its reputation was strongly positive, and its financial status was improving steadily.

The original governing body and management team achieved a monumental accomplishment in planning, constructing, making operational the new hospital, and in seeing it through its first decade of growth and challenges. As the second decade emerged, some of the leaders had died and some had chosen to step aside so that others might lead. Most notably, J. Rufus Evans, MD, retired in 1969, and Waldo Sowell succeeded him as chairman of the DeKalb County Hospital Authority.

Sowell engaged the A. T. Kearney Company to assist the trustees in developing a leadership and strategic plan to meet the needs of the hospital that had doubled its capacity in 1971. He appointed committees with assigned responsibilities that decentralized the governing body's planning and decision-making processes. The hospital brought in new executives to manage the enlarged responsibilities of the expanded facility. John Gerlach was promoted to director of Patient Services, Charles Eberhart was recruited as director of Administrative Services, and Bill Sublett was made director of Personnel. When William Thrasher became executive director of the DeKalb County Hospital Authority, Eberhart was named administrator and Douglas Buchner became director of Administrative Services.

The hospital, seeking legal counsel with expertise in hospital issues, turned to the Powell Goldstein law firm and named Ed Dorsey as hospital attorney. He was succeeded by the firm's James Rawls in 1978.

In addition to senior executive additions, the hospital added other leaders. It selected

DE KALB GENERAL HOSPITAL

Opposite: Paul Crank, MD, cardiologist and former director of Medical Affairs, examines a Patient.

During the 1970s and 1980s, DeKalb General Hospital's reputation was at its highest since the hospital opened its doors in 1961.

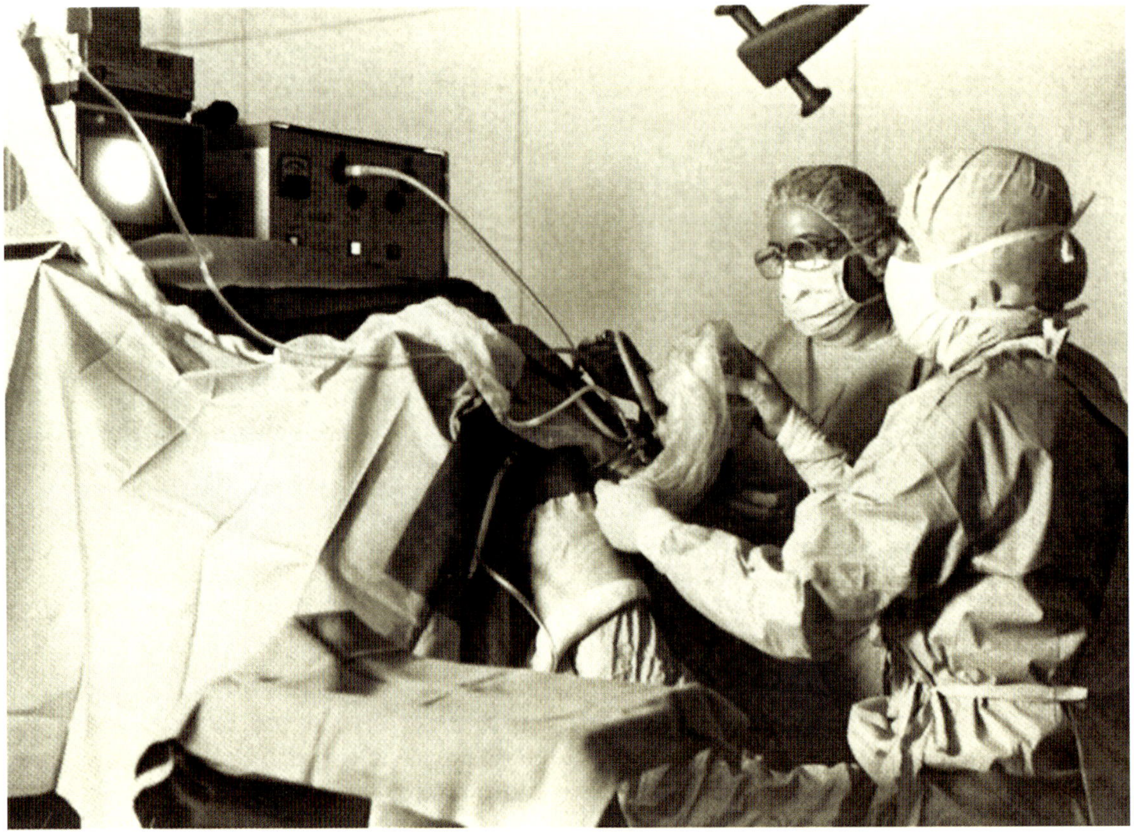

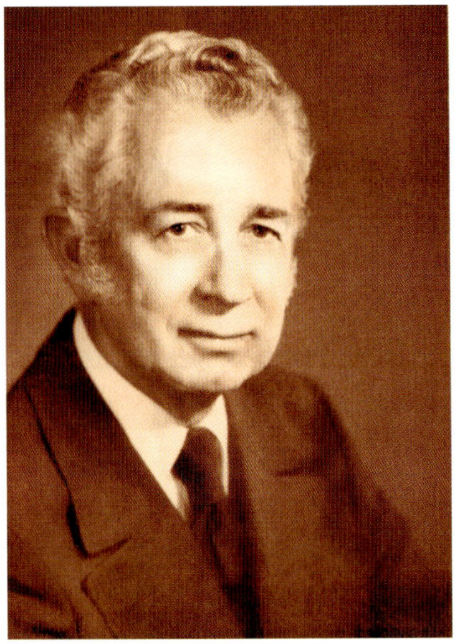

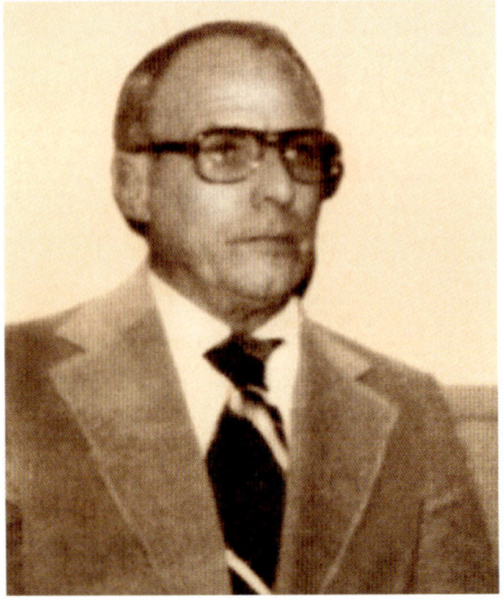

Above: A. Waldo Sowell (top) became a member of the Hospital Authority in 1964. and was elected chairman in 1969. After Sowell suffered a fatal fall in 1976, William P. Tatum (above) was elected chairman.
Above right: Arthroscopy being performed on a patient at DeKalb General Hospital.

Marilyn Gibbs (later Barry) as its medical librarian and John Harrel, MD, as its first director of Medical Affairs. It established a Physical Therapy Department with Dilys Jagger as director and a Social Services Department with Esther Russell as director.

The trustees officially launched an initiative to develop a medical facility in South DeKalb County when, in 1970, the county passed a $1,950,000 bond for that purpose. DeKalb General opened its Mental Health Unit and Skilled Nursing Facility. It expanded Radiology Services to include nuclear medicine. It established a Credit Union, expanded the Laboratory from 2,500 square feet to 10,000 square feet, established an IV (intravenous) Team, saw the beginning of regular Tuesday morning continuing medical education (CME) conferences, established a Tumor Registry, and ventured into the use of major computer systems.

When Sowell suffered a fatal fall at home in 1976, William P. Tatum was elected chairman, and Tatum maintained a major leadership role for seventeen years. During his tenure and close working relationship with Administrator Eberhart, the hospital moved forward in developing a South DeKalb medical facility with the purchase of forty acres of land, construction of the first FamilyCare Center, and the creation of a four-phase plan to fulfill the promise of a medical facility in that community.

Martha Kalember succeeded Thrasher as director of Hospital Relations, Bill Sublett succeeded Buckner as director of Administrative Services, and Bonnie Phipps succeeded Charles Anderson as chief financial officer. Wayne Spangler, MDiv, became the first hospital chaplain, and Kathy Hayes was named the first director of Volunteer Services.

The hospital created service line development teams that identified opportunities and inaugurated initiatives in cancer services, surgical services, women's and infants' services, cardiology services, and mental health services. It established a Pulmonary Function Laboratory, a Diabetes Medical Center, a Level 3 Trauma Center, a Rape Crisis Center, a Cardiac Catheterization Laboratory, and a Cancer Center. It recruited a neonatologist in 1978 and established a neonatal intensive care unit for premature newborns and those with special medical needs.

It acquired state-of-the-art technology such as computerized tomography (CT) and magnetic resonance imaging (MRI) scanners in radiology and was at the forefront of utilizing the revolutionary laparoscopic surgical technology. It added a Diagnostic and Treatment Center for non-emergency illness and outpatient procedures, an Ambulatory Surgery Center, a centralized adult Rehabilitation Center and a Pediatric Rehabilitation Center, a Diagnostic Breast Center to offer mammography services, the first hospital-based Wellness Center of its kind in the southeast, a Diagnostic Imaging Center for outpatient radiological procedures, a Central Energy Plant and Incinerator, and a Professional Office Building on campus.

In 1988 the Authority acted on the medical staff's recommendation to change the name of the hospital from DeKalb General Hospital to DeKalb Medical Center to reflect the expansion of facilities, expertise, and services provided by the institution. The hospital became a member of the Volunteer Hospital Association (VHA), an alliance of nonprofit community hospitals to realize economies of scale in purchasing and services, held its first annual Nightingala fund-raising event, and established the DeKalb Medical Center Foundation to raise funds and friends for the hospital.

Bonnie Phipps, as the new chief financial officer in 1986, and the Finance Committee initiated a creative investment strategy to build a significant financial reserve for the hospital. DeKalb Medical Center had enjoyed a period of prosperity with its rapidly growing medical staff, patient volume, new services, and the ability to collect a reasonable amount for services provided. There were indications, however, that such prosperity was not to continue indefinitely with emerging third-party-payer and regulatory restrictions. While the opportunity presented itself, Phipps led the hospital in a plan that created a healthy financial reserve that would prove invaluable in the challenging years to come.

Yet, with all this prosperity, growth, and expansion, Administrator Eberhart, Chairman Tatum, and the other trustees were concerned. They saw the need for a new governance structure that could address the opportunities and challenges that lay ahead.

The DeKalb County Hospital Authority first discussed restructuring in 1985 as part of a strategic planning process.[1] Fourteen other Georgia authority hospitals already had done so, including Northside Hospital in Atlanta, Cobb General Hospital in Austell, Memorial Medical Center in Savannah, Northeast Georgia Medical Center in Gainesville, University Medical Center in Augusta, Phoebe Putney Memorial Hospital in Albany, and The Medical Center in Columbus.[2] Authority Chairman W. P. Tatum, Administrator Charles Eberhart, hospital attorney James Rawls, consultants, and other senior executives held all-day sessions to examine the benefits, liabilities, requirements, and challenges involved in restructuring.[3] In September 1990 Eberhart sent the following memorandum to Tatum:

> *I have become increasingly concerned about the viability of the hospital authority model as the best model for the governance of the medical center in the future.*

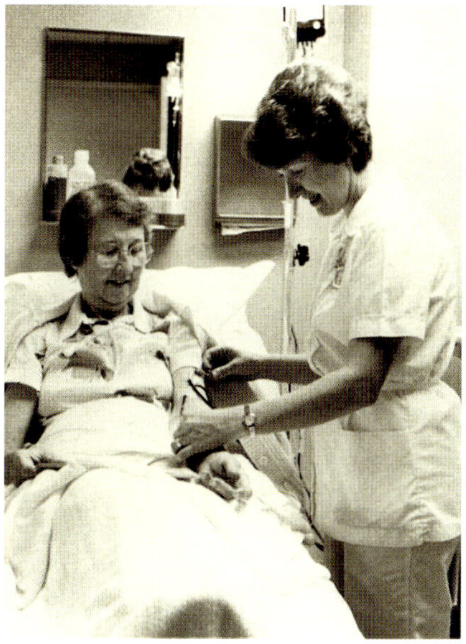

A hospital patient receives a blood transfusion.

As you know, the hospital authority law model of governance has had many advantages since its creation by the [Georgia] General Assembly in 1946. However, this model may not be capable of remaining successful in the future with the enormous competitive, economic, legalistic, and regulatory complexities that have developed in the healthcare industry especially in the last ten years.[4]

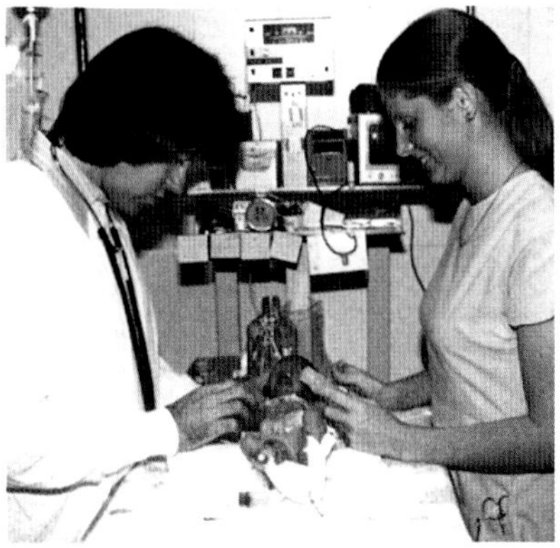

An infant is examined by J. Michael Armand, MD, and a neonatal ICU nurse.

Eberhart identified several of the problems and limitations imposed by the authority governance model:

1. Georgia hospital authorities are prohibited from electing qualified leaders who do not reside in the county.
2. While more than 35 percent of DeKalb Medical's patients originated outside DeKalb County, under authority law the hospital is prohibited from providing services outside the county's geographical boundaries.
3. An authority hospital is prohibited from acquiring or establishing a for-profit entity.
4. An authority hospital cannot create a separate, legally-distinct, subsidiary corporation.
5. An authority hospital must abide by open meeting and open records laws, a requirement to which competitors are not subject.
6. An authority hospital must limit the number of trustees to nine, even though the workload of the governing body may need additional physician and community representation.[5]

Chairman Tatum forwarded Eberhart's memorandum to all members of the authority with the following message:

I have received the enclosed memo from Eberhart, which I believe deserves very serious consideration by the Authority. I have asked Eberhart to visit with each of you to discuss this concept. Would you please study his memo at your earliest convenience and be prepared to meet with him soon?[6]

The primary reasons for restructuring were, therefore, to provide the governing body with the ability to make the most of business and service opportunities and to deal with challenges in ways not permitted by authority law. The Authority developed a white paper entitled "DeKalb Medical Center Analysis of Corporate Restructuring" that it distributed to the public, to hospital staff and physicians, and to local and state officials explaining what it was doing and why it was doing it.[7]

There were, however, other concerns that played a significant role in the Authority's decision to restructure. Those concerns involved conflicts that were taking place around the state in regard to the relationship between hospital authorities and county officials. There were disturbing instances of indifference, neglect, hostility, and openly confrontational and adversarial relationships.

The Athens-Clarke County Commission refused to act on any of the vacancy nominations submitted by the Clarke County Hospital Authority. The authority had to sue the commissioners and obtain a court order before they would appoint individuals nominated by the authority.[8]

The Gwinnett County Commission facetiously sent to its hospital authority the names of George H. W. Bush, a county secretary, and a physician for one vacancy; and Dan Quayle, another county secretary, and another physician for a second vacancy. When the authority refused to make a selection from these "stacked decks," the county commissioners publicly reprimanded the authority for not rubber stamping its physician nominees. One of Gwinnett County's state representatives called the authority's meeting a disgrace and threatened to introduce a bill into the legislature stipulating that counties need submit only one name to authorities that they would have to accept.[9]

At the request of Floyd County commissioners, one of its state representatives introduced a bill (that did not pass) that would essentially place every hospital authority under the direct supervision and day-to-day control of the county commissions.[10]

The DeKalb County Hospital Authority was well aware of those encounters around the state and would, indeed, later experience its own troubles with its county commission.

Although Georgia law states that "the authority shall make rules and regulations for its governance,"[11] the DeKalb commissioners on one occasion insisted on the specific number of members the Authority should have.[12]

The DeKalb commissioners sometimes delayed acting on Authority reappointments and vacancies for inordinate periods. In June 1997, for example, out of nine seats on the board, there were three vacancies and five expired terms. Two of the vacancies had existed for three years, two of the expired terms had existed for two years, and two had existed for one year.[13] Fortunately, members could continue serving after the expiration of their terms until reappointed or replaced. The county refused to nominate for reappointment one of the trustees because a county official had personal differences with that trustee.[14]

Nominations for the Authority became politicized. In 1993 one commissioner aggressively sought to place African Americans on the Authority and publicly said, "There should be only one qualification. That is that any person who lives in that community [South DeKalb with its predominantly black population] . . ." could be a representative.[15]

The Authority became increasingly concerned that candidates might be focused more on political or personal agendas than on the best interests of the medical center and community. The trustees were cautious about the information they should share with the new members. Administrator Eberhart wrote, "I think it is important for us to take the opportunity to . . . win over the confidence of the new individual Authority members and hopefully we can end up with nine supportive members who can make a positive and lasting contribution to the hospital. . . ."[16]

In preparation for the Authority's deliberation of restructuring, Eberhart and his team created the necessary documents and developed a set of fifty questions (with answers) that explored the issues to be considered, identified the models that might best meet the medical center's needs, and outlined the process to be followed. In March 1991 Eberhart distributed the questions to the trustees after which Chairman Tatum called a special meeting of the Authority. The trustees unanimously, with one abstention, voted to restructure.[17]

Reorganization took place in two phases. In August 1991 the Authority incorporated DeKalb Medical Center, Inc., (DMC), a new, nonprofit, private operating company. The new DMC Board of Directors consisted of eleven members, and W. P. Tatum was elected its chairman. On March 23, 1992, the DeKalb County Hospital Authority signed a lease and transfer agreement with DMC[18] that commenced on April 1, 1992, and extended for forty years, the maximum term permitted by law.[19] The Authority retained ownership but leased to DMC all of its assets and holdings except three: the undeveloped forty acres on Hillandale Road in South DeKalb County, the proceeds from the bond fund issued in 1970 for a South DeKalb hospital, and $20,000 in cash retained for operating expenses.[20] When, in November 1993, DMC began developing the Hillandale property, the Authority also

In August 1991, the hospital became a new, nonprofit private operating company with the new name of DeKalb Medical Center.

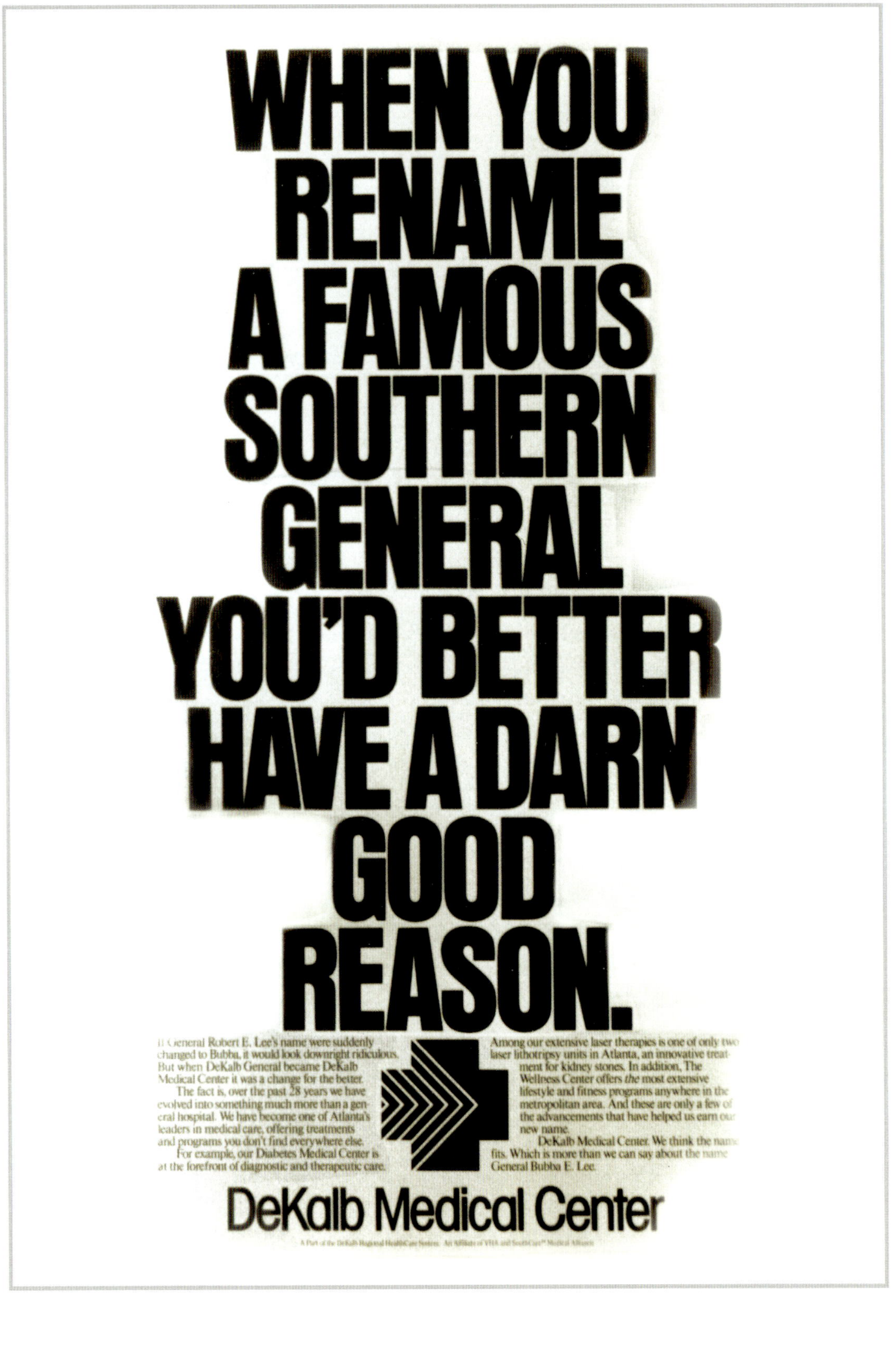
WHEN YOU RENAME A FAMOUS SOUTHERN GENERAL YOU'D BETTER HAVE A DARN GOOD REASON.
If General Robert E. Lee's name were suddenly changed to Bubba, it would look downright ridiculous. But when DeKalb General became DeKalb Medical Center it was a change for the better.
The fact is, over the past 28 years we have evolved into something much more than a general hospital. We have become one of Atlanta's leaders in medical care, offering treatments and programs you don't find everywhere else.
For example, our Diabetes Medical Center is at the forefront of diagnostic and therapeutic care.
Among our extensive laser therapies is one of only two laser lithotripsy units in Atlanta, an innovative treatment for kidney stones. In addition, The Wellness Center offers *the* most extensive lifestyle and fitness programs anywhere in the metropolitan area. And these are only a few of the advancements that have helped us earn our new name.
DeKalb Medical Center. We think the name fits. Which is more than we can say about the name General Bubba E. Lee.
DeKalb Medical Center

leased to DMC the land and transferred the proceeds form the South DeKalb bond fund.[21]

While the Authority retained ownership of its assets, DMC assumed responsibility for the day-to-day management and operation of the hospital and all facilities and services associated with it. It assumed responsibility for the Authority's contractual agreements and liabilities, such as its Hill-Burton obligations to provide for charity and indigent patients, and the hospital's participation in the Medicare and Medicaid programs. Hospital employees became employees of DMC that agreed to maintain salaries and benefits and to make payments to the Authority sufficient to meet the Authority's bond obligations.

In December 1992, during phase two of the reorganization, DMC Inc. incorporated a parent, nonprofit holding company, DeKalb Regional Healthcare System, Inc. (DRHS).[22] DRHS would oversee DMC Inc. as well as any other subsidiaries created in the future. The DRHS board held its first meeting in April 1993 and elected Charles Ginden as chairman. The DRHS board had nine members, five of whom were required to be members of the DMC board.[23]

In 2004, president and CEO Eric Norwood and the directors of DMC and DRHS once again restructured the governance of the organization. DRHS had acquired the Decatur Hospital and incorporated Decatur Health Resources Inc., (DHR) as its owner. It also was in the process of completing the new hospital at Hillandale in South DeKalb. This reorganization centralized the governance of the hospital system in the parent body, DRHS, which was renamed DeKalb Regional Health System, the system generally to be referred to as "DeKalb Medical."[24] The three hospitals would be named DeKalb Medical at North Decatur, DeKalb Medical at Downtown Decatur, and DeKalb Medical at Hillandale.

This change reduced the number of governing bodies from three to one. Under the new organizational structure, DMC and DHR would remain separate subsidiaries of DRHS and would act only on items required from a regulatory, legal or Joint Commission on Accreditation of Healthcare Organizations standpoint such as governing medical staff credentialing. The new DRHS board had thirteen directors, approximately one third of whom were physicians, an executive committee, and eight other committees. The DRHS executive committee would serve as each of the two subsidiary boards, and the officers of DRHS would be the officers of each subsidiary board.

There would be a unified medical staff for all DRHS hospitals with shared governance. Each hospital's medical staff would elect its own chief and representatives to serve on the DeKalb Medical Staff Executive Committee. Each hospital would grant its own privileges, but there would be shared medical staff organization, shared bylaws, shared clinical departments, shared credentialing process, and shared common standards for membership categories, membership qualifications, peer review, and grievance processes.[25]

In addition to the DMC and DHR subsidiaries, DRHS established a third subsidiary, DRHS Ventures Inc., to oversee future joint ventures the system might undertake or other for-profit opportunities it might pursue.[26]

The 2004 reorganization established for each hospital a Community Committee made up of community residents and DRHS directors, physicians, and members of the hospital administration. The Community Committees would provide a local community voice for each of the three hospitals.[27]

The 2004 restructuring brought an integration and efficiency to the system that reflected the growth and the services that had evolved over the twelve years since the first reorganization was undertaken.

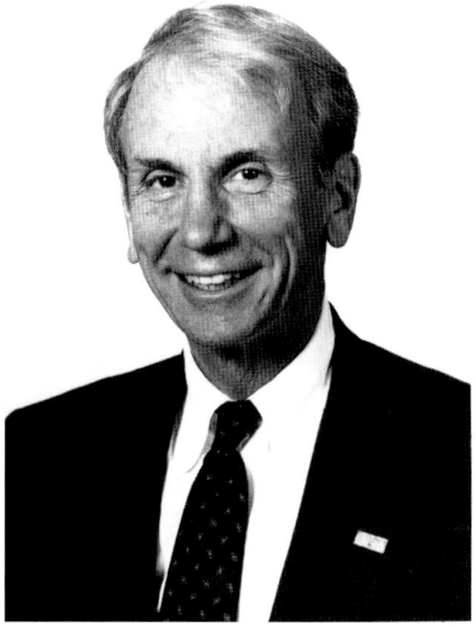

Charles Ginden, chairman of the DRHS Board.

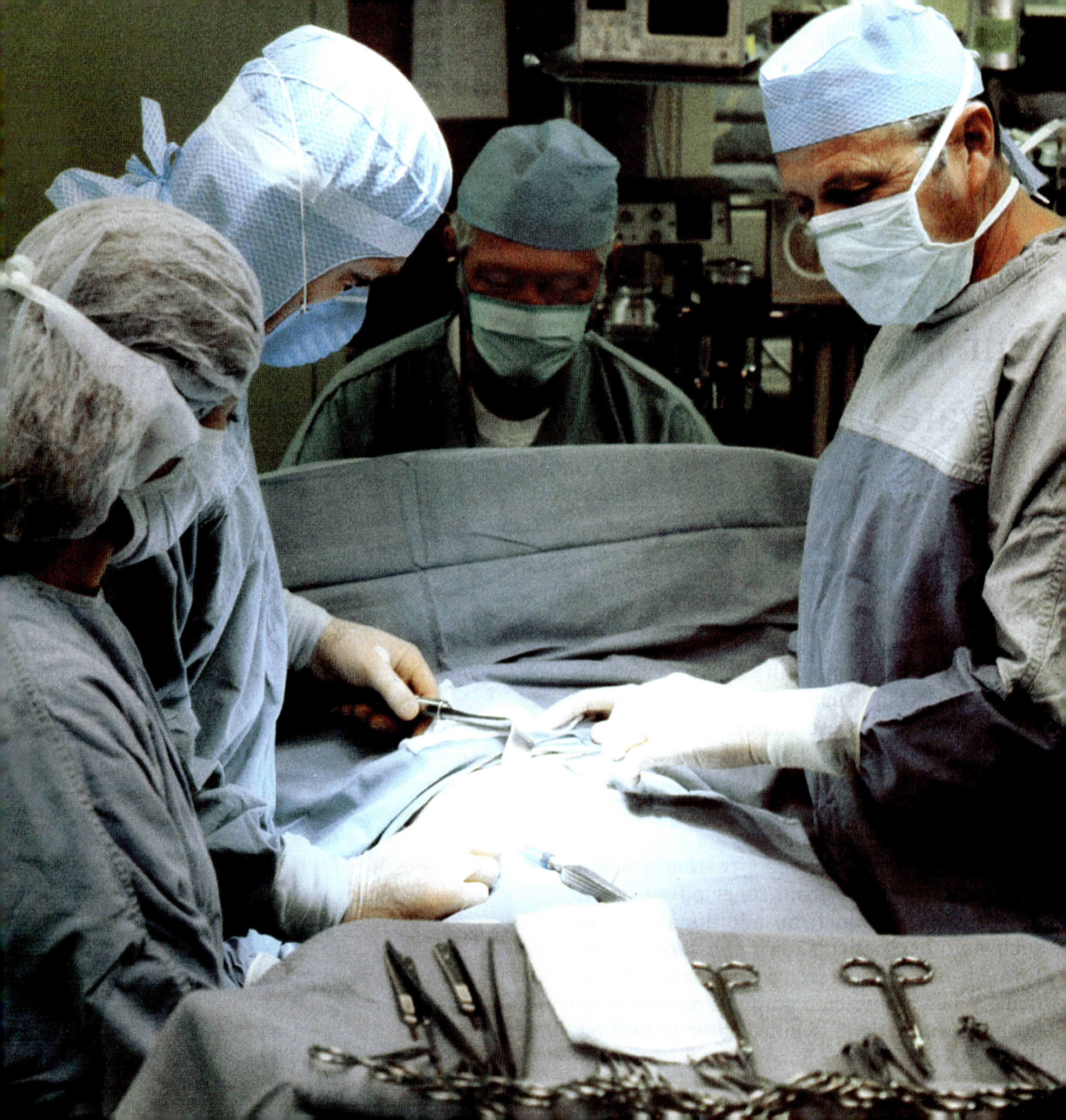

CHAPTER SIX

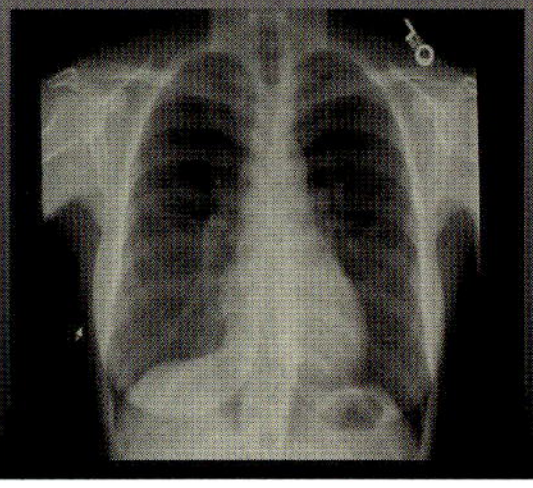

Horizontal Integration with PROMINA

IN AUGUST 1965 THE DEKALB COUNTY HOSPITAL AUTHORITY UNANIMOUSLY ADOPTED THE FOLLOWING RESOLUTION:

> *Be it resolved that the DeKalb County Hospital Authority, the governing body of DeKalb General Hospital, does herewith endorse the need for the development of Northside Hospital as planned, and we encourage the support of all community and other groups in connection with the accomplishment of this facility to help meet the great and overwhelming needs for hospital services in the greater Atlanta area.*[1]

When managed-care came to Atlanta, it gave insurers much greater power over where patients went for their medical care and what procedures would be covered.

Three decades later, the hospitals in greater Atlanta, including the newly named DeKalb Medical Center, were in a dramatically different situation. Rather than supporting the establishment of more hospitals, each was competing for patients and vying for the best possible reimbursement for its services.

The major factor that altered the healthcare environment was the explosive emergence of managed-care organizations. The managed-care industry came late to Atlanta, but once it arrived, it matured to a level of power and prominence in a brief span of time that had required years in other parts of the country. Through negotiated contracts with businesses and individuals, those insurers increasingly controlled patients' choice of physicians and hospitals. They also controlled how much hospitals, physicians, and other healthcare providers would be reimbursed for their services.

Hospitals found themselves operating with a defensive mentality. DeKalb Medical Center was no exception. Hospitals faced new questions: What did they have to do to compete with other hospitals to secure contracts for patients? How could they obtain reimbursements sufficient to stay in business? How could they achieve sufficient cost containment to be competitive without sacrificing quality of care? How could they accumulate adequate reserves in the face of the ever-increasing cost of technology, facilities, labor, and supplies?

DeKalb Medical Center, like many hospitals, focused on two solutions. First it maintained and enhanced strong ties with its physicians, including its primary care physicians, through a new type of relationship known as "vertical integration" that sought to align hospital and physician incentives. It also sought alliances with other hospitals through a relationship known as "horizontal integration" to gain collective strength and leverage for negotiating with managed-care organizations and other third-party payers. Neither initiative alone would be enough. Both horizontal integration and vertical integration seemed required to survive and thrive in the emerging competitive market.[2]

DeKalb Medical Center soon realized it needed to be an integral part of a larger entity that would enable it to compete in the new healthcare market.

Collaborating with other hospitals was not a new experience for DeKalb Medical Center. In 1986 the hospital became a member of Volunteer Hospital Association (VHA), Georgia,[3] a chapter of the national VHA organization. The Georgia chapter included eighteen nonprofit community hospitals statewide. It was a purchasing and management cooperative that returned savings to its members, and it was a successful initiative. Each year, it returned more to its members than they had invested in membership fees. In 1995 VHA Georgia shared $288,000 with DeKalb Medical Center, nearly four times the $77,000 in membership fees that DeKalb paid that year.[4]

DeKalb Medical Center continued its membership in VHA Georgia.[5] In the new competitive market, however, it determined it needed something more. It needed to be an integral part of a larger entity that would enable it to compete in the new healthcare market. What that entity would look like and which hospitals would be a part of the alliance were unknowns. But DeKalb Medical Center began exploring.

It cast a large net over wide waters. Over a period of two years, before coming to a decision, DeKalb Medical Center held discussions with Rockdale Health System, Henry General Hospital, Georgia Baptist Hospital (later known as Atlanta Medical Center), Emory University Hospital, Northside Hospital, St. Joseph's Hospital, and the PROMINA organization that included Northwest Health System (later known as WellStar), Piedmont Medical Center, and Gwinnett Medical Center.

The process began in May 1994 when Charles Eberhart announced to the DeKalb Medical Center Board of Directors that he planned to engage in discussions with Rockdale Health System.[6] Consultants analyzed the two institutions, concluded that the organizations were compatible, and advised exploring a relationship.[7] Executive teams from the two hospital systems held a series of meetings, and within six months the Rockdale board said it was receptive to a noncash merger.[8] Each system prepared a position paper that defined what it wanted the relationship to look like. Not surprisingly, those position papers exposed conflicting expectations and concerns.[9]

Despite the differences, the negotiating teams moved increasingly closer to an agreement[10] until the Rockdale chief executive officer (CEO), Archer Rose, and the chief operating officer (COO), Kim Hubbard, unexpectedly resigned.[11] At that point, Rockdale's acting CEO, William Sands, asked that discussions be put on hold "pending the stabilization of their management."[12] Meaningful negotiations never resumed. Sands observed that Rockdale seemed to be seeking a relationship where "2 + 1 = 5," and no organization was offering what Rockdale needed.[13] DeKalb Medical Center stayed in touch with Rockdale but engaged in no further discussions.

At the same time that DeKalb Medical Center was holding discussions with Rockdale, DeKalb Medical Center leaders also met with the other institutions. They held limited discussions with Henry Medical Center and Georgia Baptist Hospital, but these discussions yielded little promise. Meanwhile the PROMINA organization repeatedly urged DeKalb Medical Center to join its ranks. DeKalb Medial Center's leaders, however, felt it important to explore fully the possibility of an alliance with Northside Hospital, Emory University Hospital, and St. Joseph's Hospital, individually or collectively, before making a decision about PROMINA.

Attorney Robert Baudino of Des Moines, Iowa, assisted DeKalb in examining its horizontal integration possibilities. The board of directors defined its goals, the qualities it required in any partner(s), and the results it expected from any affiliation.[14] The board developed a profile and prioritized the characteristics it required in a candidate, what it wanted the affiliation to look like in the marketplace, the cost effectiveness of the organization, the effects an affiliation would have on the managed-care environment, the relationship it would have with physicians, and what the corporate structure and governance would look like. It used that profile as a guide in the negotiations that followed. The negotiating team charted how each candidate measured up to the profile priorities and reported those findings to the board.

In mid-1994 DeKalb Medical Center executives met individually with Emory Hospital CEO John Henry, with Northside Hospital CEO Sidney Kirschner, and with St. Joseph's Hospital CEO Ron Hogan. All three were interested in establishing a relationship with DeKalb Medical Center, but none had defined the nature of that relationship.[15] In the meantime, St. Joseph's Hospital and Northside Hospital undertook prolonged and intensive negotiations aimed at merging those two institutions. They made it clear, however, that should their merger occur, they wanted DeKalb Medical Center to join them.[16]

In May 1995 Northside and St. Joseph's broke off their merger negotiations. But each of these hospitals, along with Emory, continued to say it wanted to explore an affiliation with DeKalb.[17]

DeKalb next entered into extended discussions with Emory and St. Joseph's. Because of the vast differences in the three institutions and the special obligations Emory had as an academic institution, the three agreed that if an affiliation occurred, it would be a joint operating company in which they shared an operating statement but not one another's debt. They agreed that they would invite other hospitals to join their alliance, but Emory, St. Joseph's, and DeKalb would be the core of the system.[18]

Significant concerns arose that the group could not resolve, including how managed-care contracting would be done, the importance of primary care physicians in the system, medical school funding, and cultural differences. In addition, Emory hired a new vice president for Health Affairs, Michael Johns, MD, and Emory could not predict the direction he would want that institution to take.[19] Finally Emory made it clear that it would expect to retain significant control over such areas as human resources, operating and capital budgeting, and asset utilization.[20] DeKalb saw that those requirements compromised the essence of the affiliation it was seeking, and, further, it saw the many contingencies as major impediments. It therefore discontinued its discussions with Emory.

In November 1995 physicians from Northside Hospital and DeKalb Medical Center urged the leadership of the two hospitals to reopen negotiations.[21] The Northside board of directors also indicated a willingness to resume discussions with St. Joseph's and DeKalb.[22] DeKalb was encouraged that Northside CEO Sidney Kirschner no longer required that he be named the CEO of any alliance formed, a requirement that was a major obstacle in the earlier merger negotiations between Northside and St. Joseph's.[23]

Kirschner, however, quickly placed other obstacles on the table. DeKalb and St. Joseph's wanted the three institutions to form a joint operating company with the option of moving toward a full merger at a later time if mutually desirable. Kirschner and Northside insisted on a full merger from the beginning. DeKalb and St. Joseph's wanted only moderately restrictive conditions for withdrawal from the system. Northside insisted on stringent and punitive withdrawal conditions. DeKalb and St. Joseph's wanted the CEO of the system to be selected after the system was formed. Northside insisted that the CEO be selected in advance, that there be only three CEO candidates, that they all be internal candidates, and that each be nominated by the three hospital boards.[24]

When the DeKalb board of directors met in April 1996, the negotiating team reported that Northside CEO Sidney Kirschner remained firm in his requirements. He was so intransigent that the DeKalb team wondered if he might want DeKalb to join the PROMINA organization so that he would be free to negotiate an alliance with the Columbia/Hospital Corporation of America (HCA) organization.[25]

Regardless of Kirschner's motives, DeKalb decided it could not go forward with an affiliation with Northside. It appeared left with two options: continue pursuing a relationship with St. Joseph's with the hope of eventually bringing into that affiliation Rockdale Hospital, Henry Medical Center, South Fulton Hospital, and possibly others; or join PROMINA. One of the obvious problems of an affiliation with St. Joseph's without Northside was the small market share. Even if the alliance brought in Rockdale, Henry, and South Fulton, their collective market share would be little more than half of what DeKalb would enjoy as a part of the PROMINA organization.[26]

In the meantime, DeKalb learned that PROMINA was holding discussions with Emory. If Emory joined PROMINA, there would be no place for DeKalb. Emory would cover the geographical area that DeKalb could provide and would eliminate any need for DeKalb in the system. This new information added some urgency to DeKalb's decision.[27]

DeKalb identified a number of advantages in joining PROMINA. It would enjoy the strength and leverage of PROMINA's centralized managed-care contracting capability. It would be a part of a system that had an attractive geographical coverage in metropolitan Atlanta. It should realize significant cost savings from PROMINA's centralized services and mass purchasing. PROMINA was already an established system, having been created in 1994, and was clearly ahead of other alliances in the Atlanta area.[28] DeKalb had a long history of good relations and distinct cultural affinity with the leaders of the PROMINA hospitals. While PROMINA theoretically could exercise certain controls, it had demonstrated a willingness to permit each member considerable autonomy regarding its operations, strategic planning, and the development of local physician organizations. Finally, the cost of joining PROMINA and supporting the projected operating expenses seemed reasonable and cost effective.[29]

DeKalb also recognized disadvantages and contingencies. By joining PROMINA, DeKalb would leave Northside and St. Joseph's free to negotiate with Columbia/HCA, thus creating a strong competitor in DeKalb's service area. DeKalb would abandon any possibility of forming an affiliation with St. Joseph's, Rockdale, Henry, South Fulton, and possibly other hospitals that would offer metropolitan Atlanta an important counterbalance to PROMINA, Emory, and Columbia/HCA. Many of DeKalb's physicians were strongly opposed to a PROMINA affiliation. Finally the PROMINA organization was already established, and DeKalb would have a limited opportunity to develop the system's structure or its strategic plans, or to provide leadership in its management team.[30]

DeKalb realized it needed to make a decision soon. Otherwise, the PROMINA option might be gone.[31] PROMINA CEO Bernard Brown told DeKalb that if it submitted a letter of intent to join PROMINA by the next PROMINA board meeting on April 10, 1996, PROMINA probably would choose DeKalb over Emory. If DeKalb delayed, he could not give DeKalb that assurance.[32] That may have been a bluff, but DeKalb saw it as a real threat to its future.

On April 1 the DeKalb Regional Healthcare System Inc. (DRHS), Board of Directors voted 6-to-1 to submit a letter of intent to affiliate with PROMINA.[33] PROMINA's board of directors accepted the DRHS letter of intent and proposed proceeding in four phases.[34] In phase 1, the two organizations would define issues to be examined and resolved, during which period each could continue negotiating with other parties should it choose to do so. Phase 2 would consist of a "due diligence" process in which nine study groups and a Liaison Committee would explore areas of mutual interest and develop a list of issues and concerns to be negotiated and resolved. During this phase, both systems would cease negotiating with other parties. In phase 3, the two systems' boards would negotiate and seek to resolve the issues and concerns identified in phase 2. In phase 4 the parties would consummate the affiliation.[35]

PROMINA and the DRHS board were concerned about the DeKalb physicians opposition to the affiliation. PROMINA said it wanted the system to be physician friendly and physician driven, with physicians filling up to 49 percent of the board seats.[36] The contracts that PROMINA signed depended upon its physicians delivering the services and abiding by the terms agreed upon.[37] Each member of PROMINA would form a Local Integrated Delivery System (LIDS) that would review proposed contracts and grant PROMINA permission to sign those contracts. Once signed, hospitals and physicians would be obligated to deliver what PROMINA promised.[38] Physician support, therefore, was essential.

DeKalb physicians were not convinced that PROMINA was physician friendly or physician driven. The physicians felt it had not demonstrated that commitment in action.[39] They contended PROMINA had squeezed some private physicians out of business when it employed 170 primary care physicians and had contracts with 165 specialists.[40] They recalled that in 1995 PROMINA required its Cobb County physicians to sign an amendment to their contracts that restricted them to providing services only to PROMINA's managed-care contract patients. Many Cobb County physicians refused and formed their own independent practice association.[41]

DeKalb physicians had other concerns. They deemed as unsatisfactory the LIDS agreement that PROMINA wanted DRHS to sign, as inadequate the service area PROMINA proposed for DRHS, as significant the potential loss of autonomy by the hospital and physicians, as inadequate the physician representation in PROMINA's leadership, and as unacceptable the lack of trust between DeKalb physicians and PROMINA.[42]

The DeKalb physicians formed one of the nine phase 2 study groups, and when it made its report to the DRHS board in August 1996, sixteen out of the twenty physicians in the group voted against DeKalb's affiliating with the PROMINA system.[43]

On June 12, 1997, the DeKalb Regional Healthcare System, Inc. signed an agreement to become affiliated with PROMINA.

The DRHS board took the physician vote seriously, but agreed to move into phase 3 to see if it could resolve not only the physician concerns but also those identified by other phase 2 study groups.[44] Indeed PROMINA agreed to all of the DRHS recommendations except for minor modifications to the DRHS service area proposal.

Given PROMINA's agreement to its conditions, the DRHS board authorized PROMINA to apply for antitrust clearance from the Federal Trade Commission for the pending DeKalb-PROMINA affiliation,[45] which the commission approved.[46] In February 1997 the DRHS board voted to accept the PROMINA affiliation agreement[47] and to provide $900,000 as its share to fund the PROMINA Health Plan, PROMINA's managed care contracting entity.[48]

DRHS and PROMINA officially signed the affiliation agreement on June 12, 1997.[49] DRHS board members H. Duane Blair, MD, and Oliver Lee were named to the PROMINA Board of Directors, and Catherine Huggins, MD, DeKalb Medical Center's chief of staff, became an ex officio

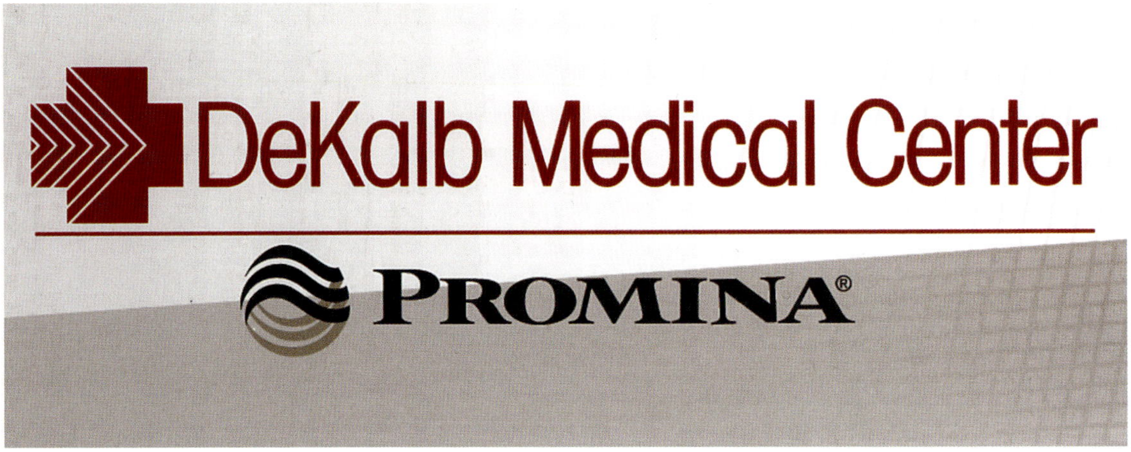

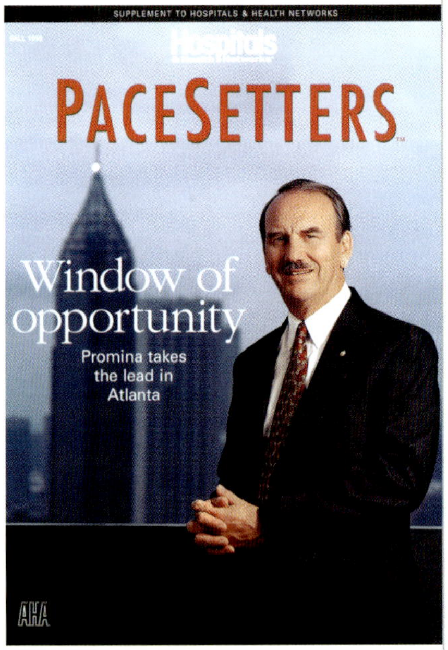

Top right: The DeKalb Medical Center logo once it became affiliated with PROMINA. **Above:** Bernard "Bernie" Brown, first CEO of PROMINA, on the cover of *Hospitals and Health Networks* magazine in 1998.

member.[50] DRHS thus became a part of Georgia's largest community-based health system.

With DRHS in its ranks, PROMINA consisted of five hospital systems: DRHS, Gwinnett Health System, Northwest Health System (later WellStar), Piedmont Health System, and Southern Regional Health System. Those five systems represented fourteen hospitals, 2,500 staffed beds, seventy satellite and mobile health centers, 18,000 employees, and more than 2,500 physicians. Each of the five systems incorporated the PROMINA name into its signage and logo. PROMINA's 1998 operating budget, including the operating budgets of its five systems, was $1.26 billion.[51]

The PROMINA structure was not a merger of the members, but a holding company with five operating units—the five member systems. The Local Integrated Delivery Systems (LIDS) actually owned PROMINA. PROMINA retained only reserve powers. Each of the five members had equal representation on the PROMINA board regardless of its size or the value of its assets. As PROMINA CEO Bernard Brown described it, "We're a case of reverse evolution. We have children (the hospitals), parents (the LIDS), and a grandparent (PROMINA). But in our family, the parents give birth to the grandparent."[52]

In addition to its board of directors, PROMINA had four permanent councils, each with representatives from the five systems. The Operations Management Council dealt with hospital and operational issues, the Managed Care Council handled centralized contracting, the Medical Services Council managed medical issues, and the Executive Council dealt with recommendations received from the other three councils.[53]

Each LIDS retained its own assets, its own medical staff and physician-hospital organization (PHO). Each LIDS provided its own healthcare services and oversight of the care provided by its physicians. The one thing that was centralized from the beginning was single-signature managed-care contracting. PROMINA sent all contract proposals to each LIDS for review and input, but when PROMINA CEO Bernard Brown signed on the dotted line, all fourteen hospitals and LIDS physicians were bound by the terms of that contract.[54]

The five member systems agreed that it made good business sense to standardize as many things as possible for the sake of efficiency and cost effectiveness. Early on, PROMINA standardized employee benefits at all its facilities, making the benefits portable should employees move from one system to another. It made employee policies uniform, created a corporate compliance program to reduce the likelihood of violating regulations and healthcare laws, and centralized the members' liability insurance coverage and purchasing contracts.

DRHS was optimistic about its decision to join the PROMINA system. CEO John R. Gerlach described the decision to affiliate with PROMINA as "one of the biggest decisions we have faced in our thirty-five-year history." He added that "in the first year alone, we expect to save more than $500,000 on twenty purchasing contracts in addition to other savings we'll receive by consolidating accounting, auditing, and risk management contracts at the PROMINA level. Another major advantage to affiliating with PROMINA is centralized managed-care contracting, which is expected to bring us more business."[55]

In the beginning, the decision to become a part of PROMINA appeared to be a good one for DRHS. There were physicians who contended they could have done better on their own, but the majority conceded that PROMINA was obtaining more managed-care contracts at better rates than they could have secured individually.[56] There were departments that said they were getting better prices on drugs and supplies before joining PROMINA, but most agreed that the member hospitals were benefiting from the cost savings of bulk buying. CEO Bernard Brown reported that PROMINA saved $25 million to $30 million annually in supplies and services through centralized purchasing.[57] Gerlach said that in DRHS's first year in PROMINA, it saved $1.7 million on supplies, equipment, and services and shared significantly in the nearly 200,000 covered lives secured by PROMINA's managed-care contracts.[58] In its second year, the total PROMINA savings amounted to $12.3 million, PROMINA's managed-care organization claimed 225,000 covered lives, and the cost savings and managed-care contracting benefits continued to evolve and improve.[59] There was a general enthusiasm in being part of a new and powerful organization that supported and benefited the hospitals, physician practices, and the communities they served.

But there also were major challenges, some of which had been anticipated. From the outset, the CEOs of the member systems admitted that it was a tall order to expect each hospital system to put the interest of the PROMINA system above its individual interests. The challenge of getting the members to function like an integrated system as opposed to a federation of independent states was a daunting one. DeKalb's Gerlach acknowledged, "There's a loss of power, and you can feel personally threatened. It's hard to change overnight from a stand-alone system to a partner with your former competitors."[60] WellStar CEO Thomas Hill predicted, "We probably have not yet really tackled the tough issues, such as the relative roles of the LIDS and the parent organization. I think that our congenial little group of LIDS executives is in for some tough debates. How we work through them will be Promina's ultimate test."[61] The late Robert Lipson, MD, who succeeded Thomas Hill as president and CEO of the WellStar Health System, observed, "Theoretically, we've given everyone a voice. But it could be ten years or more before we know if this is really working."[62] Frank Rinker, president and CEO of the Gwinnett Health System, predicted that "it remains to be seen whether we can pull together to create a common culture that will enable PROMINA to think and act as a single company when it needs to."[63]

They were right. PROMINA was described in the March 1997 issue of *Hospital and Health Networks* magazine as America's most integrated system.[64] PROMINA CEO Bernard Brown described the organization as "a hybrid of vertical, horizontal and virtual integration."[65] But those who knew PROMINA well knew it was far from integrated. The concept that it could voluntarily act like an integrated system while maintaining local autonomy proved to be unrealistic. While managed-care con-

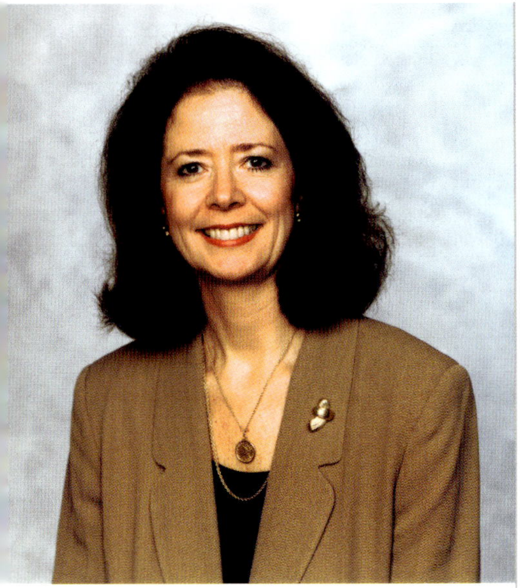

Bonnie Phipps, DeKalb's former chief financial officer, became the CEO of PROMINA in June of 2001.

tracting was centralized from the beginning, while benefits and human resources policies were standardized early on, and while compliance policies were adopted uniformly across the system, other initiatives never materialized despite the investment of considerable resources, time, and energy.

Systemwide "clinical integration," in which physicians across the system accepted and utilized identified best practices, never replaced traditional local practices of providing health services. Shared information systems and shared medical information never materialized. Efforts to introduce certain service excellence programs across the system met with a lack of readiness or willingness on the part of members. Despite the desire, commitment, and dedicated effort to attain the goal of integration, the task proved greater than the capacity of those seeking to make it happen.

PROMINA experienced multiple changes in leadership. One of the distinct advantages that attracted DRHS to PROMINA was the common culture shared by its members and the long-standing collegiality of its leaders. Charles Eberhart and John Gerlach at DeKalb, Thomas Hill at WellStar, Frank Rinker at Gwinnett, Richard Hubbard at Piedmont, Eugene Leblond at Southern Regional, and Bernard Brown formerly at WellStar all knew, respected, and trusted one another. As Piedmont CEO Richard Hubbard observed, "PROMINA's glue is mutual trust."[66]

All of that changed in rapid fashion. In April 2000 the Southern Regional board of directors asked Eugene Leblond to resign.[67] A year later, in June 2001, PROMINA CEO Bernard Brown retired to be replaced by Bonnie Phipps. Phipps, DeKalb's former chief financial officer, was president of the PROMINA Health Plan.[68] She resigned her PROMINA position one year later to become CEO of St. Joseph's Hospital.[69] In December 2001 Piedmont CEO Richard Hubbard retired to be replaced by R. Timothy Stack.[70]

PROMINA began to lose members. Soon after DRHS joined, WellStar expressed dissatisfaction with some of PROMINA's decisions and initiatives. In October 1998 the WellStar board voted to withdraw.[71] WellStar had been the instigator of PROMINA and its first member. Its withdrawal was a major blow to the image and the effectiveness of the organization, fracturing the system's dominance in the market and leaving PROMINA without a significant presence in northwest Atlanta.[72]

WellStar's withdrawal was a contentious one. PROMINA bylaws provided for only three conditions under which a member could leave the system: (1) when continued membership posed an imminent legal and/or financial threat to the member; (2) when changes in the law or the economics of the healthcare industry made the PROMINA affiliation obsolete; and (3) when PROMINA had breached its obligations regarding the powers the bylaws granted the member.[73] It is unclear on what condition WellStar based its withdrawal, but there was a major disagreement as to how much money WellStar owed the organization.[74] PROMINA eventually sued WellStar before a settlement was finally reached.[75]

Next Piedmont left. In the spring of 2002, Piedmont CEO Timothy Stack stated publicly that his system was reassessing its role in PROMINA and that it also might leave the organization.[76] In October 2002 Piedmont proposed two options for remaining a member. The first was that Timothy Stack be named PROMINA's CEO and sole director.[77] The other was that Piedmont manage PROMINA for two years after which Piedmont could continue that arrangement or could walk away with no penalty.[78] DeKalb, Gwinnett, and Southern Regional rejected both proposals. In November 2002 Piedmont issued a letter of intent to withdraw from PROMINA. PROMINA reached a final settlement with Piedmont in August 2003.[79]

PROMINA, which once boasted five strong members and fourteen hospitals that covered nearly the entire metropolitan market area, now had three members with five hospitals and only partial geographical coverage. Yet, these three remaining members—DeKalb, Gwinnett, and Southern Regional—pledged to continue working together on integrated quality initiatives, contracting, and purchasing. They agreed to going forward with a $40 million clinical information system known as QUEST (an acronym for Quality, Uniformity, Efficiency and Safety through Technology), designed to make patient care safer and more effective by reducing medical errors and to attract managed-care contracts.[80]

Finally PROMINA struggled financially. It lost substantial sums on its managed-care contracts, especially on its venture into at-risk contracts.

The ability to negotiate attractive managed-care contracts on behalf of its member hospitals and physicians was one of the keystones of the PROMINA organization. There was every reason to think that, with the strength of its members, the geographical coverage it enjoyed, and the experience of its leadership, PROMINA would be able to contract effectively on behalf of it constituency.

In 2002, Georgia Insurance Commissioner John Oxendine singled out PROMINA for not paying physicians in a timely manner for services provided, and in some cases, not paying them at all.

In 2002, however, Georgia Insurance Commissioner John Oxendine singled out PROMINA for not paying physicians in a timely manner for services provided, and in some cases, not paying them at all.[81] Those delays primarily involved "global, capitated at-risk" contracts that PROMINA negotiated with insurance carriers such as Blue Cross, Cigna, Humana, Coventry, and Aetna.[82] PROMINA agreed to provide care for the insurers' members at a predetermined rate. The insurers agreed to pay PROMINA a per-member, per-month rate or a per-procedure rate, and PROMINA was responsible for providing needed services and paying its hospitals and doctors. The hospitals and physicians, in turn, agreed to provide services according to the terms of the contracts. In exchange for those agreed-upon rates, insurers steered their members to the participating PROMINA hospitals and physicians.

With those contracts, if medical costs were higher than expected, PROMINA absorbed the losses. If medical costs were lower than expected, PROMINA reaped the financial benefits. Such risk arrangements were common when PROMINA was formed in 1994, but increasingly healthcare systems across the county ceased participating in them.[83]

PROMINA began losing money on its contracts as early as 1998. Some hospitals and physicians owed PROMINA money because they had exceeded the cost limitations to which they had agreed in their contracts. PROMINA kept tabs on these deficits but delayed calling on the hospitals and physicians to pay what they owed.[84] As a result, PROMINA was unable to pay complying hospitals and physicians such as the DeKalb LIDS. PROMINA began asking hospitals and physicians with deficits to pay up.[85] In addition, PROMINA asked its member systems to accept financial liability for a line of credit needed to meet its claims payment obligations,[86] and it asked them to make PROMINA a loan to use for working capital.[87]

In addition to its existing debt, PROMINA's cash-flow deficits increased at a rapid rate.[88] Member systems were asked to provide more funds to cover additional losses that were discovered.[89] The total financial deficit eventually found was enormous.[90]

PROMINA discontinued all risk-based, capitated insurance contract arrangements in favor of traditional fee-for-service contracts. The process of working through the risk-managed contract commitments already in place, however, would require months.[91]

This development was threatening to PROMINA's viability. Its ability to negotiate favorable managed-care contracts on behalf of its members had been at the heart of the system's reason for being. Instead of providing financial benefits, the organization became a heavy financial burden.

Prior to joining PROMINA, DeKalb was an organization that the insurers needed. After PROMINA, DeKalb was an organization that needed the insurers.

PROMINA reduced its workforce from three hundred to sixty personnel[92] and launched a new initiative to negotiate fee-for-service contracts with insurers based on demonstrated quality of performance by its member hospitals and physicians. It called its new initiative "Rewards for Quality."[93] It would be based on the QUEST clinical information system involving a multiyear project to install a Computerized Physician Order Entry (CPOE) system and pharmacy information system in each of its hospitals at a cost of $40 million.[94] PROMINA counted on being able to market demonstrated quality service in the belief that employers were willing to pay top dollar in exchange for demonstrated quality.[95]

PROMINA, however, found that insurers were not buying what it was selling. It was unable to negotiate favorable contracts based on "demonstrated quality care." In the fall of 2003, PROMINA announced that its efforts to negotiate favorable contracts based on quality had met "with significant resistance" and it had been unsuccessful in getting managed-care plans to embrace PROMINA's Rewards for Quality program.[96] PROMINA then relinquished altogether its responsibility for managed-care contracting. As of November 1, 2003, that function reverted back to the local hospitals and the doctors within the system.[97]

The PROMINA board continues to exist, and the three remaining CEOs serve as a management group.[98] PROMINA as once structured, however, no longer exists. PROMINA bylaws were revised to make PROMINA essentially a joint venture of its remaining three members.[99] They participate in a group-purchasing organization known as Partners Cooperative Group Purchasing Organization, Inc.,[100] but the remaining member systems assumed responsibility for their own liability insurance.[101] None of the hospitals any longer bear the PROMINA name. There are only rare references to the once-prominent organization.

Joining PROMINA was a watershed event in the history of DeKalb Medical Center. The decision to join was made with good reasons and thoughtful, diligent, thorough deliberation. From nearly every perspective, it seemed the right thing to do at the time. It was an appropriate defensive decision as well as a proactive one. There appeared to be a clear need to become a part of a strong, collegial, geographically dispersed alliance given the managed-care environment and other market factors that catapulted onto the Atlanta scene, and PROMINA appeared to be DeKalb's best option.

There was a benefit from joining PROMINA. That benefit consisted of a new appreciation of the role that physicians must play in the future of healthcare systems. The PROMINA experience revealed the need, as never before realized, for a collaborative relationship between hospitals and physicians and for a new decision-making role physicians must have in health systems that thrive in the future.[102]

Yet joining PROMINA was costly. It imposed a financial loss far greater than any realized savings or return on investment. Those losses came at a time when DeKalb already faced other financial strains. Joining PROMINA also was costly in terms of the drain of leadership, energy, time, and focus that were diverted from the needs and opportunities of the local organizations. It was costly in terms of the alienation that developed between institutions, its leaders, and its physicians that had enjoyed a long history of friendship, respect, trust, and collegiality.

Joining PROMINA may have increased DeKalb's vulnerability to the will of managed-care organizations and other insurers. When the once formidable alliance came apart, it left each member on its own. Prior to joining PROMINA, DeKalb was an organization that the insurers needed. After PROMINA, DeKalb was an organization that needed the insurers.

THE PROMINA NEWS TRAIL

DeKalb medical Board Seeks OK of PROMINA Link
Atlanta Business Chronicle, Sept. 2, 1996

DeKalb Doctors Worry PROMINA Alliance Would Hurt Private Practice
Atlanta Business Chronicle, Aug. 16, 1996

PROMINA Northwest Recruits 165 More Doctors
Atlanta Business Chronicle, Oct. 14, 1996

Georgia Could Soon Have 50 Managed-Care Companies
Atlanta Business Chronicle, June 9, 1997

PROMINA Expects $63 Million Surplus This Year
Atlanta Business Chronicle, June 23, 1997

PROMINA Launches HMO, Aiming for 100,000 Members
Atlanta Business Chronicle, August 22, 1997

PROMINA is Atlanta's Grand health Care Experiment
Bernard Brown, *Pacesetters*, Hospitals and Health Networks, Fall 1998

Window of Opportunity: PROMINA Takes the Lead in Atlanta
Pacesetters, Hospitals and Health Networks, Fall 1998

PROMINA's CEO Says Integrated Delivery Works
Atlanta Business Chronicle, January 18, 1999

PROMINA Takes Bigger Role in Health Network
Atlanta Business Chronicle, June 15, 1999

PROMINA Flexes its Muscle in Managed Care
Atlanta Business Chronicle, August 25, 2000

Hospital CEOs Say Goodbye
"The friendships that forged PROMINA would suffer a blow"
Atlanta Business Chronicle, Dec. 21, 2001

Hospital Systems' $9M Dispute Now a Lawsuit
"Suing former partner Wellstar"
Atlanta Business Chronicle, Sept. 17, 2001

PROMINA CEO Quits, Joins St. Joe's as CEO
Atlanta Business Chronicle, July 19, 2002

PROMINA Restructures, Drops Managed Care Contracting
"Delegating the managed care contracting function to the local hospitals"
Atlanta Business Chronicle, Oct. 31, 2003

The Rise and Fall of an Empire
Bernard L. Brown Jr., *Lessons Learned on the Way Down*, 2008

Joining PROMINA made DeKalb part of a failed endeavor. Despite DeKalb's best motives, its best efforts, and its loyalty to the organization to the end, PROMINA was a failure. The reasons were many. Regardless of the reasons, the members had to live with the realization that they had given of their best when their best was not enough to achieve success. Many of the physicians who opposed the alliance continue to say, "We told you so."

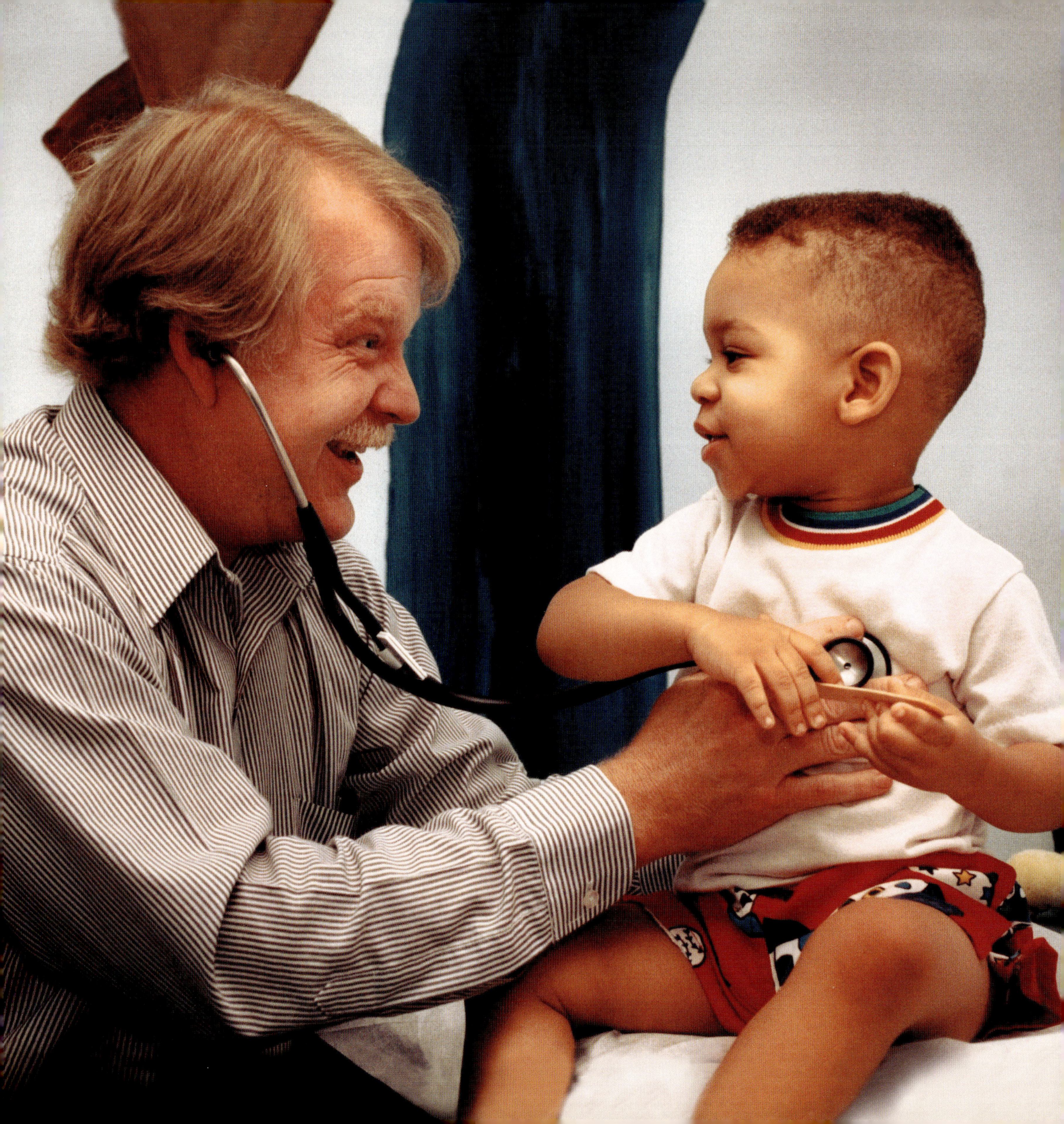

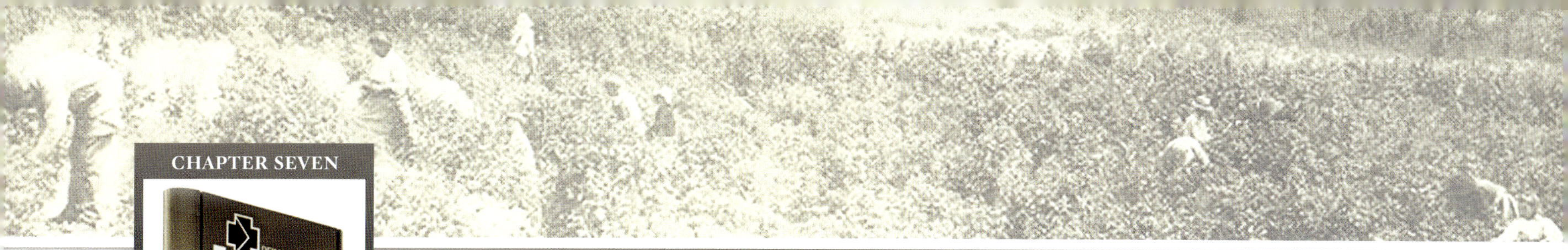

CHAPTER SEVEN

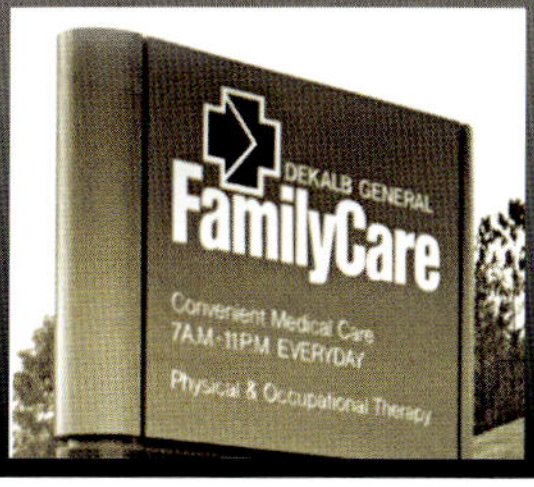

Vertical Integration: Primary Care and a Physician-Hospital Organization

DeKalb Medical Center was one of the few hospitals with a very strong primary care base. As managed care played a more active role in Atlanta, it became very important for the hospital to maintain and protect that base. Duane Barclay, DO, (opposite) a family physician, succeeded Andy Morley, MD, as director of the Primary Care Division for DeKalb Medical Center.

DeKalb Medical Center needed horizontal and vertical integration if it was to compete and thrive in the newly defined marketplace. It joined PROMINA to achieve horizontal integration, and it addressed the issue of vertical integration to align hospital and physician incentives on two fronts: protecting and enhancing its primary care physician base and creating a physician-hospital organization.

Protecting and Enhancing Its Primary Care Physician Base

Primary care physicians include family physicians (formerly known as general practitioners), general internists, obstetricians/gynecologists, and pediatricians. When managed care came to metropolitan Atlanta, DeKalb Medical Center was one of the few hospitals that had a strong primary care base that included general internists and family physicians. Emory Hospital, Piedmont Hospital, Crawford Long Hospital, Georgia Baptist Hospital, St. Joseph's Hospital, and Grady Memorial Hospital all had internists on their medical staff, but none had family physicians. All primary care physicians, on the other hand, had been an integral part of DeKalb Medical Center from its inception. J. Rufus Evans, MD, a general practitioner (family medicine did not become a specialty until 1969), spearheaded the creation of the hospital and was the first chairman of the DeKalb County Hospital Authority. Homer Allen, MD, a general practitioner, served as chairman of the DeKalb Medical Society's Medical Advisory Committee that wrote the hospital's first medical staff bylaws and its medical staff rules and regulations and that processed the first applicants to the medical staff. Floyd Sanders, MD, a general practitioner, was the second chief of staff and the second physician member (after Evans) to be elected to the Hospital Authority. Of the sixty-six original members of the medical staff, twenty-four were general practitioners and sixteen were general internists. The four physicians who served as DeKalb's first full-time emergency department staff were prominent general practitioners. A third of DeKalb Medical Center's chiefs of staff have been primary care physicians.

DeKalb Medical Center established three FamilyCare centers to provide primary care services to the community. In 1986 it opened FamilyCare South DeKalb and purchased FamilyCare Tucker. In April 1988 it opened FamilyCare Decatur at the corner of Church and Sycamore streets on the edge of the hospital campus.[1]

In 1990 DeKalb Medical Center contracted with four internists to become the first "hospitalists" in the state of Georgia.[2] DeKalb referred to these physicians as the Medical Emergency Associates, or MEAs. They admitted and managed patients who came to the Emergency Department needing hospital admission without a personal physician or without a physician on the hospital's medical staff. When those patients were ready for discharge, the MEA physicians referred them to a primary care physician for follow-up care.

In the 1990s managed-care organizations and other insurers looked at a hospital's base of primary care physician as a key factor in deciding which hospitals would receive favorable contracts. Many Atlanta hospitals and medically-related groups found themselves severely wanting. DeKalb Medical Center was in a strong negotiating position but at risk to be raided. In July 1993 CEO Charles Eberhart warned the DeKalb Medical Center Board of Directors:

> *As you may know, there is a virtual stampede going on in this market by a host of different entities, including venture capital organizations like American Health Care Groups, stock companies like Pacific, and others including Emory, Aetna, Decatur Hospital, Georgia Baptist Medical Center, and others to acquire primary care practices (mainly family practice and general internal medicine). There is a very real possibility that we could discover soon that the best and the brightest primary care practices that were supporting our specialists and hospital have been acquired by others and that the patients they were referring to us will be diverted to others.*[3]

"There is a very real possibility that we could discover soon that the best and brightest primary care practices that were supporting our specialists and hospital have been acquired by others and that the patients they were referring to us will be diverted to others."

— CEO Charles Eberhart to DeKalb Medical Center Board of Directors in July of 1993

Three weeks after Eberhart sent that memorandum to the board, one of DeKalb's busiest family physicians brought to him a letter that he and many members of the medical staff had received from Frank Hauser, MD, Emory's director of External Affairs, which said in part:

> *. . . The Emory University System of Health Care is considering the development of a network of doctors and hospitals across the metropolitan Atlanta Area. I am writing to you to explore the possibility of your involvement with us. . . . If you are interested in joining us in this venture, please complete the preliminary application enclosed and return it to me.*[4]

Emory, Georgia Baptist Medical Center, Decatur Hospital (prior to its being acquired by DeKalb Regional Healthcare System) and other hospitals began purchasing primary care practices and courting DeKalb's most supportive physicians. DeKalb took action to retain and increase its primary care physician base.

First it purchased the practices of physicians who wanted to be employed by the hospital. In July 1993 the DeKalb Medical Center Board of Directors approved a plan to purchase up to twenty of the most productive practices whose physicians had an interest in being acquired.[5] The board ranked that project as number one on its priority list and authorized more than $5 million to begin the initiative.[6] By 1996 DeKalb Medical Center had acquired ten practices that included eighteen physicians.[7] In addition to protecting its existing primary care base, DeKalb recruited additional physicians. By 1996 it had recruited and employed eleven new physicians.

DeKalb Medical Center established new primary care centers throughout its service area. It constructed or purchased facilities at Stone Mountain, Embry Hills, Snapfinger Woods, Candler Road, Chapel Hill, Killian Hills, Jimmy Carter Boulevard, Virginia Highland Avenue, Buford Highway and downtown Decatur.[8] It staffed those facilities with employed physicians and with private practice physicians who wished to relocate or expand their existing practices. By 1997 DeKalb had twenty-five practice sites staffed by over forty employed physicians and ten private practice physicians.[9]

It established an International Medical Center on Buford Highway with Tong Huynh, MD, as medical director to provide primary and urgent-care services to a diverse population that included African American, Korean, Vietnamese, Chinese, and Hispanic citizens. The center leased space to Scottish Rite Children's Medical Center to provide pediatric services.[10] DeKalb Medical Center also opened a Senior Health Center to provide senior citizens with primary care services, geriatric assessments, and consultative services.[11]

Owning and managing physician practices was a new experience for DeKalb Medical Center. Historically the relationship between the hospital and physicians had been one of mutual support with "no strings attached." In fact, one of the early requirements for membership on the medical staff was that the physician must be in the private practice of medicine and not salaried or employed by any institution. DeKalb Medical Center, therefore, had much to learn in a short period of time.

In December 1993 CEO Charles Eberhart and members of his staff visited Floyd County Hospital in Rome, Georgia. Floyd County Hospital had acquired twenty-five practices. The administrator told Eberhart's team that their experiment had been a happy one for the hospital and for the doctors because they had followed one cardinal principle: "Where things already are going well in the practice, the hospital left well enough alone and did not meddle with the management of the practice."[12]

DeKalb Medical Center, however, could not follow that advice. Unlike Floyd County Hospital, DeKalb had to coordinate and manage newly recruited physicians and newly established practices as well as experienced physicians and their existing practices. Eberhart named Andy Morley, MD, one of the community's family physicians, as director of the Primary Care Division. Morley provided oversight to the practices and physicians, negotiated with other physicians who wished to sell their practices, recruited new physicians, managed the primary care sites, developed new sites as needed and provided support services to hospital-owned practices as well as to physicians in private practice. Morley assembled a staff and created Network Medical Services, a management service organization.[13]

It was an expensive and complex undertaking that required a large support staff. The cost of providing Network Medical Services and other support to the primary care practices understandably resulted in a net operating loss in each of the early years.[15] In addition, some physicians who were accustomed to autonomy in operating their practices as they deemed appropriate, were unhappy with the new rules by which they had to operate and the perceived inefficiencies the rules entailed.

Hospital systems around the country began rethinking the value of hospital-owned practices. In 2002, the Hospital Corporation of America (HCA) divested itself of all its physician-owned practices.[16] In 2000, Southern Regional Medical System sold its practices after sustaining a $5 million operating

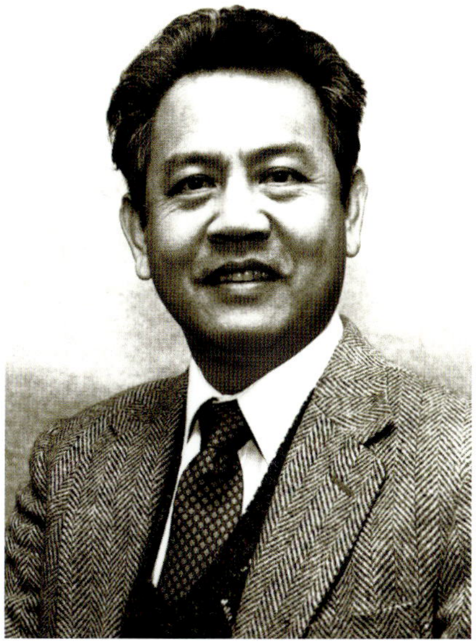

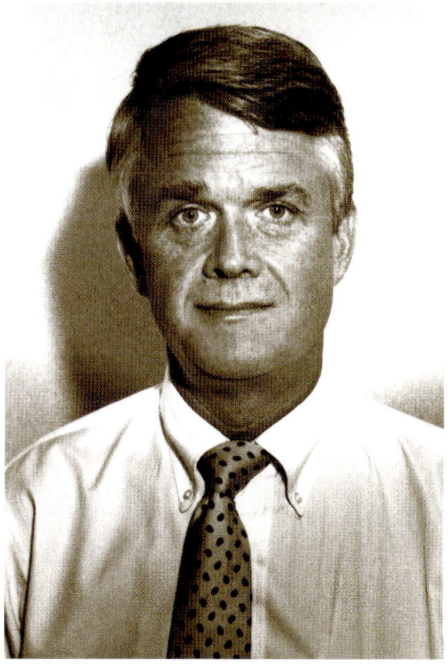

Top: Tong Huynh, MD, a family physician, was medical director at the International Medical Center. **Above:** Andy Morley, MD, a family physician in the community, was named director of the Primary Care Division for DeKalb Medical Center. Morley assembled a staff and created Network Medical Services, a management service organization.

loss in fiscal year 1999.[17] Furthermore, in addition to the cost of maintaining primary care networks, the healthcare market was changing. Insurers ceased ranking hospital systems according to the size of their primary care base. The keen competition between hospitals for primary care physicians, one of the primary reasons for DeKalb's getting into the business, was disappearing.

Despite the operating losses, DeKalb believed its Primary Care Division provided a positive value. The community still looked to primary care physicians as the main source of its medical care. Specialists who admitted patients to the hospital and used most of the hospital's services depended on primary care physicians' referrals.[18] DeKalb, therefore, elected to take a middle course and a modified strategy. It ceased acquiring existing practices or creating new primary care centers. It sold some of its acquired practices to physicians who wanted to return to private practice. It sold its FamilyCare Tucker center and its International Medical Center on Buford Highway.[19] And it looked for ways to economize its remaining operations. Duane Barclay, DO, succeeded Morley as director of the Primary Care Division and instituted a new business model.[20] The new model reduced the support staff and scope of support services[21] and instituted a more incentivized physician pay scale.[22]

DeKalb, still appreciative of the enormous value of primary care physicians, continues to actively recruit them to establish their own practices or to join existing practices in the community and to support them in a variety of ways to enhance their practices and their relationship with the DeKalb Medical system.

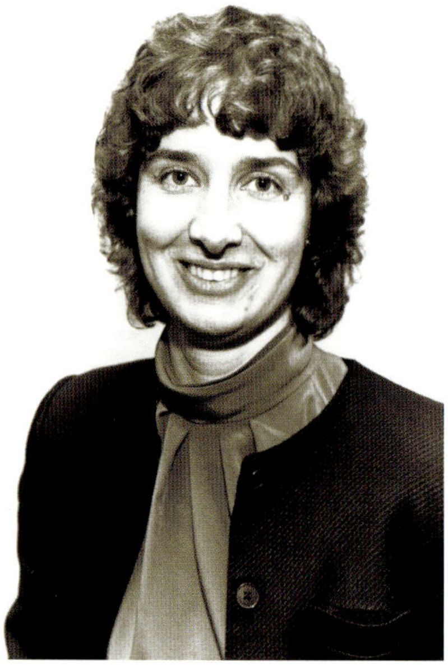

Martha Crenshaw, MD, is a family physician and past recipient of DeKalb Medical Society's Julius McCurdy Citizenship Award.

The Physician-Hospital Organization

For the first two decades, the hospital and physicians enjoyed a relatively happy and symbiotic relationship. Each benefited the other. Physicians used the hospital for its special care and services and as a place they could provide their own care and services. Hospital and physicians were reimbursed for the services each provided by out-of-pocket payments by patients, by insurance reimbursements, or by a combination of the two.

The hospital benefited from physicians' orders. The longer physicians kept patients in the hospital and the more care and services they ordered, the more the hospital was paid. And the longer patients remained in the hospital and the more care and services physicians provided, the more they were paid. Medicare and Medicaid initially paid physicians and hospitals on the basis of the specific care and services provided, even if they were paid at a reduced rate.

All that changed in the mid-1980s. In October 1983 Medicare instituted what was known as the Prospective Payment System that classified hospitalized patients according to diagnosis, type of treatment, age, and other criteria. Hospitals received a predetermined payment for each patient according to those criteria. Medicare paid physicians for procedures they performed or services they provided based on a national uniform value scale.[23]

Under the new system, if the physician ordered tests and services that cost the hospital more to provide than Medicare paid, the hospital absorbed the loss. The physician's ordering pen, therefore, became one of the most powerful factors in the hospital's financial viability.

Other insurers followed Medicare's lead and began paying predetermined amounts according to a patient's diagnosis or procedure. Expectant mothers were given only an allotted amount of time to deliver their babies and recover.

Eventually insurers negotiated "capitated" contracts with hospitals and physicians in which the insurer paid a given amount of money per patient, per month, in return for which physicians and hospitals agreed to provide all the medical services required for that insurer's patients. If the enrolled patients required few medical services, the contracting physicians and hospitals realized a profit. If those patients required care and services that cost more than the insurer agreed to pay, the physicians and/or hospitals had to absorb the loss.

These changes drastically altered the symbiotic relationship that once existed between physician and hospital. Instead of consistently benefiting from the physician's orders, those orders could now place the hospital at financial risk. The more care and services the physician ordered, the more the hospital was at risk for financial loss.

In addition to imposing financial constraints, the public and payors began looking at the quality of care provided by physicians and hospitals, the outcomes achieved, patient safety data, and patient satisfaction scores.

The hospital had to do a better job of aligning hospital and physician incentives. As a first step, the hospital and physician leaders took an educational approach and informed physicians about these changes and the crucial role the physician played in the hospital's financial viability. They provided physicians with confidential reports on the cost of providing care for their patients as compared with that of their colleagues. They also shared with physicians their mortality rates, infection rates, and other quality, safety, and patient-satisfaction data.

Physician leaders developed and recommended to their colleagues "best-practice" models for high-quality, cost-efficient care of major diagnoses such as pneumonia, heart attacks, strokes, and commonly performed surgical procedures. Those educational, voluntary efforts enhanced physician awareness, altered some practice patterns, and generally improved the efficiency and quality of patient care. Yet, more was needed.

In 1993 CEO Charles Eberhart proposed that DeKalb Medical Center and its physicians form a physician-hospital organization to move the physician-hospital relationship to a higher level.[24] Julian "Fred" Fuerst, MD, chief of staff, appointed an ad hoc committee that included physicians, administrators, and board members to study the concept.[25] Physicians strongly endorsed the idea[26] and voted 118-to-1 to go forward with its development.[27] A permanent fifteen-member committee was appointed, chaired by Michael Kinstler, MD,[28] that created the instrument for true vertical integration, the DeKalb Physician-Hospital Organization (DPHO).[29]

The DPHO was incorporated in February 1994 and became operational the following August.[30] Its board of directors was composed of three primary care physicians, three specialty physicians, and three hospital representatives. The DPHO board elected Kinstler as its first chairman[31] and named Judy Mitchell, the hospital's director of Managed Care, as its first chief executive officer.[32]

The DPHO had a membership fee of $250 each for primary care physicians and $1,000 for specialty physicians. DeKalb Medical Center matched the physician fees, and the DeKalb Medical Center Board of Directors advanced the DPHO a five-year line of credit of $2,000,000 for start-up expenses.[33] Out of 179 eligible primary care physicians, 93 joined; and out of 160 eligible specialty physicians, 144 joined.[34] The membership included twenty-nine hospital-based physicians.[35]

The DPHO was a collaborative initiative between the hospital system and physicians to negotiate contracts with managed-care organizations, other insurers, and employers. It was a single, integrated negotiating entity to compete for contracts more effectively than physicians or hospitals could negotiate individually and to align physician-hospital incentives.[36]

By November 1994 the DPHO had contracts with U.S. Healthcare, MetLife, and United

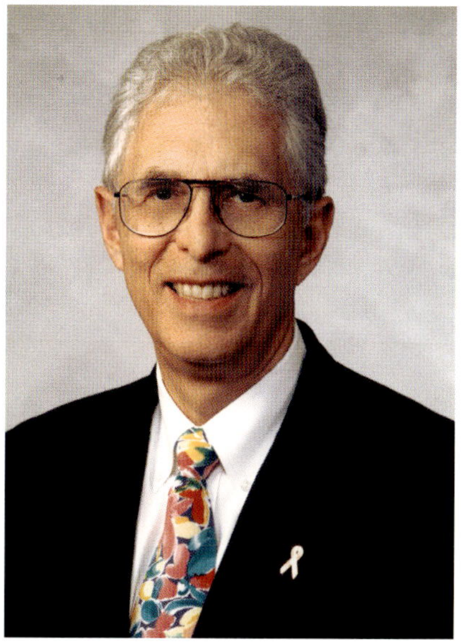

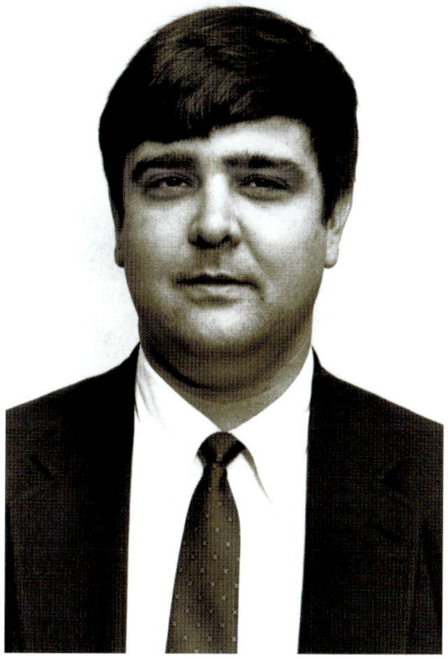

Top: Julian "Fred" Fuerst, MD, was chief of staff and responsible for appointing the committee to study the DeKalb Physician-Hospital Organization concept. **Above:** Michael Kinstler, MD, was the first chairman of the DeKalb Physician-Hospital Organization. The organization was incorporated in February of 1994 to negotiate more favorable contracts than individuals could obtain on their own, and to align physician-hospital incentives.

Healthcare of Georgia,[37] and it entered into a capitation contract with U.S. Healthcare involving between three thousand and five thousand individuals.[38] In 1996 it developed its own DPHO Health Plan for DeKalb Regional Healthcare System employees.[39]

Early in 1996 the DeKalb Medical Center Board of Directors became concerned about the financial viability of the DPHO. The DPHO had hired nine full-time staff members, had used all the physician membership fees and hospital matching funds, had drawn down more than $500,000 of the $2 million line of credit extended by the hospital, and still had not generated positive revenue.[40] In March of 1996, however, the DPHO reported a profit.[41]

One of its early sources of revenue was its contract with the DeKalb Medical Center to provide clinical oversight of the hospital's Medical Management Program, a program that monitored the efficiency and effectiveness of the patient care provided.[42] The DPHO monitored and encouraged cost-effective, high-quality medicine.[43] It reviewed inpatient care to assess the appropriateness of the assigned level of care, treatment plans, discharge plans, and other clinically related issues. DPHO physicians interacted with admitting physicians when problems were identified. The hospital paid the DPHO $25,000 a month for the service and shared with the DPHO a percentage of the savings achieved.[44] In the first five months of its contract, the DPHO saved the hospital $2 million[45] and, with the fees and bonus earned, repaid the entire line of credit loan advanced by the hospital.[46] The DPHO subsequently continued seeking to sustain a positive financial performance.[47]

One impediment to profitability was the difficulty of collecting what it was owed by PROMINA. When DeKalb Regional Healthcare System joined PROMINA, it was required to have a Local Integrated Delivery System (LIDS) to review and approve PROMINA's proposed managed-care contracts and to manage those contracts once signed. The DPHO became DeKalb's LIDS. It was successful in implementing and managing even the at-risk contracts that PROMINA negotiated in which hospitals and physicians were responsible for needed services to a population of patients for a predetermined amount of money.[48] When PROMINA encountered financial problems due to deficits incurred by other LIDS, however, it was unable to pay the DPHO what it was owed. DPHO showed a profit of $7.8 million, but PROMINA was able to pay DPHO only $3.6 million.[49] DPHO finally reached a settlement with PROMINA, but received only a portion of the remainder it was owed.[50]

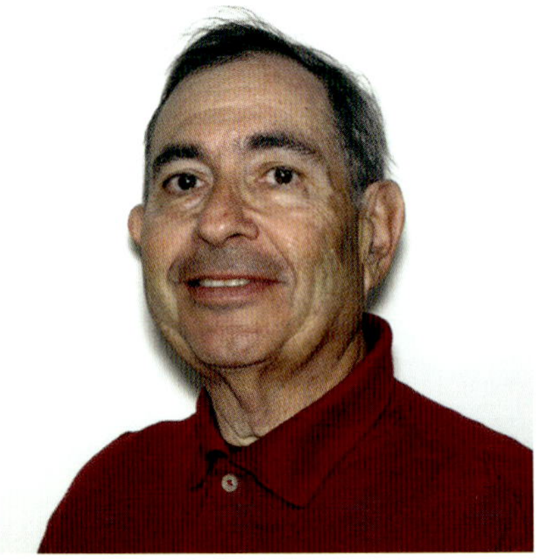

The DeKalb Physician-Hospital Organization chose Albert Wildstein, MD, to be its second chairman in 2001.

In 2001 the DPHO board elected Albert Wildstein, MD, as its second chairman.[51] In 2003, after PROMINA relinquished to its members responsibility for negotiating their own contracts, Wildstein led the DPHO in creating a new type of agreement with Blue Cross called "pay for performance."[52] Physicians supported the agreement, and DeKalb Medical Center and Decatur Hospital subsequently became participants. It was a joint clinical integration concept designed to achieve reimbursement based on demonstrated quality, efficiency, and safety of patient care.[53]

To document and demonstrate its quality and efficiency, DPHO agreed to document its patient care and compare it against recognized benchmarks. To measure its performance, CEO Eric Norwood and his team established the DeKalb Quality Institute and named Steve Meurer, PhD, as its first director. Cathleen Wheatley, RN, later succeeded Steve Meurer. The institute collected and analyzed data, identified best practices in the health industry, helped develop new standards, and measured and reported DeKalb's performance to the hospitals, the physicians, and the insurers.[54]

The nationally recognized Health Care Advisory Board named DPHO's clinical integration model as its top pick of best practices for physician-hospital relationship development.[55] DPHO is

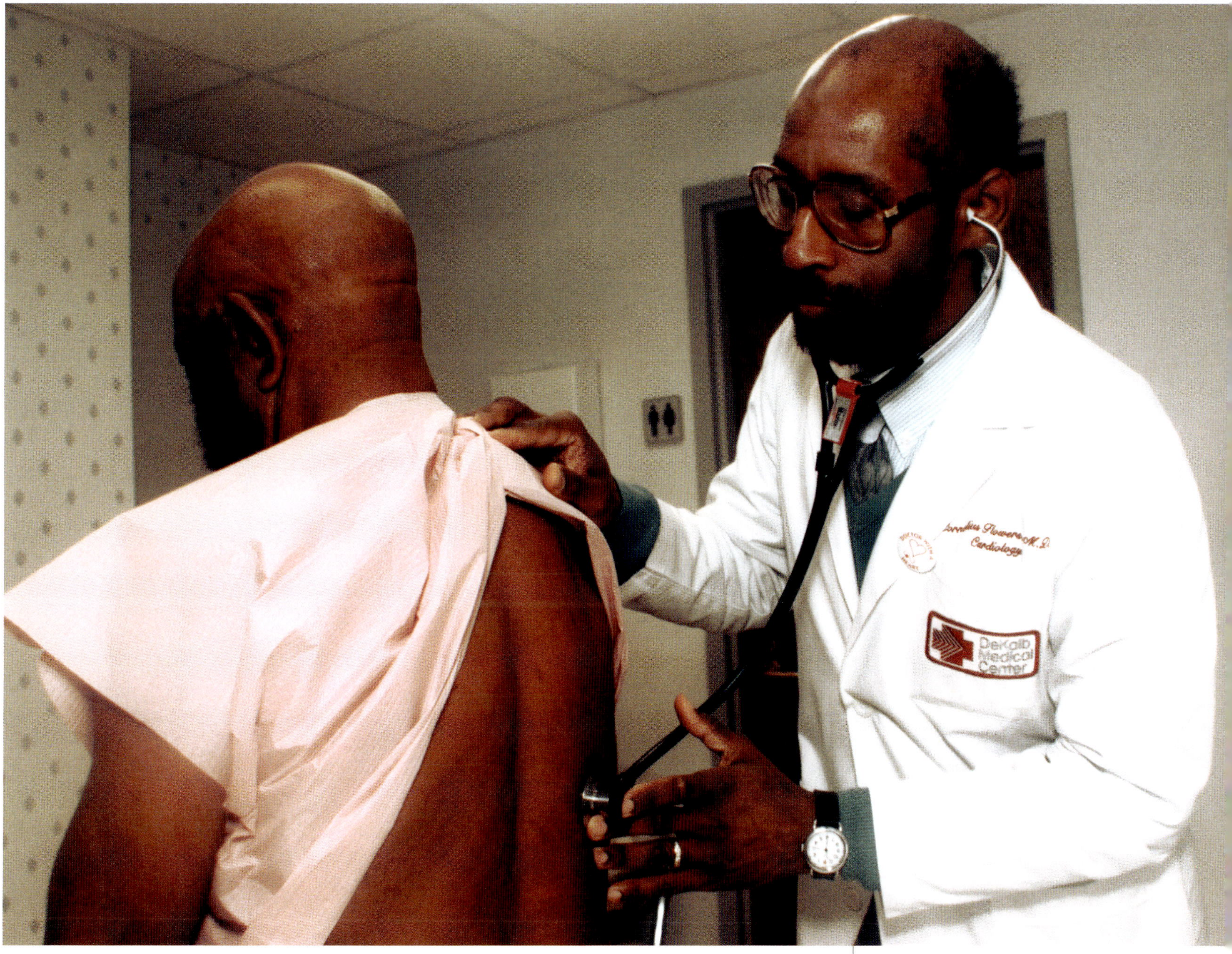

recognized as one of the strongest and most effective physician-hospital organizations, not only in the region, but in the nation. It has had extraordinary physician, staff, hospital, and governing body leadership and support. It has operated like a business with decisions and rules not always popular. But it has achieved a remarkable degree of service to the community, DeKalb Medical, and physicians and has taken vertical integration a giant step forward in aligning physician and hospital incentives.

Cornelius Flowers, MD, a cardiologist internist at DeKalb Medical, examines an adult patient.

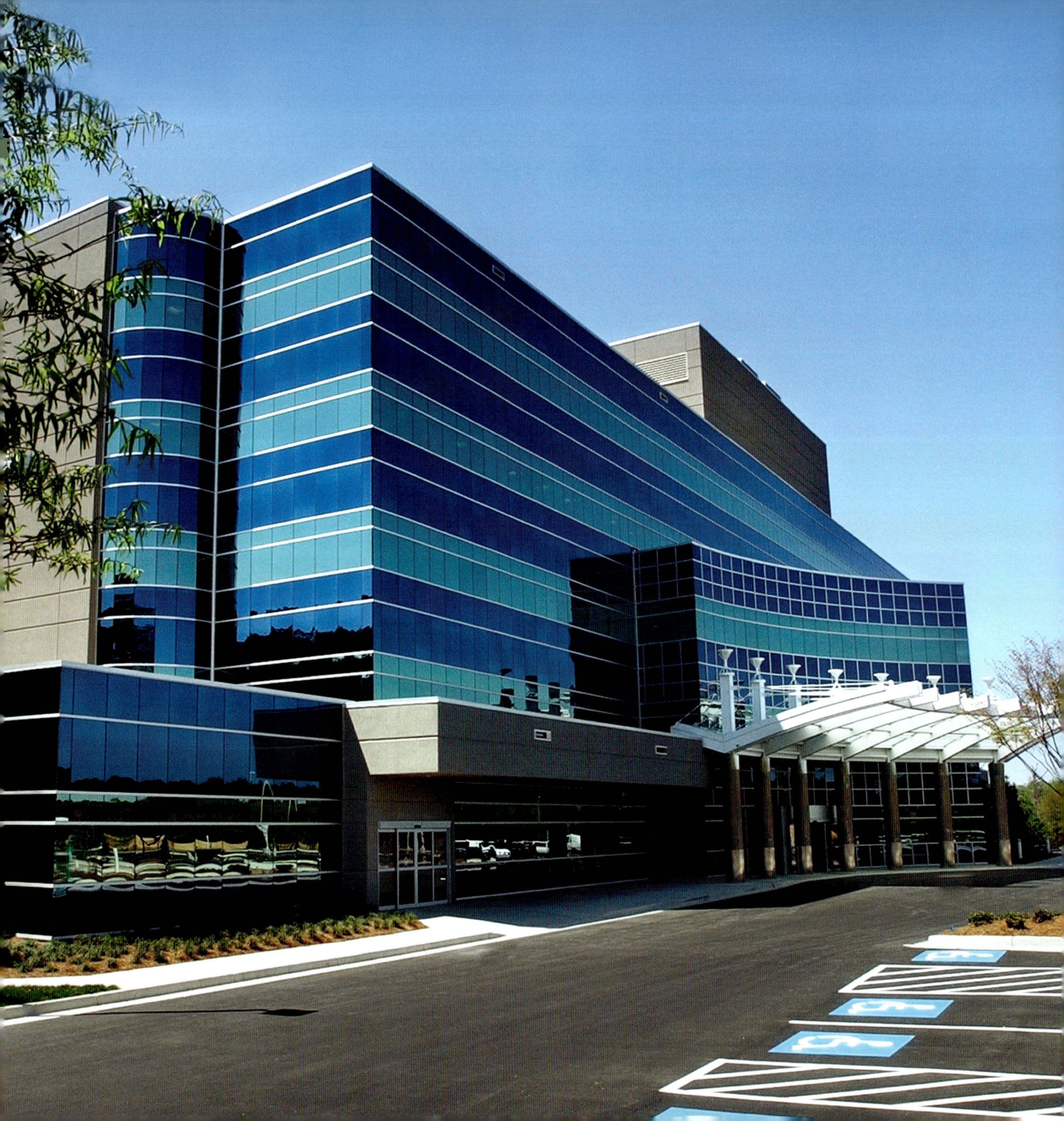

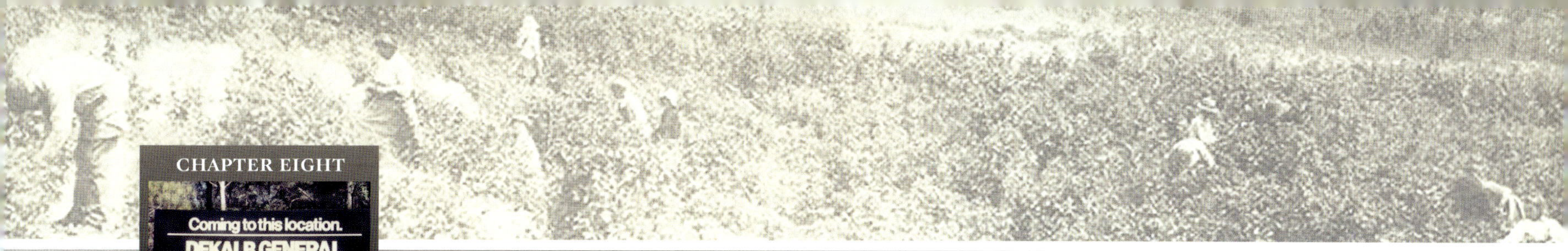

CHAPTER EIGHT

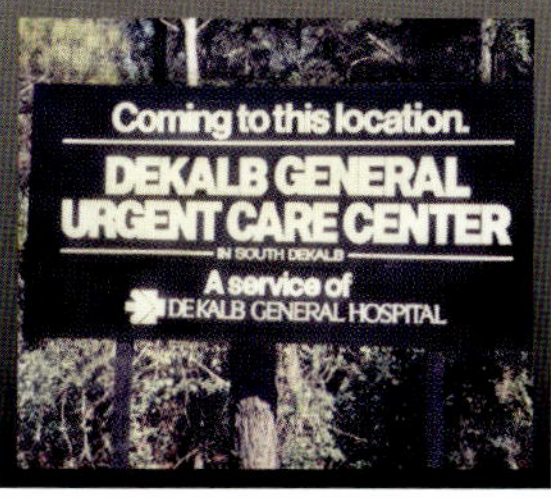

DeKalb Medical Adds Two Hospitals

THE 1957 CONSTITUTION OF THE DEKALB COUNTY HOSPITAL AUTHORITY STATED THAT

> *The general purpose of the Authority shall be to erect and operate one or more hospitals for the care of the sick in the county. For the better execution of this general purpose, the Authority may provide and operate hospitals and sanitariums, dormitories, clinics, housing accommodations, or other public buildings for the use of patients and officers and employees of any institution under the supervision and control of the Authority. . . .* [1]

Opposite: DeKalb Medical at Hillandale Hospital.

The Authority and the ensuing governing bodies responded to that commission by adding two hospitals to the DeKalb Medical system, DeKalb Medical at Downtown Decatur and DeKalb Medical at Hillandale.

DeKalb Medical at Downtown Decatur

Decatur Hospital (now known as DeKalb Medical at Downtown Decatur) was established when DeKalb General Hospital was going through a period of growth, renovation, and expansion that limited its capacity and services. In its first decade, DeKalb General experienced an explosive growth in the volume of patients. The population and the number of physicians in its service area grew exponentially. The demand for beds, services, and operating time exceeded the hospital's capacity and led to a renovation and expansion that more than doubled the number of beds and added a skilled nursing facility and a mental health unit.

This project offered desperately needed relief to the growing demand for hospital services, but getting there was long, painful, and costly. Construction required three years, from July 1968 to July 1971. It involved closing existing beds already in short supply; curtailing even more the hospital's surgical capacity; forcing the support staff to work out of temporary quarters; and creating noise, dust, and inconveniences that staff, physicians, and patients had to endure. A mass resignation of nurses in 1969 further curtailed beds and services.

Physicians had difficulty admitting patients to the hospital or scheduling them for surgery. Emergency admissions had first priority, urgent cases could be admitted only when rarely available space permitted, and elective admissions and surgical procedures were essentially nonexistent.

Against that background, a group of physicians and oral surgeons saw an opportunity to build and operate a private, for-profit hospital in Decatur. They formed a limited partnership known as the Decatur Professional Investors with three general partners and approximately ninety limited partners. Limited partners purchased interest in the partnership at $11,000 a share.[2] It was not only an opportunity for a good financial return; it was also an answer to the shortage of hospital beds and surgical services.

A group of physicians and oral surgeons saw an opportunity to build a private, for-profit hospital in Decatur. It was not only an opportunity for a good financial return; it was also an answer to the shortage of hospital beds and surgical services. Decatur Hospital opened in 1973.

Many of the investors were physicians on the DeKalb General medical staff, which caught the attention of the DeKalb Hospital Authority. The Authority, concerned about a conflict of interest, asked its Professional Service Committee to meet with three of the investors who were DeKalb General Hospital-based physicians. The committee met with each of the physicians and asked three questions:

1. Was the physician financially invested in Decatur Hospital?
2. Did the physician plan to remain at DeKalb General Hospital?
3. Did the physician feel there was a conflict of interest?

Each physician answered "yes" to the first two questions and "no" to the third question.[3] The Authority accepted their answers and did not raise the issue again.

Decatur Hospital opened in 1973. It was a six-story facility that contained 120 licensed beds, including 91 medical-surgical beds, 4 intensive care beds, and 25 substance abuse beds. The hospital eventually focused on three key services: outpatient surgery, substance abuse, and rehabilitation medicine. Ophthalmologists, orthopedists, otolaryngologists, plastic surgeons, urologists, oral surgeons, general surgeons, and podiatrists found the hospital convenient and efficient for outpatient procedures. A substance abuse unit was directed by Charles Allard, MD; and rehabilitation services that served patients with head injuries and other conditions resulting in neurological impairment were provided by Meadowbrook Atlanta Neurobehavioral Center.[4]

In 1977 Decatur Professional Investors contacted the DeKalb County Hospital Authority to say the hospital might be for sale.[5] The Authority appointed a committee to investigate the matter. Neither side, however, made an offer, and the discussions were suspended.[6]

In 1979 OrNda Healthcorp (OrNda), a for-profit hospital management company, signed a twenty-year lease with Decatur Professional Investors to manage and operate the hospital. OrNda paid slightly less than $62,000 a month for a lease that included the right to purchase the building and an option to buy the land on which Decatur Hospital was constructed.[7]

In 1991 OrNda contacted the newly named DeKalb Medical Center (DMC) to say it was interested in selling its Decatur Hospital operation. OrNda was restructuring its holdings, and Decatur Hospital was its only medical facility in Georgia. It would either sell its operation or enter into some type of joint venture with an interested partner.[8]

DMC saw several advantages in acquiring Decatur Hospital. Doing so would expand DMC's ambulatory surgery business, including the services of podiatrists who were on staff at the Decatur Hospital. It would add a significant substance abuse service and would broaden DMC's rehabilitation marketshare with Meadowbrook's neurobehavioral program. It would acquire 120 additional licensed hospital beds without having to go through the certificate of need (CON) process as would be required by the state for adding new beds to an existing facility; and though small in volume, Decatur Hospital's inpatient medical and surgical business would also be a good addition. Finally, as a defensive measure, acquiring Decatur Hospital would prevent it from falling into the hands of one of DMC's major competitors such as Georgia Baptist Hospital, Tenet Healthcare Corporation, or the Hospital Corporation of America (HCA).[9]

In the meantime, in 1992 the DeKalb County Hospital Authority approved a restructured governance plan that created DeKalb Medical Center Inc. (DMC) and its parent body, DeKalb Regional Healthcare System Inc. (DRHS). In July 1993 the DMC Board of Directors made an offer of $9 million to OrNda to buy its operation, the hospital building, and the option to purchase the land.[10] OrNda, of course, did not own the building or the land. It only owned the operational rights, equipment, supplies, inventory, goodwill, business relations, the name of the hospital, and other items related to the operating business of the hospital, and an option to purchase the building and the land. DMC's offer would require OrNda to exercise its right to buy the building and retain the option to purchase the land.[11]

OrNda rejected the offer of $9 million, saying it was too low.[12] DMC then offered OrNda $9 million for its current holdings and an additional $3,650,000 to purchase the building and the option to buy the land. The offer stipulated that if OrNda could buy the building and the option to buy the land for less than $3,650,000, it could keep half of the savings.[13]

In 1991, DeKalb Medical Center saw several advantages in acquiring Decatur Hospital. On June 10, 1994, after much negotiation, the right to operate the hospital was purchased for $6 million.

In December 1993 DMC's parent company, DRHS, decided that DMC was not the proper vehicle to acquire Decatur Hospital because of several issues that included its Hill-Burton obligations, differences in medical staff bylaws, and differences in salary scales and benefits. It therefore created Decatur Health Resources Inc. (DHR) as a new, nonprofit, tax-exempt entity to purchase and operate Decatur Hospital. DHR was incorporated in May 1994 with DRHS as its parent company,[14] and DHR made the same offer to OrNda.

DMC/DRHS CEO Charles Eberhart expected the deal to close by the end of December 1993 or mid-January 1994 at the latest.[15] The closing, however, did not take place on either of those dates. OrNda attributed the delay to some "unresolved problems on their end,"[16] but Eberhart was concerned that OrNda was shopping around for a better offer. OrNda insisted that that was not the case. OrNda said their "problems" involved several mergers and acquisitions that it was negotiating and associated capital gains tax issues. OrNda wanted to show the Decatur Hospital sale as a financial loss to offset profits from its other transactions, but it did not want to reveal the loss until after an upcoming shareholders meeting.[17]

In the meantime, other information came to light. OrNda was not able to reach an agreement with Decatur Professional Investors to buy the building. DRHS said that reduced significantly the value of OrNda's Decatur Hospital operation. In March 1994 Eberhart sent a revised purchase agreement to OrNda that changed DHR's offer from $9 million to $6 million and that removed the requirement that OrNda purchase the facility and land option.

OrNda made no response. On April 13 attorney Robert Baudino, on behalf of DHR and DRHS, wrote to OrNda saying that if OrNda did not respond in writing with an acceptance or rejection of the offer by the end of the business day on April 14, DHR's offer would be withdrawn.[18] OrNda accepted the revised offer of $6 million, and DHR closed the deal on June 10, 1994.[19] The DeKalb Regional Healthcare System now included another 120 licensed beds and approximately 190 new employees.[20]

DHR spent an additional $1 million purchasing clinical and other equipment for Decatur Hospital. It still had to decide what to do about the building. Eberhart recommended purchasing the building from Decatur Professional Investors. He said the purchase price would be only slightly more than lease payments. The directors, however, elected to sign a five-year lease.[21]

DHR retained Carol Nikola, OrNda's chief executive officer, to remain in that position. She served for two years.[22] Richard T. Schmidt succeeded Nikola in 1996 and served as executive director until he retired in 2002.[23] Schmidt was followed by H. "Skip" Wright, III, who became executive director in 2002 and remained in the position until the position was discontinued in 2007 as part of a DRHS reorganization.[24]

Owning the new hospital was not easy. DeKalb Medical Center and Decatur Hospital, long-time competitors that were now part of the same family, found it challenging to work together as partners. Communication and collaboration did not come easily. At one meeting of the DRHS board of directors, CEO Carol Nikola identified thirty-one operational and communication issues that needed to be addressed to make the partnership work more smoothly.[25]

But the greatest problem in operating Decatur Hospital was financial. Operating losses persisted for DHR's first two years of ownership, totaling as much as $300,000 a month.[26] During Executive Director Richard Schmidt's tenure, Decatur Hospital changed from being a general medical/surgical facility to a specialty hospital. While continuing to provide its outpatient services, its ambulatory surgery services, and its specialties in ophthalmology, podiatry services, and primary care services to senior citizens, the hospital developed three new specialty services: the Wound Care Center, the Atlanta Laser Vision Center, and a long-term acute care (LTAC) service.[27] The addition of these services was to improve the hospital's image and its financial status.

The results, however, were not as positive as anticipated. The Wound Care Center offered outpatient care to patients with chronic wounds from a variety of sources including diabetes, cancer, burns, insect bites, pressure ulcers (bed sores), poor circulation, nonhealing surgical sites, swelling, and immunological disorders. The center provided a service to the hospital and to the community, but its financial picture was never encouraging. By the year 2000, it was losing $300,000 annually.[28] In the spring of 2002, the center was relocated to the second Professional Office Building on the North Decatur campus.[29] In its new location, it had greater exposure to members of the medical staff and their patients and the potential for a more favorable financial performance.[30]

In November 1996 Decatur Hospital contracted with the Atlanta Laser Vision Center to perform keratectomy surgery for nearsightedness using the hospital's new VISX excimer laser instrument that it had purchased for $575,000.[31] Twenty-two ophthalmologists underwent training to perform the procedure.[32] Patient volume for this service, however, never met expectations.[33] In November 1997 the hospital discontinued its contract with the Atlanta Laser Vision Center, renovated the space, and signed an agreement with The Laser Center, an international refractive surgery company with over forty surgery centers, to take over eye surgery in the hospital. The Laser Center made the facility open to all ophthalmologists on the staff.[34] It had a strong referral relationship with optometrists, and it paid Decatur Hospital $10,000 a month to use the hospital's space and equipment, plus an additional fee for each patient in excess of forty per month.[35] That arrangement was more successful. In 1998 Decatur Hospital sold its VISX Excimer laser to The Laser Center which relocated it to The Laser Center's Buckhead site.[36] It had been used very sparingly, and the sale enabled the hospital to recover at least a portion of its investment.

The most successful of the three innovations was the LTAC service that Decatur Hospital established in October 1996 under the medical direction of Thomas DeMarini, MD. The LTAC Unit provided care for medically stable patients who required daily physician management, six to eight hours of intensive nursing, and respiratory care. Many of the patients were on ventilators and cardiac monitors.

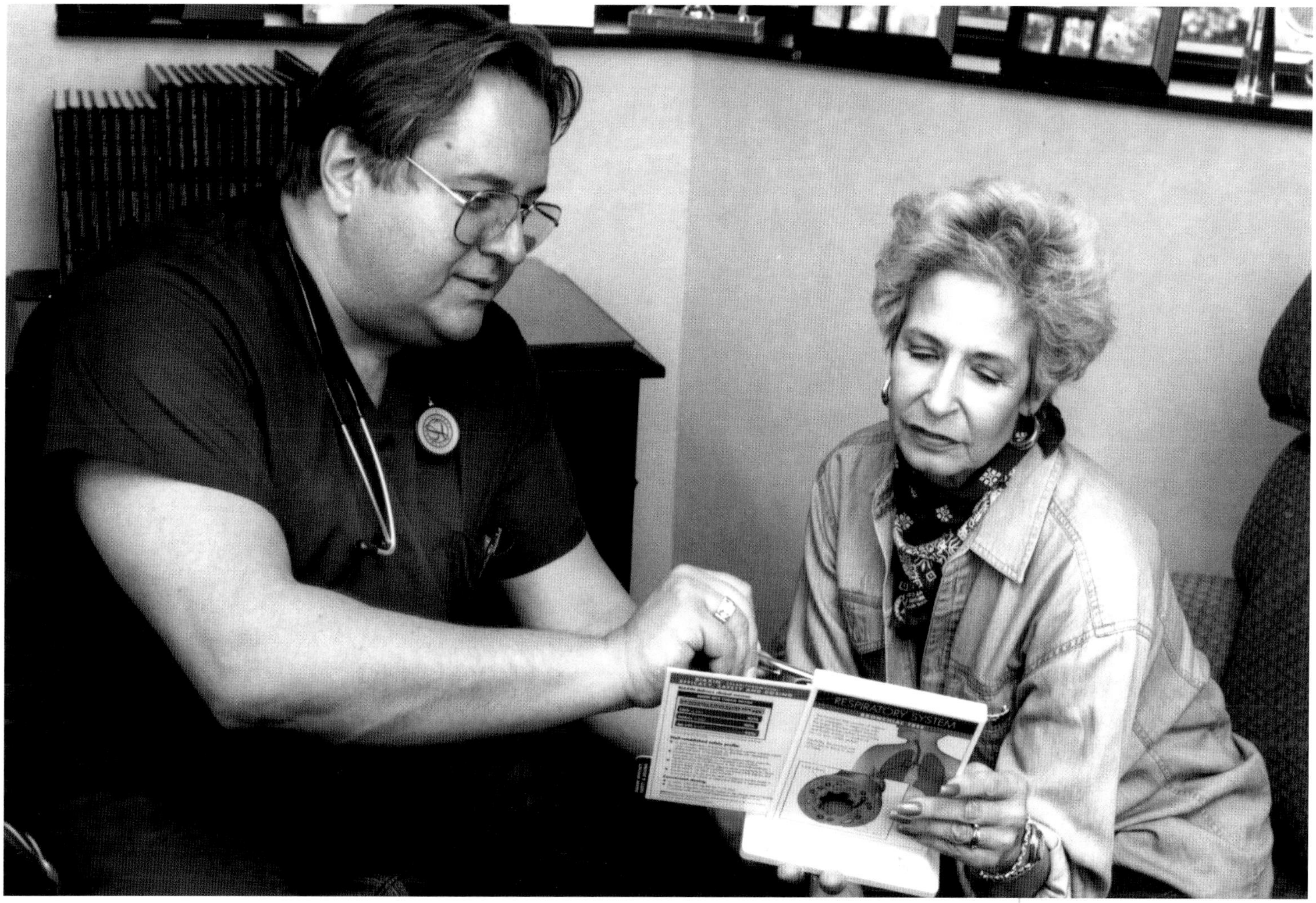

In 1996 Thomas DeMarini, MD, pulmonologist, became medical director of the Long-Term Acute Care service at the Downtown Decatur Hospital.

Patients remained on the service for an average of seven weeks.[37] With good medical management and attention to proper nutrition, the service helped patients become independent of ventilators.[38] The unit opened on the fifth floor of the hospital with six beds.[39] It expanded to twenty-one beds in 1997[40] and then to twenty-nine beds.[41] In 1997 Decatur Hospital received certification as an LTAC hospital.[42] By the spring of 1998, there were as many as nine patients at a time on the admission waiting list,[43] which, in 1999, prompted the hospital to expand the unit to forty-four beds at a cost of $1,110,000.[44] LTAC's advanced metabolic and nutritional assessment proved to be a key factor in patients' becoming independent of the ventilator.[45]

The LTAC Unit not only rendered a significant service to the community, but it promised to be one of the more profitable services for Decatur Hospital. In July 1997 Medicare declared the service to be exempt from fixed payments and eligible for reimbursement on the basis of the actual cost of providing care.[46] In 1999, however, Medicare changed its reimbursement rules and began paying on a per diem ($773 per day) basis regardless of the services required, with a cap of $38,600 per patient.[47] Finally, in 2003, Medicare instituted the Prospective Payment System (PPS) for LTAC, reimbursing the hospital a fixed amount according to the patient's diagnosis regardless of the services or the length of stay required.[48] In the meantime Decatur Hospital opened a new, six-bed Special Care Unit equipped to provide specialized patient care that permitted the LTAC Unit to admit and retain patients with a greater intensity of illness for whom there were enhanced Medicare reimbursements.[49]

In addition to reductions in reimbursement, there was a reduction in the source of its LTAC patients. Traditionally 40 percent of LTAC patients came to Decatur Hospital from outside DeKalb Medical's service area. In 2003 Southern Regional Medical Center and South Fulton Hospital each opened their own LTAC unit[50] with a subsequent decline in LTAC patients at Decatur Hospital.[51] Despite its reduction in patients and revenue, the unit continued to remain financially viable and to serve a major community need. In 2006 Decatur won the Joint Commission on Accreditation of Healthcare Organization's seal of approval as the first hospital in the nation to receive certification for working with patients diagnosed with respiratory failure and ventilator dependence.[52] The hospital is seeking certification in two more areas—diabetic retinopathy and cataracts—and is planning to have all-private rooms to enhance the appeal of the LTAC Unit.[53]

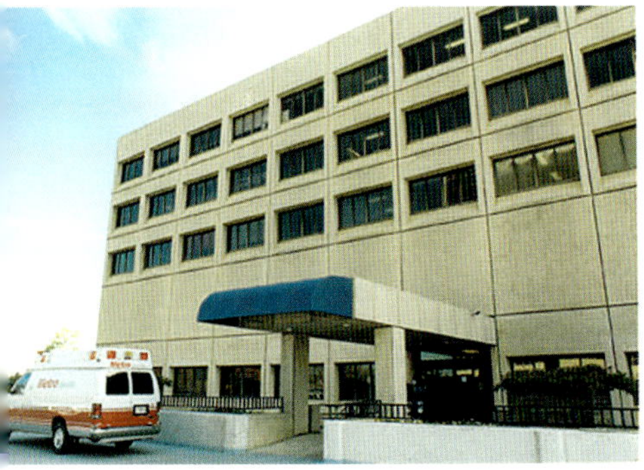

DeKalb Medical at Downtown Decatur.

In 1997, two years before the building lease was to expire, the directors of DRHS and DHR again faced the question of what to do about the Decatur Hospital building. The boards basically had five choices.

1. They could extend the present lease agreement to maintain the operation of the hospital with the option to buy the building and land, in which case they had to give notice of their intent to extend the lease six months before the current lease expired.
2. They could negotiate a new lease arrangement that would have to be finalized by the end of the current lease on January 31, 1999.
3. They could exercise a formal purchase option by which DHR would be obligated to buy the building at the fair market price agreed upon by three appraisers.
4. They could engage in informal purchase negotiations.
5. They could do none of the above and vacate Decatur Hospital at the end of its lease on January 31, 1999.[54]

The DRHS directors elected to follow the fourth option. They authorized DHR to initiate informal negotiations with Decatur Professional Investors.[55] The owners rejected DHR's first two offers, and DHR rejected the counter offers from Decatur Professional Investors. It appeared that an agreement was not possible and that DHR might walk away from Decatur Hospital.[56] Finally, Decatur Professional Investors accepted an offer of $6 million for the operation, the facility, and the land option. The closing took place on September 29, 1998, and Decatur Hospital became the property of DHR, a subsidiary of DRHS.[57]

In August 2007 the DeKalb Medical system's new strategic plan determined that DeKalb Medical at Downtown Decatur (the new name it gave Decatur Hospital) would focus on post-acute care services such as those provided by the LTAC Unit, home health services, and rehabilitation services.[58] It will relocate all Downtown Decatur surgical services to the North Decatur campus.[59]

DeKalb Medical at Hillandale

In July 1967, when DeKalb General was only six years old, the Hospital Authority published a "Long-Range Plan" that it submitted to the Georgia Department of Public Health. The plan described three phases of development.[60] Phase 1 called for the immediate expansion of DeKalb General to meet the urgent need for additional space and services. Phase 2 called for establishing "a satellite hospital and related hospital services for the South DeKalb area." Phase 3 proposed building a hospital in the north DeKalb area. The Authority included phase 3 in response to the state health department's pressure for it to assume responsibility for the vacated Veterans Administration Hospital on Peachtree Road as discussed in chapter 3.

In support of the phase 2 proposal, the Authority cited the steady growth of population and resources in South DeKalb and the need for additional medical services. The plan called for a two-hundred-bed general hospital, a one-hundred-bed long-term care facility, a thirty-bed mental health community center, and a medical office building. The project would be funded by a combination of county bonds, hospital reserved resources, and Hill-Burton funds. The plan identified a portion of the old federal prison "Honor Farm" in Panthersville as a site for the project. Construction could begin in 1969 and be completed by 1972.

As early as 1967, the Hospital Authority had planned to provide medical facilities and services in South DeKalb County.

As early as 1967, therefore, the Hospital Authority planned to provide medical facilities and services in South DeKalb County. In January 1969 Hospital Authority Chairman Rufus Evans asked the DeKalb County Bond Commission to include money for a South DeKalb hospital in an upcoming bond election.[61] Clark Harrison was the new county commission chairman, and he was committed to having a hospital in South DeKalb operated by the Authority. When, in the spring of 1969, he learned that a private group considered building a hospital in the area, he engaged architect Gene Bothwell to prepare plans for a two-hundred-bed hospital and secured an option to buy thirty-five acres of land on American Field Drive at $4,000 an acre. He met with the Authority in June 1969, outlined what he had done, and transferred the land option to the Authority. He and the trustees agreed that the first priority was to expand DeKalb General Hospital and to secure land in South DeKalb, but defer for the time being the construction of medical facilities there.[62]

In May 1970 DeKalb County citizens approved a $1,950,000 bond for land and a hospital in South DeKalb.[63] The county commissioners wanted the Authority to buy a portion of the federally owned Honor Farm for the South DeKalb hospital instead of the American Field Drive property.[64] The Honor Farm included 580 acres, and the federal government said it would make available a portion of it for a medical facility. The commissioners passed a resolution that assured the DeKalb General Hospital trustees that the county stood behind the Authority's acquiring land and developing a medical facility in South DeKalb. The commissioners also promised to turn over to the Authority the $1,950,000 bond money as soon as the bonds were sold.

The bonds were sold and the county turned the bond fund over to the Authority in February 1971.[65] With the money in hand, the Authority applied to the U. S. Secretary of Health, Education, and Welfare (HEW) for approximately forty acres of the Honor Farm.[66] Fourth District Congressman Ben Blackburn supported the Authority's application.[67] In August 1971 HEW conveyed to the Authority a deed for 39.25 acres of the Honor Farm with the stipulations that the Authority build a hospital there within the next eight years and that it make annual interest payments of $4,232.[68]

While the county leaders enthusiastically favored a hospital in South DeKalb, the Authority encountered reluctance elsewhere. The DeKalb Medical Society urged the Authority to proceed with caution. It said the bond money was insufficient to buy land and build a hospital, and it said the medical manpower needed to staff another hospital was not available.[69] In addition, the Metropolitan Atlanta Council conducted a survey in June 1971 that said there were already too many hospital beds in metropolitan Atlanta. The report predicted an excess of 1,500 beds by 1973 and 2,500 beds by

1975.[70] With the council's report on record, the Authority knew the state would not approve a hospital in South DeKalb County unless it could demonstrate a specific need.

To identify such a specific need, the Authority engaged the services of Hamilton and Associates consultants in 1972 to conduct a feasibility study.[71] The consultants, however, concluded that there was no current need for a hospital in South DeKalb. They recommended that, instead of a hospital, the Authority should build one or more ambulatory centers in the area.[72] They also strongly recommended that the Authority look for a site more centrally located than the Honor Farm. They suggested looking for land east of interstate highway I-285 and along highway I-20. Hamilton and Associates provided an updated report a year later that reaffirmed their earlier findings and recommendations.[73]

"One promising concept being evaluated is a free-standing ambulatory/emergency/outpatient unit which could later be expanded by the addition of other hospital services as needed."

— Waldo Sowell
Hospital Authority Chairman
to Commission Chairman
A. C. Guhl

The citizens of South DeKalb, however, wanted action, and they applied pressure to the elected officials for a hospital. In September 1974 the new commission chairman A. C. Guhl asked Authority chairman Waldo Sowell to send him a letter outlining the Authority's plans.[74] Sowell sent the following letter that was couched in general terms:

> *As you know, the DeKalb County Hospital Authority is continuing its interest and efforts with regard to the health needs of South DeKalb.*
>
> *At the present time, the Authority is working toward the acquisition of land in the South DeKalb area. In addition, our Planning and Development Committee has been working on this project for some time. It is studying health delivery systems in operation in other communities to recommend the most appropriate facilities for South DeKalb. One promising concept being evaluated is a free-standing ambulatory emergency/outpatient unit which could later be expanded by the addition of other hospital services as needed.*
>
> *The Authority would welcome an expression of support from the board of commissioners as we move ahead on this project and as we continue working together for DeKalb County.*[75]

Sowell intended to provide the commissioners with a general statement, but the commissioners interpreted his letter in very specific terms. They publicly declared that Sowell's letter meant "the Hospital Authority has developed a concept for phased construction of the South DeKalb Hospital which would include as its first phase a free-standing ambulatory emergency/outpatient unit, as its second phase the addition of a general hospital services facility, and as its third phase an expansion of basic services as well as the addition of specialized services as community health needs may warrant."[76] The commissioners urged the Hospital Authority to proceed as expeditiously as possible at least with phase one.[77]

The local press became aware of the commissioners' interpretation and reported the news with bold headlines. The *Atlanta Journal* said, "After nearly four years of silence, the DeKalb Hospital Authority has started unveiling tentative plans for a South DeKalb area hospital."[78]

In the meantime, the Authority, following Hamilton Associates' 1972 recommendation, began looking for another site while holding on to the forty acres in the Honor Farm. It took much longer than anticipated to find and acquire desirable land. Trustee Wash W. Lively and Administrator Charles Eberhart evaluated several pieces of property before recommending in February 1976 that

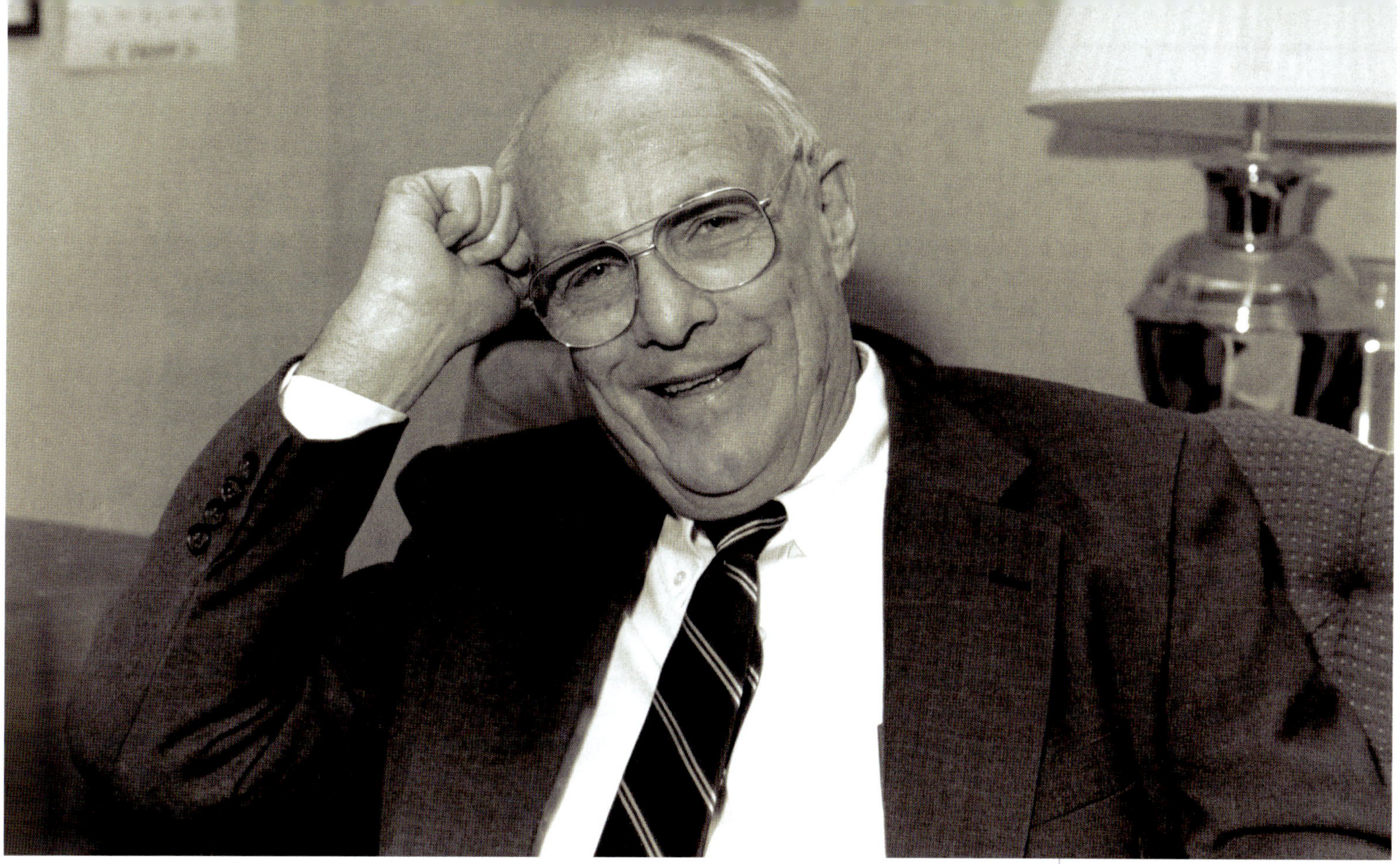

the Authority buy forty acres owned by Southeast Properties Inc. on Hillandale Road. It was, as recommended by Hamilton and Associates, located east of I-285 and along I-20.[79] After prolonged negotiations, in July 1976 the Authority signed a contract for 41.83 acres on Hillandale Road at a cost of $327,000.[80] The accumulated interest from the 1970 South DeKalb bond fund was more than enough to pay for the land.[81]

While the Authority was looking for land, a private group once again showed interest in building a medical facility in the area. The South DeKalb Homeowners Association welcomed the idea of a private hospital and encouraged the state and county officials to give it their support. When the Authority learned about this initiative, it sent a resolution to the county commissioners and the Georgia Department of Human Resources reaffirming its commitment to build a hospital in South DeKalb. It also sent a letter to the state reminding it of the county's commitment to support the Authority's plan to build a medical facility in the area.[82] Despite public support, the state rejected the private hospital's proposal.

Now that it had forty acres on Hillandale Road, the Authority had to dispense with the federal Honor Farm property. After exploring several options, in June 1977 it returned the property to the federal government with the recommendation "that this property . . . be passed to DeKalb County."[83] The hospital's only financial investment in the property had been the annual interest of $4,232.

With the site finally settled, the South DeKalb community and elected county officials pressed for action.[84] South DeKalb citizens and the commission chairman-elect Manual Maloof called for at least a free-standing emergency center. In September 1976, two months after purchasing the Hillandale property, Hospital Authority Chairman Waldo Sowell suffered a fatal accidental fall at home, and

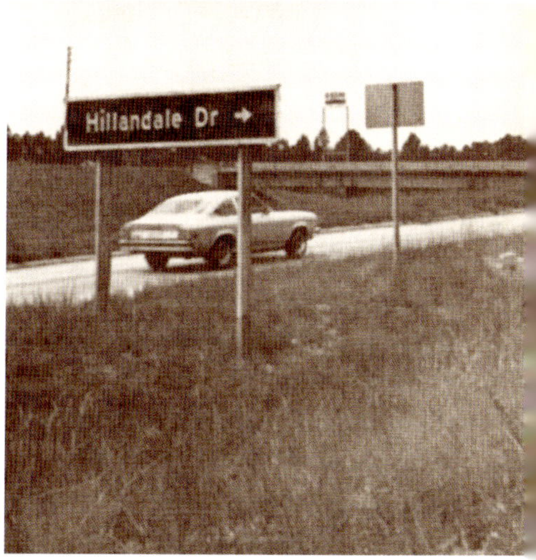

Top: When W. P. Tatum succeeded Waldo Sowell as the Authority Chairman, he reactivated the South DeKalb Development Committee. **Above:** In 1976 the Authority signed a contract to purchase nearly forty-two acres on Hillandale Road for a new hospital to be built.

the Authority elected W. P. Tatum as his successor. Chairman Tatum reactivated a South DeKalb Development Committee "to study the healthcare and facility needs in South DeKalb."[85] The committee found, however, that the demographic and economic data still did not support building a hospital. In addition, the DeKalb Medical Society openly opposed building any kind of facility and urged, instead, recruiting new physicians into the area. The Authority still had no persuasive information to show the direction it should take and no clear indication when that information would come. As Authority member Ralph Birdsong observed, "the Authority was in a dilemma between compassion versus economics."[86]

Yet another issue entered the Authority's deliberations in the fall of 1980. The Grady Memorial Hospital contract with Fulton County and DeKalb County would expire at the end of 1983. Some DeKalb citizens and elected officials argued that the county should not renew the contract but let DeKalb General Hospital and the county government assume responsibility for providing medical services for its indigent population. County attorney George Dillard urged the Authority to be cautious in doing anything in South DeKalb until a decision was made on the Grady contract.[87] The county eventually renewed its contract with Grady, but the time required to make that decision imposed yet another delay on the South DeKalb project.

In the summer of 1984, National Medical Enterprises Inc. (NME), a California-based, for-profit hospital chain, submitted a certificate of need (CON) application to the state to build a 140-bed hospital on a forty-acre tract of land on Covington Highway near Panola Road. NME called it the Community Hospital of DeKalb.[88]

DeKalb General Hospital, Decatur Hospital (still privately owned), Doctors Hospital (later renamed Northlake Regional Medical Center), Georgia Baptist Hospital (later called Atlanta Medical Center), Rockdale Hospital, and others immediately opposed NME's application. South DeKalb residents, on the other hand, overwhelmingly supported it.[89] They said that at last they would get their long-dreamed-of hospital.

Despite the community's support, the state rejected NME's application[90] based on the fact that several hospitals were within a thirty-minute drive of the proposed hospital site, that many of those hospitals were operating at less than capacity,[91] and that the South DeKalb service area would have an excess of seven hundred hospital beds by 1988.[92]

The ardent community support for NME's failed effort created a renewed sense of urgency for the Authority. In October 1984 Charles Eberhart recommended that the Authority purchase additional land in the area and build an urgent care center.[93] In April 1985 after looking at three possible sites,[94] the trustees purchased fourteen acres on Covington Highway near Panola Road, appointed Mary Hollis, RN, as project development coordinator,[95] and held a groundbreaking ceremony in November.[96] The center was a 6,000-square-foot facility designed to provide medical services for minor illnesses and injuries as well as a place for community health and education programs.[97] FamilyCare South DeKalb opened its doors on July 21, 1986.

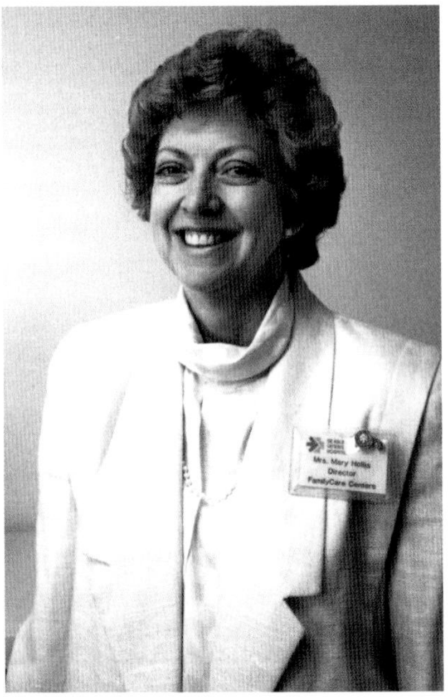

Mary Hollis, RN, was appointed project development coordinator for building the 6,000-square-foot medical facility, FamilyCare South DeKalb.

The facility opened with a celebration, but not everyone was happy with it. Some thought it too much, and some thought it too little. Some physicians in private practice saw the center as competition. John Heard, MD, long-time family practitioner in Decatur and one of the county's more articulate physicians, saw the hospital's half page newspaper ad. It pictured a child holding a teddy bear with a caption that read, "Whether it's you or your children, a fever or sore throat, a rash or the flu . . . the quick help you can count on is now very close to home." Heard responded with an article in the

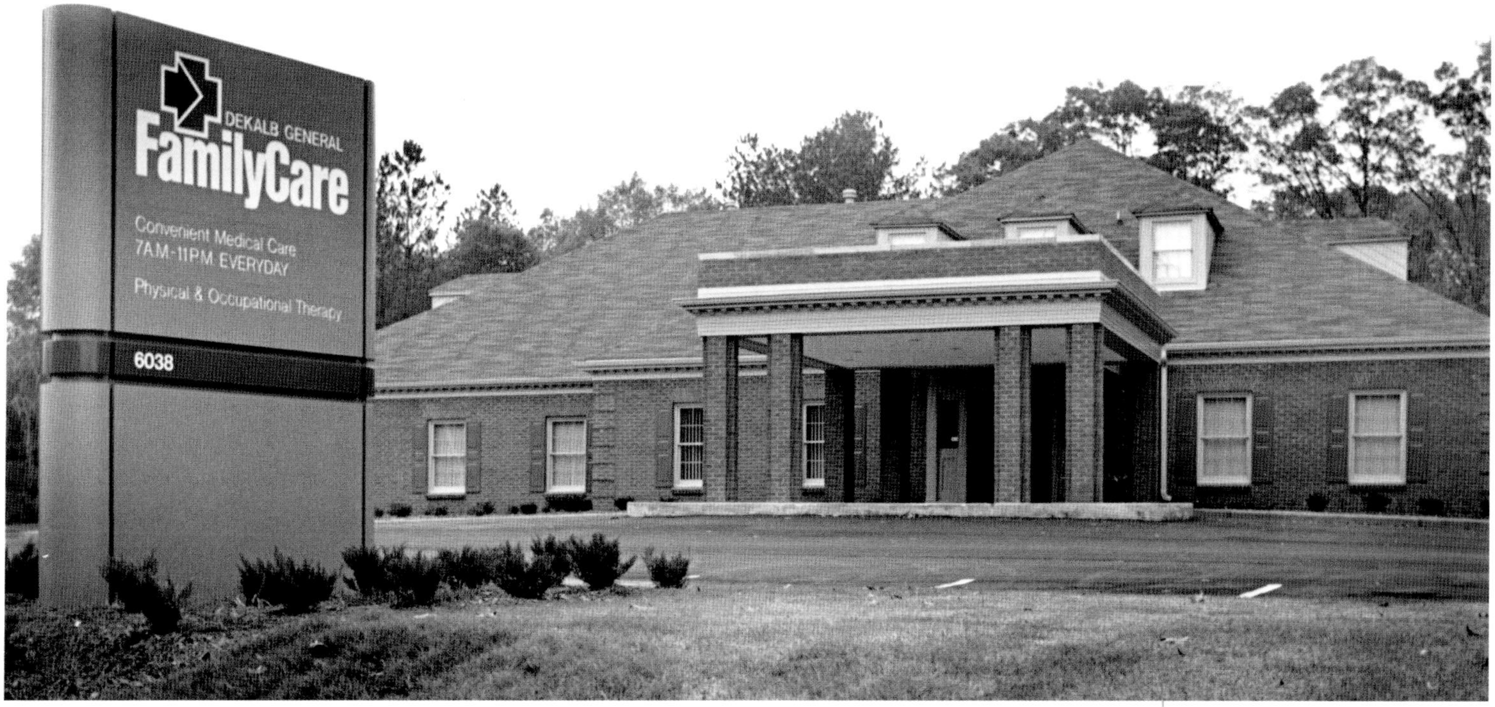

DeKalb General Hospital newsletter entitled, "Et Tu, DeKalb General?" reminiscent of the words of Julius Caesar when he saw his friend Brutus among his assassins.[98]

Some South DeKalb citizens saw it as too little. They wanted more than a facility that provided medical services for minor illnesses and injuries. Before the center was built, State Representative Ken Workman sponsored a resolution that was passed by the House of Representatives in March 1985 "urging DeKalb General Hospital to plan for, develop, and operate a full emergency care facility in southeast DeKalb County which will be able to treat serious emergencies as well as minor illnesses and injuries."[99] He secured petitions signed by thousands of South DeKalb residents supporting his plea for a full emergency facility. He urged DeKalb General not to build an urgent care center, contending that it would delay even more the possibility of getting what was "really needed" in the area.[100]

The Authority was keenly aware of South DeKalb's impatience and the growing clamor for a hospital with a full-service emergency facility. Therefore, in February 1986, while FamilyCare South DeKalb was still under construction, the Authority filed a CON application with the state for a one-hundred-bed, 85,000-square-foot, three-story hospital on its Hillandale property at a cost of $18 million.[101] It would have eighteen beds for obstetrics and gynecology, a nursery with twenty bassinets, thirty-five surgical and medical beds, seven intensive care beds, five pediatric beds, and a twenty-four-hour Emergency Department.[102] To neutralize the state's concern about excessive beds in the area, the Authority agreed to transfer to the South DeKalb hospital one hundred of its DeKalb General licensed beds.[103] The Authority proposed to call the facility "South DeKalb Hospital."

Rockdale Hospital, Henry General Hospital, Newton General Hospital, and Decatur Hospital (still privately owned) opposed the Authority's application, and the state had its own concerns.[104] The state contended that even with the transfer of one hundred existing licensed beds, the new hospital would contribute to the problem of excessive hospital beds since DeKalb General was not currently using those beds. It was staffed for only 411 of its 525 licensed beds.[105] While the South DeKalb

Above: FamilyCare South DeKalb opened its doors on July 21, 1986. **Below:** John Heard, MD, a long-time family practitioner, felt the new facility was competition. He wrote an article for the DeKalb General Hospital newsletter entitled: "Et Tu, DeKalb General?"

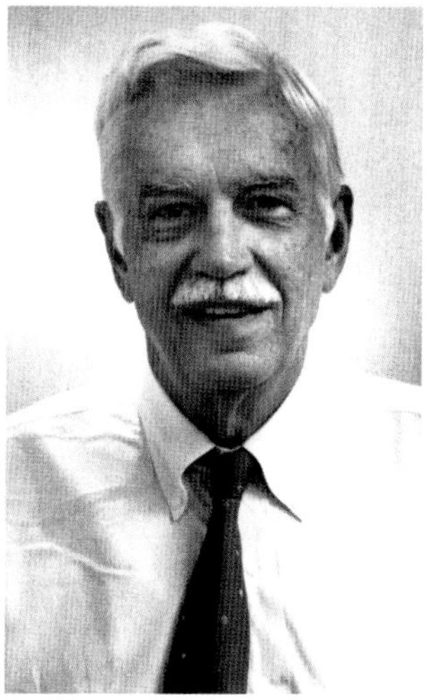

Hospital would not increase the actual number of licensed beds in the area, the state said it would in fact increase the number of functional, operational beds.

The state also rejected the Authority's claim that the new hospital would meet the needs of an underserved population.[106] It contended that DeKalb General, Rockdale, Henry General, Newton General, and other hospitals were all within thirty minutes driving time from the area that South DeKalb Hospital would serve.

Finally, the state was concerned about the added cost of a new hospital. One member of the state's review committee said, "The major thing is the cost. . . . We have to take a look at the whole ball of wax. Even though there will be no increase or addition of [licensed] beds in the area, we have to see if the alleged need for accessibility outweighs the cost."[107]

In May 1986 the state rejected the Authority's application.[108] The state acknowledged that its bed criteria was based on historical data that failed to take into account the rapid growth of South DeKalb. In a letter of support for the project, DeKalb County Commissioner Robert Lanier reminded the state that "the southeast quarter of DeKalb [County] is growing at a faster rate than Gwinnett County, the fastest growing county in the United States."[109] Nevertheless, the state said it was bound by existing rules.[110] The Authority now at least could say to the citizens of South DeKalb, "We made a good-faith effort to build a hospital and emergency facility, but the state prohibited us from doing so."

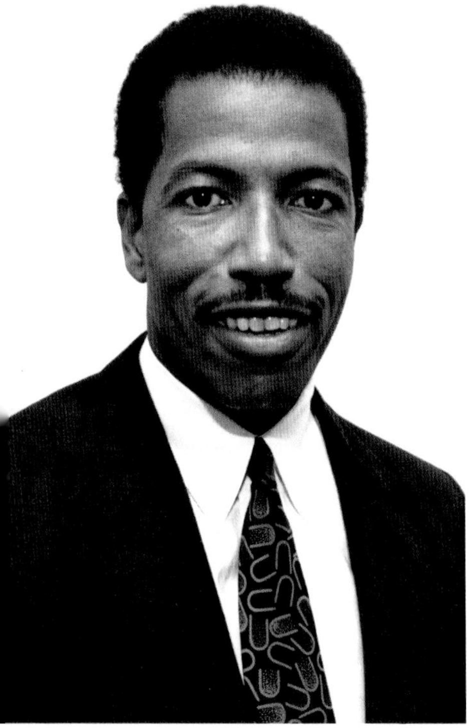

In December of 1991, Oliver Lee was named chairman of a newly appointed committee that would proceed with the South DeKalb study and planning.

The Authority and the community were relatively quiet on the subject of a hospital for the next five years. Then in December 1991, the press ran a letter to the editors urging DeKalb Medical Center to build not just one but two hospitals in the southern part of the county.[111] In January 1992 Hospital Authority Chairman W. P. Tatum placed the South DeKalb project back on the active agenda and "appointed a standing Committee on South DeKalb . . . to proceed with the South DeKalb study and planning." He named Oliver Lee as chairman of the committee,[112] and Administrator Charles Eberhart named Julia Hunter Jones director of the South DeKalb project.[113]

In 1993 the Authority transferred to DeKalb Medical Center Inc. (DMC) all of the South DeKalb bond funds and the forty-acre Hillandale property.[114] The DMC board approved the development of South DeKalb in four phases: phase 1, a combined medical office building and outpatient diagnostic center; phase 2, expanded outpatient services and additional medical office building space; phase 3, an inpatient hospital with a true emergency facility; and phase 4, a long-term care facility.[115]

Many South DeKalb citizens were unhappy with DMC's four-phase plan. They wanted a hospital, and they wanted it soon. At a South DeKalb prayer breakfast, county commission candidate Lou Walker called on all citizens in South DeKalb to sign a petition to help make the hospital a reality.[116] Former DeKalb commissioner John Evans assembled a public hearing on the question of why South DeKalb still did not have a hospital twenty-three years after the county issued a bond for that purpose.[117] He had a packed house with nearly two hundred people attending a standing-room-only, "two-to-a-chair" meeting.[118] He focused on the fact that the state threw a roadblock in the Authority's efforts to build a hospital in 1986 using obsolete criteria. He urged the citizens of South DeKalb to make their voices heard in the state legislature to change "the [obsolete] criteria which currently includes drive times, bed-to-population ratios in the county and other factors."[119]

In the meantime, Charles Eberhart was actively pursuing plans for a hospital in South DeKalb. In April 1992 he outlined for the trustees thirteen reasons why they should plan and prepare (though not file) another CON application for a hospital. He cited the current support of physicians, the six years that had elapsed since their previous application, the growth of the population in the area, the

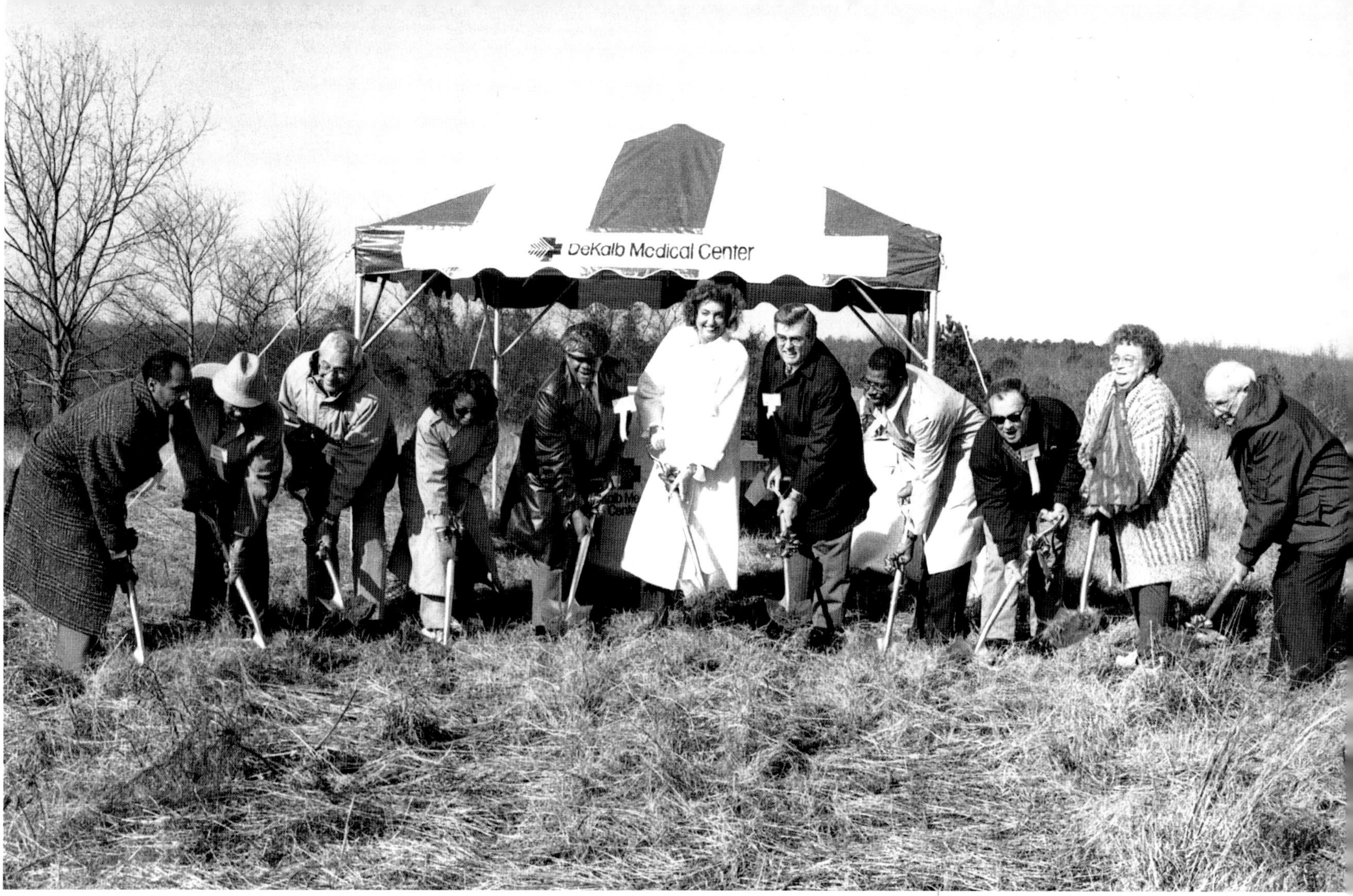

DeKalb Medical Center broke ground for the phase I outpatient diagnostic medical center building in December 1993.

possibility of changes in the state's criteria, and the risk that a competitor might file another CON application.[120] Eberhart pleaded with the Authority, "Please, please, please don't discuss this with anyone as timing will be critical . . . [and] competitors might be listening."[121]

Eberhart engaged Jennings, Ryan and Kolb consultants to conduct a feasibility study for a hospital[122] and engaged attorney Pamela Stephenson, formerly with the State Health Planning Agency that evaluated and approved or rejected CON applications, to serve as a consultant to assist in preparing the application.[123] The application was prepared, but the feasibility study still did not support building a hospital, and a CON application for a hospital would not be filed for another nine years.

The consultants did conclude that the phase 1 medical office building and outpatient diagnostic center was feasible, and they recommended going forward with that project. The state approved the CON application in October 1993.[124] Northlake Regional Medical Center filed a letter of objection with the state but never filed a formal appeal, and DMC broke ground in December 1993.[125]

The project progressed well except for relocating Bidez Road, which ran across the HIllandale property. DMC wanted it moved to the east side of the property to allow for the full development of the land. Julia Hunter Jones met with representatives from the DeKalb County Planning Department to discuss the project and encountered stiff opposition. She described that meeting in a memo to Charles Eberhart:

> *[It] felt like a small ambush. They all appeared to be fine-tuned to saying "No." No money. No interest. No way. . . . [I said] we [DMC] would have the engineering work done, and we would like the county to do the grading and the state to do the curbing and paving. (The laughter began at that point.). . .[They] insisted that the county has absolutely no money, and we should pay for everything ourselves.*[126]

Fortunately, DeKalb County CEO Leane Levetan agreed for the county to provide the clearing and grading work, and she persuaded the state to do the paving. DMC provided engineering and other services.[127] The hospital hosted a grand opening ceremony for the facility in October 1994.[128]

The three-story facility cost $7.5 million and included 41,550 square feet. The medical office component occupied the top two floors and accommodated fourteen physician offices. The outpatient diagnostic center occupied the ground floor and included a laboratory, imaging center, rehabilitation service and a wellness center.[129] Of the total cost, DMC used $3.5 million of the $10 million that had accrued in the bond fund to pay for the first-floor diagnostic center. DMC paid for the top two floors with $2 million of its own unrestricted hospital reserves and $2 million in commercial loans.[130]

In 1994 DMC converted the standing Committee on South DeKalb into the South DeKalb Advisory Committee. Oliver Lee remained chairman, and he and the project director Julia Hunter Jones selected physicians and citizens from the South DeKalb area to serve with them. The advisory committee was a creative, active, and aggressive group that assessed community needs, processed proposals, and made recommendations to the DMC board.

Since phase 1 was a success,[131] in 1998 the advisory committee determined the time was right to move forward with the next step. It proposed combining phase 2 and phase 3 into what it called an "Alternative Healthcare Model" to include an ambulatory surgery center, a birthing center, a short-stay inpatient unit, a twenty-four-hour emergency facility, and additional physician offices.[132] DMC asked the state to exempt the proposed facility from the CON process.[133] The state, however, denied the request.[134]

With that denial the advisory committee was back to "square one,"[135] but it did not remain idle. In January 1999 it asked DMC to file an application for an "Outpatient Hospital," the first such facility in Georgia.[136] The plan included a three-story, 63,000-square-foot building. The top two floors would be for physician offices; and the 22,750-square-foot first floor would house an outpatient surgery center, observatory and recovery beds, rehabilitation services, and a minor emergency center that would be open twenty-four hours a day, seven days a week. The new outpatient surgery center would offer state-of-the-art video laparoscopic surgery, contain three operating rooms, and be equipped for orthopedic, gynecological, podiatric, ear-nose-and-throat, and general surgical procedures.[137]

DMC filed its application in April.[138] Rockdale Hospital and Eastside Hospital submitted letters of opposition, but neither filed a formal appeal[139] and the state approved the application in the fall of 1999.[140] Construction got underway in October,[141] and DMC opened the state's first Outpatient Hospital in August 2001.[142] It cost $11.3 million.[143] DMC used $6.3 million of the $15.3 million remaining in the South DeKalb bond fund for the first floor and paid the remaining $5 million for the

South DeKalb Hospital

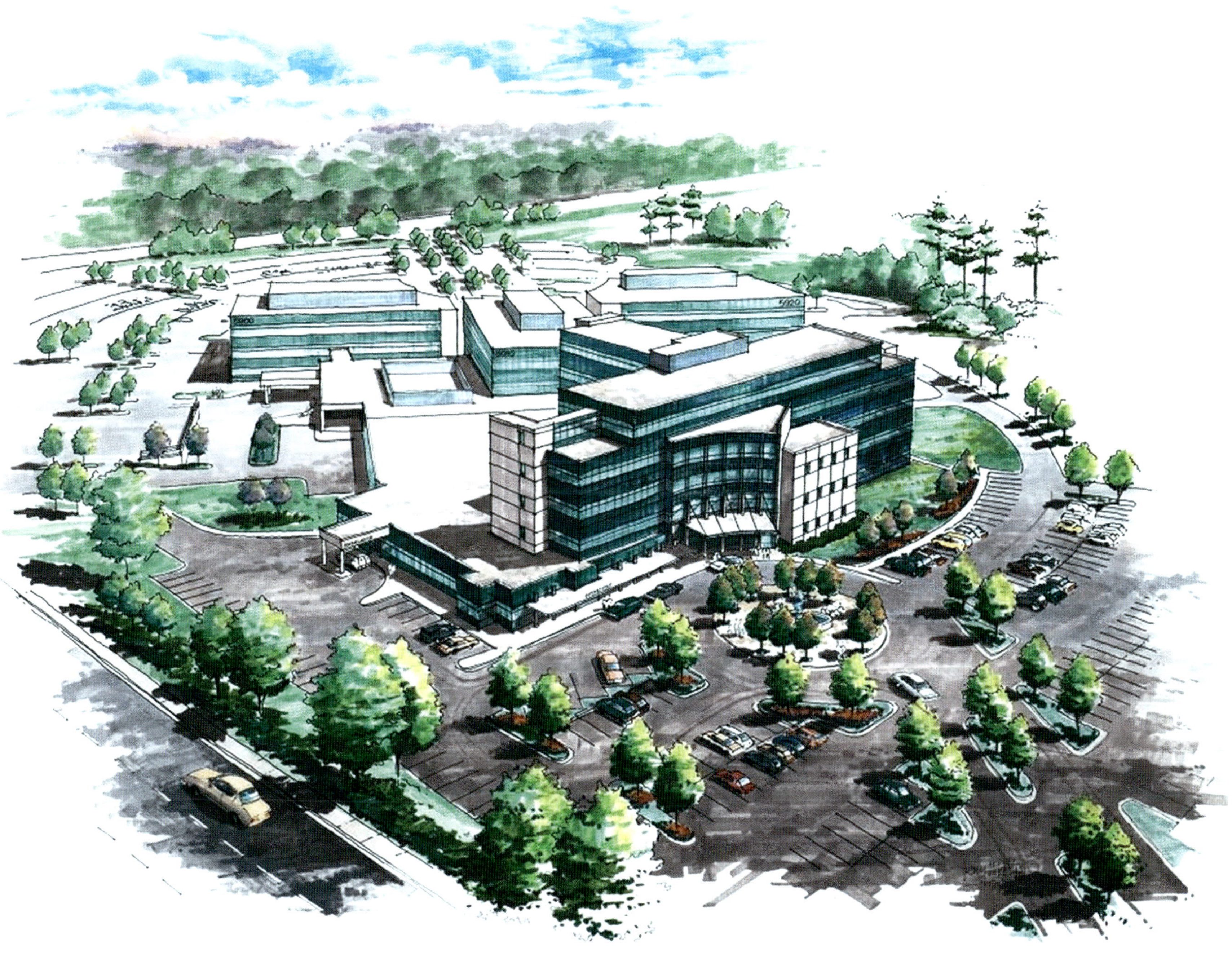

second and third floors with commercial loans. FamilyCare South DeKalb on Covington Highway relocated to the new facility. The authority sold the vacated FamilyCare building and the surrounding fourteen acres to a retail shopping center for $1,550,000.[144]

DMC continued looking for the opportunity to build a hospital at Hillandale. In 2000 it once again retained Jennings, Ryan and Kolb consultants to conduct another feasibility study. This time they presented a favorable financial proforma for a South DeKalb hospital. They projected a positive net income by the third year of operation.[145] DMC Chief Financial Officer Bonnie Phipps cautioned the board that a hospital in South DeKalb must develop its own marketshare rather than depend on transfers from DeKalb Medical Center and Decatur Hospital lest those latter facilities suffer.[146] Her caution would prove prophetic.

DMC filed a CON application with the state in August 2001. It called for a one-hundred-bed, five-story building that would cost approximately $65 million.[147] It stipulated that DeKalb Medical Center would transfer seventy-four of its licensed beds and Decatur Hospital would transfer twenty-six of its licensed beds to provide the proposed one hundred beds.[148] The Authority agreed to issue bonds to pay for the facility.[149]

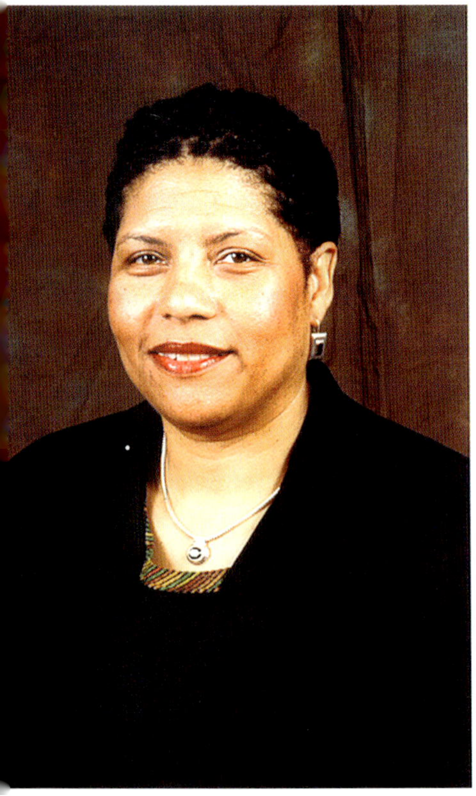

Delphyne Lomax, a South DeKalb resident and business owner, was named chairperson of the South DeKalb Hospital Planning Board in 2002.

Two months after DeKalb Medical Center filed its application, Tenet Healthcare Corporation filed a CON application to build Stonecrest Medical Center at the new Stonecrest Mall located between DMC's Hillandale site and the town of Lithonia.[150] Tenet proposed a $90 million, one-hundred-bed hospital. It matched DeKalb Medical Center's offer to give up one hundred of its existing licensed beds for the Stonecrest facility.[151]

Tenet Healthcare Corporation was a for-profit conglomerate based in California that owned Atlanta Medical Center (formerly Georgia Baptist Hospital), South Fulton Regional Hospital, North Fulton Regional Hospital, and Spalding Hospital in Griffin, Georgia.[152] National Medical Enterprises (NME), which had unsuccessfully applied for an application to build a one-hundred-bed hospital in South DeKalb in 1984, was one of Tenet's predecessor companies.[153]

The state approved DeKalb Medical Center's application in February 2002.[154] Fifteen hundred local citizens, civic leaders, hospital leaders, and local dignitaries joined in a victory celebration on the Hillandale campus,[155] and DMC hosted a gala groundbreaking ceremony in March 2002.[156] With the prospects of a hospital near at hand, DeKalb Medical Center broadened the mission of the South DeKalb Advisory Committee in 2002 and renamed it the South DeKalb Hospital Planning Board to reflect the group's expanded responsibilities. Delphyne Lomax, a South DeKalb resident and business owner who had served on the South DeKalb Advisory Board since its inception in 1994, was named chairperson. The new board membership included physicians, residents, civic volunteers, business members, and church leaders who lived and worked in the South DeKalb community.[157]

To no one's surprise, Tenet filed both an appeal and a request to "remand" (send back) to the state both hospital applications for further review based on the allegation that the state had committed two technical, procedural errors in granting a certificate of need to DMC.[158] First it said DMC's financial plan did not meet state standards. In addition it said DMC's proposed hospital did not meet the state's required ten-mile distance from Rockdale Hospital. (DMC pointed out that Tenet's site at Stonecrest Mall was only five miles from Rockdale Hospital.)[159] Tenet also implied that DMC's application had received "hometown political favoritism" by the state.[160]

The state agreed to review these complaints, but in September 2002 reaffirmed its decision to approve DMC's CON application. Once again Tenet appealed the decision and requested a second

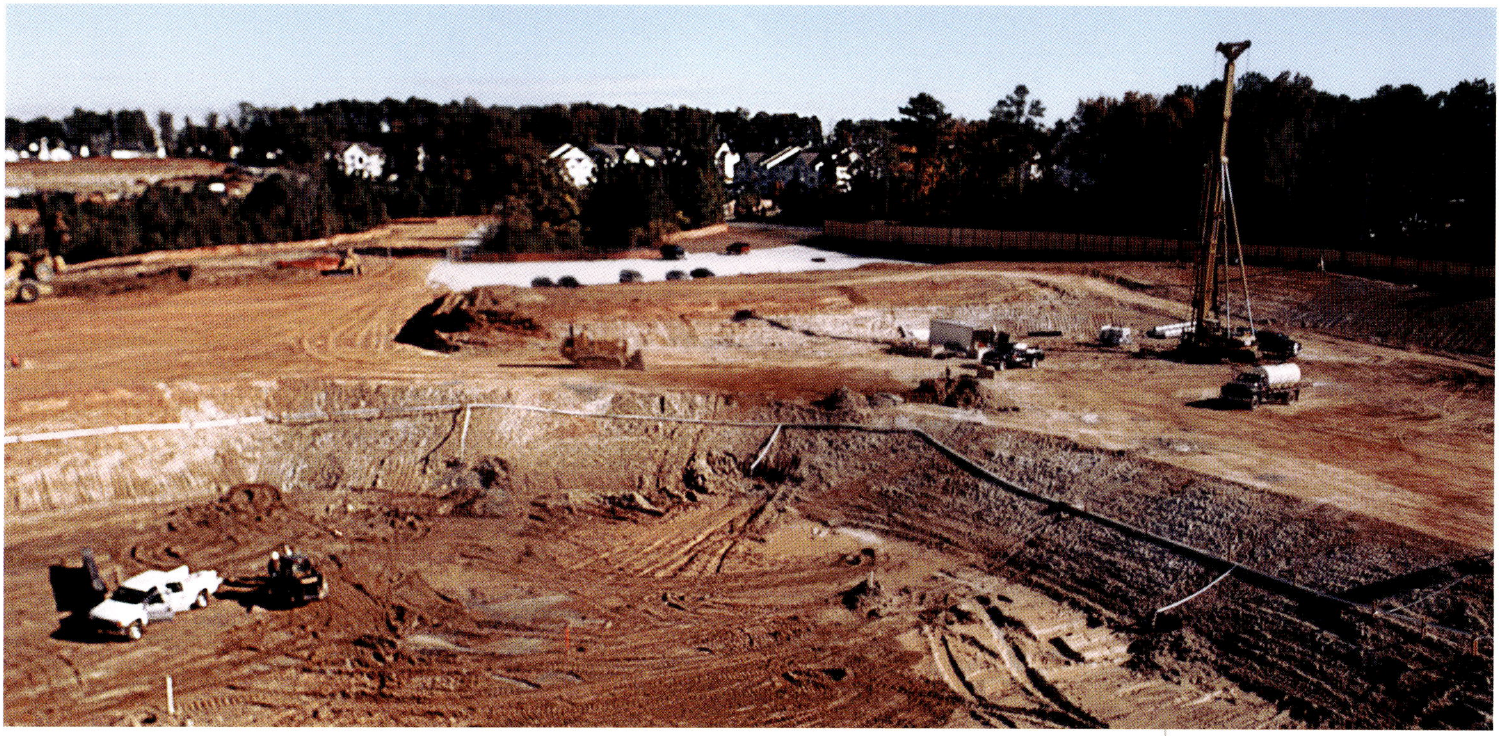

Excavation began in preparation for building the new hospital.

remand, filing two new legal complaints. In January 2003 the state approved DMC's application for the third time only to have Tenet, Rockdale, Northlake Regional Medical Center, and Eastside Hospital each file an appeal.

DMC CEO John Gerlach, who had succeeded Charles Eberhart following Eberhart's death in May 1995, urged the public to respond, and more than five thousand individuals sent letters to the state in support of DMC's application.[161] The state observed that DeKalb Medical Center planned to have all private rooms, offer more neonatal services than Tenet, and would construct its hospital at a cost of $65 million, which was less than the $90 million that Tenet proposed.[162] Finally the state outlined in its nineteen-page decision how DMC's plan was "superior in virtually every respect," including location, affordable patient charges, and a local governing board with decision-making authority.[163]

Behind the scenes, CEO Gerlach facilitated a crucial maneuver. He negotiated an agreement with Tenet that finally brought an end to Tenet's repeated appeals. Tenet agreed to withdraw its objections and permit DMC to have the CON if DMC could secure its financing within twelve months. DMC agreed, in turn, to step aside and let Tenet build its hospital if DMC did not obtain financing within that time frame. In August 2003 the Authority approved the issuance of $103 million in bonds and revenue certificates, $65 million of which was designated for the construction of the Hillandale hospital.[164] DMC would use a portion of the remaining funds to retire existing bond indebtedness and leave $7 million in the bond fund for working capital purposes.[165] DMC met the financial challenge that Tenet laid down.

Publicly, Tenet's representative said, "We recognize the critical need for a hospital in South DeKalb and will not appeal the state's decision to allow DeKalb Medical Center to move forward with providing this facility to the community." On behalf of DMC, Julia Hunter Jones responded, "We appreciate the community spirit shown by Tenet Healthcare Corporation."[166] Neither party acknowledged publicly Gerlach's behind-the-scenes negotiations that allowed the process to go forward.

Rockdale Hospital agreed with the terms worked out with Tenet.[167] Hospital Corporation of America (HCA), parent company of Northlake Regional Medical Center, would not negotiate a separate agreement even when DeKalb offered to support its efforts to obtain certain managed-care contracts.[168] The state nevertheless rejected Northlake's appeal and in June 2003 notified DMC for the fourth and final time that its application was approved.[169]

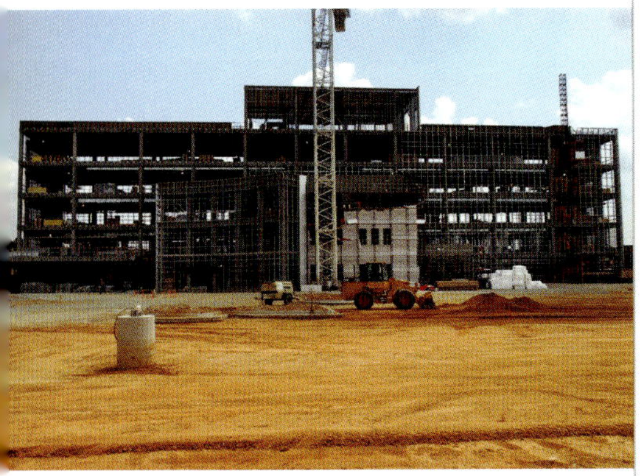

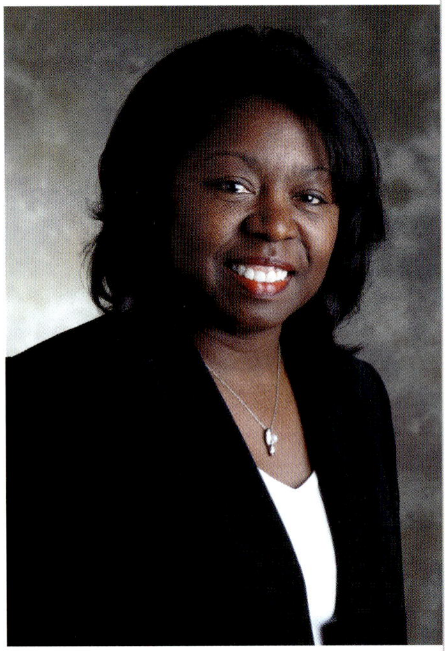

Top: Construction on the hospital began in September 2003. **Above:** Julia Hunter Jones, who had served as the director of the South DeKalb project, was named hospital administrator for DeKalb Medical at Hillandale.

DMC selected Brasfield and Gorrie as general contractor[170] with the stipulation that it utilize significant minority participation.[171] Approximately 32 percent of the work was performed by minority contractors.[172] The Collins Project Management firm managed the design and construction process, and Wilson Consulting Company headed the medical equipment process.[173] Construction began in September 2003. The Imaging Center was the first department to open in January 2005,[174] and the hospital officially opened for business in July 2005.[175]

The hospital is a six-floor, 191,000-square-foot facility that cost nearly $66.6 million. It features two "VIP" suites, one hundred private rooms, including sixty-two medical and surgical beds, twenty-five postpartum mother/baby beds, a five-bed antepartum unit for expectant mothers needing hospitalization, and eight intensive care beds. It houses twenty-two Emergency Department examination rooms, four operating suites, two gastroenterology procedure rooms, nineteen post-anesthesia recovery bays, eight labor and delivery rooms, ten special care nursery beds, and state-of-the-art imaging services.[176]

DMC initially selected "DeKalb Medical Center at Hillandale" as the hospital's name to capture both the importance of its location and its relationship to DeKalb Medical Center, the flagship of DeKalb Regional Healthcare System. DRHS later renamed it "DeKalb Medical at Hillandale" when the name "DeKalb Medical" was chosen as the term to identify the DRHS system.

DMC named the street leading up to the hospital the Lou Walker Drive in honor of the former DeKalb County commissioner who was a leading advocate for a hospital in South DeKalb and who died in August 2004 from injuries sustained in an automobile accident.[177]

Julia Hunter Jones was named hospital administrator, and Cornelius Flowers, MD, was elected by the medical staff as the hospital's first chief of staff. When, in 2007, Jones resigned to accept a position with Children's Healthcare of Atlanta at Hughes Spalding,[178] Clay Fowler, a native Atlantan with fifteen years of hospital management experience was chosen from among more than four hundred applicants as the new vice president and administrator of DeKalb Medical at Hillandale.[179]

At the opening ceremony, Administrator Jones recalled the 1992 challenge Charles Eberhart offered her when he said, "I have forty acres of red Georgia clay, and I want you to build a hospital there."[180] CEO Eric Norwood congratulated Jones for not only building a hospital but also building a culture.[181]

The hospital opened its doors at 7:00 AM on July 18, 2005. Just two minutes later, the first patient arrived in the Emergency Department. At 7:30 AM, surgeons Rogsbert Phillips, MD, and Michael Quinones, MD, performed the hospital's first surgeries. At 9:43 AM, Eldred Taylor, MD, delivered the first baby, Sophy Grace Bryant. By noon the Emergency Department had seen twenty-three patients.[182]

When the hospital opened, it was staffed for fifty-one of its one hundred beds. Administrator

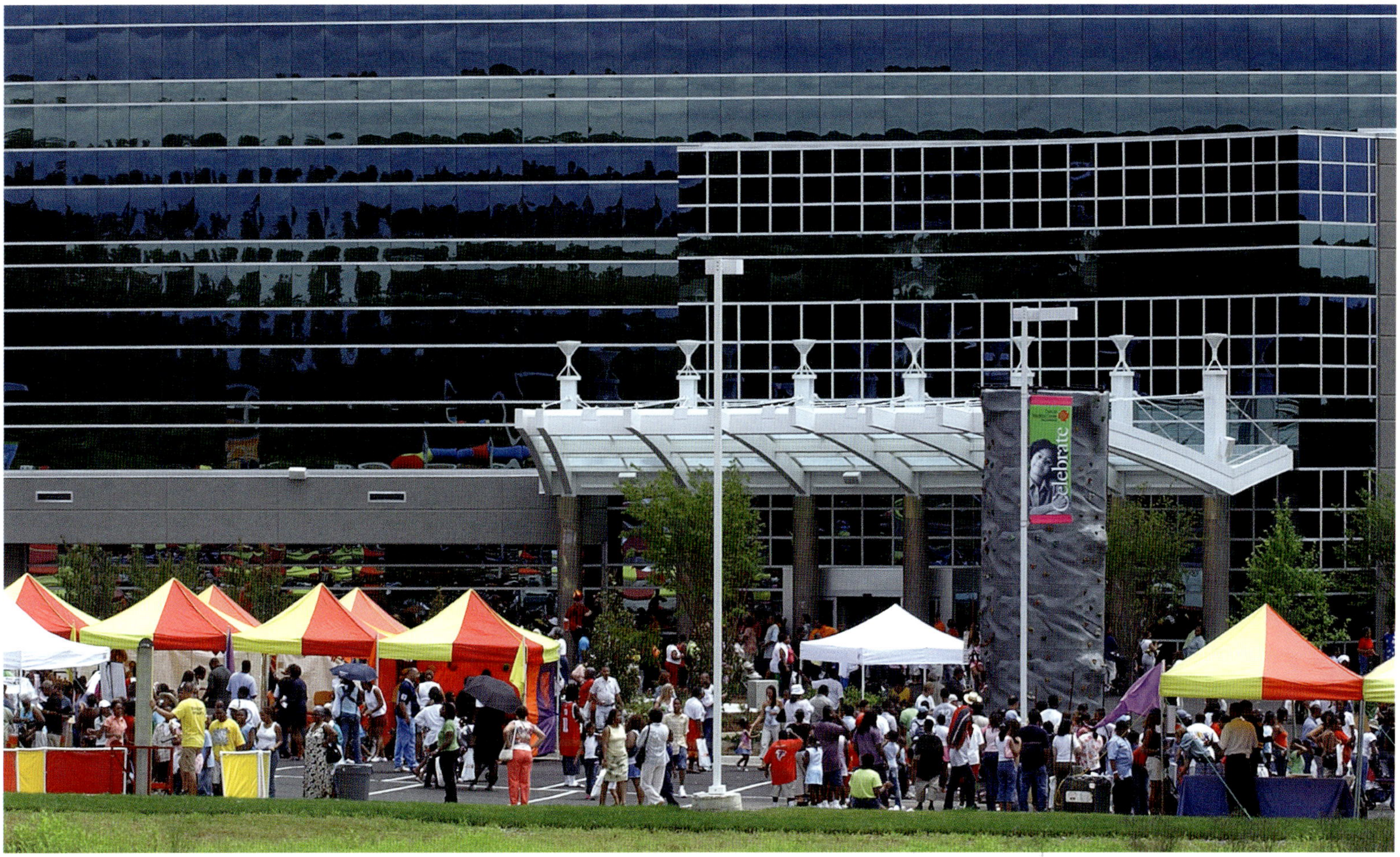

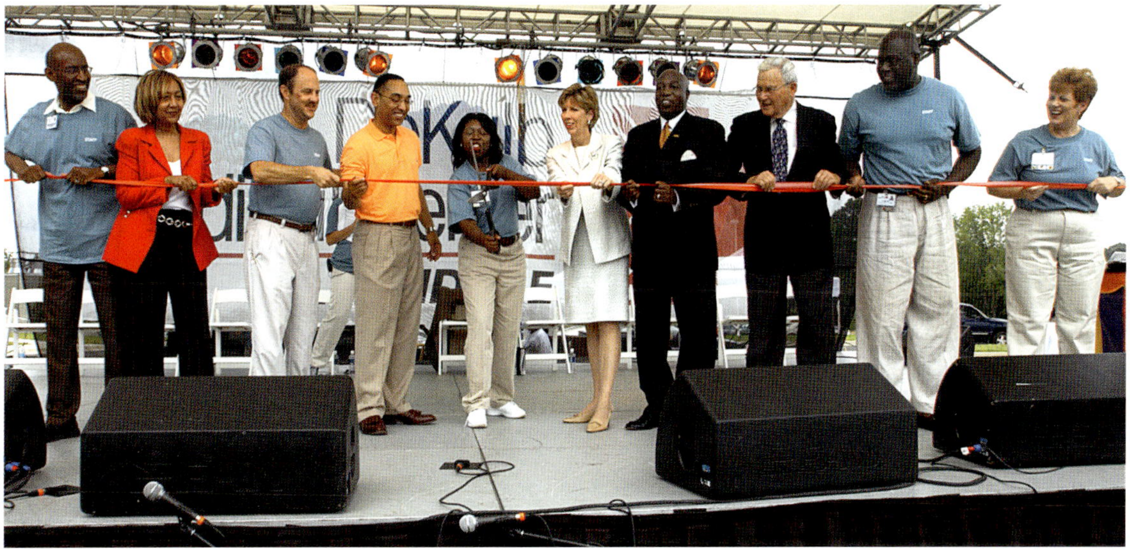

Above and left: The opening celebration for DeKalb Medical at Hillandale was well attended with a celebratory ribbon-cutting ceremony. The hospital opened its doors at 7:00 AM on July 18, 2005. The first baby was born at 9:43 AM and by noon the Emergency Department had seen twenty-three patients.

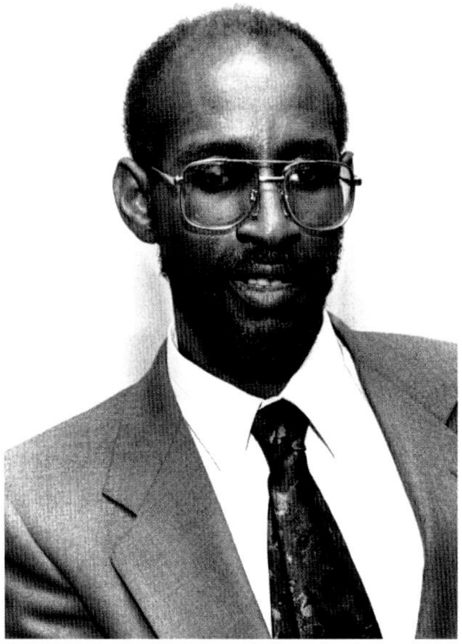

Cornelius Flowers, MD, was the first chief of staff at Hillandale and chairman of the Hillandale Advisory Board.

Jones predicted 2,955 annual admissions, 1,224 deliveries, 1,860 surgeries, 25,000 Emergency Department visits, and 37,000 outpatients visits.[183] By its one-hundredth day of operation, the hospital had delivered 247 babies, treated 12,000 patients in the Emergency Department, and doubled its opening day staff to handle the increasing workload.[184] In its first year of operation, the hospital admitted 2,632 patients, treated more than 26,000 patients in the Emergency Department, performed 1,677 surgeries, and delivered 1,149 babies.[185]

The consultants in 2001 had presented a financial feasibility report that predicted the hospital should have a positive net operating income within three years. That projection was sufficiently encouraging to go forward with the project.[186] The first five months of operation at Hillandale, however, were alarming. Whereas projections had predicted 8 percent bad debts for the first year, bills that were sixty-to-ninety days past due were running at 18 percent, amounting to bad debts of $1 million a month.[187] The majority of bad debt was originating in the Emergency Department where a significant portion of patients had no insurance.[188]

By the end of the first fiscal year, the financial picture improved somewhat, showing a net operating loss of only $500,000 greater than the budgeted loss.[189] By the end of 2007, the hospital was ahead of budget, showing a net operating gain of $570,000 versus a budgeted net loss of $493,000.[190] Those improvements were the results of a larger percentage of insured patients, educating the community to use primary care physicians rather than the Emergency Department for nonurgent medical needs, a continued increase in patient volume and recruiting more physicians for the hospital. Financial viability, however, remains a concern for the hospital due in large part to its payer mix that remains heavily weighted with Medicaid and uninsured patients.

DeKalb Medical at Hillandale was recognized as the first planned digital hospital in Georgia and one of only 2 percent of hospitals in the nation to implement successfully a computerized physician order-entry system and computerized clinical documentation. It was a major factor in DeKalb Medical's being listed as one of the twenty-five "most wired" hospital systems in the nation by *Hospitals & Health Networks* magazine, the official journal of the American Hospital Association.[191]

In 2007 Dale McCord, MD, of Atlanta Oncology Associates and Bruce Feinberg, DO, of Georgia Cancer Specialists initiated plans to construct a 10,000-square-foot full-service Cancer Treatment Center on the Hillandale campus. DeKalb Medical agreed to lease the land for the facility with the option of becoming an investor in the real estate or the operation of the center.[192] McCord received the state's approval to transfer his radiation oncology unit from the Northlake Regional Medical Center location to Hillandale.[193] That project remains in the planning stage.

In 2007 DeKalb Medical established the Hillandale Advisory Board that named Cornelius Flowers as chairman. The board included physicians, administrative staff, and members of the DeKalb Medical at Hillandale Community Committee. The board was charged with making DeKalb Medical at Hillandale one of the nation's "top 100 Hospitals."[194]

DeKalb Medical at Hillandale was a dream that finally came true. From the time in 1967 when the Authority included a South DeKalb hospital in its long-range plan, to 1970 when the county issued a $1,950,000 bond to build a hospital, to 1976 when the Authority acquired forty acres of land at Hillandale, to 1986 when the Authority opened FamilyCare South DeKalb and submitted its first unsuccessful certificate of need application for a hospital, to 1994 when DMC established the South DeKalb Advisory Committee and opened its phase 1 Medical Office Building and Outpatient Diagnostic Center, to 1998 when the state rejected its proposed CON-exempt Alternative Healthcare

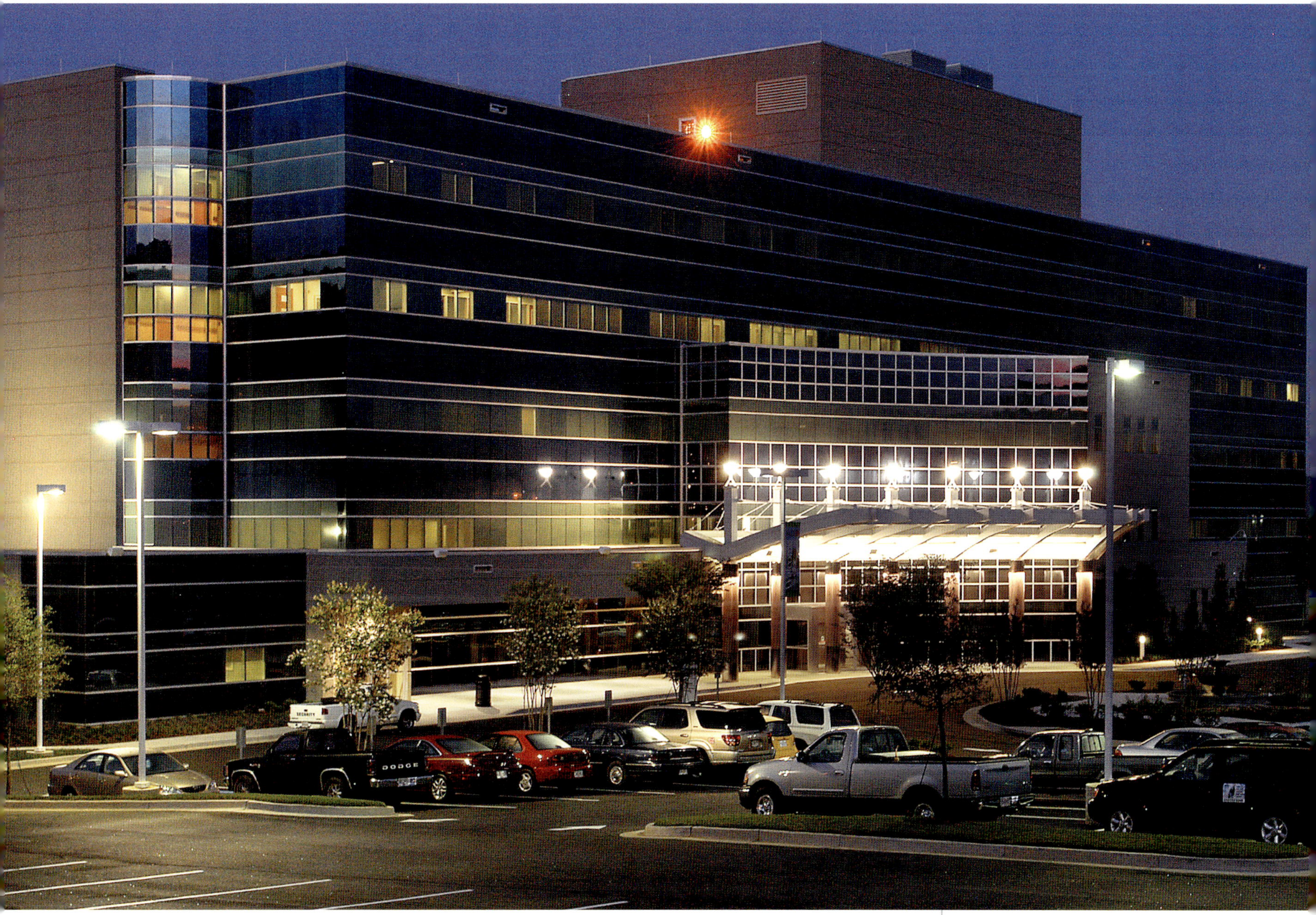

Model hospital, to 2001 when it opened its "Outpatient Hospital" as an outpatient surgery/medical urgent-care center, to 2002 when DMC converted the South DeKalb Advisory Committee into the South DeKalb Hospital Planning Board, to July 2005 when DeKalb Medical Center at Hillandale opened, the thirty-eight-year-old dream and labor of many became a reality.

The challenge remains to recruit more physicians to use the hospital, to attract more of the citizens of the community who dreamed of and pleaded for a hospital in their community, to continue meeting the health needs of the community, and to sustain the hospital's financial health.

DeKalb Medical Center at Hillandale was a thirty-eight-year-old dream come true.

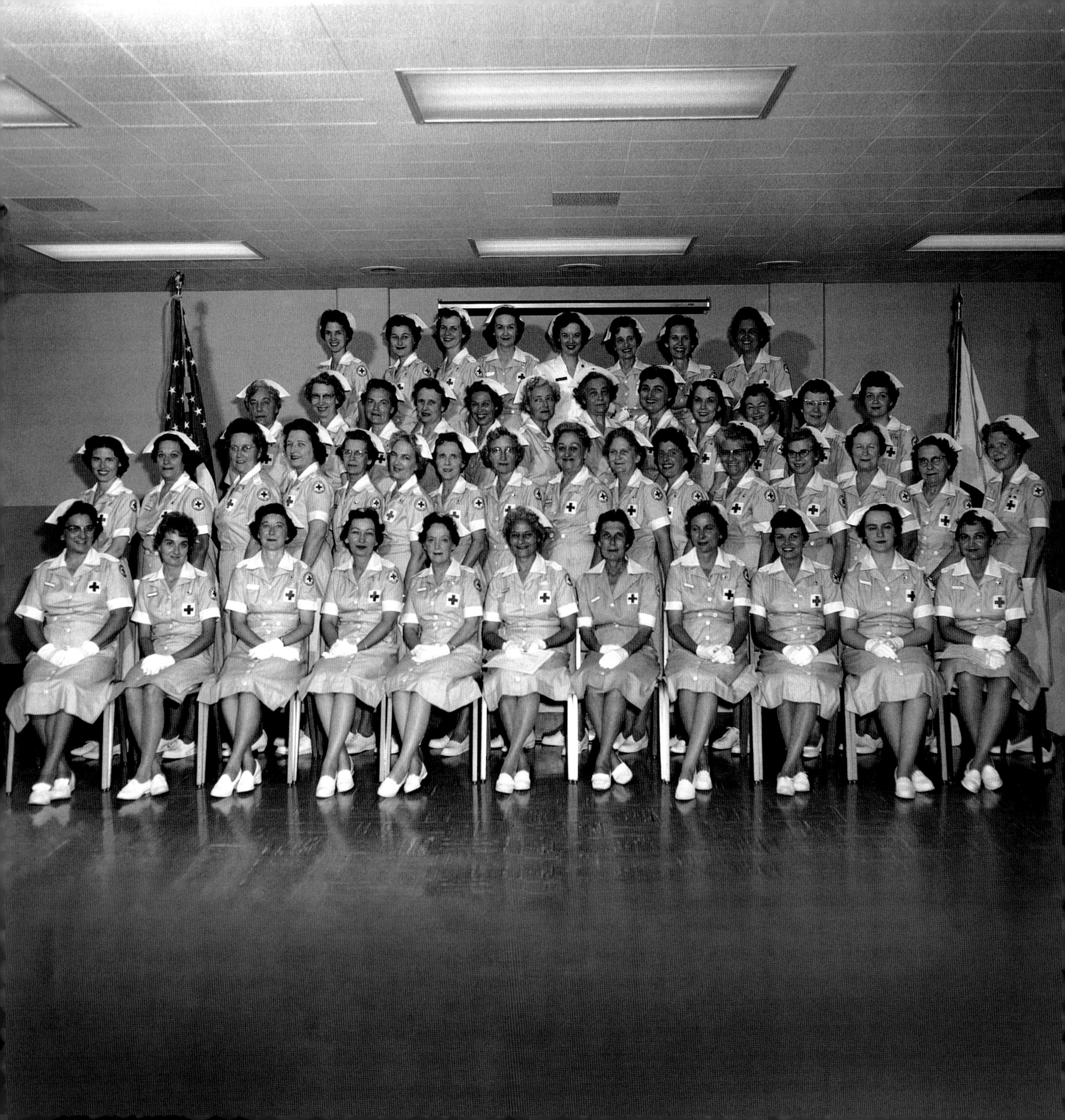

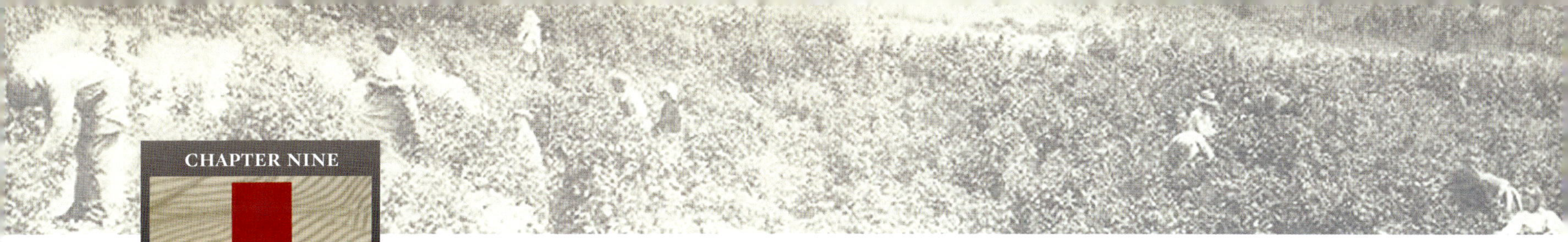

CHAPTER NINE

Volunteers and the DeKalb Medical Foundation

Opposite: Gray Ladies Red Cross Volunteers in 1961.

Volunteers

Administrator William Thrasher knew from the beginning that there would be a place and need for volunteers at DeKalb General Hospital. A 1959 newspaper quoted him two years before the hospital opened as saying:

> *We are hoping to use volunteer workers and have provided an office for the director of Volunteer Services, plus locker and lounge rooms for volunteer workers.*[1]

He had no way of knowing the extent of personal service, goodwill, and financial support that volunteers would contribute. Those contributions came from Red Cross Volunteers, the DeKalb Junior League, the DeKalb Medical Auxiliary, and a host of other organizations and individuals (see Appendices M and N).

Red Cross Volunteers

Frances Stukes was chairman of the DeKalb County Red Cross. In February 1961 she called on Thrasher and offered to provide DeKalb General Hospital with the services of Red Cross "Gray Ladies" volunteers,[2] the name coming from the gray dress that was their original official uniform. Their organization originated in 1918 when a group of women volunteered to assist patients at Walter Reed Army Hospital in Washington, DC. Other hospitals heard about their work, requested similar services, and the Red Cross Gray Ladies organization emerged.[3] In 1965 the American Red Cross changed the group's name to Red Cross Volunteers, and the blue uniform replaced the gray dress.[4]

When DeKalb General Hospital opened in May 1961, Stukes had 40 volunteers trained and ready to work.[5] There were 56 volunteers by the end of the following month, and within a year DeKalb General had 113 Red Cross Volunteers.[6]

Those volunteers were a service organization, not a fund-raising group. Stukes said the Gray Ladies would "serve as guides to new patients; write letters for, read to, and do small errands for patients; and try whenever possible to contribute to their comfort and recovery."[7] Initially they were assigned to the Emergency Department, the Recovery Room, the Intensive Care Unit, the Information Desk, and "Visiting." When "visiting," volunteers at first did just that:

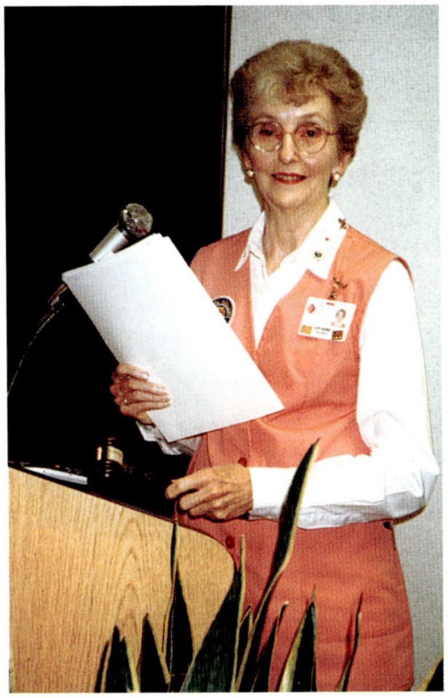

Above and right: Ann Hord, a Red Cross Volunteer, organized blood drives for the hospital and in 1999–2001 was president of the DeKalb Medical Auxiliary.

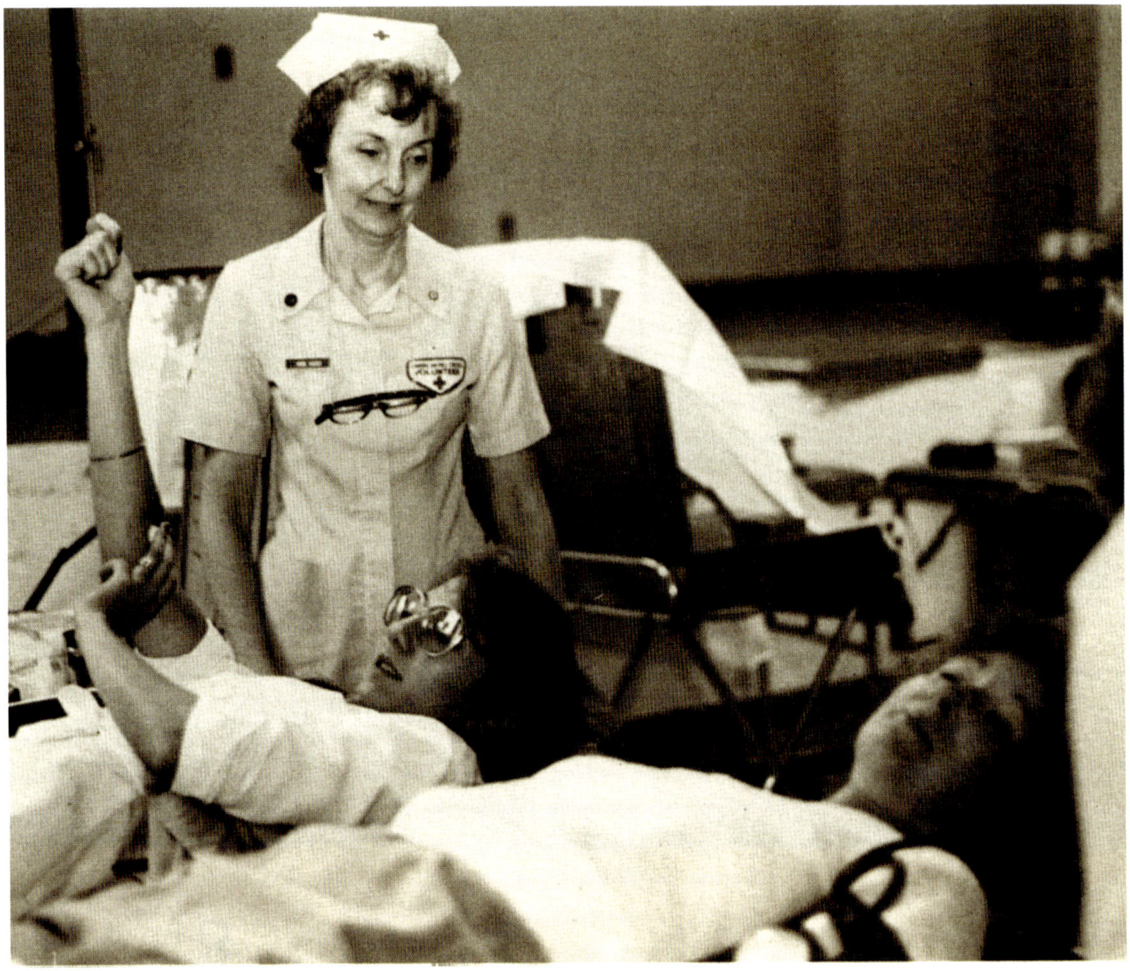

they visited with patients to befriend and comfort them. Eventually visiting volunteers assumed some of the duties usually assigned to nursing aides, such as taking temperatures and emptying bedpans. Following the hospital's major expansion in 1971, Red Cross Volunteers were assigned to other departments. In the hospital's first year, 150 volunteers gave 20,500 hours of service.[8] By 1991 members of the Red Cross Volunteers were working in thirty areas of the hospital and had given more than 300,000 hours of service.[9]

In addition to the adult program, teenage Red Cross Youth Volunteers donated thousands of hours of service to the hospital. Many gained such meaningful experience as volunteers that they eventually pursued a variety of health-related careers.[10]

The hospital depended on having blood and blood products for its patients, using approximately 1,200 units every month for which it depended on outside sources.[11] Red Cross Volunteer Ann Hord organized DeKalb General Hospital's own blood drives. They were held six times a year. The Red Cross processed donated blood and returned it to DeKalb General's blood bank. In the 1990s DeKalb Medical Center drives collected more than two hundred units of blood annually.[12] In 2004 it collected more than any hospital in metropolitan Atlanta;[13] and in 2006 its participants contributed 515 units, ranking number one in the nation among the "largest number of pints donated" for hospitals with one thousand or more employees.[14]

In 1995 the American Red Cross disbanded all its hospital-based volunteer programs nationwide. At that time the DeKalb Medical Center unit was the largest in the United States.[15] Volunteers with the Red Cross Volunteers were working in thirty areas of the hospital.[16] Sixteen of the 1995 volunteers had served twenty or more years, and thirty-two had served ten or more years.[17] In light of the Red Cross decision, DeKalb Medical Center administration elected to restructure the hospital's unit and unify its volunteer services. It encouraged the Red Cross Volunteers to join the already-established DeKalb Medical Center Auxiliary and offered to pay the first year's membership fee as well as assist in the cost of new uniforms. Despite the disbanded status of the national Red Cross program, some volunteers wanted to retain their DeKalb Medical Center Red Cross identity and were disappointed—even unhappy—at having to make the change.[18] Nevertheless, over 90 percent of the Red Cross Volunteers joined the DeKalb Medical Center Auxiliary and continued their valuable volunteer service.[19]

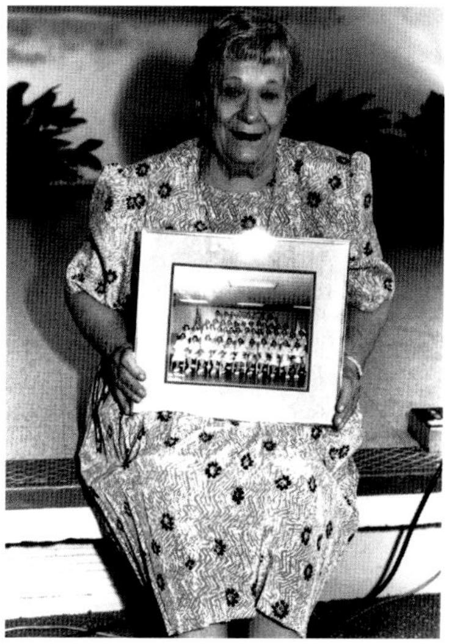

Peg Kaiser, Red Cross Volunteer and DeKalb Medical Auxiliary member, retired after giving forty years, and 12,000 hours of service and answering 610,500 phone calls.

The DeKalb Junior League

The DeKalb Junior League was another volunteer organization that offered its services and resources to the hospital. The local organization was founded in 1934 as the Decatur Junior Service League. In 1960 it changed its name to the DeKalb Junior Service League,[20] and in 1971 it became the DeKalb Junior League when it joined its national organization.

The league donated $3,000 toward a chapel when the hospital was under construction in 1960.[21] When the hospital opened, it offered to operate a gift shop. William Thrasher accepted the offer and gave the group a small room on the first floor near the snack bar. Some described the room as "a broom closet."[22] They sold candy, magazines, cigarettes, and some personal items. In one of the employee newsletters, the league advertised: "You can even replace hosiery torn on filing cabinets or one of the many other places waiting to rip your last pair of stockings."[23]

The league made it clear from the beginning that the gift shop would be a fund-raising enterprise to support several of its projects and that only a portion of the gift shop profits would go to the hospital.[24] In its second year, the gift shop netted nearly $2,900[25] of which the league donated $500 to DeKalb General.[26] In 1963 the league added a "Cheer Cart" that sold items from the gift shop to patients and their families in patient rooms.[27] In 1970 the hospital relocated the league's gift shop to the lobby on the first floor near the main entrance.[28]

The league, however, had to give up the gift shop, a change that eventually led to the formation of the DeKalb Medical Auxiliary. That change occurred in 1971 when the DeKalb Junior Service League applied to the National Association of Junior Leagues to become a member. Its application was approved, and it became the DeKalb Junior League.[29] Sarah Looper, president of the restructured league, informed Administrator Thrasher that regrettably the governing body of the national organization would no longer permit them to operate the gift shop because they were not "trained personnel."[30]

At the hospital's request, the DeKalb Junior League established a semi-independent Hospital Guild that recruited volunteers to operate the gift shop. The guild renamed the gift shop the Dogwood Shop.[31] In 1973 the Hospital Guild officially separated from the DeKalb Junior League, joined the Georgia Hospital Association's Council on Auxiliaries, developed its own bylaws, and became the DeKalb General Hospital Auxiliary.[32]

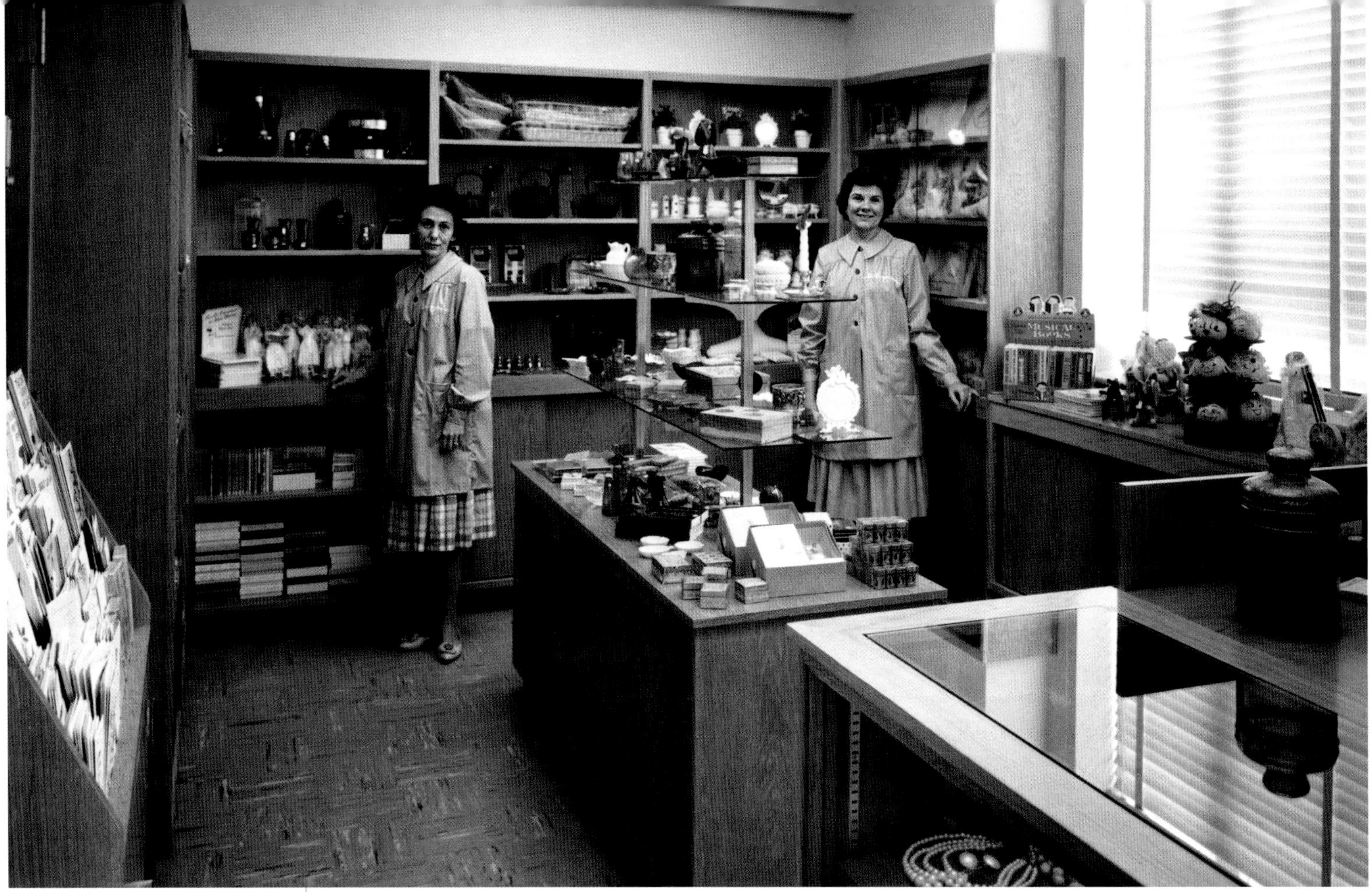

Above: The original gift shop opened by the Junior League at DeKalb General Hospital in 1961. **Right:** In 1990, Paula Austin managed the Dogwood Shop, which replaced the original gift shop.

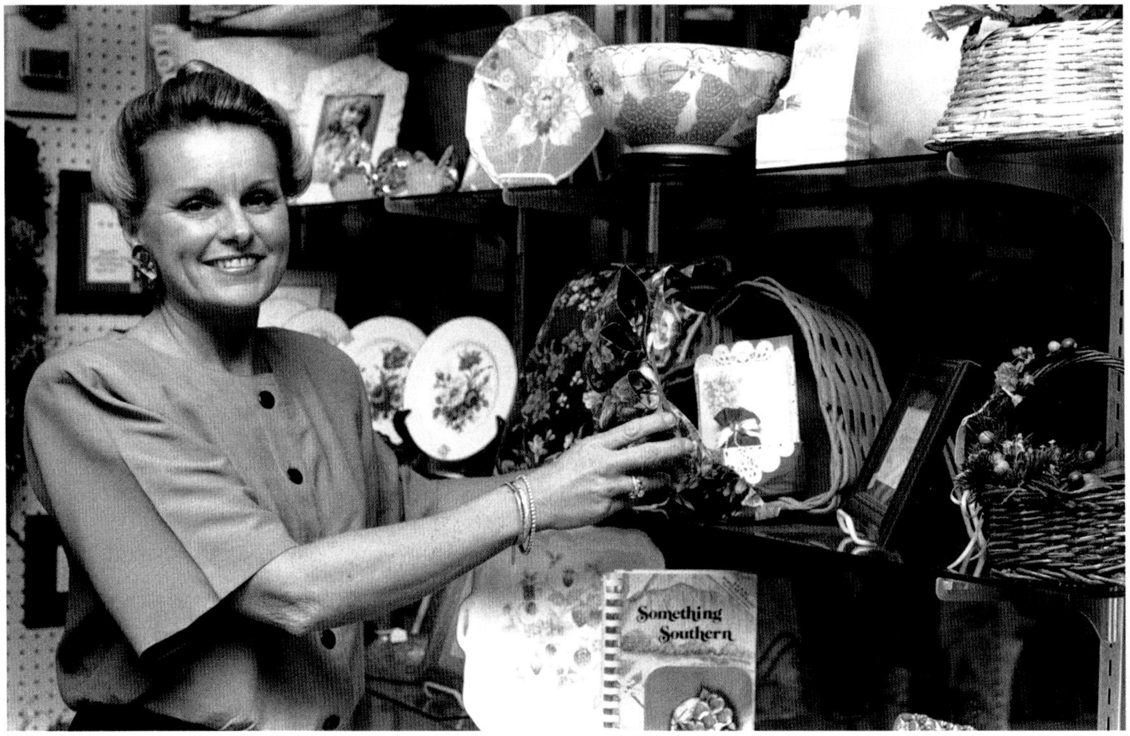

The DeKalb Junior League's services to DeKalb, however, did not end with the gift shop. in 1990 it played a decisive role in the formation of the DeKalb Rape Crisis Center in DeKalb Medical Center's Emergency Department. The league encouraged the hospital to house and support the center, and it recruited many volunteers who continue to play an important role in its services.[33]

The DeKalb Medical Auxiliary

Once the DeKalb General Auxiliary was established in 1973, Ree Stamps was elected as its first president. Jackie McCloud was vice president, Frances Thibadeau secretary, and Grace Lindley treasurer.[34] Annie Ruth Anderson (later Brown) became the auxiliary's second president.[35]

Ladies in the auxiliary wore blue smocks until 1975 when they chose pink as their official uniform. Dressed in pink, they were unofficially referred to as "Pink Ladies."[36] That title, of course, did not apply to the many male volunteers who became vital members of the auxiliary.

Unlike the Red Cross that did not try to raise money, the auxiliary described itself as a fund-raising as well as a service group.[37] And unlike the DeKalb Junior League that divided its profits among other causes, the auxiliary dedicated all its profits to the hospital and hospital-related services.

While most of the auxiliary's income originated in the Dogwood Shop, it created numerous other fund-raising enterprises. It held sales of books, linens, jewelry, watches, leather, sportswear, trinkets, quilts, toys, flowers and plants, handmade crafts, handbags, uniforms, and shoes. In 2006–2007 alone, the auxiliary generated $36,000 in ten special sales.[38] (Anyone who has attempted to pass an auxiliary booth during one of these sales knows what persuasive salespersons these volunteers can be.[39]) It also sold pictures of infants born at DeKalb Medical Center and instituted the Love Light Tree in 1980 for individuals to make donations in honor or in memory of others.[40]

The auxiliary's financial contributions have been remarkable. In its first year, it donated $5,000 to purchase a surgical table,[41] and a year later it raised $12,000 for mammography equipment.[42] In 1976 auxilians donated $20,000 to equip the hospital's first pulmonary function laboratory.[43] They paid for a beautiful, peaceful, wooded Dogwood Park on the northwest corner of the hospital campus that eventually became the site of the first Professional Office Building.[44] They purchased a C-Arm Imaging Intensifier for the operating room[45] and ultrasound equipment for Radiology.[46] They contributed $50,000 to help establish the DeKalb Rape Crisis Center in the Emergency Department, donated a van for the Mental Health Unit,[47] installed clocks in each room in the Skilled Nursing Facility,[48] and made a $155,000 donation toward the purchase of a Wellness on Wheels van to provide free services to schools, businesses, and underserved communities.[49]

In 1980 the auxiliary established a nursing scholarship fund to which it pledged $40,000 a year.[50] By 1995, in fifteen years, it had contributed $640,000 to assist 348 nursing students. By 2007 it had awarded $855,000 in scholarships.[51]

The auxiliary annually donated $35,000 to the Cancer Center.[52] In 2002 it established the Auxiliary Wish List Fund for community outreach projects or to make it possible for departments to purchase items needed to serve patients and their families. In the first five years, the Auxiliary Wish List Fund contributed over $121,000 to fifty-one department projects.

Once the DeKalb Medical Foundation was established, the auxiliary channeled most of its money to the foundation in support of its projects. By 2007 the auxiliary had raised a total of approximately $4.5 million of which approximately $1.8 million went to the foundation.[53]

The services provided by auxilians have been enormous. Auxilians work in nearly every hospital

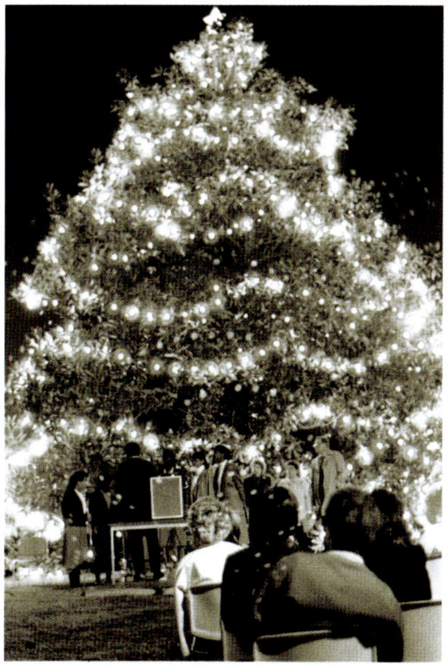

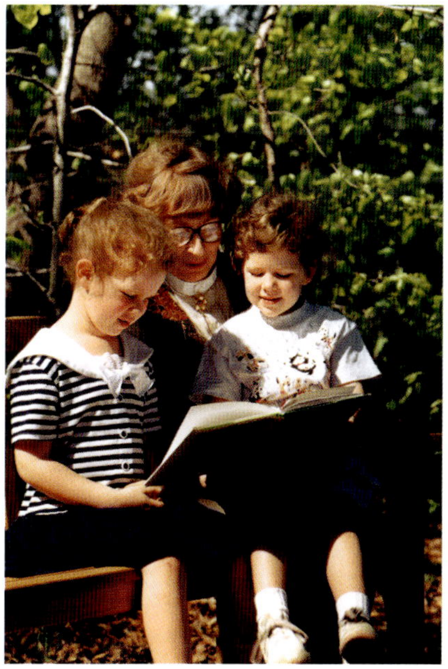

Top: The lighting of the Love Light Tree, 1988. **Above:** Kay Brown, a long-time administrative assistant to the chief financial officer, with her granddaughters enjoying Dogwood Park.

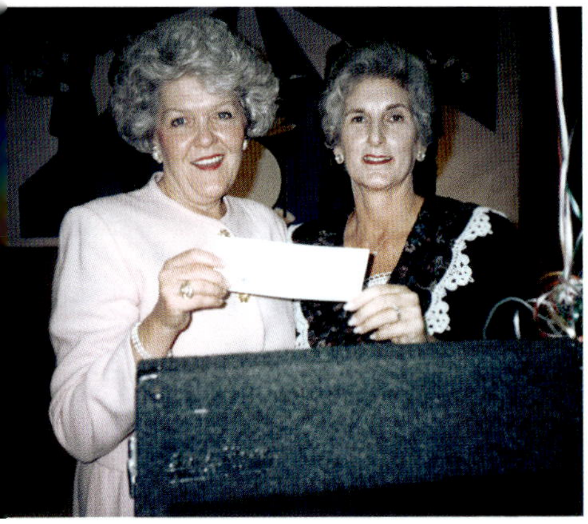

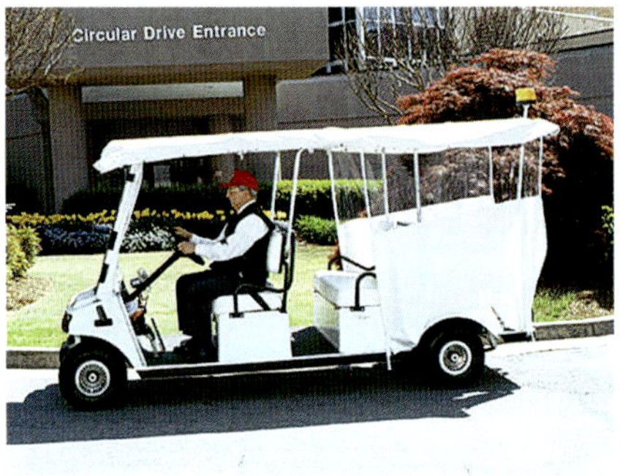

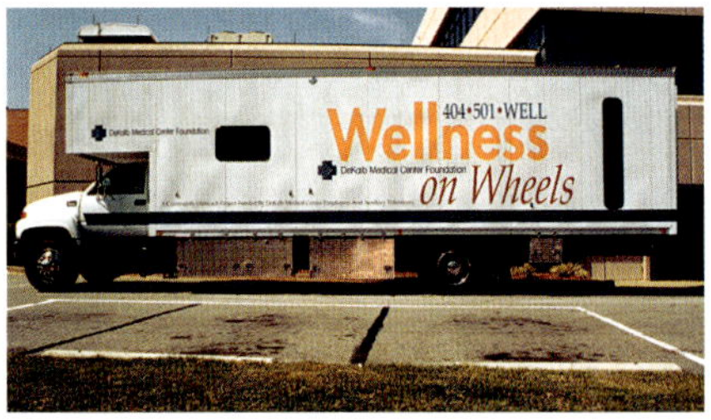

Top: Claire Peterson, (right) president of the DeKalb Medical Auxiliary, presents a check for $155,000 to Judy McMahan, chairperson of the DeKalb Medical Center Foundation. **Center:** The DeKalb Medical Auxiliary courtesy car. **Above:** The Wellness on Wheels van. **Right:** The volunteer "Knit Wits" knitting baby hats and blankets for the DeKalb newborns.

department. They manage the Dogwood Shop, assist in sorting and delivering mail, answer the phone and give directions at the Information Desk, prepare Emergency Department stretchers for patients, escort patients, provide clerical work and patient support in the critical care units, sort materials and make copies of requested information in the Health Sciences Library, provide coffee and tea to visitors in waiting rooms, drive the courtesy car to transport visitors and staff around the campus, receive and deliver flowers to patient rooms, assist with patient transport in the Diagnostic and Treatment Center (DTC), help the staff prepare for presentations in Education Services, assist in registration in the Breast Center, help with mass mailings in the DeKalb Medical Foundation, and assist with equipment and care of babies in the Mother/Baby unit.[54]

They make mastectomy pillows for breast cancer patients. They helped establish and continue to assist in the Consumer Health Library.[55] In 2002 the auxiliary began sponsoring DeKalb Medical's participation in MedShare International, a nonprofit organization that collects and sends surplus medical supplies and equipment to healthcare institutions in developing countries such as Haiti, Kenya, and El Salvador. In 2007 the three DeKalb Medical hospitals donated over 5,000 pounds of surplus medical supplies and equipment to MedShare International.[56]

Auxilians also work at the Downtown Decatur and Hillandale hospitals and with the Wellness on Wheels van.[57] They coordinate with a group affectionately known as "The Knit Wits," which gathers once a week to knit caps and make blankets for newborns. The Knit Wits produce over one thousand caps a year in a project begun twenty-three years ago by former DeKalb Medical Nursery's Gertrude Weiser, RN.[58]

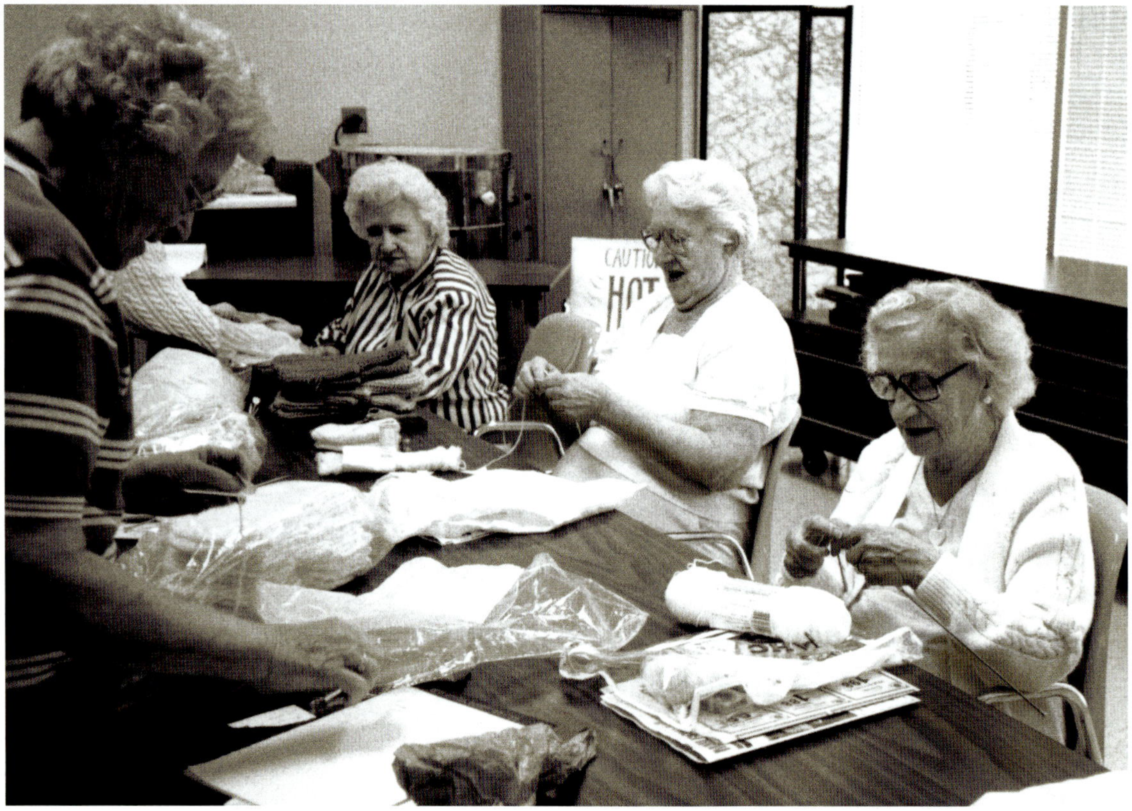

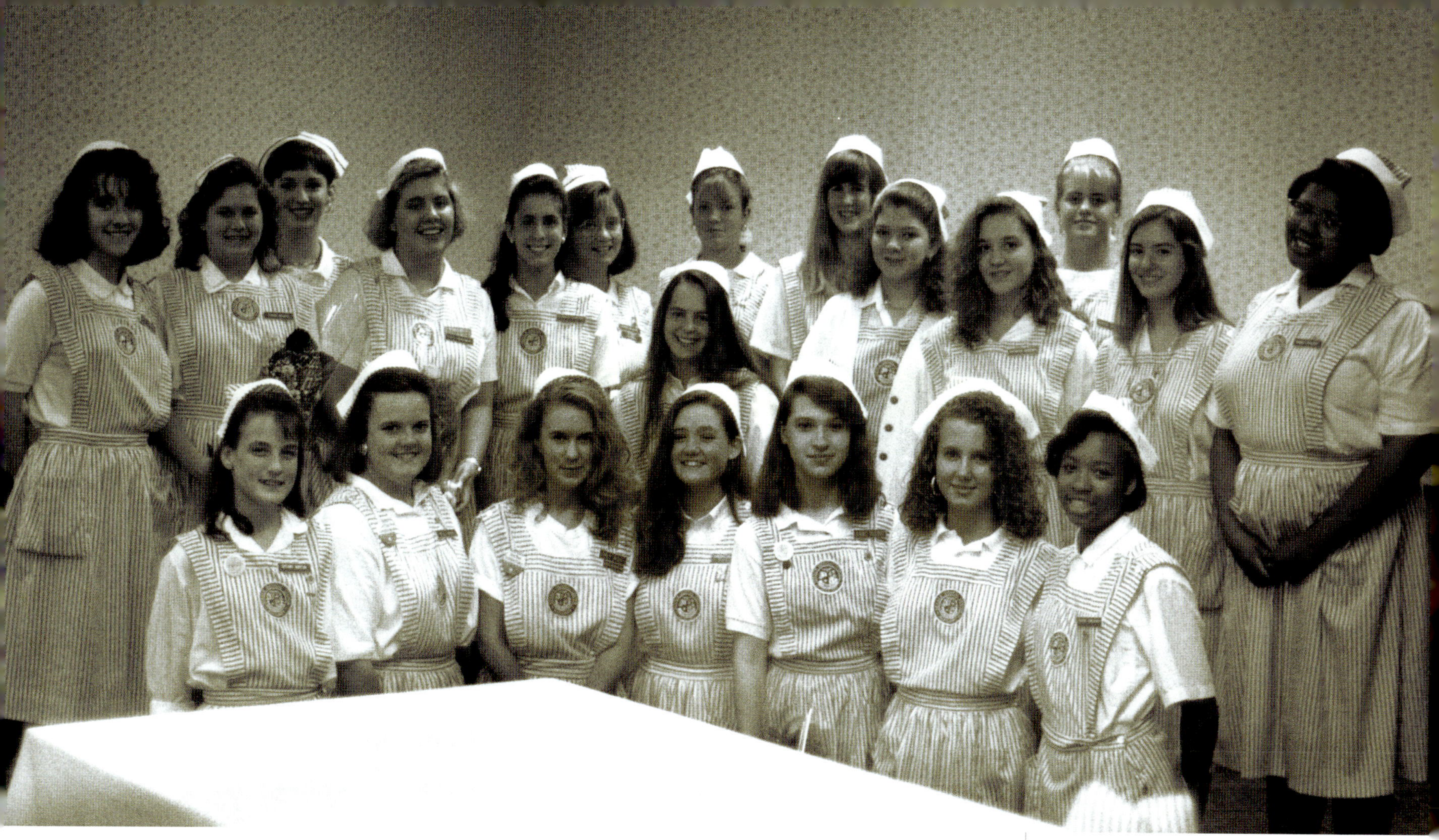

Adult auxilians recruit, organize, mentor, and encourage college-age volunteers and teen Candy Stripers. Through their volunteer work with the auxiliary, these young people have rendered valuable service, have learned the value of giving, and have been introduced to the possibility of future health-related careers.

Each auxilian contributes a minimum of one hundred hours of service a year. By the end of its first year, the auxiliary had 127 adult members who contributed 12,000 hours and 8 summer junior volunteers who donated over 1,000 hours.[59] In 2001, the fortieth anniversary of the hospital, the auxiliary celebrated its one million hours of service.[60] By 2007 auxiliary members had donated nearly 1.25 million hours. The hours contributed by the auxilians translate into millions of dollars in salaries that the hospital would have had to pay employees to perform those services freely given.[61]

In 2007 alone, the auxiliary's 130 active members, 25 associate members, 18 life members, and 24 new members donated 38,401 hours of service.[62] The dedication and contributions of these members is legendary. When Peg Kaiser retired in 2001 after forty years and 12,000 hours of service as both a Red Cross volunteer and an auxilian, she estimated that she had answered the phone 610,500 times.[63] Those volunteers heroically and unselfishly serve the institution, support the staff, and minister to patients with the gifts of their time, their talents, and their love.

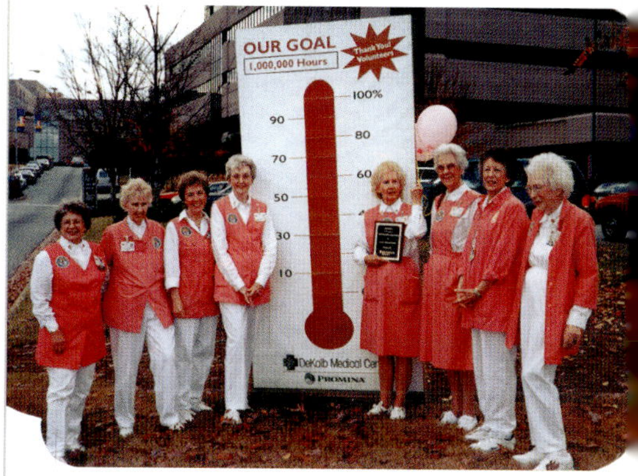

Top: All Youth Volunteers at the 1992 banquet.
Above: DeKalb Medical Auxiliary members celebrate 1,000,000 hours of service in 2001.

Other Volunteers

Members of the medical staff, the hospital staff, and the community volunteer in a variety of other worthy service endeavors. The Good Will/Good Works Program places individuals without established job skills into volunteer positions that allow them to gain on-the-job experience and skills to qualify for employment.[64] College students, many of whom are enrolled in premedical or nursing programs, volunteer for duties that provide a meaningful service and firsthand clinical experience.[65] DeKalb Medical physicians, nurses, and other employees staff the Physicians' Care Clinic that offers services to uninsured DeKalb citizens. Physicians and others professionals donate their vacations and pay their own way to provide medical care in Kenya, South Africa, Haiti, and other underserved areas of the world.[66] DeKalb volunteers build homes for Habitat for Humanity. They conduct physical examinations for youth sports teams. In one year members of the Care Corps, another organization that chooses specific projects to support each year, contributed over 6,000 hours in a variety of volunteer activities.[67] First Steps identifies and works with pregnant women at risk. Health Adventures mentors young people who have an interest in health careers. Volunteers participate in runs, walks, and marathons to raise money and awareness for health-related causes.

In addition to providing direct patient care, physicians, hospital staff, and community volunteers thus play a vital role in supporting and enhancing DeKalb Medical's mission to "partner with our community to improve lives by providing excellent healthcare services."[68]

The DeKalb Medical Foundation

DeKalb General looked to the community for financial support even before the first brick was laid. The trustees tried in several ways to encourage donations. They advertised that a donor could memorialize a room with a gift of $2,500 or more[69] or could have a plaque mounted on a hospital room door by

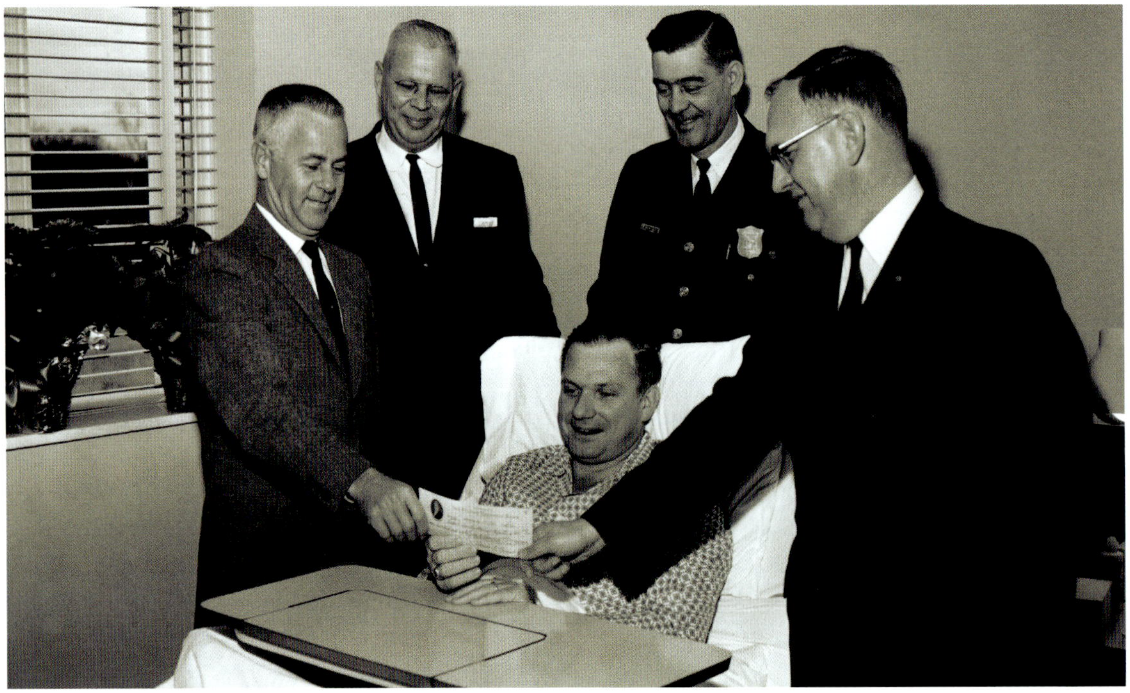

The DeKalb County Masonic Association presenting a check to William Thrasher to furnish a solarium at the hospital. Left to right: Horis A. Ward, Norman E. Turner, Leon Freeman (patient), David Clayton, and William Thrasher, administrator.

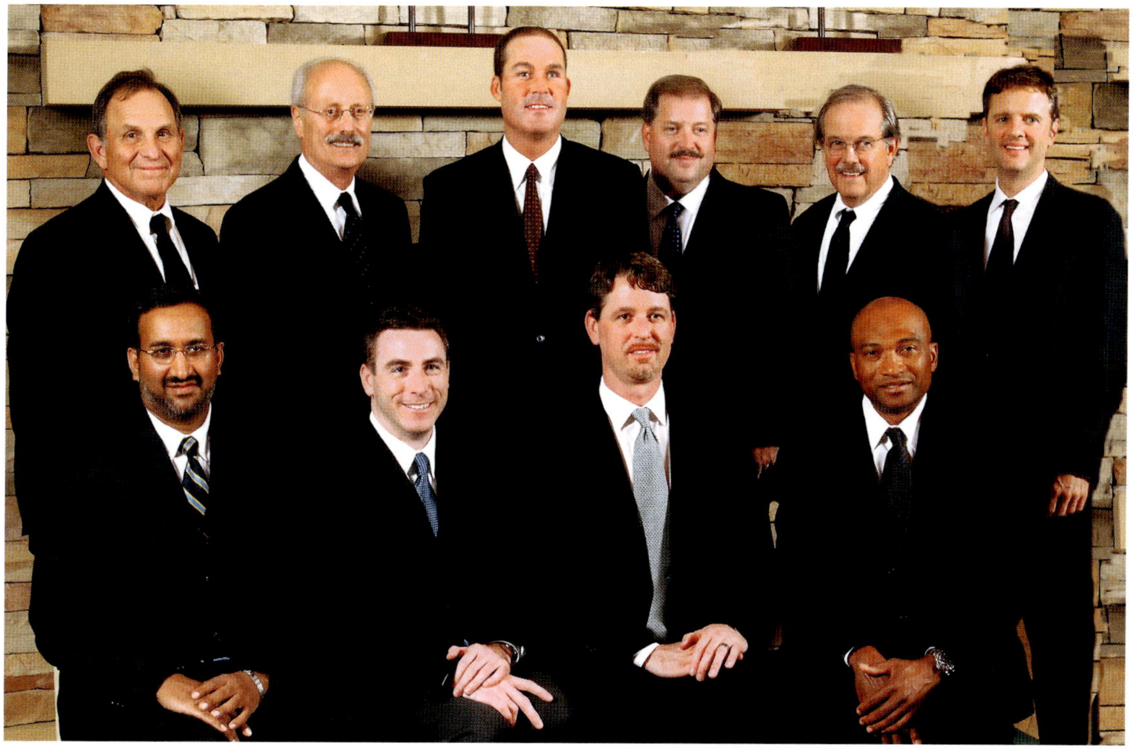

Radiology Associates of DeKalb, P.C. were major donors to the 2006–2009 campaign. Left to right top row: Jay S. Coffsky, MD, Gary M. Laskey, MD, John C. Reid II, MD, Gordon L. Hixson, Jr., MD, Robert L. Davies, MD, Linton W. Eberhart IV, MD, bottom: Pramod K. Kaila, MD, Christopher J. Krebs, MD, Steven C. Storey, MD, Kelvin K. Belcher, MD. Not pictured is William G. Whitaker, MD.

giving $1,000 to furnish a room.[70] They asked civic organizations to sponsor scholarships for students enrolled in the nursing program at the Smith-Hughes Vocational School with the hope scholarships would help employ nurses when DeKalb General opened.[71] The DeKalb County Hospital Authority launched a campaign to raise $100,000 for all-electric hospital beds and other equipment not originally budgeted.[72] It conducted a direct-mailing solicitation campaign.[73] Trustees called on the Woodruff Foundation, the Whitehead Foundation, the Campbell Foundation, and the Doraville General Motors plant executives to request $25,000 from each organization.[74]

Their efforts bore fruit in varying sizes. Among the donors, the General Motors Doraville plant contributed $25,000,[75] the Whitehead Foundation made two gifts of $10,000 each,[76] the DeKalb County Board of Commissioners donated $55,000,[77] the Junior Service League gave $3,000 for the chapel,[78] Mrs. T. W. Robinson donated $2,000 to furnish two rooms,[79] the Decatur Lions Club contributed $1,000 to furnish a room,[80] the Decatur Pilot Club held a fund-raising spaghetti supper,[81] the Cotillion Club gave $500 for a "Mood-Master" taped music system for the hospital,[82] and the Happy Grandmother's Club donated a Bible for the chapel.[83] Contributions continued to come after the hospital was built.

But not every lead paid off. One physician told the trustees that one of his patients wanted to make a sizeable donation to the hospital.[84] The Authority immediately dispatched Administrator William Thrasher and trustee Ross McCain to call on that potential donor. They reported back at the Authority's next meeting that, unfortunately, the individual did not have any spare money.[85]

Over the years many individuals and organizations have made substantial financial contributions to the hospital and its services. In 1961 hospital employees established the Good Samaritan Fund to

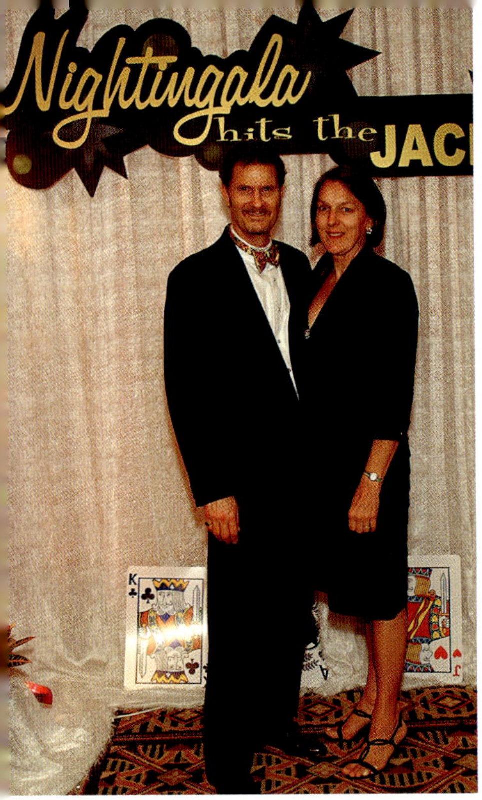

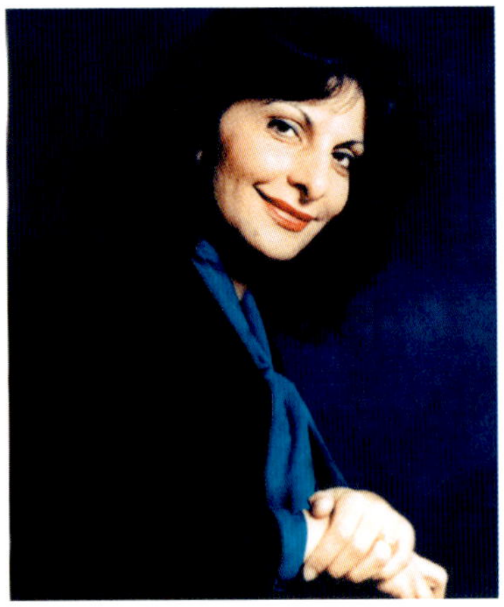

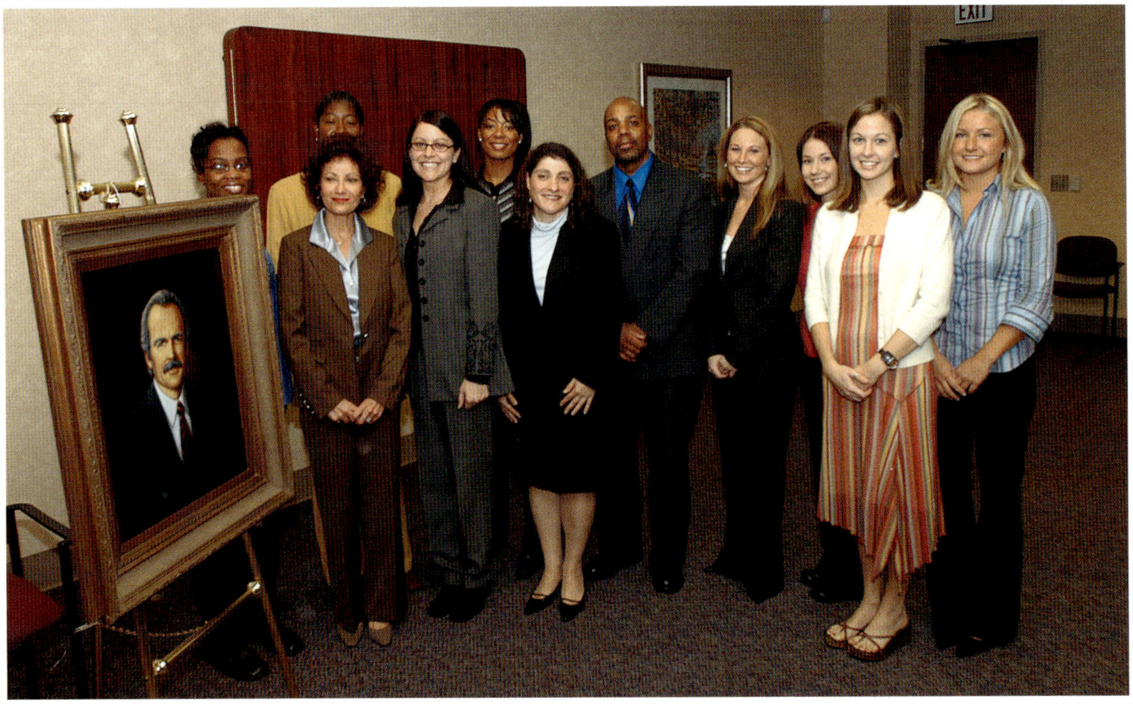

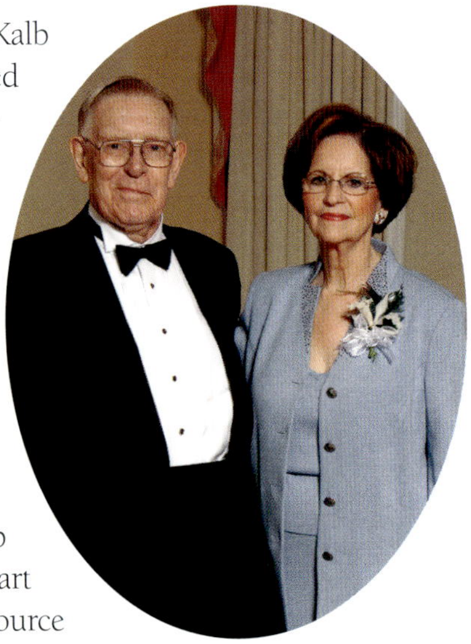

Top: Robin Dretler, MD, and his wife Muffie Michaelson originated the idea of a Nightingala to raise money for the hospital. **Above:** Gulshan Harjee, MD, internist and member of the DeKalb Medical Board of Directors, established a scholarship program for high school seniors interested in pursuing a medical career. **Top right:** Jean Coppage White stands next to a portrait of Mark Coppage, MD, in whose memory the Coppage Nursing Scholarship was created. Standing with Jean are recipients. **Right:** Jack and Audrey Morgan are generous donors who established a scholarship enabling DeKalb Medical employees to further their education in health-related fields.

benefit patients with financial needs.[86] In 1971 employees established the Good Neighbor Fund, later named the Friendship Fund, to benefit some of the more-than-fifty charitable organizations in the greater Atlanta area.[87] The Friendship Fund later was merged with W.H.A.T., still another employee-sponsored charitable fund (see below).

In 1989 Robin Dretler, MD, and his wife Muffie Michaelson conceived an annual Nightingala extravaganza to raise money and goodwill for the hospital. Some thought it would never work. They were wrong. The very first Nightingala was a "roaring" success, provided great fun, and raised $7,000 for nursing scholarships.[88]

In 1993 the family of Mark Coppage, MD, a highly regarded DeKalb Medical anesthesiologist who died in an automobile accident, established a nursing scholarship in his memory. Jean Coppage White and her husband Glenn White match all funds contributed by supporting donors.[89] As of 2007 the fund has awarded 103 scholarships totaling $246,400 to nursing students.[90]

Audrey and Jack Morgan established a scholarship for DeKalb Medical employees seeking to further their education in a health-related field.[91] Gulshan Harjee, MD, created a scholarship fund for high school seniors who wish to pursue a career in medicine or allied health care.[92] William P. Tatum, long-time chairman of the Hospital Authority, and his daughter Susan established a scholarship in memory of Mrs. Tatum to encourage excellence in oncology nursing at DeKalb Medical.[93] Dee Keeton organized the charitable Charles B. Eberhart Memorial Golf Classic.[94] The auxiliary, as described above, was a major source

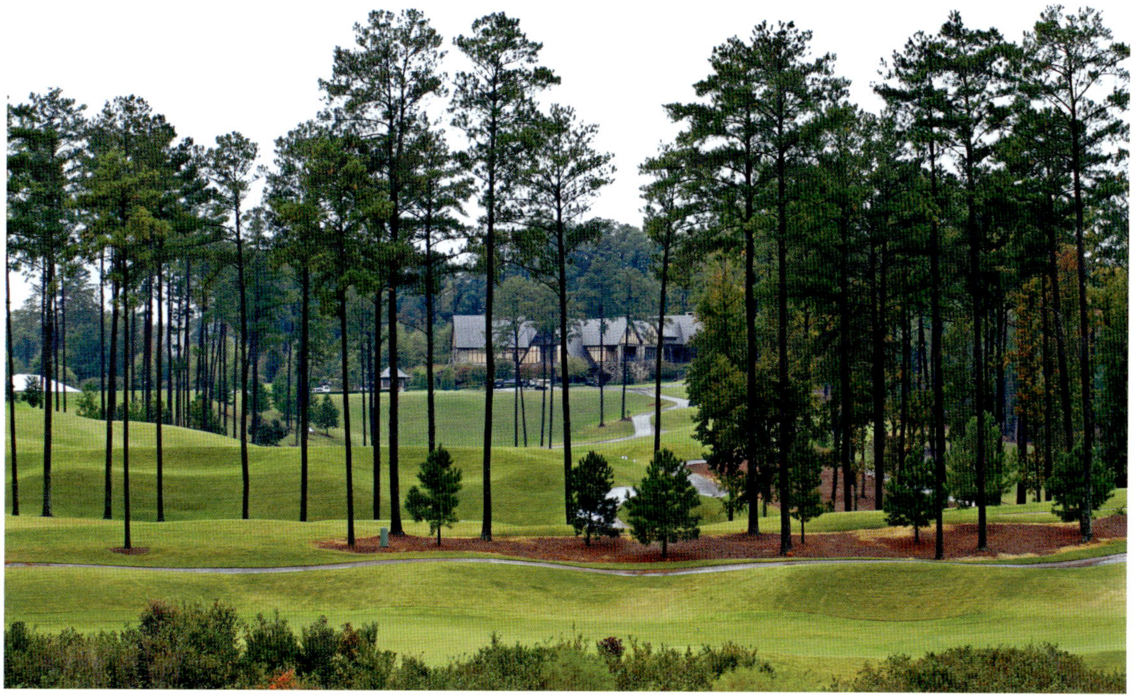

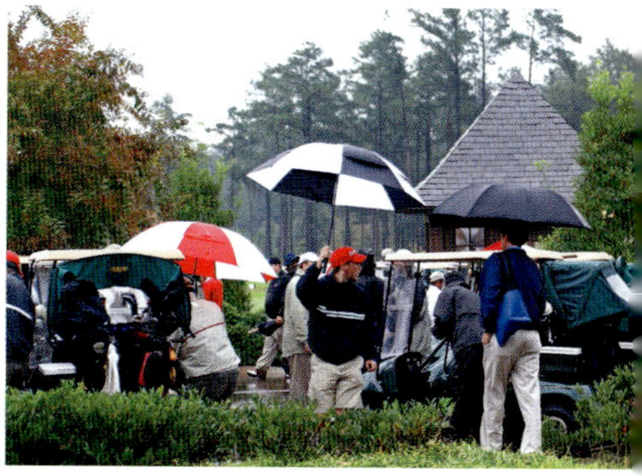

Left and above: Dee Keeton organized the Charles B. Eberhart Memorial Golf Classic, which has been a major source of financial support since it began in 1973.

of financial and personal service support from the time it was established in 1973.

In the spring of 1988, DeKalb General Hospital Authority member Judy McMahan urged Administrator Charles Eberhart and the trustees to establish a development organization to "raise friends and raise funds" for the hospital.[95] McMahan was persistent, and eventually Eberhart and the trustees liked the idea. Eberhart and McMahan attended a seminar to learn more about creating such an organization. They recommended the foundation model with its own governing board of trustees.[96] The Authority retained the services of Lyons Associates to assist in its development and approved foundation bylaws and articles of incorporation in the summer of 1990.[97] Charles Eberhart, William P. Tatum, and Judy McMahan were named as the three original trustees.[98] Judy McMahan also was asked to serve as the first DeKalb Medical Foundation chairperson, and Dana Jackson (later Rawls) was named its first executive director.[99]

The mission of the foundation was to strengthen the linkage between DeKalb Medical and the community through communication, education, service, and philanthropy; and to improve the standard of health in the community by raising friends and funds for the healthcare initiatives offered through DeKalb Medical.[100]

In 1992 DeKalb Medical employees created a voluntary giving program to support the foundation and other causes. They called their program "W.H.A.T.," originally an acronym for "We Help Achieve Tomorrow," and later "Working, Healing, Achieving Together."[101] In addition to contributing more than $2 million to the foundation,[102] W.H.A.T. merged with the employees' Friendship Fund in 1992 and has given support to as many as twelve or more community service organizations, including the DeKalb Rape Crisis Center, the Atlanta Union Mission, the Atlanta Community Food Bank, and the Brain Tumor Foundation for Children.[103] W.H.A.T.'s membership includes more than nine hundred employees, over half of whom make their donations through regular payroll deductions.[104]

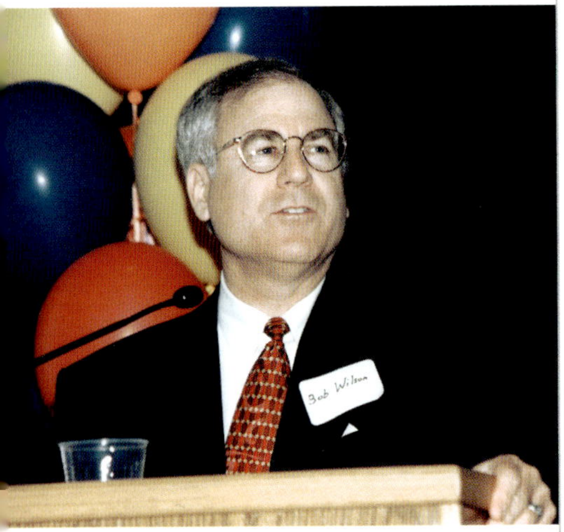

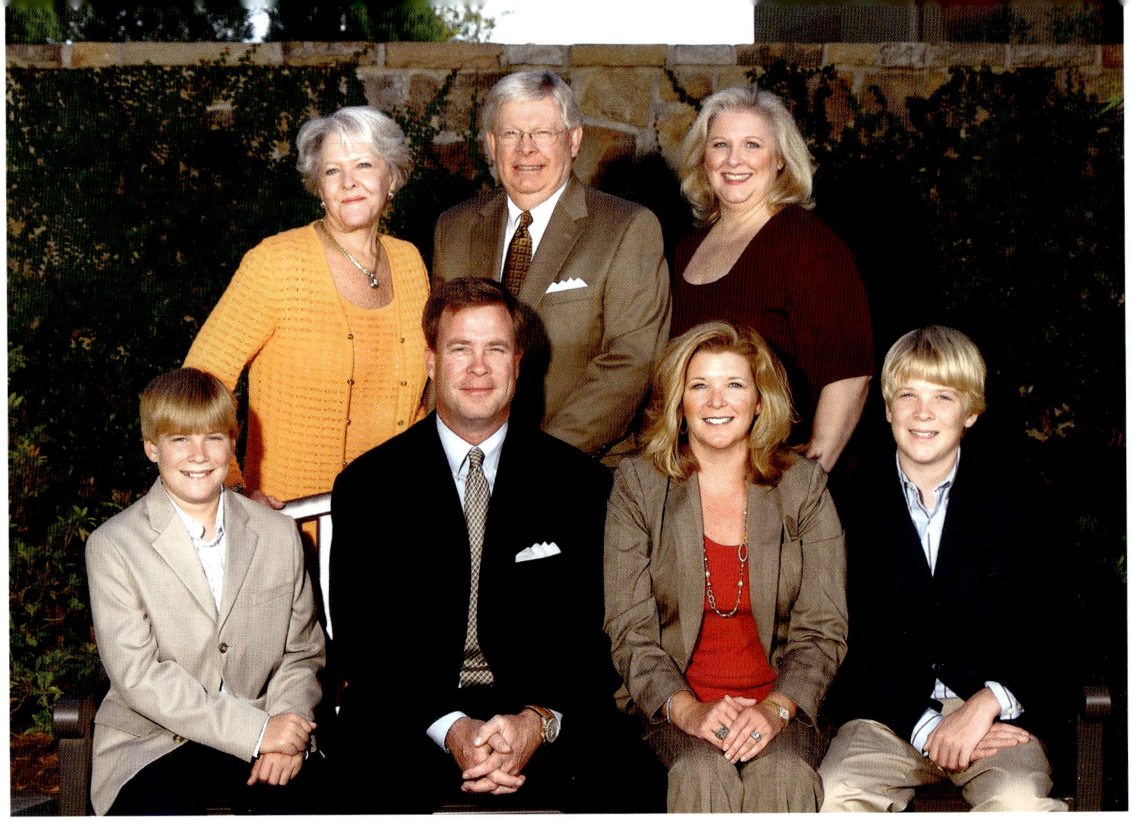

Above: Robert E. "Bob" Wilson is DeKalb Medical Foundation's fourth and present chairman, and a member of the DeKalb Medical Board of Directors. **Above right:** Robert and Judy McMahan helped make it possible to renovate and expand the Emergency Department and the critical care units. Their portraits hang in the Hall of Heroes and the Atrium in the Women's and Surgery Center has been named in honor of their family.

Once the foundation was established, many of the existing fund-raising initiatives came under its umbrella and donated most if not all of their funds to foundation projects. The DeKalb Medical Auxiliary has contributed over $1.8 million, the Nightingala more than $1.5 million,[105] and the Golf Classic more than $500,000 to the foundation.[106]

The foundation became a major factor, as McMahan predicted, in creating personal and financial support for DeKalb Medical. From its inception through 2007, it completed four major fund-raising campaigns and initiated a fifth. Judy McMahan served as foundation chairperson through the first two campaigns, Maureen Vandiver became chairperson in 1996, J. Randall "Randy" Carroll in 1999, Sarah Sloan in 2000 and Robert E. "Bob" Wilson in 2001. The directors of the foundation who succeeded Dana Jackson Rawls include Heather Van Sice, Rhonda Davidson, Mendy Nord, and Leigh Minter who was named executive director of the DeKalb Medical Foundation in 2007.

The 1991–1994 campaign raised $1.5 million to renovate, expand, and equip the Surgery and Maternity Center.

The 1994–1996 campaign raised $1.6 million to renovate and expand the Emergency Department and the Critical Care units.[107] It was supported by major donations from Robert McMahan in honor of his wife Judy for whom the new coronary care unit was named; from Audrey and Jack Morgan in honor of Audrey Morgan's sister, Bobbie Bailey, for whom the Emergency Department waiting area was named; and from the auxiliary and W.H.A.T.

The 1996–2001 "Community Partnership/2000" campaign raised $5 million for the Charles B. Eberhart Cancer Center, including the expansion of the Kann Outpatient Treatment Center and the acquisition of radiosurgery software; the Wellness on Wheels to provide health care, screening, and educational activities to the underserved members of southwest DeKalb County and the Buford Highway corridor; the Physicians' Care Clinic for underinsured and uninsured citizens of DeKalb County; and a $500,000, three-year pilot project in partnership with the City of Decatur schools to provide school nurses for on-site health services in the schools and education for students and their families, and to link every student with a primary care physician.[108] For its support of this innovative school project, the foundation received the Atlanta Business Chronicle's Healthcare Hero Award.[109]

The 1996–2001 campaign was supported by major contributions from the Lou Morris and A. Worley Brown Foundation to establish an endowment fund for the Cancer Center's free cancer-counseling, educational, and screening activities;[110] from William L. "Pete" and Jerri Pike to redesign and renovate the DeKalb Medical at North Decatur chapel;[111] and from the auxiliary and W.H.A.T.

The 2003–2005 "Diagnosing the Future" campaign raised more than $5 million to purchase a PET/CT scanner in the Imaging Center, two digital mammography machines, stereotactic radiosurgery equipment and software, and contributed to the expansion of the cancer center endowment for its free services, and the Wellness on Wheels services. The campaign exceeded its $5 million goal due to major contributions from former CEO John R. "Jack" and Barbara Gerlach, Duane and Emy Blair,[112] Lou Brown Jewell in honor of Betty Castellani,[113] Bobbie Bailey,[114] Jack and Audrey Morgan,[115] the sixteenth annual Nightingala, W.H.A.T., the DeKalb Medical Auxiliary, and the Susan G. Komen Foundation.

The 2006–2009 "Building a Healthier Tomorrow" campaign raised $5.5 million for all-private beds for the North Decatur and Downtown Decatur hospitals, diabetes and cancer health education, continued support of the Physicians' Care Clinic and replacement of the Wellness on Wheels van. The campaign received major donations from William L. "Pete" and Jerri Pike for the chapel at DeKalb Medical at Hillandale, Gregory B. and Betty Levett Sr., for the Emergency Department reception area at Hillandale, Neil and Jackie Christman for the new Wellness on Wheels and the Physicians' Care Clinic,

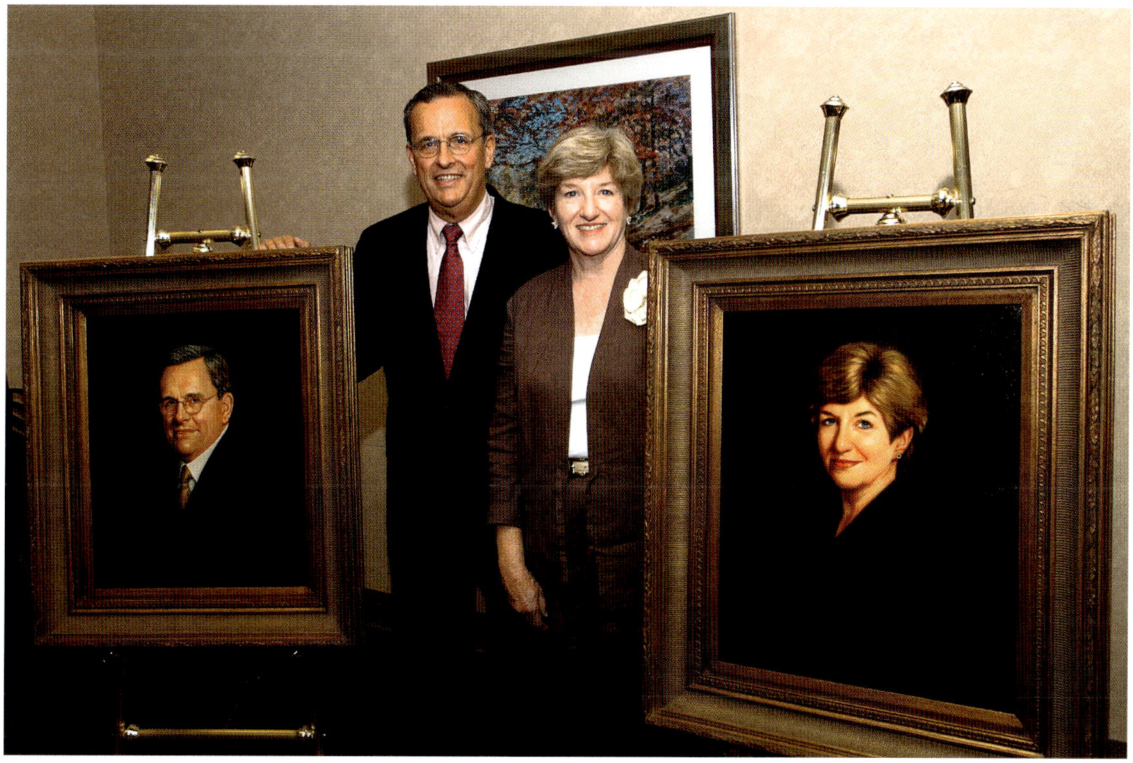

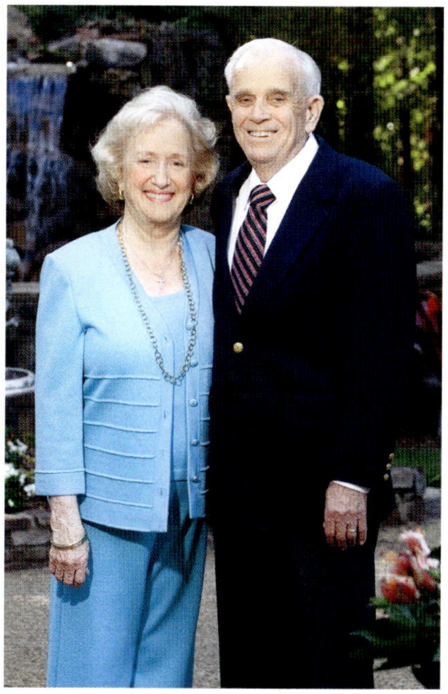

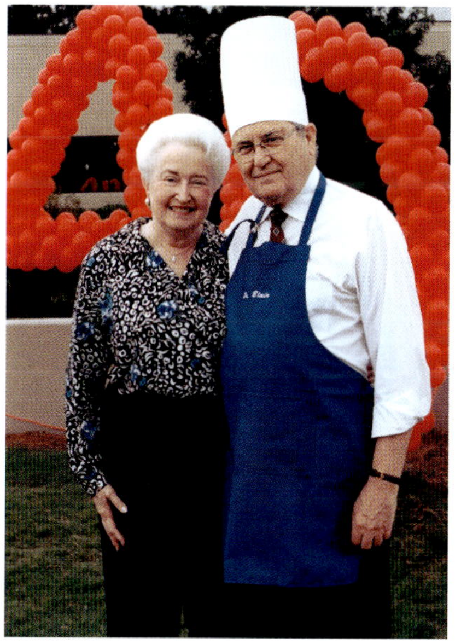

Left and above: Former CEO John R. (Jack) Gerlach and his wife Barbara standing near their portraits, and Duane Blair, MD, and his wife Emy were all major donors to the 2003–2005 Foundation campaign "Diagnosing the Future."
Top: William L. (Pete) and Jerri Pike made major donations for the chapels at the North Decatur and the Hillandale hospitals.

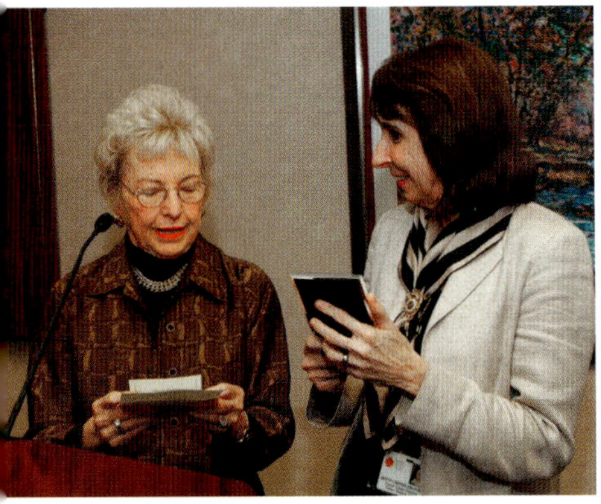

Top: Lou Brown Jewell, left, made a major gift to the Foundation in honor of Betty Castellani. **Right and far right:** Neil and Jackie Christman and Gregory and Betty Levett Sr. all were generous donors to the foundation campaign.

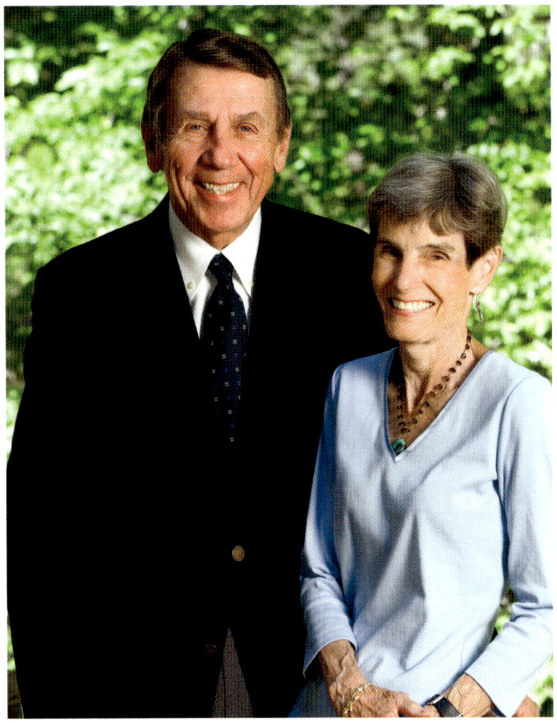

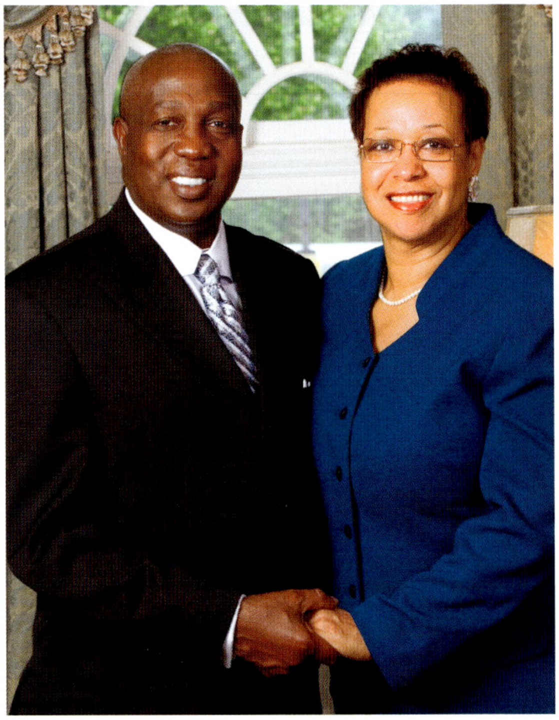

Radiology Associates of DeKalb, PC, for the Diagnostic Imaging Center Reception Area, the Robert and Judy McMahan family for the Atrium in the Women's and Surgery Center, Jack and Audrey Morgan for the Physicians' Care Clinic, the Dorothy B. Stretcher Estate, Neal and Joan Pope, the DeKalb Medical Auxiliary, the Nightingala, the Charles B. Eberhart Memorial Golf Classic, and W.H.A.T.

The 2006–2009 campaign achieved early success due a to a $3.3 million gift by Bobbie Bailey, already a major contributor to the foundation. A portion of her gift, $1.8 million, closed the current "Building a Healthier Tomorrow" campaign, and the remaining $1.5 million launched the foundation's next campaign that includes acquiring state-of-the-art robotic surgical technology and a dedicated breast MRI.[116]

At a time when DeKalb Medical simultaneously faced increasing financial challenges and growing service needs, the DeKalb Medical Foundation has made an invaluable contribution to the life and mission of the institution. It not only has provided funds to support the organization's mission and services, it has welded DeKalb Medical to the hearts and minds of a host of community volunteers and employees who have become its goodwill ambassadors as well as its benefactors.

On the occasion of her retirement from the DMC and DRHS boards in 2005, Judy McMahan was recognized for her special contributions to DeKalb Medical and to the foundation. Her roots were described as deep and wide. She delivered her first child at DeKalb General Hospital in 1964. She became a member of the Red Cross Volunteers in 1976 and the DeKalb Medical Auxiliary in 1995. She served as a member of the DeKalb County Hospital Authority from 1985 to 1996 and as a member of the DMC Board of Directors and the DRHS Board of Directors from 1992 to 2005. She was chairman of the DMC Board from 2000 to 2004.

Judy McMahan jokingly said that when she first introduced the idea of a hospital foundation,

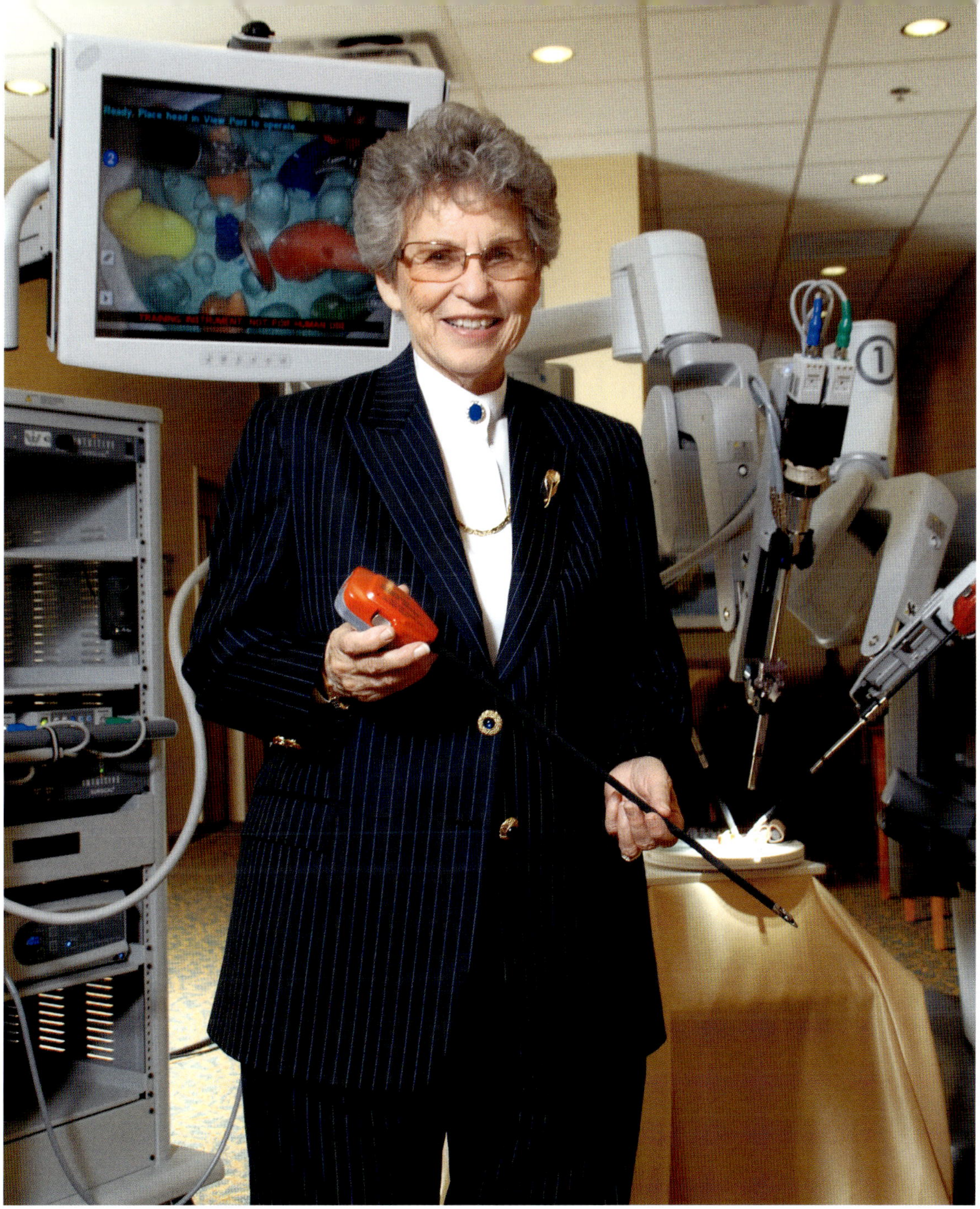

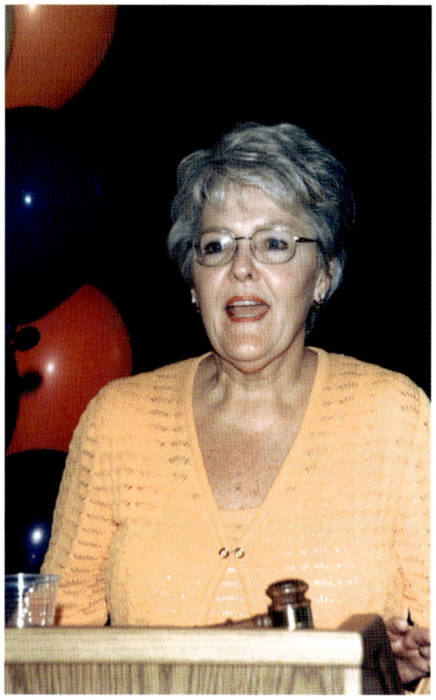

Left: Bobbie Bailey donated $3.3 million, which completed the 2006–2009 campaign "Building a Healthier Tomorrow" and launched the next campaign that purchased the surgical da Vinci robot. **Above:** Judy McMahan is founder and first chairperson of the DeKalb Medical Foundation.

there were only two people whom she was sure would give any money: her husband and Charles Eberhart.[117] She greatly underestimated the esteem in which she is held and her persuasive powers.

One supporter said "her presence is enough to turn strangers into friends, and her energy can ignite even the stuffiest of crowds."[118] Her vision of a foundation that could bring personal and financial support to her hospital became a reality and exceeded all expectations. At the time of her retirement, the foundation had raised over $14 million and created a climate of sharing and caring.[119] The legacy of the service, energy, love, and leadership she has given to DeKalb Medical, and the financial support she and her family have given to DeKalb Medical are immeasurable and invaluable.

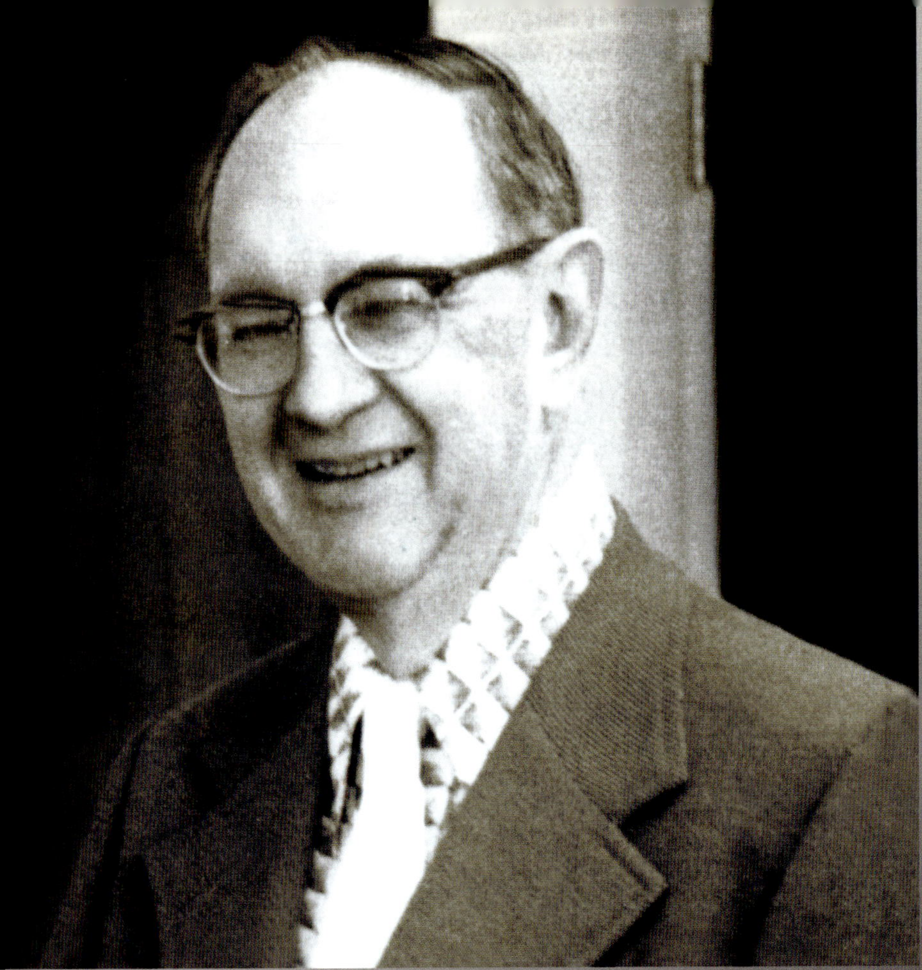

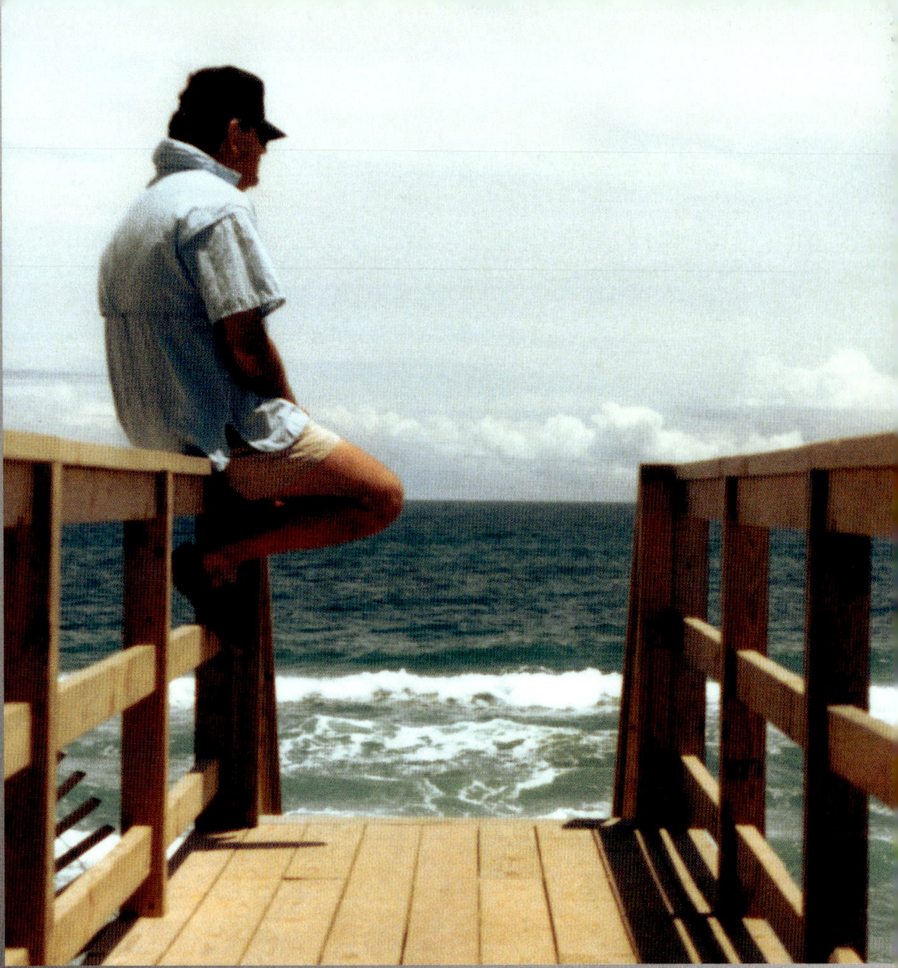

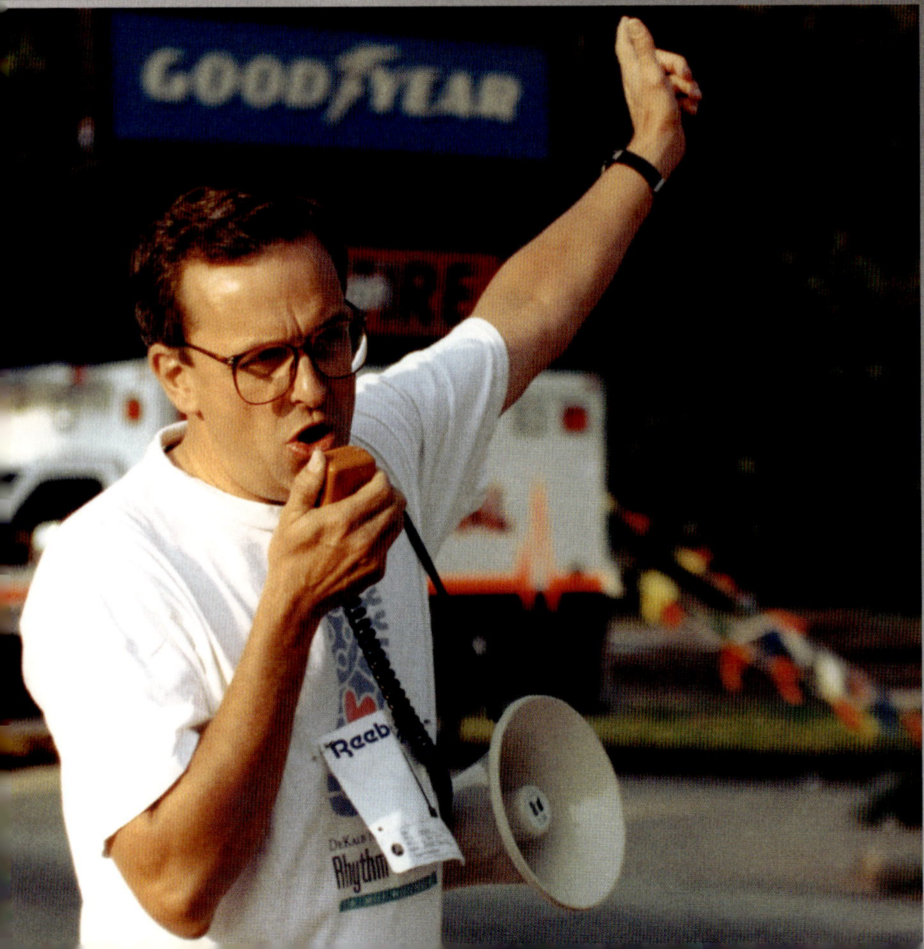
GOODYEAR

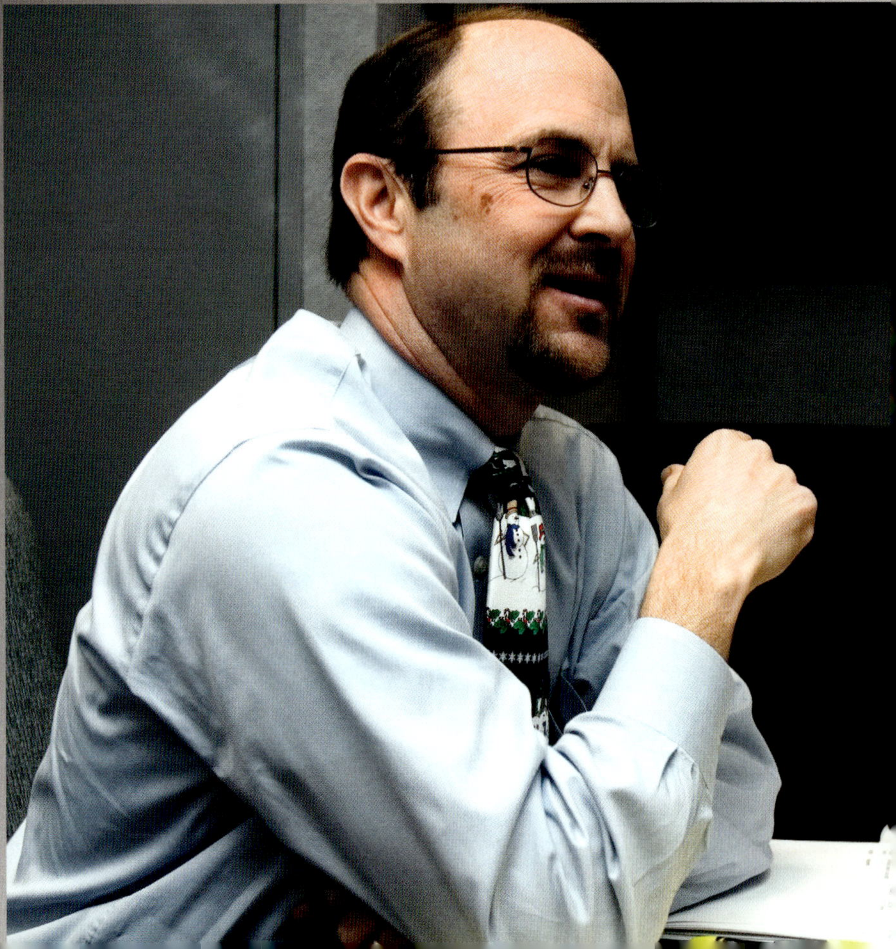

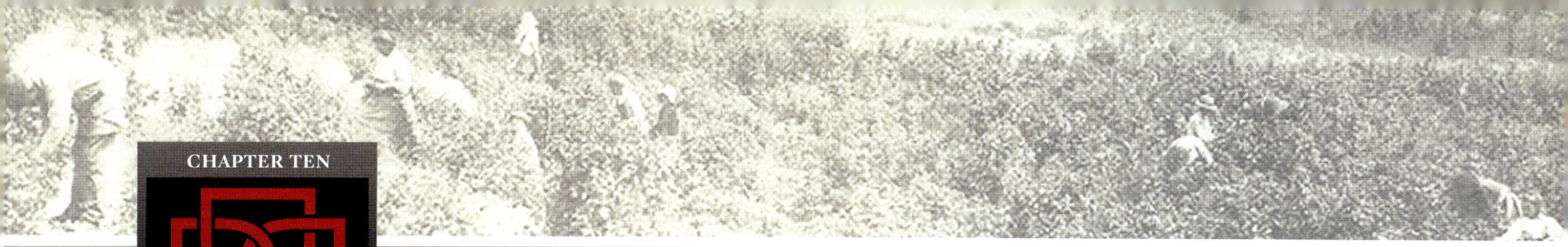

CHAPTER TEN

The Legacy of the Leaders

Lives of great men all remind us
We can make our lives sublime,
And, departing, leave behind us
Footprints in the sands of time.

— "A Psalm of Life" by
Henry Wadsworth Longfellow

DeKalb Medical has benefited from the leadership of four strong administrators/chief executive officers: William Harwell Thrasher (1958–1973), Charles Barr Eberhart (1973–1995), John Richard Gerlach (1995–2003), and Eric Paul Norwood (2003–present).

Each has left his individual, indelible mark on the community, the lives he touched, and the institution he served. Though retired from the helm of DeKalb Medical, John Gerlach continues to contribute and serve. While still at the helm, Eric Norwood is contributing daily to the DeKalb Medical story.

Opposite: Clockwise beginning at top left: William Harwell Thrasher, Charles Barr Eberhart, Eric Paul Norwood, and John Richard Gerlach. **Right:** William Thrasher as a young student.

William Harwell Thrasher

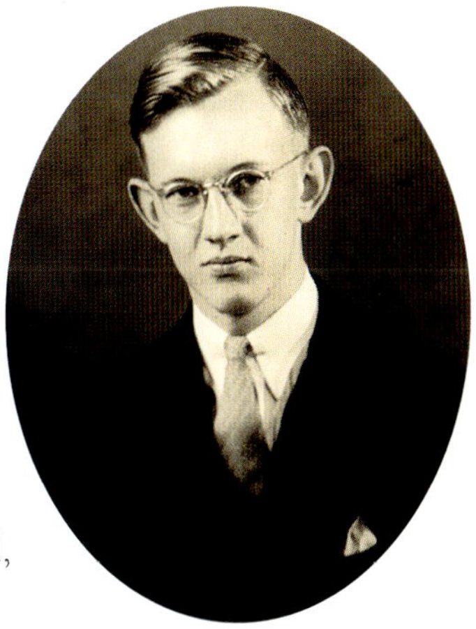

William H. Thrasher became DeKalb General Hospital's first administrator in 1958. He was born in Watkinsville, near Athens, Georgia, in 1917. He obtained his first three years of elementary education in Plains, Georgia, before moving with his family to Decatur, Georgia, where he attended Winnona Park Grammar School, Decatur Junior High, and Decatur Boys High. He received a bachelor's degree in business administration from Emory University in 1939. He married Mary Helen Finger in 1947, and they had five children: William Harwell Jr., Jo Anne, Donald, Douglas, and Mary.

William Thrasher with his wife Helen and two of their children Harwell (left) and Joanne (right).

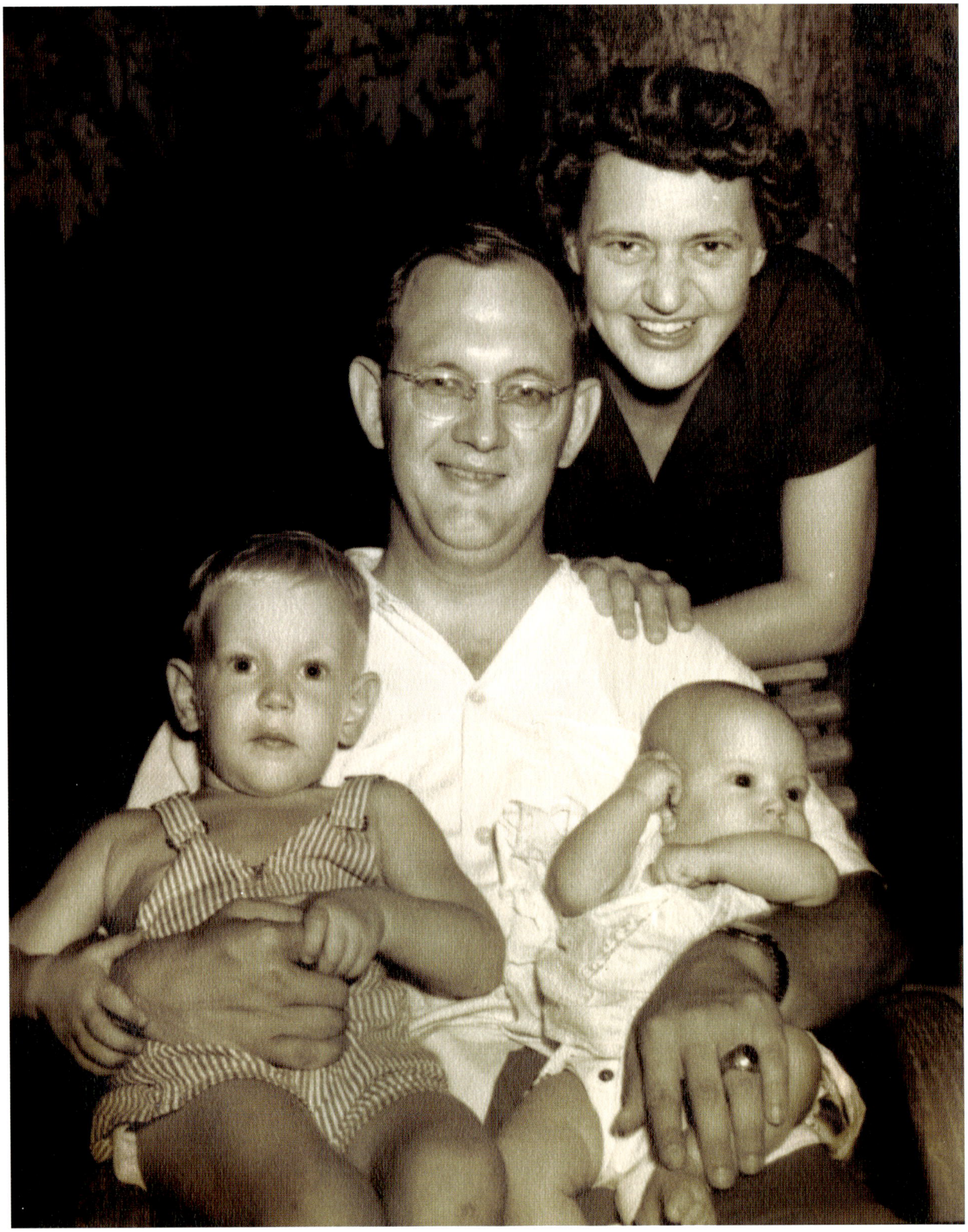

Following his graduation from Emory, Thrasher worked in the insurance industry and then served in the War Department's Army Counter Intelligence Corps in World War II. At the end of the war, he returned briefly to the insurance industry before taking a position with the Georgia Department of Public Health and later becoming director of the John D. Archbold Memorial Hospital in Thomasville, Georgia. As a result of his health-related experiences, Thrasher decided to enter the field of hospital administration.

He received a master's degree in hospital administration at the University of Minnesota in 1955 and served three years as administrator of Athens (Georgia) General Hospital. He was at Athens when he became a candidate for the administrator's post at DeKalb General Hospital which was still in the planning stage.

As described in chapter two, the DeKalb County Hospital Authority was sufficiently impressed with Thrasher's ideas about planning and operating a hospital, ideas he had to provide without the benefit of seeing the architectural plans or meeting with the governing body, that in 1958 it offered him the job as employee number 0001.

Thrasher was respected for his integrity. He was known to be truthful and trustworthy, and he looked for those values in others. He revealed a great deal about his own value system in the staff he selected. He sought individuals who were competent and experienced but who demonstrated something more. He chose Ted Barner as his first assistant administrator because he had worked with Barner in Athens and knew he would bring character as well as competence to the job. Charles Anderson was chosen as the hospital's first chief financial officer because he "was of good character and fully qualified to do the work." He named Opal Hopkins Fyffe as his director of Nursing over other highly qualified candidates because he knew she could do the job, but also because he "liked her" and knew they could work well together.[1] In Thrasher's estimation, one's values were as important as one's training, experience, and expertise.

For Thrasher, the Hospital Authority was both a blessing and a challenge. The trustees were a blessing because they were committed "heart and soul" to the hospital. What they gave to their responsibilities as trustees—the time, talent, and energy—was legendary. They were totally committed to its success. The hospital was their "baby," and they were determined to see it thrive and grow. And they provided a strong balance of expertise that included medical experience, business acumen, financial knowledge, legal proficiency, and a background in education, all of which contributed to planning and managing a new hospital. They had strong ties with the political and business leadership of the community; and they enjoyed the unqualified respect of the community, public officials, physicians, and the media, again valuable assets. They were proven leaders.

When Thrasher brought to the trustees an idea that they liked or presented them a need that they approved, he could be confident that his idea would get done and his need would be met. His challenge was to get them to like and approve his ideas and needs. They were a "hands-on" governing body. They were not inclined to build the hospital and then turn it over to someone else to run. They appreciated Thrasher's ability, but they also appreciated the challenges and pitfalls involved in managing a hospital with its financial, regulatory, service, and operational complexities and requirements. They felt obligated to be closely involved with its operation and management. When Thrasher once asked the trustees to show him a vote of confidence by granting him authority in such matters as purchasing equipment, travel expenses, salary adjustments, and hiring personnel, they gracefully declined.[2] Authority Chairman Rufus Evans met with Thrasher almost every morning

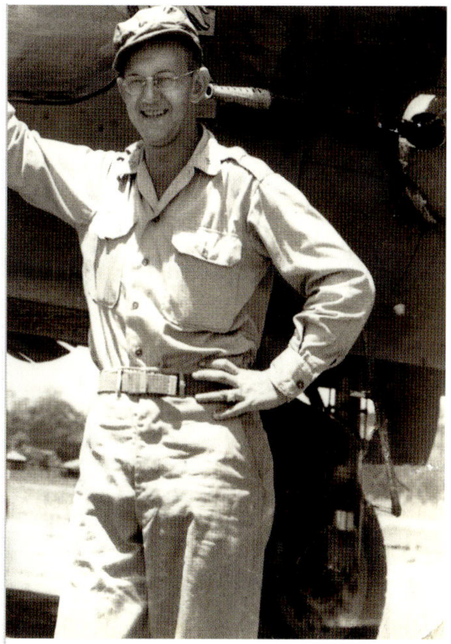

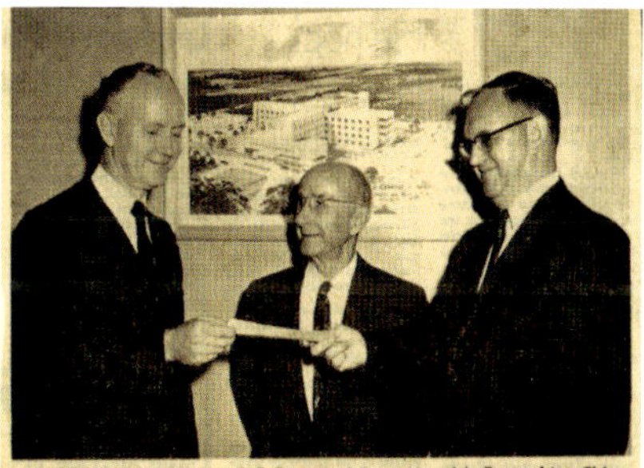

$1,000 GIFT TO HOSPITAL -- F. E. Patterson, left, president of the Decatur Lions Club, presents a check for $1,000 to William H. Thrasher, administrator of the DeKalb General Hospital. Looking on is Lion Eugene Sanders, in whose honor the club gave the money to furnish a hospital room.

Decatur Lions Raise $1,000 For DeKalb General Hospital

When President F. E. (Pat) Patterson of the Decatur Lions Club presented a check for $1,000 to Administrator William H. Thrasher of DeKalb General Hospital, he remarked that it represented the fulfillment of a wish for a hospital in DeKalb County which was made twenty years ago by the Decatur Lions. The presentation took place October 7 in the temporary administrative offices of the hospital at 125 Atlanta Avenue in Decatur.

The Decatur Lions Club is the first organization to contribute in the current drive to raise $150,000 in supplementary funds for equipping the hospital. Mrs. T. W. Robinson, Sr. of Avondale Estates was the first individual to contribute, when she donated two rooms in memory of her late husband last year.

The room furnished by the Lions Club will be given in honor of Lion Eugene Sanders. It was under his leadership that the Lions raised $10,000 in 1939-40 for the enlargement and development of the DeKalb County Clinic. Lion Sanders was president of the club at that time, and during 1944-45 he was Georgia District Governor of Lions International. At the Georgia State Lions Convention in Macon in 1949 he was voted the most distinguished Lion in Georgia. During his 22 years in Lionism he has been a constructive leader, was chairman of four Georgia State Lions conventions, has helped organize over 35 new Lions clubs, and is now sering as an International Counselor of Lions International. Lion Sanders has been head of the science department at Henry Grady High School in Atlanta for many years and is considered an outstanding leader in the science field in Georgia.

The new $4,500,000 hospital, located at 2701 North Decatur Road near Decatur, will have 200 beds and will be up-to-date in every respect. It will be one of the few hospitals in this section offering progressive patient care. The opening of the new facility is planned for the spring of next year.

Top: William Thrasher serving in World War II. **Above:** The president of the Decatur Lions Club, F. E. "Pat" Patterson, offers the first donation by an organization toward the DeKalb General Hospital in the form of a $1,000 check to William Thrasher.

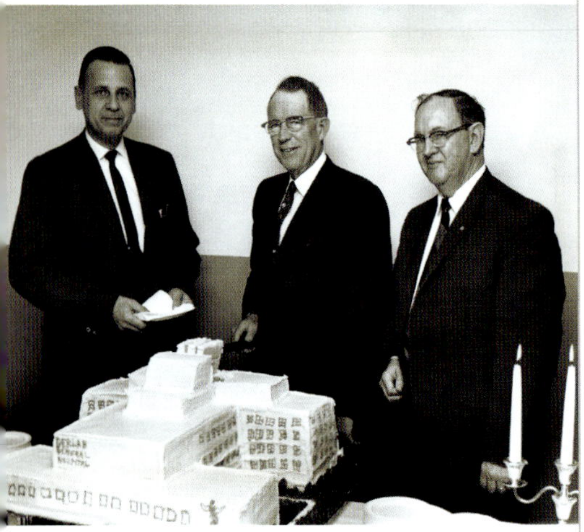

Above: Left to right: Chief of staff L. C. "Buck" Buchanan, MD, Authority member Wash W. Lively, and hospital administrator William Thrasher celebrate the first anniversary of DeKalb General Hospital. **Right:** In supervising the design and construction of DeKalb General Hospital, William Thrasher incorporated one of the first intensive care units to be included in any hospital in the nation.

to review hospital issues and the administrator's plans for the day. Decisions, large or small, were not made without Evans' knowledge, involvement and approval.

Thrasher's lack of delegated authority may have contributed to the resignation of one hundred nurses in January 1969. The nurses looked to him to convey their needs and concerns to the trustees. He looked to the trustees to respond to the concerns he brought to them. He was a kind and gentle person who was unable to convince the governing body of the need to address the nurses' grievances in a proactive, timely, and effective manner.

While his relationship with the Authority may have been a challenge, Thrasher did not share that concern with others. The medical staff, the employees, and the community saw him as an effective leader who brought to the hospital the values and the environment that made it special, and his accomplishments were extraordinary. He entered the DeKalb General Hospital scene when the trustees needed his knowledge, experience, and guidance in planning a new hospital, a task that was new to all of them. He advised the architects on the design of the hospital, including such innovative features as one of the nation's first intensive care units. He oversaw the construction project. He was the key person in determining the thousands of pieces of equipment needed and which equipment manufacturer to choose. He chose the key personnel needed to open and operate the hospital. He was the trustees' ambassador and spokesman to the media and the community, advising them of the hospital's status and plans and enlisting their support. He managed the birthing of the hospital and its emergence into adolescence with all the challenges associated with such a massive undertaking. He saw the institution through the dramatic mass resignation of 100 of its 130 nurses to a postresignation period of recovery and stability. He headed the major 1968–1971 expansion project that more than doubled the size of the facility. As one leader observed, he was Chairman Rufus Evans's "right hand and left hand."[3]

His unique leadership and contributions were recognized widely in the community. In 1972 he was named one of the five outstanding hospital administrators in Georgia by the very same Georgia State Nursing Association that he had challenged in 1969 when the association attempted to be DeKalb General nurses' bargaining agent. The Decatur Rotary Club named him a Paul Harris Fellow. The Stone Mountain Rotary Club gave him the Rufus Evans Community Service Award. The Decatur Lions Club named him the Senior Citizen of the Year.

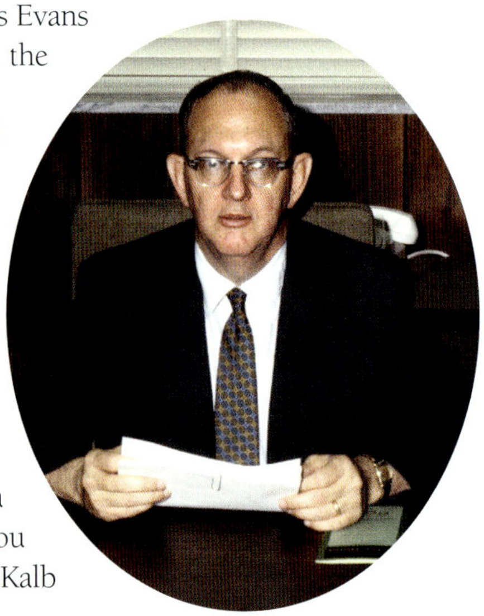

He was especially appreciated for his values and his personal example that created an environment of compassion and competence. He loved the members of the hospital staff and openly showed his trust and appreciation for them. "He saw the good in everyone."[4] He often was heard to say, "We care about those who come to this hospital for care, and we care about those who provide their care." At the dedication ceremony, he said to those assembled, "The medical staff and personnel of DeKalb General Hospital are here to comfort and help you until you can help yourself, because you are not just another case to us. You are a human being in trouble, sick, and lonely, and taking care of you comes first. You are our reason for being here."[5] He coined the DeKalb General Hospital slogan, "Open 24 hours, and we deliver."[6]

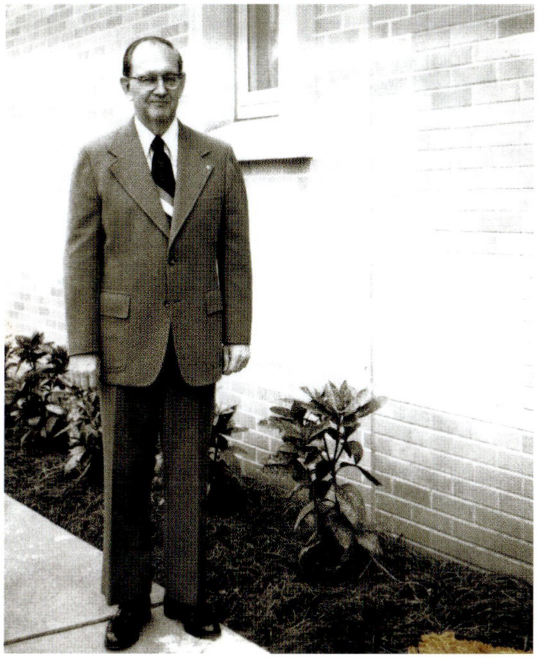

PAGE 6 A THE DEKALB NEWS/SUN 6/29/83

Thrasher Gets Annual 'SCOTY' Award

William H. Thrasher, the director of hospital relations at DeKalb General Hospital, has been named the 1983 winner of the Decatur Lions Club's annual "SCOTY" (Senior Citizen of the Year) award.

The "SCOTY" award has been made each year for 21 consecutive years to honor an outstanding senior citizen of the Decatur area. It is made to show appreciation for the contribution the recipient has made to the community through church, civic and other community organizations and through professional services.

Mr. Thrasher was born in Watkinsville, Ga. August 25, 1917. He has lived in Decatur most of his life. After graduation from Decatur Boys High, he finished Emory University with a Bachelor of Business Administration degree. He received his masters degree in Hospital Administration from the University of Minnesota.

Mr. Thrasher has been in hospital administration for more than 30 years. He was formerly the administrator of John D. Archbold Memorial Hospital, in Thomasville, Ga., and the Athens General Hospital, Athens, Ga.

Previously, he was associated with the Georgia Department of Public Health, the Georgia Association of Insurance Agents and the Retail Credit Company. During World War II he was a special agent in the Central Intelligence Corps of Military Intelligence.

HE RETURNED to Decatur in 1958 as administrator of the proposed DeKalb General Hospital. In this capacity, he was responsible for supervising the design and the construction and staffing of the hospital. He incorporated into the design the first intensive care unit to be included in any hospital in the nation.

After the hospital was opened in 1961, he continued as the administrator until January 1, 1973 when he was made executive director of the DeKalb County Hospital Authority, which is the governing body of the DeKalb General Hospital.

In October 1974 he became the Director of Hospital Relations at DeKalb General Hospital.

In this capacity, most of the patient related problems, complaints and incidents which occur at the hospital are referred to him for handling. He also works with the insurance company's representatives and lawyers in the handling of liability claims.

Mr. Thrasher has been active in local, state and national hospital association work. He has served on many committees and is past president of the Metropolitan Atlanta Hospital District.

In 1972, the Nursing Association of Georgia selected him as one of the five outstanding administrators of the state.

HE ALSO HAS been active in community affairs.

He served as foreman of the DeKalb Grand Jury for one term, and is a member of the DeKalb Grand Jury Association. He is member of the Decatur Rotary Club and has served as a member of its board of directors. The Rotary Club recently designated him as a Paul Harris Fellow in recognition of his community service.

He and his wife, Helen, have three sons and two daughters and four grandchildren.

The oldest son is in research and development with Control Data Corporation. The two younger sons, who are twins, are both ministers. The older daughter has a masters degree in early childhood education and is in church work. The younger daughter is a graduate of the University of Georgia, and is administrative secretary to the director of development in the business college at the University of Georgia.

Mr. and Mrs. Thrasher are members of the Decatur First Methodist Church. Mr. Thrasher has served on the administrative board of the church.

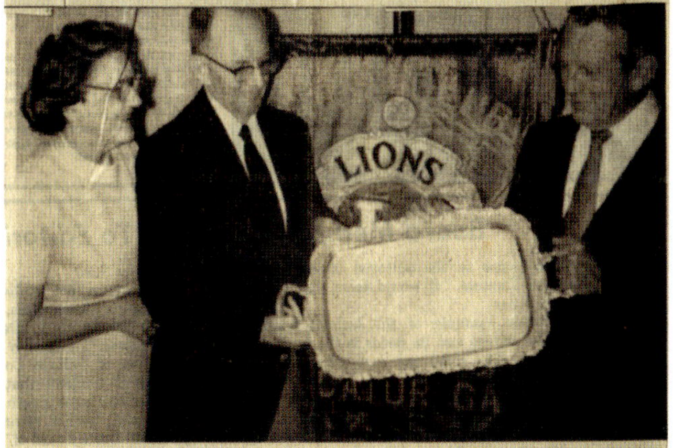

'SCOTY' Award To Thrasher

William H. Thrasher and his wfe, Helen, accept the Decatur Lions' "SCOTY" award from club member Steadman Burgess.

Thrasher "walked the talk" and demonstrated each day in his work and life the purpose and values he articulated. He knew the physicians and the employees by name. He visited with patients and wanted to know if their needs were being met. He came to the hospital at night and circulated among the various departments and service areas. He listened to concerns from physicians, employees, and patients, and he was responsive to those concerns.

Charles Eberhart succeeded Thrasher as administrator in 1973 when Thrasher became executive director of the DeKalb Hospital Authority. In 1974 Administrator Eberhart asked Thrasher to serve as the director of Hospital Relations because of his "people skills." He held that position until he died on November 12, 1983.

The William H. Thrasher Good Samaritan Award was established in 1984, and it is presented each year to the hospital employee who has demonstrated in his or her life and work the attitude of the Good Samaritan. It is awarded to employees who go beyond the minimum requirements of duty and reach out to others with love, compassion, and generosity. The award is named for the man who set such an example and left such a legacy. (See Appendix K for a list of the recipients.)

As DeKalb General Hospital's first administrator, Thrasher stamped the hospital with the seal of respect, appreciation, caring, and compassion for its employees, its physicians, and its patients. By his example he helped make DeKalb General Hospital a place where employees found joy and pride in their work, where physicians wanted to bring their patients, and where patients found competence and compassion in their care.

Top left: A man of true compassion and dedication to all members of the hospital and its patients, Thrasher lived the values he spoke of and believed in. He also coined the hospital slogan, "Open 24 hours and we deliver!" **Above:** William Thrasher is awarded the coveted "Scoty" award by the Decatur Lions Club.

Charles Barr Eberhart

A prayer is framed and hangs in the Building Services Department on the North Decatur campus that reads:

> *O Lord, hold us in the palm of your hand and direct us in the care of our patients, our neighbors, and each other.*
>
> *Lead us together forward through the difficulties, complexities, and pain that all organizations must continually experience to thrive, grow, and change.*
>
> *Help us constantly to lift up the best that we have to offer now but never be satisfied.*
>
> *Create in us an insatiable curiosity and desire to always be better than we have been.*
>
> *Help us to find focus and purpose to our endeavors on behalf of our patients. We are grateful for the resources you have made available to us for the carrying out of our mission.*
>
> *In our impatience with life and circumstances, help us always to remember that we are on your time and not our own.*

"Help us to find focus and purpose to our endeavors on behalf of our patients. We are grateful for the resources you have made available to us for the carrying out of our mission."

— Charles B. Eberhart
Hospital Administrator

It is "My Prayer for DMC" that Charles Eberhart wrote at 5:30 AM on the morning of October 17, 1994, two months after he was diagnosed with a malignant brain tumor and at the conclusion of six weeks of radiation therapy.[7]

His prayer not only hangs in the Building Services Department. It may be found in other offices throughout the hospital, cradled in desk drawers, kept in files marked "special items to keep," or folded and reverently carried about in personal wallets. It is a reminder of one who touched lives and impacted DeKalb Medical in a special way. It is a reminder of Charles Eberhart's leadership, his courage, his spirit, his compassion, and his integrity that impregnated the institution with a spirit that made others feel it was a unique place to be as a patient, to work as an employee or physician, and to support as a member of the community.

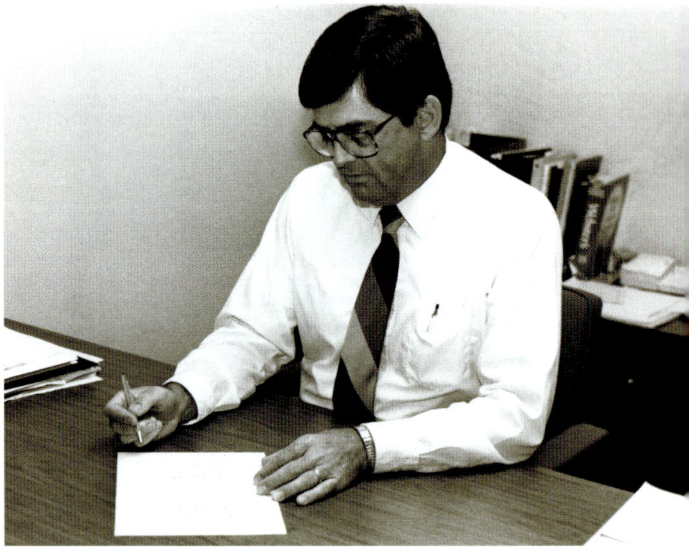

Opposite and right: Charles Barr Eberhart was selected hospital administrator in 1973.

Charles Eberhart was born in Atlanta on September 2, 1938. He attended Morningside Elementary School, Grady High School, Emory University, and the University of Montevallo in Alabama where he received his bachelor's degree in business administration in 1961. He received his master's degree in hospital administration from George Washington University in 1964. He married Helen Gene Smith, and they had two children, Charles and Margaret.

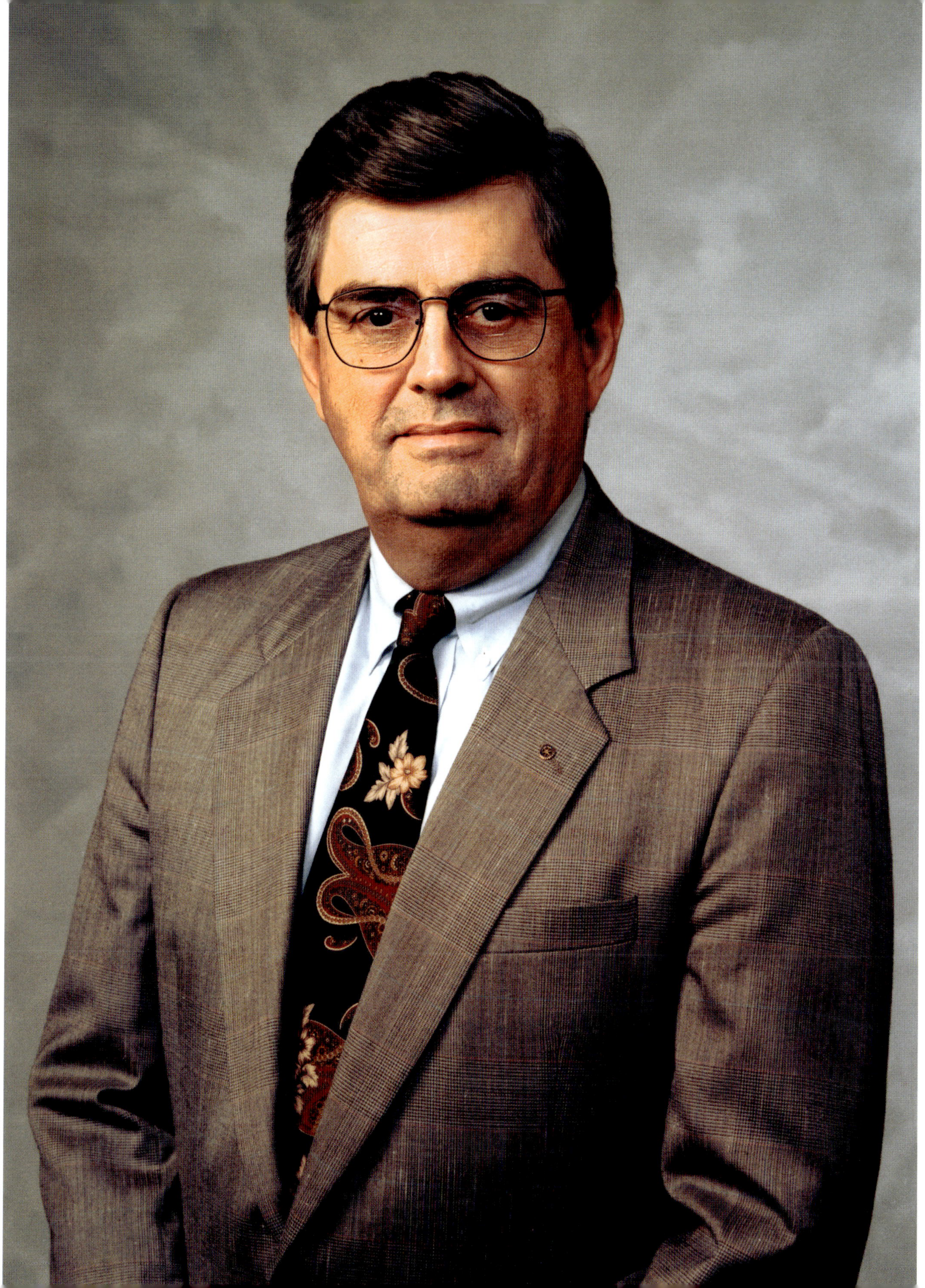

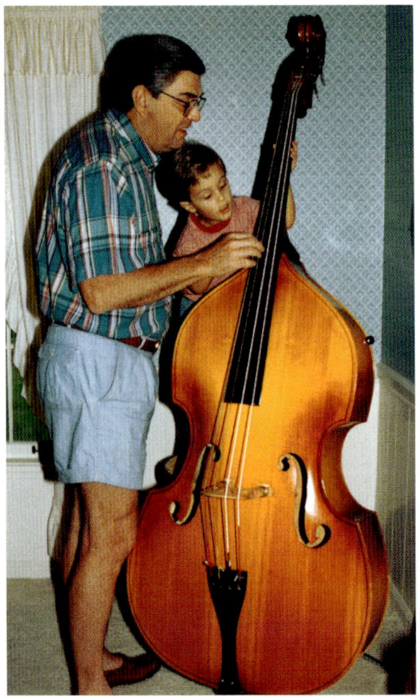

Above: Charles Eberhart adored sharing his love of music with his family. **Below:** "Catch-and release" fishing was one of his favorite pasttimes.

He was a master woodcarver, having learned the art from his father "as soon as I was able to cut myself."[8] He also was an avid fisherman who faithfully practiced the "catch-and-release" approach to fishing—a hobby that he shared with his wife whom he admitted "owned the family record for the biggest and the most fish caught."[9] They enjoyed making music together with Charles on the bass fiddle and Helen Gene on the banjo.

With a father who was a noted Atlanta physician and a mother who was a nurse, Eberhart had an early interest in medicine and hospital work. He often went with his father to see patients in the hospital. During the summer months of his undergraduate college years, he worked as a central supply technician and operating room scrub nurse at Atlanta's Crawford Long Hospital and as a male nursing assistant at Shelby Memorial Hospital in Alabaster, Alabama.[10] He often said that those early hands-on experiences gave him a great appreciation for the important role and contribution of all hospital employees.[11]

Eberhart attributed his decision for a career in hospital administration to an interview he had with William Thrasher in 1958 when Thrasher enthusiastically shared with him the plans for DeKalb General Hospital. Eberhart was then a student at Emory University, and the DeKalb General Hospital plans were still on the drawing board. He kept with him through the years a picture of himself as a young student and Administrator Thrasher looking at the plans for DeKalb General Hospital before it was ever built. Eberhart said it was that interview with Thrasher that helped him realize hospital administration was the part of health care that interested him most. He said he never regretted his decision, and in later years exclaimed, "I really can't think of anything that would be more fun than this. I really can't."[12]

After receiving his master's degree in hospital administration, he became assistant administrator of Floyd General Hospital in Rome, Georgia. He was working in that capacity in 1970 when DeKalb General Hospital invited him to accept its new position of director of Administrative Services to work with the very man who had influenced his career decision.

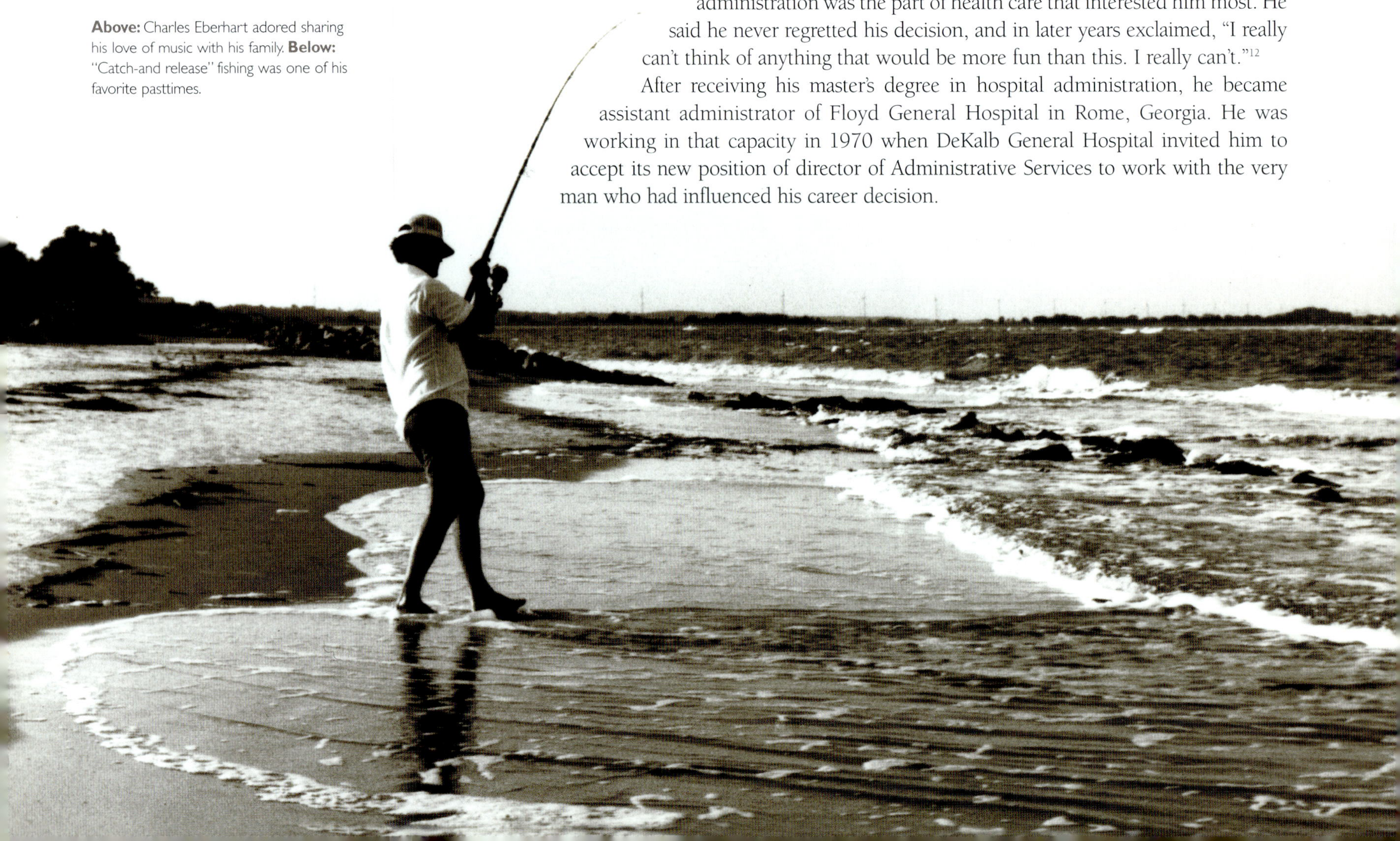

When William Thrasher became the executive director of the DeKalb County Hospital Authority in 1973, the Authority selected Charles Eberhart as administrator. When the organization was restructured in 1992, Eberhart became chief executive officer (CEO) of DeKalb Medical Center Inc., (DMC) and DeKalb Regional Healthcare System, Inc. (DRHS).

Eberhart led the institution from being a small community DeKalb General Hospital into a prominent medical center and healthcare system with regional recognition. The hospital's budget grew from $16.5 million in 1975 to $169 million in fiscal year 1994–1995.[13] He guided the system in acquiring neighboring Decatur Hospital. He led the Hospital Authority in restructuring the organization. He worked with the Authority to acquire the land for a medical campus in South DeKalb County, began developing the facilities, and laid the foundation for a hospital in South DeKalb that would open its doors ten years after his death.

In 1985 he established the first hospital-based wellness center in the southeast,[14] shepherded the hospital through a series of major expansions, and instituted the construction of the first professional office building that brought many of the hospital's physicians onto the North Decatur hospital campus.

He was often described as a "thinker" who looked beyond the horizon and saw what was not apparent to most. Seeing the impact that managed care would have on the hospital, physicians, and patients, he led the organization in its horizontal integration negotiations with other institutions and in its vertical integration initiatives with primary care physicians and a strong DeKalb Physician-Hospital Organization (DPHO). He recognized the need and helped implement a strategy to build a substantial financial reserve in preparation for financial rainy days that he saw coming over the horizon.

He focused on what was good for the hospital and the community. He led in the establishment of a Trauma Center and a Rape Crisis Center in DeKalb Medical Center's Emergency Department. Both met with significant challenges and resistance, but he recognized the community need for both these services and saw to it that they became a part of the hospital's outreach.

He appreciated the critical importance of education and helped create a formal educational program for hospital managers. He conducted a series of medical staff leadership retreats, encouraged the governing body to attend leadership conferences, and helped establish in partnership with a local university an on-campus master's degree program in business administration for hospital staff and physicians. He insisted that his administrative team read and apply Peter Senge's book, *The Fifth Discipline*, the theme of which is that "every vital institution is a learning organization."

He regularly sought the counsel of his friend and hospital attorney, James Rawls. He spent nearly every Friday afternoon with his close friend, William P. Tatum, chairman of the Hospital Authority and the DMC Board of Directors to share with the chairman detailed information about what was going on in the hospital and to solicit Tatum's advice.

He recognized the need for a partnership of the hospital, physicians, and community. He supported Judy McMahan in establishing the DeKalb Medical Foundation to raise funds and friends for the medical center. He created a series of service line development teams that brought administration, staff, and physicians together on a regular basis to explore the needs of and develop plans for women's and infants' services, surgical services, cancer services, cardiology services, and mental health services.

Charles Eberhart was diagnosed as having a brain tumor in August 1994. Following the completion of radiation therapy that fall, Eberhart undertook a course of chemotherapy. The chemotherapy created significant side effects and showed no evidence of effectiveness. He elected to

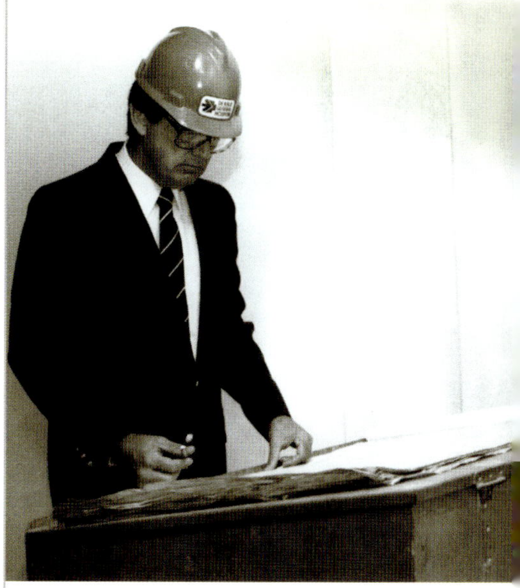

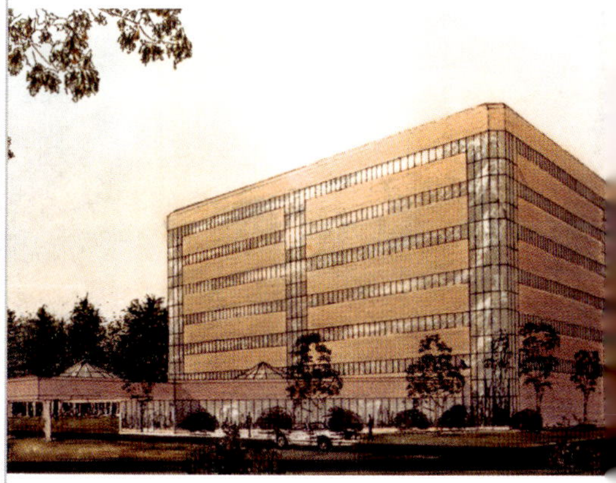

Charles Eberhart oversees the construction of the first Professional Office Building that brought many physicians onto the hospital campus.

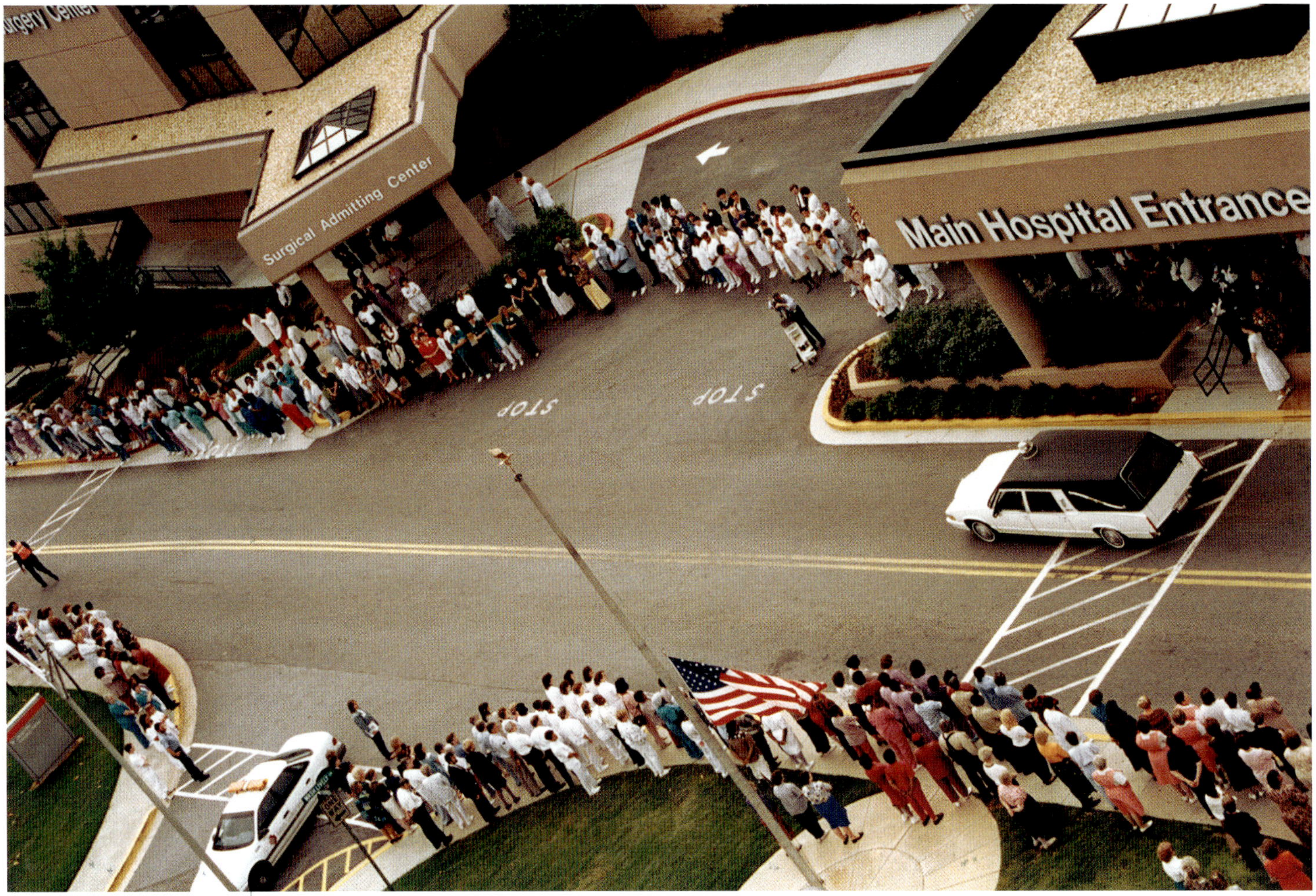

A hearse carries the body of Charles Eberhart in front of the hospital and the people he loved.

discontinue chemotherapy and also chose to forego surgery because of the potential mental impairment it might produce. He turned most of his leadership responsibilities over to his close friend and chief operating officer, John Gerlach, but continued working at home and at the hospital as his condition permitted. He died at DeKalb Medical Center at 4:00 AM on Sunday, May 28, 1995.

When the severity of Charles Eberhart's illness became apparent, many struggled with two unknowns. The first was trying to understand why such an illness should befall such a special individual. The second was trying to imagine DeKalb Medical Center without his leadership.

There were numerous public acknowledgements of the community's appreciation for Charles Eberhart's accomplishments and influence. In 1994 the DeKalb Medical Society presented him with the distinguished Julius McCurdy Citizenship Award; he was the first nonphysician to receive that award in its twenty-one year history.[15] He received the Volunteer Hospital Association Leadership Award that also was named in his honor. In 1994 the governing body named the hospital's cancer center The Charles B. Eberhart Cancer Center.[16] The cancer center established the annual Hero Award in recognition of those who, like Eberhart, demonstrated unusual courage and strength in dealing with life and cancer. The DeKalb Medical Foundation established the annual Charles B. Eberhart Award in his memory for those who had made outstanding contributions to the community, the foundation, and the medical center. Dee Keeton and Decatur Hospital instituted the annual Charles B. Eberhart Golf Classic as a fund-raiser in his memory. The Georgia Hospital Association presented the 1996 Distinguished Service Award posthumously to Charles Eberhart.[17] The foundation established the Charles B. Eberhart Fund to provide leadership and management training for the hospitals' physicians and employees.[18]

Eberhart is remembered for his personal qualities and for what those qualities meant to the organization and its people. They remember his remarkable sense of humor and his ability to "pull" stories and humorous anecdotes out of his memory bank to fit almost any occasion, always on target even if at times a little off color. They remember his pride in the hospital and its appearance and his attention to the smallest detail. As a woodcarver, he often checked the sharpness of his wood carving tools under the microscope;[19] as a CEO he looked at the hospital under the microscope as well as in its big picture. No piece of tape stuck to a hospital door, no smudge on a corridor, no piece of trash on the floor, and no weed in a flower bed went unnoticed or unattended. Director of Administrative Services Bill Sublett recalled Eberhart's habit of placing a piece of blue tape with the date on it next to a flaw he might observe to see how long before the flaw was corrected.[20] He was convinced that attention to the smallest details reflected the institution's true commitment to excellent patient care.

Those who worked with Eberhart remember his honesty, his integrity, and his trustworthiness. They remember his loyalty to his staff and his devotion to the institution. They remember his compassion and caring. They remember his desire that every person who worked at DeKalb Medical feel a sense of ownership and know that they were appreciated and valued, and that every patient know that his or her care was the hospital's first and foremost concern.

On the occasion of Eberhart's death, Mark Davis, MD, one of DeKalb's prominent physicians wrote:

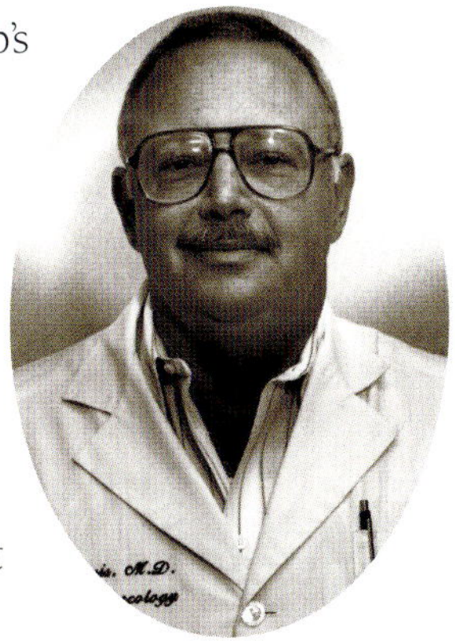

> *I did not realize it until today, but Charles Eberhart was my teacher for two decades. In the early days of my practice, my wife would say, "It takes you so long to get home from DeKalb General; why can't you practice at one of the hospitals closer to home on the northwest side of town?" My answer was, "Because they really care about the patients at DeKalb. I've never seen a hospital like it." I know that this quality of caring came from Eberhart and from the special people that he surrounded himself with.*[21]

Julia Hunter Jones, long-time DeKalb employee and former administrator of DeKalb Medical at Hillandale, found Eberhart's greatest leadership strength to be his mentoring. "He had the uncanny ability to assign you responsibilities you knew were far beyond your ability [and] then to support you, prod you, encourage you, and guide you until you achieved what you thought was beyond your reach but what he knew all along was in you." Then she added, "He was a person you always could trust. If he said, 'Julia, let's jump off this cliff together,' you would jump without hesitation. Then, halfway down, you would say, 'All right, now, Charles, what's your plan?'"[22]

After being diagnosed with a brain tumor, Charles Eberhart wrote to the boards of directors, "All I ever wanted was a hospital that I could devote myself to, heart and soul."[23] He did that, indeed, and in doing so he created a DeKalb Medical with heart and soul.

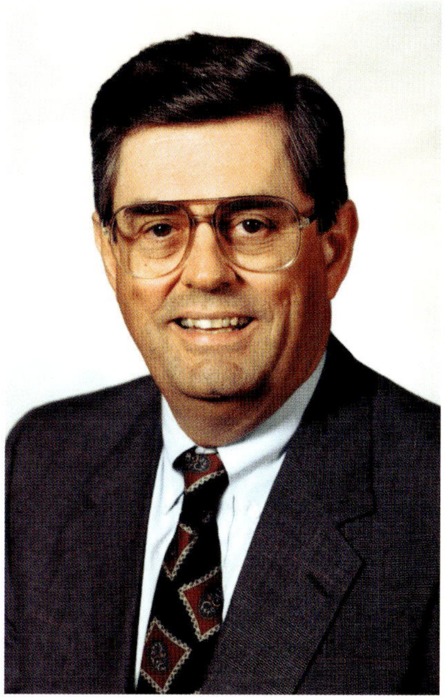

Above: Charles Eberhart will always be remembered for his integrity, his humor, and his great attention to detail. **Left:** Mark Davis, MD, worked with Eberhart for two decades and was one of many to feel grateful for having known him.

“Our burdens should never prevent us from remembering that we are, in fact, a hospital with a soul, . . . that we are incredibly privileged to come to work each day to a place where healing can take place, and that . . . we all are a part of the healing process”

— John R. Gerlach
Hospital Administrator

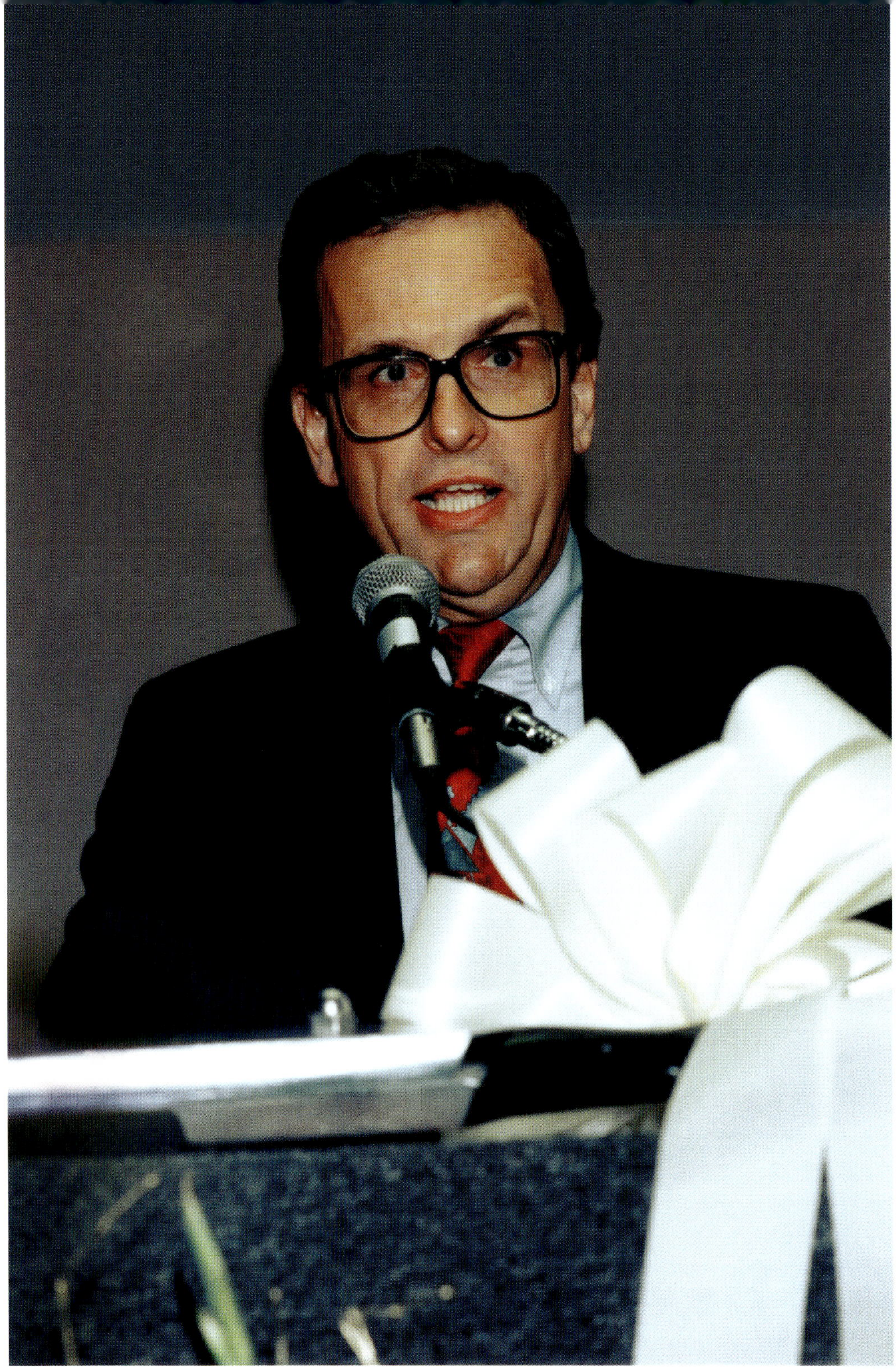

John Richard Gerlach

Following Eberhart's death, the boards of directors selected John R. "Jack" Gerlach to be the new president and CEO of DMC and DRHS. Eberhart realized the severity of his illness and endorsed Gerlach as his successor should he not be able to continue leading the organization.[24] The boards considered John Gerlach to be the most qualified of their candidates. He had been a member of the senior executive staff since 1968, he knew the inner workings of the hospital, he had been a major contributor to its development, he knew and was respected by the staff and the community, and he possessed the character and competence the boards wanted in their new leader.

John Gerlach was born in Fargo, North Dakota, in 1941, where he attended grade school and high school. He chose pharmacy as his first career and received his bachelor's degree in pharmacy from North Dakota State University in 1963. Following one year of apprenticeship in pharmacy, he entered the U.S. Army and served as pharmacy officer at Fort McPherson in Atlanta. While at Fort McPherson, he enrolled in Georgia State University's master's degree program in hospital administration and came to DeKalb General to work part-time as a registered pharmacist while he completed his graduate studies. In October 1968, after receiving his master's degree and completing an administrative residency at Indiana University Medical Center, he dropped by DeKalb General just to speak to Thrasher and was offered the position of assistant to the administrator at DeKalb General Hospital.[25] He accepted the offer and came to DeKalb with his wife, Barbara, and their three children, Jeff, Beth, and Christie.

He arrived on the scene as the hospital was facing two major issues. The first was the expansion project that would increase the capacity of the hospital from two hundred beds to six hundred beds and expand its services. Gerlach was hired to oversee the construction project and the purchasing of all its furnishings and equipment. He said he thought the job would last for only a few months after which he would go to something else.[26] Little did he know that he would remain with the institution for more than thirty-five years.

The second critical issue he faced on arrival was a growing discontent on the part of the hospital's nurses. Many had signed on with the Georgia State Nurses' Association (GSNA) for the association to serve as their bargaining agent in dealing with DeKalb General salaries, benefits, and professional issues. The Authority and administration refused to recognize GSNA as the nurses' bargaining agent. Their impasse led to the resignation of 100 of its 130 nurses in January 1969. Coping with the loss of most of its nurses was one of the most significant challenges the hospital and Gerlach would ever face.

A third unexpected challenge occurred when Administrator Thrasher suffered a heart attack in the spring of 1969. Gerlach served as acting administrator until Thrasher returned to work later in the summer.

In 1970 he was promoted to the position of director of Patient Services with a wide array of administrative, operational, and clinical oversight duties. In 1981 he was named associate administrator, and in 1991 became the chief operating officer and associate administrator. In 1994 he became administrator of DeKalb Medical Center and chief operating officer of the hospital system under a corporate reorganization. In 1995, after Eberhart's death, the boards named him president and CEO of DMC and DRHS.

Those who visited Gerlach in his office stood in awe at the height to which piles of documents on his desk could rise, but were equally in awe of his ability at a moment's notice to find just the item in those stacks that he needed. They also were amazed at his talent for multitasking—to simultaneously and effectively manage multiple responsibilities. He had an encyclopedic knowledge

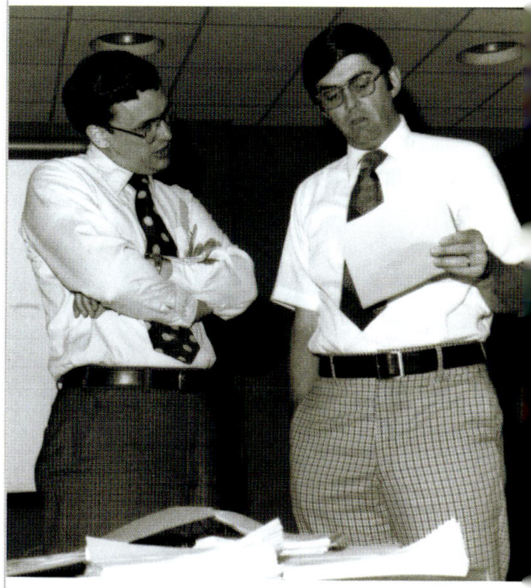

John Richard Gerlach, left, with Charles Barr Eberhart. Gerlach was selected as the system's president and CEO upon Eberhart's death. It was what Eberhart wanted, and the directors agreed.

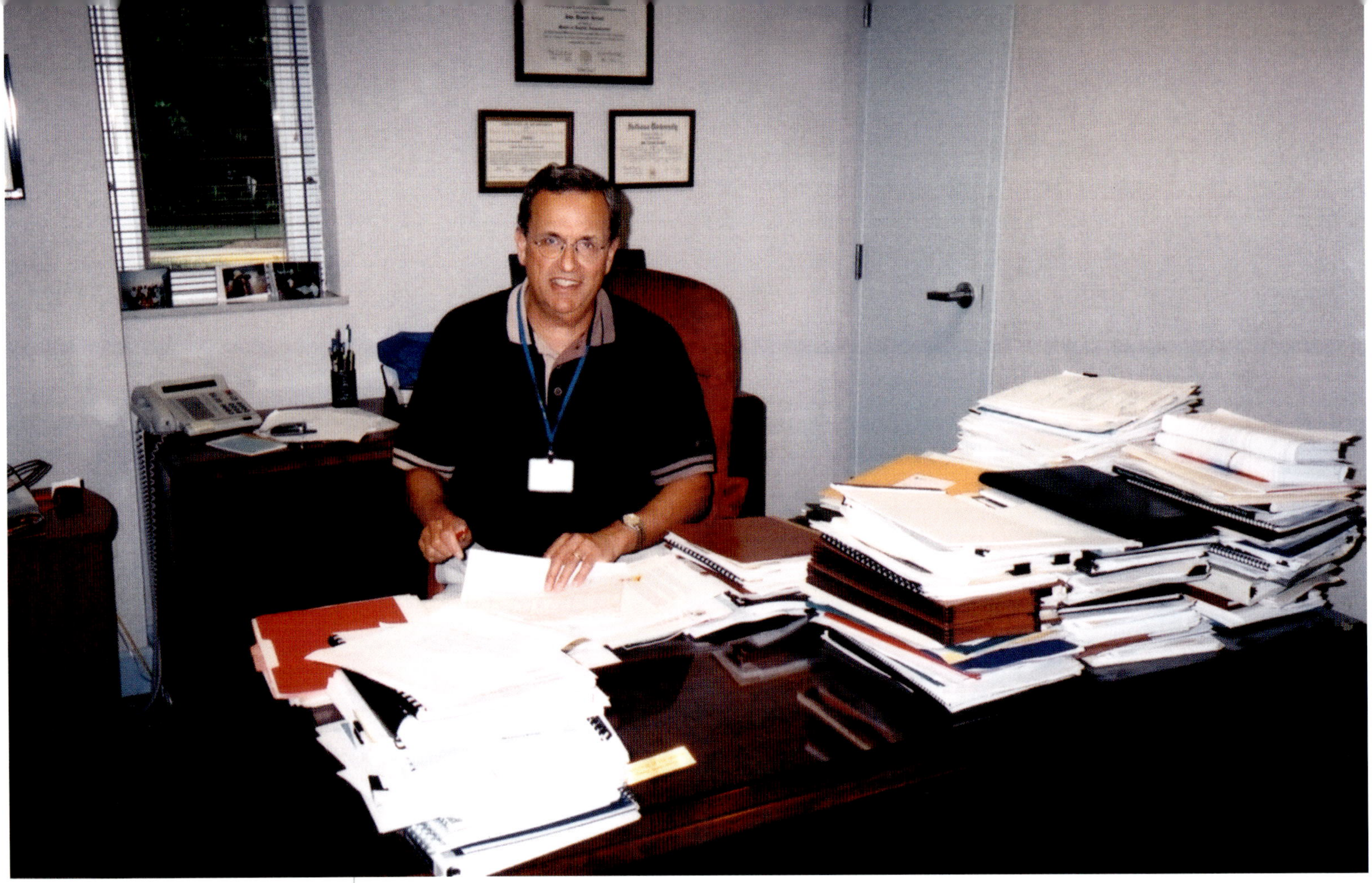

Above: Following in Eberhart's shoes could have been a daunting task. But Gerlach became known and admired for his patience, understanding, professionalism, dignity, and competence.

of details pertaining to the organization, its finances, its activities, and its people. He saw the organization grow from a tightly knit family of 800 employees to "more of an extended family of some 3,700 employees on the three campuses and in other neighborhood locations,"[27] nearly 1,000 physicians, and 400 volunteers. DeKalb Medical served more than 300,000 patients in 2002 including approximately 24,500 inpatients, 204,500 outpatients, 74,500 emergency patients, and 6,000 births while providing the community with $43 million in uncompensated care.[28]

When Gerlach was named president and CEO in 1995, he faced many challenges, but two stood out among the rest. The first was to gain the trust and confidence of the organization and community following the death of Charles Eberhart who was considered by many to be unique and irreplaceable. The second challenge was PROMINA. Shortly after John Gerlach became president and CEO, DRHS joined PROMINA as the best choice available for a hospital alliance and horizontal integration. He would help shape PROMINA in its efforts to deliver on the hopes and promises for which it was created. He later had to deal with its demise.

John Gerlach rose to both these challenges admirably. He appreciated the widespread insecurities that followed Eberhart's death, and he joined in acknowledging his predecessor's gifts. He recalled the time when he and Charles Eberhart both applied for the job of administrator when Thrasher transferred to another position. Said Gerlach, "We both won—Charles got the job, and I got the chance to work with him and learn from him. It was one of the most positive experiences of my career."[29]

Through such situations, Gerlach demonstrated understanding and patience but also the dignity,

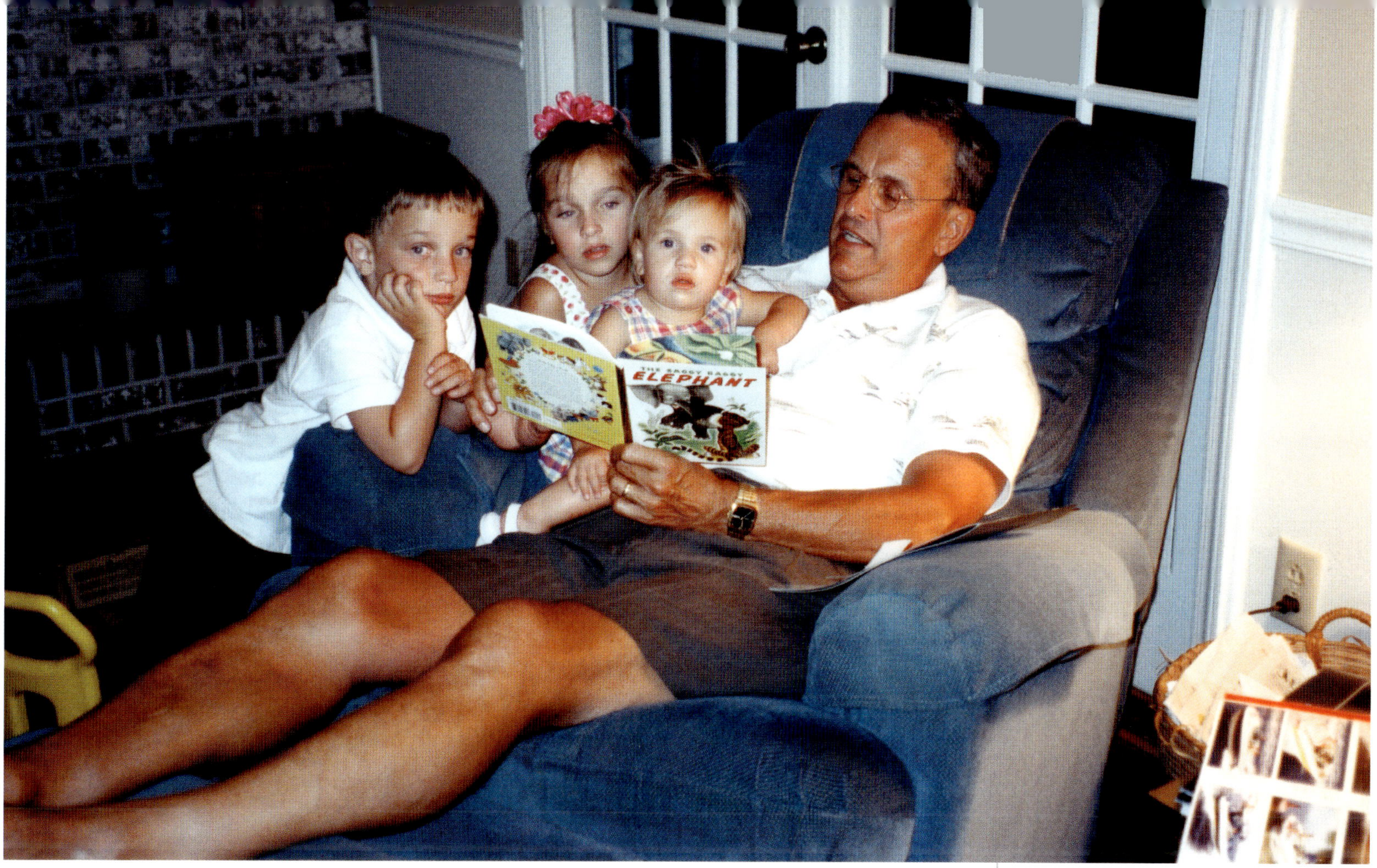

professionalism, and competence that proved to the organization that he was worthy of the mantle left to him and capable of moving the organization forward. As president and CEO, he added the second professional office building on the North Decatur campus with its new Wellness Center, new Diagnostic Breast Center, the new Charles B. Eberhart Cancer Center, the Herbert E. Kann Outpatient Cancer Treatment Center, and the Radiation Oncology Center. He completed the construction of a new Emergency Department, a new Intensive Care Unit/Coronary Care Unit (ICU/CCU), a new Diagnostic Treatment Center, a new Laboratory, a renovated and expanded Outpatient Surgery Center, an expanded parking facility, and a pedestrian bridge. He oversaw the establishment of a forensic toxicology laboratory. He was instrumental in DeKalb Medical's participation in the 1996 Olympic Games Hospital Network, in establishing an International Medical Center, in acquiring a home health service, in expanding the services of the Wellness on Wheels van, and adding MRI technology to the Diagnostic Imaging Center.[30]

At DeKalb Medical at Hillandale, he constructed a second medical office building with an outpatient surgery center and a twenty-four-hour emergency center, and he obtained the state's approval on the certificate of need (CON) application to build the DeKalb Medical at Hillandale hospital. He led DeKalb Medical in developing a new five-year strategic plan for 2003–2008 and in launching the major QUEST/FOCUS comprehensive information technology initiative.[31]

Gerlach had to deal with new financial and customer-service issues as a result of more complex federal regulations, shrinking reimbursements, and an increased demand for patient services. While

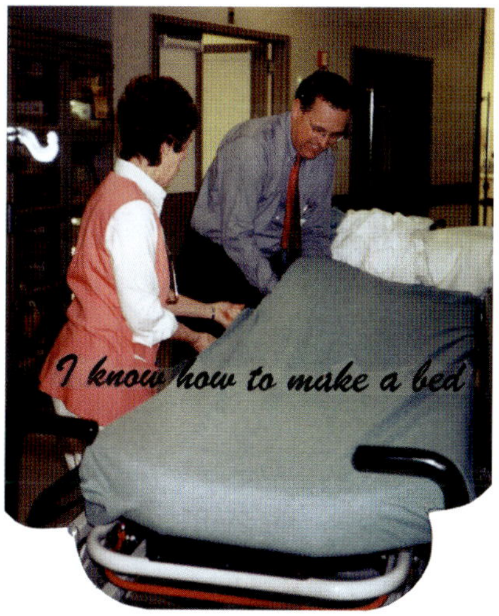

Top: Gerlach reads a story to his grandchildren. **Above:** Gerlach helps a volunteer make up a hospital stretcher, corners and all.

remaining financially strong, DRHS had to call on its investment income to cover some of its operational costs.[32] He engaged the services of Healthcare Management Services to undertake a complete assessment of the organization's operations and to make recommendations for improvement; and he engaged another firm to conduct a similar assessment of the organization's revenue-improvement opportunities.[33] With both assessments in hand, he and his team embarked on initiatives to address ten areas of operation and performance improvement; to implement a new labor management plan that "right-sized" departments;[34] and to create a new revenue enhancement initiative to improve the organization's reimbursement for services provided.[35]

Gerlach saw the need to elevate the institution's ability to understand and demonstrate the quality of its services, and led the organization in elevating its quality initiatives. He enhanced the hospital's relationship with its physicians and the role and effectiveness of the DeKalb Physician-Hospital Organization. He recognized the necessity for enhancing the organization's performance improvement processes, not only to satisfy the demands of the public and regulatory agencies but also to demonstrate and improve the quality of the services that DeKalb Medical provided. To that end he established the Quality Council (later the Performance Improvement Council) to provide a mechanism to measure performance and to achieve higher levels of performance and customer satisfaction. The council laid the foundation for the DeKalb Quality Institute that was to follow.[36]

When DRHS joined PROMINA, Gerlach was a key leader in the new organization's efforts to provide quality services to the greater Atlanta community and support to its five hospital-system members. When PROMINA experienced the rapid turnover of its once-collegial leaders, the withdrawal of two of its most prominent hospital systems, and its insurmountable financial losses, he remained loyal to the restructured organization and gave it creative leadership as long as a potential for valued services existed.

Of John Gerlach's many contributions to the organization, none was more important than his keeping DeKalb Medical focused on its reason for being. In the face of financial challenges, the pressure to cut costs and services to improve "the bottom line," and the temptation to compete with other institutions, he remained committed to providing the personnel, the technology, and the services for the best possible patient care to the people of the community. He remained focused on meeting the needs of patients as the institution's reason for being.

He also never lost sight of the healing role that was at the heart of the institution. In one of the employee newsletters, he related the story of a young woman physician who developed metastatic cancer shortly after joining the hospital's medical staff. She had an eleven-week-old son. She found an experimental drug that looked promising in clinical trials, but it required her to make weekly trips to Connecticut to obtain it. Gerlach recounted how the hospital community donated one million frequent flyer miles to make it possible for her, her husband, and their son to travel to Connecticut for those weekly treatments; and he reflected, "Our burdens should never prevent us from remembering that we are, in fact, a hospital with a soul, . . . that we are incredibly privileged to come to work each day to a place where healing can take place, and that . . . we all are a part of that healing process. It is my hope that we never lose sight of why we are here and what we are trying to accomplish as a source of healing for all the members of our community."[37]

In every responsibility and relationship, John Gerlach demonstrated personal values that reinforced his leadership ability. He showed a loyalty to the institution and to others that engendered a sense of security and well-being; an integrity that engendered respect and trust; an appreciation for oth-

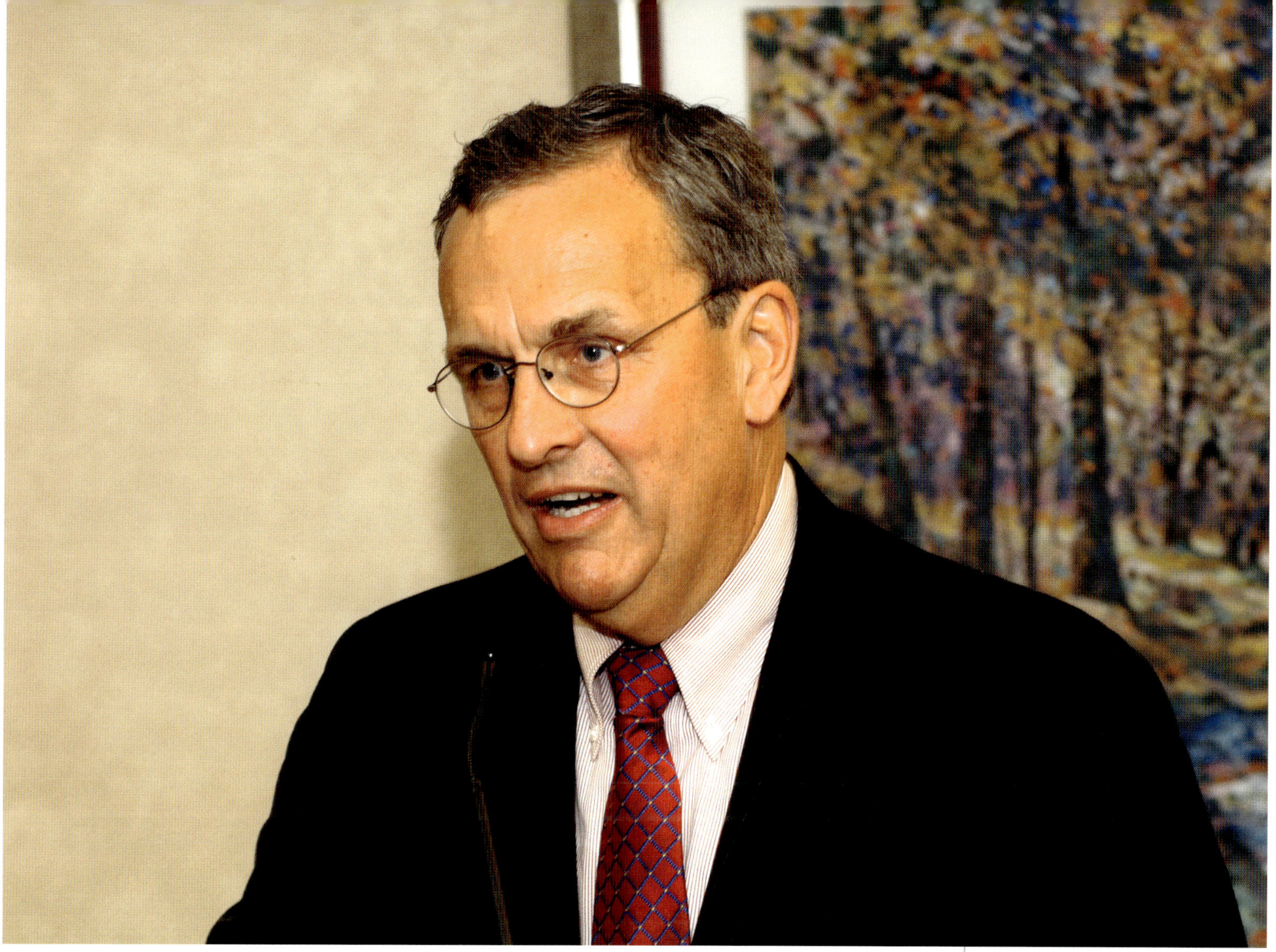

ers that engendered a sense of self-worth and that inspired initiative and creativity; a kindness and compassion that engendered a sense of being understood and valued; a servant mentality that inspired others to serve; a wisdom that engendered confidence; and a sense of humor that created an environment of fun and joy.

On the occasion of his retirement, employees, physicians, board members, elected officials, volunteers, friends, and admirers gathered to thank him for his thirty-five years of dedicated service and for what he had meant to them personally. Betty Castellani spoke for all who had known "Jack" Gerlach and who had had the privilege of working with him. She closed her remarks by saying,

> *Thank you, Mr. Gerlach, for leading us through many glorious accomplishments and standing in front of us when the stormy times raged. Thank you for being a leader who cared and a human being we are proud to know. Thank you for all you have given to DeKalb Medical Center.... The depth and breadth of your gifts are visible today, but ... as the years go by, the wisdom of your leadership and the endurance of your contributions will become more apparent with all the generations that will follow.*[38]

For thirty-five years, Gerlach proved a compassionate and powerful leader who believed the patients—not the bottom line on a balance sheet—always came first.

Eric Norwood knew from his teen years that he wanted a career in hospital administration. He chose DeKalb Medical when he personally witnessed their professionalism, competency, ethics, and a unique calling to serve.

Eric Paul Norwood

Eric Norwood was named president and chief executive officer of DMC and DRHS following John Gerlach's retirement in 2003, and he continues in that role.

Norwood was born in Wilmington, North Carolina, received his bachelor's degree in business administration from the College of William and Mary in 1978 and his master's degree in hospital administration from the Medical College of Virginia in 1981. He is a fellow in the American College of Healthcare Executives.

In 2002 CEO John Gerlach invited him to be the organization's executive vice president and chief operating officer (COO). Before coming to DeKalb, Norwood served as assistant administrator of Scotland Memorial Hospital in Laurinburg, North Carolina; as vice president and administrator of Joan Glancy Memorial Hospital in Duluth, Georgia; as senior vice president of Gwinnett Health System in Lawrenceville, Georgia; as vice president for systems development in the PROMINA Health System; and as interim president and CEO of Southern Regional Health System in Riverdale, Georgia.

In Norwood's early years, his family moved to Virginia where he attended elementary and high school and where he found his lifelong sweetheart, Nancy. They were married between his junior and senior year at William and Mary and have six children: Daniel, David, Rachel, Stephen, Christopher, and Jonathan, for all of whom Nancy Norwood provided a successful experience in home schooling.

Eric Norwood knew from his teen years that he wanted a career in hospital administration.[39] When asked what made him want to take a position at DeKalb Medical, he said that through the years he had come to know and like a number of its leaders, and he had participated in some of the organization's leadership retreats. In addition, a decade before he was invited to become the COO, he had a dramatic experience at DeKalb Medical Center that convinced him there was something special about the hospital.

On that occasion one of Eric and Nancy Norwood's closest friends was hospitalized by Paul Browne, MD, a specialist in maternal and fetal medicine. Their friend was in the twenty-fifth week of her eighth pregnancy and was in the terminal stages of multiple myeloma. Despite the advanced stage of her cancer, she was determined to live and see her baby. After long deliberation, Browne advised her that the one chance to save her baby was to perform a cesarean-section delivery from which she might not survive. She consented, still convinced she would make it. The baby survived, but she did not. Norwood said that everyone in the hospital surrounded that family with a compassion he had never seen in another hospital. He and his wife came away convinced that the people who worked at DeKalb Medical were not only professional, competent, and ethical, but they also had a unique calling to serve.[40]

Norwood succeeded John Gerlach as president and CEO as DeKalb Medical was emerging from the demise of the PROMINA alliance and when the hospital faced significant and growing challenges. Some of those challenges were intensified by the time, energy, resources, and focus that PROMINA had siphoned away from the local organization. DeKalb Medical's leaders had been called on to spend a vast amount of time in Cobb County "trying to make PROMINA work" while important issues awaited their attention at DeKalb Medical.

He faced several physician-related challenges. There was a shrinking number of surgical and obstetrical/gynecological specialists on whom the hospital depended to perform procedures that produced much of its revenue. In addition, many of the remaining surgical specialists increasingly were performing outpatient procedures in nonhospital settings. That trend appeared likely to increase with the state's recent decision to allow general surgeons to establish outpatient surgical centers without

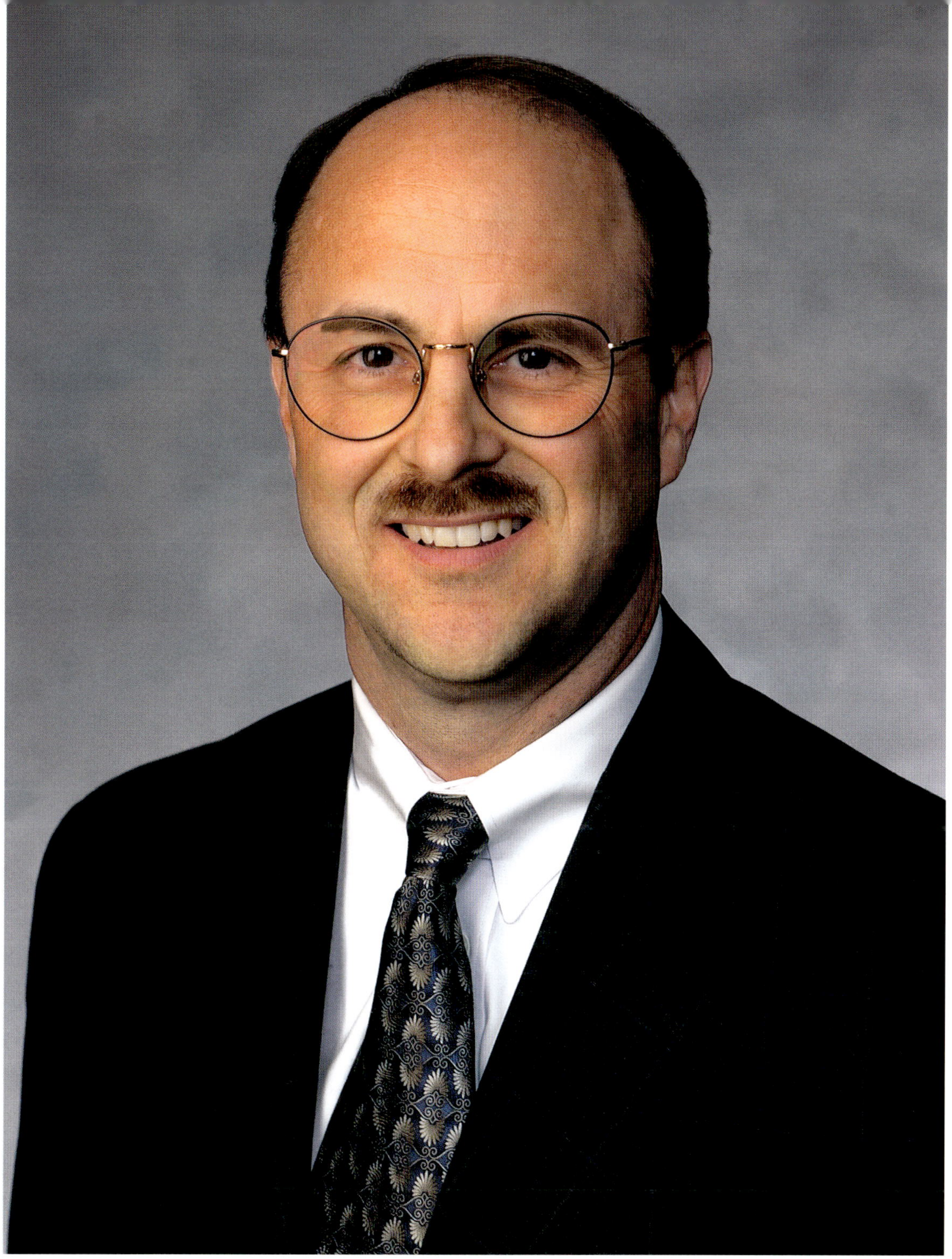

Eric Norwood faced an unprecedented number of challenges upon taking the helm at DeKalb Medical. With difficult finances at the top of his list, he was determined to increase revenue and at the same time enhance the quality, efficiency, and safety of patient care.

prior certificate of need (CON) approval. As a result of the reduced number of specialists and the trend to perform outpatient procedures away from the hospital, DeKalb Medical Center had seen the annual number of its surgical procedures drop from 18,000 to 12,000.[41]

Norwood saw the loss of a close relationship between the hospital and its primary care physicians. Most primary physicians, due to shrinking and disappearing reimbursement for their services to hospital patients, referred their patients to specialists or to hospital-based physicians for hospital care.

Norwood faced the need to reassess the hospital's relationship with the DeKalb Physician-Hospital Organization (DPHO). The DPHO very successfully managed contracts that PROMINA had negotiated on behalf of its members. In its demise PROMINA relinquished all contract negotiations back to its remaining members. Without PROMINA, the question remained as to DPHO's role and DeKalb Medical's relationship to the DPHO.

In addition to physician-related challenges, major projects were in the works or on the drawing board. Among these:

- In 2003 under Gerlach's leadership, the state gave its final approval to build a hospital at Hillandale, a dream of South DeKalb County residents since the county approved a $1,950,000 bond in 1970, and the time had come to bring it to fruition.
- The Women's Tower was an overdue commitment in the eyes of the obstetricians/gynecologists, some who had given up on its ever becoming a reality.
- QUEST, a complex and expensive electronic medical record project, had been launched in 2002 and required additional planning, staffing, funding, activating, training, and physician involvement.

At the top of Norwood's list was a difficult financial situation. Expenses were rising and revenue was falling. The combined Hillandale hospital and the Women's Tower required capital expenditures approaching $130 million. The initial operating cost of each would be substantial, and their interest and depreciation would adversely affect the system's net operating results in the short run. The electronic medical record project also required a major investment of time, energy, creativity, and money. Coupled with those increased expenses, the dramatic decline in procedures performed by the hospital's specialists had created a major loss of net income.

One of the most significant sources of financial strain, however, was the decline in reimbursement for services rendered. An increasing percentage of DeKalb Medical's patients were insured by Medicaid or not covered by any form of insurance. It was difficult enough to realize a positive net operating income with payments received from Medicare, managed-care contracts, and commercial insurers. Medicaid, however, paid little more than 80 percent of the actual cost of services provided, and those patients without insurance paid only a fraction of that amount.[42] The losses were frustrating and threatening. DeKalb Medical experienced a net operating loss of $26.5 million in fiscal year 2005–2006[43] and then $33.1 million in fiscal year 2006–2007.[44]

DeKalb Medical, of course, was not alone in facing financial difficulties. A 2007 Wall Street Journal study revealed that more than 2,000 of the nearly 3,900 acute-care hospitals in the nation sustained net operating losses.[45] Locally, Fulton County's South Fulton Hospital filed for Chapter 11 bankruptcy protection.[46] Rockdale Medical Center (at the time of this writing) is seeking a buyer because of its inability to meet all the requirements of the bond covenants for its debt.[47] Atlanta's Grady Memorial Hospital had a $55 million deficit in 2007 and faced the specter of closure or drastic reduction in services until it agreed to relinquish its governance to a new, private, nonprofit organization with the promise of multimillion dollar supplemental grants.[48]

DeKalb Medical was in the fortunate position that it could cushion its operating losses with interest earned on investments, with the use of reserves and with funds generated by the DeKalb Medical Foundation. However, its investment income was at risk due to declining market trends; it faced the unacceptable risk of failing to meet the requirements of its existing bond covenants; and it realized the

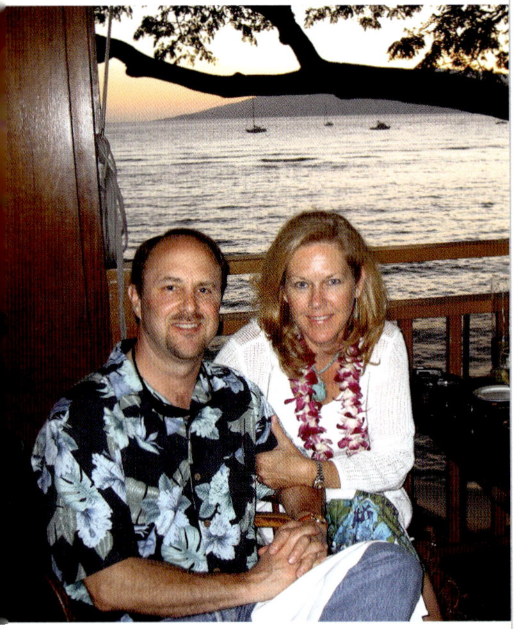

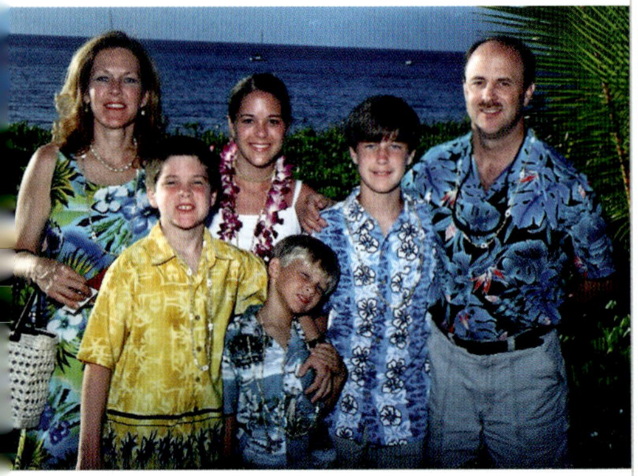

Eric and his wife Nancy with their family in Hawaii in 2003. Children in back left to right, Rachell and Daniel; in front left to right, David and Stephen.

good-business need to reverse its recent, negative financial trend.

Norwood challenged the challenges. He made tough decisions to reduce expenses. He eliminated or reduced the hours for 159 staff positions, including several on the administrative level.[49] His team outsourced services such as nutrition, emergency physicians, hospitalist physicians, environmental services, and bioengineering technical services. He discontinued DeKalb Medical's designation as a Level 3 trauma center in the state trauma network. He established a system to verify the need for hospital services for those with Medicaid coverage and those without any insurance.

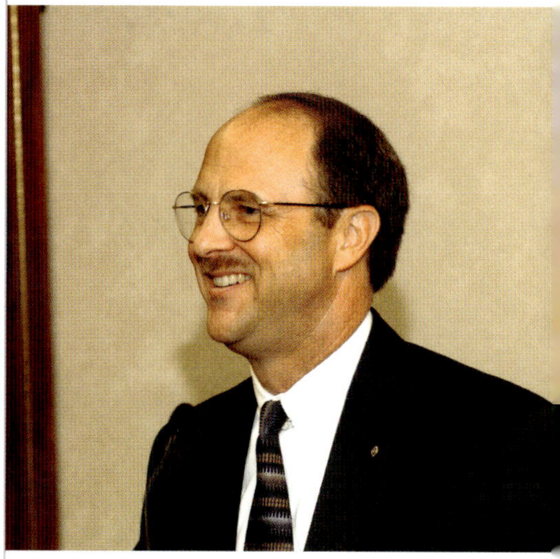

He took steps to improve quality, attract patients, and increase revenue. He joined with the physicians in the DPHO's clinical integration initiative to demonstrate quality, cost-effective patient care. He championed information technology advancements such as the Computerized Physician Order Entry (CPOE) system to enhance the quality, efficiency, and safety of patient care. He established the DeKalb Quality Institute to monitor and improve the quality of patient care, service excellence, and patient safety and to demonstrate objectively DeKalb Medical's quality of performance. As a result of these initiatives, HealthGrade, an independent healthcare rating company, analyzed nearly forty-one million Medicare hospitalization records at approximately five thousand U. S. hospitals from 2005 to 2007 and found that only 5 percent met quality standards to warrant HealthGrade's designation as a Distinguished Hospital for Clinical Excellence. DeKalb Medical was one to receive that designation with a five-star rating for its treatment of stroke, heart attack, hip replacement, hip fracture repair, peripheral vascular bypass, pneumonia, and sepsis. HealthGrade ranked DeKalb Medical as number one in Georgia for the treatment of stroke.[50]

He oversaw the completion of DeKalb Medical at Hillandale hospital and the patient tower on the North Decatur campus, determining that it would be not just a women's tower but a Women's and Surgery Center. He helped negotiate a three-year contract with Kaiser Permanente that permitted its 70,000 DeKalb County patients to receive hospital and diagnostic services at DeKalb Medical's three campuses and that gave Kaiser patients access to more than four hundred DeKalb Medical physicians.[51]

He led DeKalb Medical in a new strategic planning process that identified the primary strengths and opportunities of each of its three campuses,[52] chose the new name of "DeKalb Medical" to encompass the concept of the total health system, and created a new logo to symbolize that identity. DeKalb Medical at North Decatur would remain the main service area with special emphasis on oncology, orthopedics, and heart and vascular services; would partner with physicians to develop disease-focused initiatives in each of the service areas; and would establish development teams for each of the services to be made centers of excellence. DeKalb Medical at Downtown Decatur would focus primarily on post-acute services, including long-term acute care (LTAC), home health, and rehabilitation services. DeKalb Medical at Hillandale would work with the Hillandale Advisory Board to help make it a "top tier" community hospital.

He adopted the slogan, "Pushing Beyond" to proclaim that the new DeKalb Medical would be pushing beyond traditional expectations.[53] He initiated new marketing programs, new periodicals, new electronic communications, and continued his town hall meetings to carry the message of "Pushing Beyond" to the staff and the community,

His team recruited new specialists and primary care physicians to the medical staff. He enhanced communication with DeKalb Medical's physicians, partnered with them, and hosted meetings with them to learn their needs and to explore ways DeKalb Medical might support them in their practices. His team actively enlisted physicians for leadership roles in the development teams and advisory

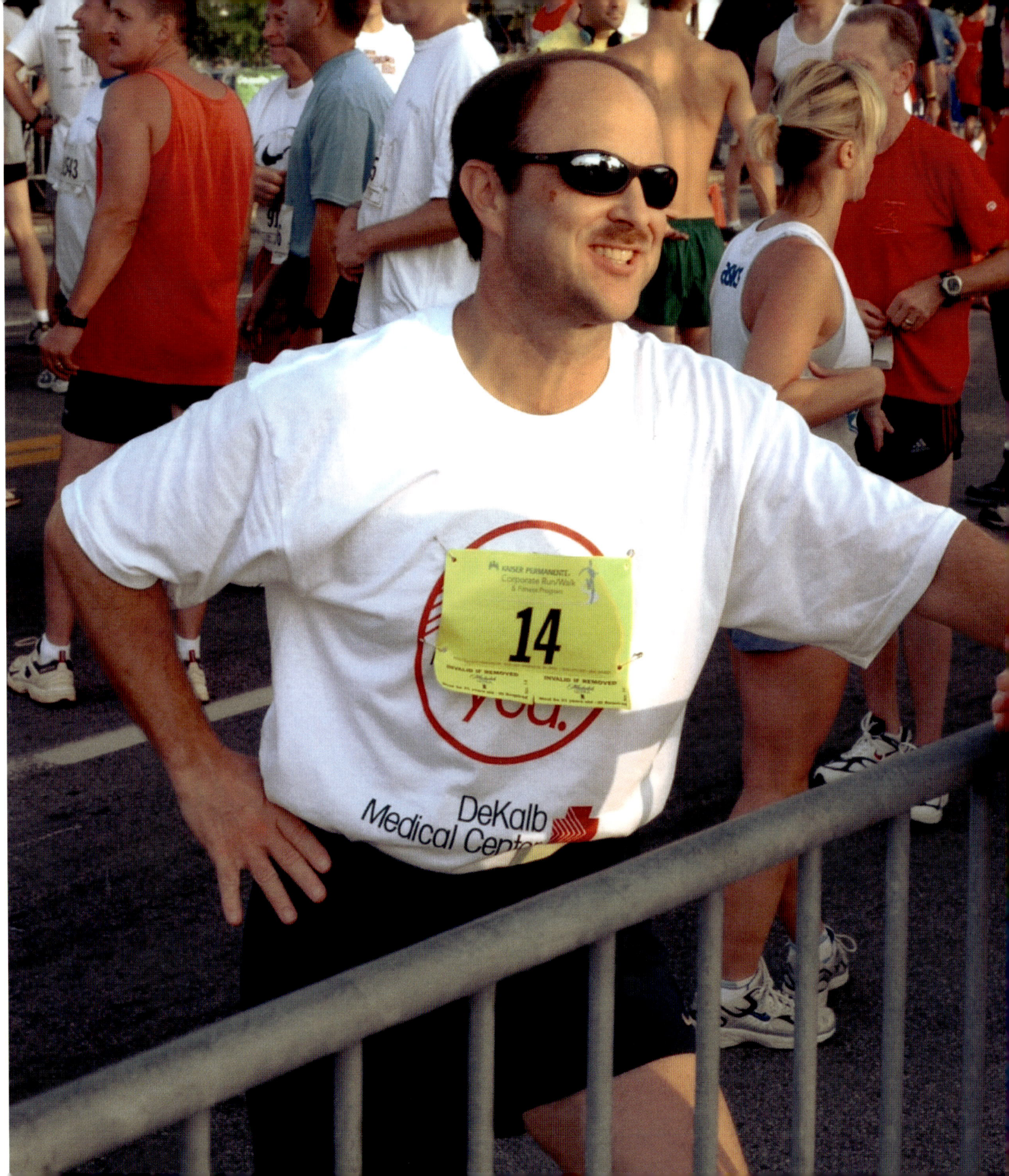
KAISER PERMANENTE.
Corporate Run/Walk
14
INVALID IF REMOVED
INVALID IF REMOVED
DeKalb

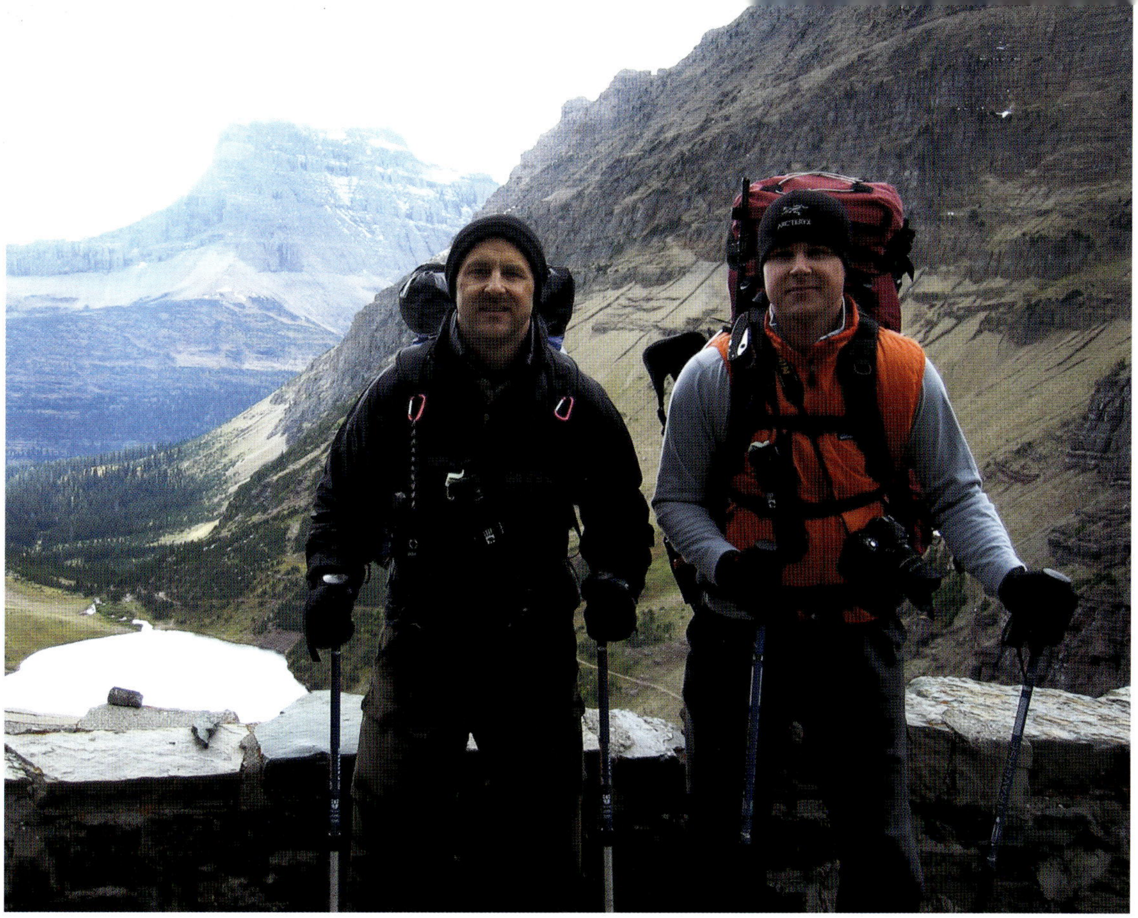

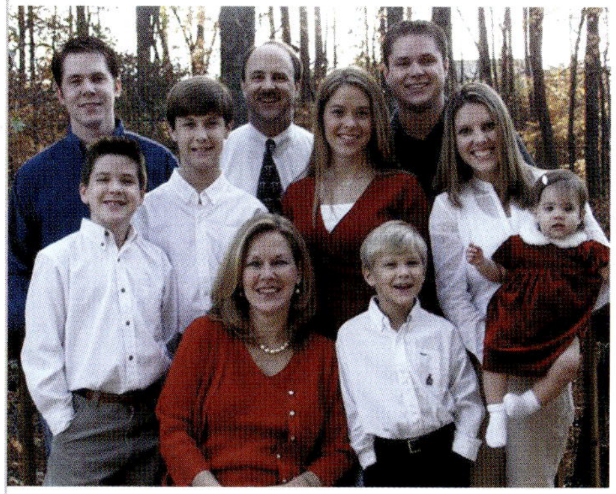

Above left: Eric and his son Daniel.
Above: Eric and his family with new granddaughter, Adalae. Back row left to right: David, Eric, and Daniel. Middle row left to right: Stephen, Rachel, and Christina holding Adalae. Front row left to right: Christopher, Nancy, and Jonathan.

boards and created joint ventures with physician partners.

Despite its financial and operational challenges, Norwood, like his predecessors, maintained a focus on the institution's mission of service to the community and the calling to serve that he had witnessed in the care given his friend in 1993. He reminds every new class of employees of the institution's heritage and of their unique opportunity to make a difference in people's lives every day. He calls on them to provide the best healthcare service in Atlanta.[54] He speaks of the organization's vision to be the recognized leader in clinical and service excellence and to be known as the best place in town to work.[55] He emphasizes DeKalb Medical's values of respecting diversity as a strength; of healing minds and spirits as well as bodies; and of serving others.[56]

Eric Norwood assumed the leadership post as DeKalb Medical faced major, unprecedented challenges. He has taken significant measures to meet those challenges while preserving the institution's heritage, mission, and values. Reflecting on the legacy of leadership at DeKalb Medical, Norwood always reminds his colleagues that they are standing on the shoulders of those who have gone before them to lay the foundation for the culture of caring for, and indeed loving, those whom the organization serves.

Conclusion

DeKalb Medical has had four leaders, each of whom has brought his own unique gifts to the institution at a time when those gifts were needed. Each has created his own legacy. Each has demonstrated leadership, integrity, devotion, and commitment; and each has built upon the foundation laid by the one going before. Each has understood that at DeKalb Medical, there will always be "miles to go" but that, in making that journey, each will leave his own "footprints in the sands of time."

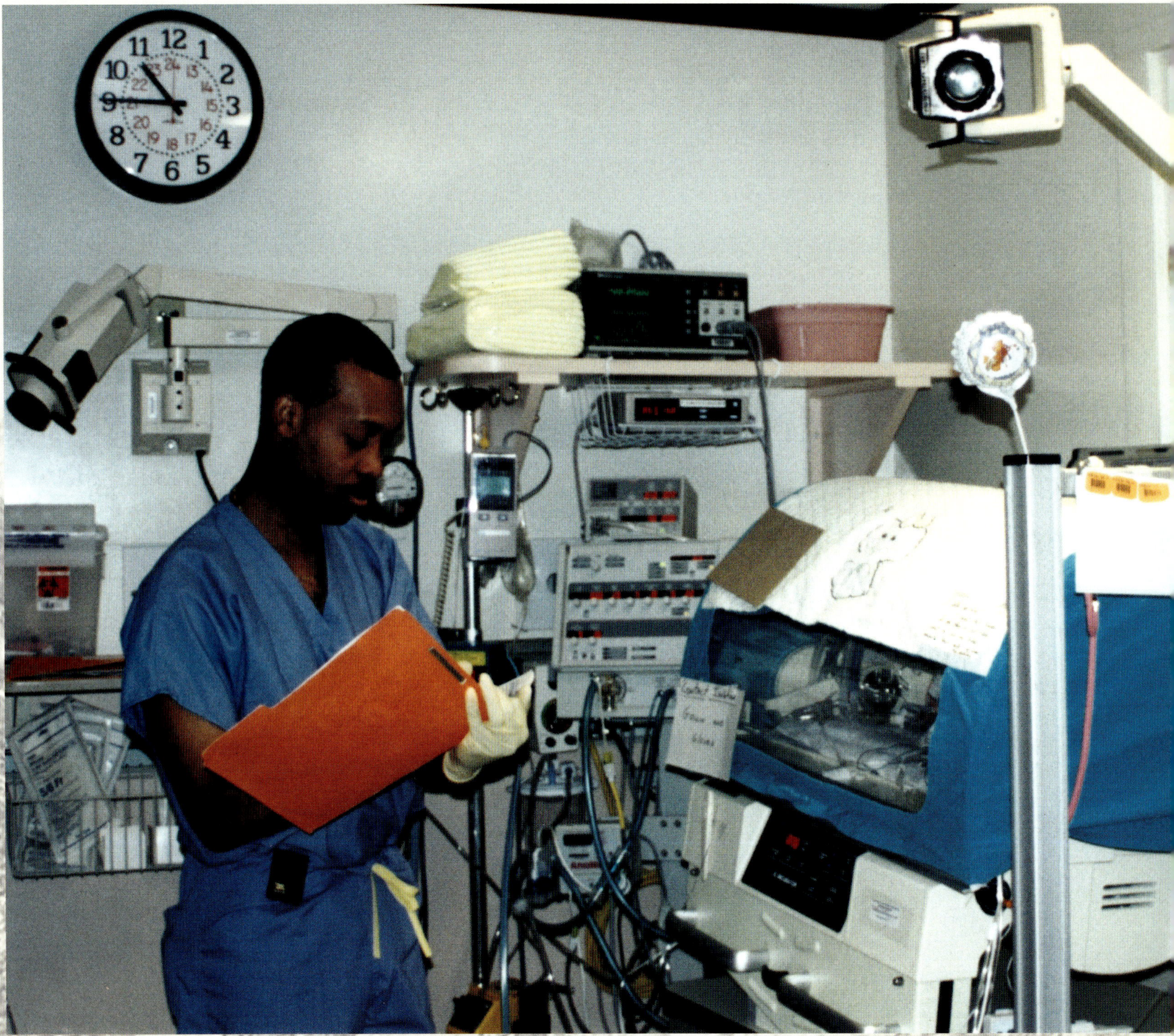

Above: Lawrence Wade, RRT, supervisor, neonatal ICU Respiratory Care.

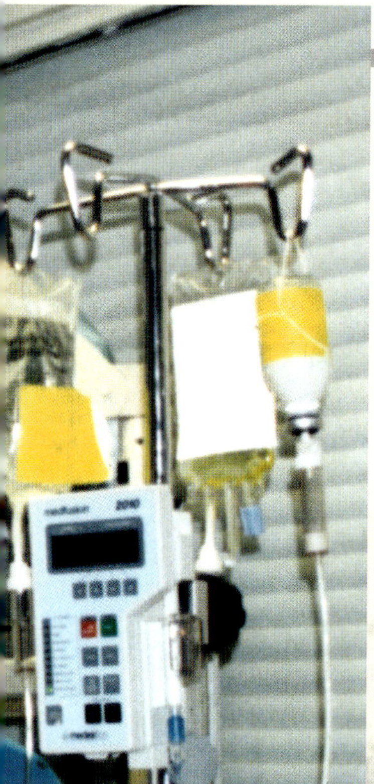

DeKalb Medical's Departments and Services at Work

Their stories, their accomplishments, their celebrations, and their challenges.

"Far and away, the best prize that life offers is the chance to work hard at work worth doing."

—Theodore Roosevelt

Anesthesia Services

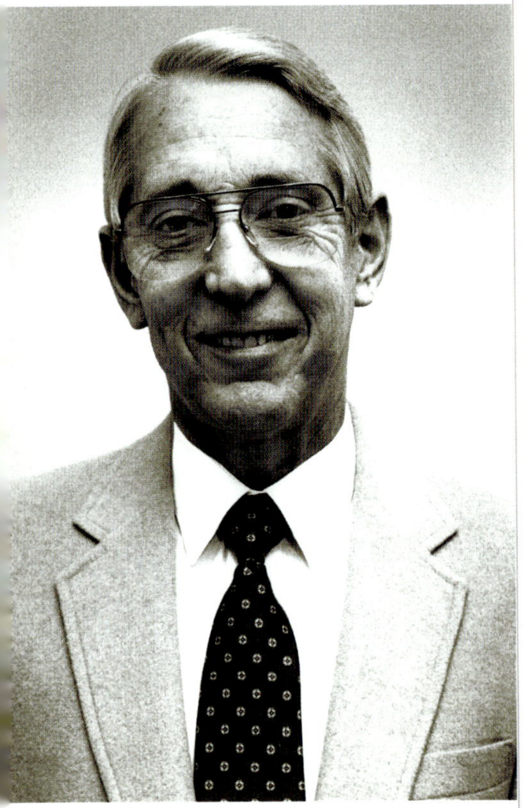
George Session, MD, was DeKalb General Hospital's first anesthesiologist.

George Sessions, MD, brought anesthesia services to DeKalb General Hospital. A native of Dawson, Georgia, Sessions attended Georgia Southwestern College and the University of Georgia for his undergraduate studies. He received his doctor of medicine degree at the Medical College of Georgia and did his residency in anesthesiology at Charity Hospital in New Orleans.

He wanted to come back to Georgia to practice medicine and thought Atlanta would offer the best opportunities. To his surprise he found that Atlanta was a "desert" for the practice of anesthesiology.[1] Some Atlanta surgeons wanted only nurse anesthetists to provide anesthesia services for their procedures. The head of the anesthesia department in one hospital wanted his staff to use only nitrous oxide and anectine drip regardless of how they were trained or what they thought to be the best agents for patients. At another hospital, the anesthesiologists were employed by the hospital and under the control of administration. One group in the late 1950s offered to hire him at a salary of $800 a month, but he observed some of its members to be engaged in poor anesthesia practices and declined the offer.

About that time, Emory anesthesiologist John E. Steinhaus, MD, was establishing a new training program at Grady Memorial Hospital, partly in response to a series of investigative reports by the *Atlanta Journal Constitution* newspaper regarding anesthesia deaths that had occurred in the Grady operating room. Sessions joined Steinhaus as an anesthesia instructor in his new program. When, however, Sessions learned that DeKalb General Hospital was nearing completion, he met with Administrator William Thrasher to explore the possibility of setting up the hospital's anesthesia program. Three other anesthesia groups also applied for the position,[2] but Thrasher liked Session's commitment to quality care and his plan to be financially independent of the hospital, which meant he would do his own billing and collecting. He was selected for the job. Sessions also suspected that two of the new hospital's leading surgeons, L. C. Buchanan, MD, and Richard Smoot, MD, spoke on his behalf.

Once Sessions was named as the hospital's anesthesiologist, he hired Sarah Brockman, CNA, as his first nurse anesthetist. Brockman had worked in the Grady Memorial Hospital Anesthesia Department for a number of years. He then asked Anibal "Andy" Adan, MD, to be his first associate, and Adan readily accepted. Adan had trained at Duke University, and he and Sessions had become acquainted at Saturday-morning anesthesia conferences.

Sessions admitted that the two of them were a little uncertain there would be enough work at DeKalb General for them to make a living. After all, it was a new hospital, and it was located a great distance from downtown Atlanta. They became reassured, however, when they learned that Buchanan and Smoot each planned to take all of their patients to DeKalb and that Lawrence P. Matthews, MD, a very busy obstetrician who delivered most of his patients under general anesthesia, also would practice there.

The hospital's agreement with Sessions stipulated that he would be responsible for his own revenue and expenses. The trustees did advance him an interest-free loan of $500 a month for the first two months, which he used to pay Brockman's salary.[3]

The hospital had five operating rooms and a cystoscopy room, but initially it used only two operating rooms, rarely a third, because of the small size of the anesthesia staff. And because there were only two anesthesiologists, Sessions and Adan were on call every other night. In February 1962, their workload increased enough to allow Sessions to hire Guillermo "Bill" Nadal, MD. Nadal's addition allowed them not only to expand their services but also to reduce their on-call schedule to every third night.

Ezequiel Fernandez, MD, and Earl Fuller, MD, joined the group in 1967, and Katherine Stuckey, MD, joined in 1969. That same year, Fuller resigned, and Jack Perkins, MD, took his place in 1970. David Nikola, MD, and Tom Robinson, MD, joined in 1971, followed by Ernest Guy, MD, in 1972, C. O. Maxey, MD, in 1973, and William Keeton, MD, in 1973.

In the mid-1960s, orthopedist Wood Lovell, MD, asked the group to provide anesthesia services at the Scottish Rite Crippled Children's Hospital, which was then located in south Decatur. Lovell (whom Sessions described as "a walking saint") and his staff operated only two days a week. The anesthesia group accepted the invitation and continued working there until Scottish Rite relocated in the 1970s to its present location in north DeKalb County.

When Decatur Hospital opened in 1973, shortly after Scottish Rite moved, the DeKalb Anesthesia Associates, as the group was then known, agreed to provide its anesthesia services. Administrator Thrasher and members of the DeKalb County Hospital Authority were concerned that their hospital-based anesthesia group was investing in and providing service for a competitor. Sessions explained to Thrasher that Decatur Hospital gave the community physicians operating room time and admitting opportunities that had not been available at DeKalb General during its decade of rapid growth and its prolonged renovation; and on top of this, his group promised not to compromise its commitment to DeKalb General Hospital.

Sessions recalled the general atmosphere in surgical services at DeKalb General to be "delightful." He had been accustomed to fighting with the surgery residents at Charity Hospital in New Orleans and with those at Grady Memorial Hospital. He said, "I was prepared to fight for the rest of my life."[4] To his pleasant surprise, there was none of that with the DeKalb General surgeons. They were easy to work with, and the fighting "just ended."

Sessions recalled that there were many dramatic moments in surgery and anesthesia, but one that stood out occurred when a child developed a sudden spike in temperature at the end of a minor eye procedure. Sessions had recently read and saved an article in the *Journal of the American Medical Association* about three children who died from a newly recognized condition known as "malignant hyperthermia" after receiving anesthesia for surgery. He was called back to the operating room one day to observe a child who immediately became cyanotic (turned blue) each time oxygen was removed. Sessions touched the child's skin and detected unusual warmth. His temperature registered 103°, and shortly thereafter, 105°. Sessions recalled the article on malignant hyperthermia. He ordered a cooling blanket, administered sodium bicarbonate to counter the child's possible acidosis, and the team worked with the child for hours. The child recovered with no apparent damage.

Two years later, that child's father was scheduled to undergo surgery at another hospital. At the request of the man's wife, Sessions called that hospital's operating room to alert them to the child's earlier experience before they began surgery on the father. Two hours into surgery, the child's father went into malignant hyperthermia and died. Later the child who had survived malignant hyperthermia and his sister were examined at a research center. There it was discovered that the father and his children shared a gene that made them prone to that rare syndrome.[5]

Sessions served as department chief until 1981 when he was succeeded by William Keeton.[6] When the anesthesia group met to select their new chief, the vote was a tie between Keeton and Mark

Coppage, MD. Sessions suggested that those two go have a beer and decide between themselves who would be chief and who would be vice-chief. When they arrived at the bar, Keeton asked how they were going to settle the matter. Coppage said that would be easy because he didn't want to be chief.[7] One of the anesthesia group's more painful losses, professionally and personally, was the untimely death of Coppage in an automobile accident in 1989.

Keeton grew up in Jackson, Mississippi, attended the University of Mississippi in Lafayette for his undergraduate work, and then went to medical school at the University of Mississippi Medical Center in Jackson. He did his anesthesia residency at Parkland Hospital in Dallas, Texas, after which he spent two years in the United States Air Force.

He decided while in the service that he would like to practice medicine in Atlanta. He had interviews with Sessions at DeKalb General and with John Patton, MD, chief of anesthesia at Northside Hospital. He decided to take the position at Northside and wrote Sessions of his decision. He was surprised to receive a gracious response from Sessions, saying that if he ever changed his mind, he would like for him to consider again a position at DeKalb General. After being at Northside for two years, Keeton did change his mind. Because of Sessions's kind offer, he returned to DeKalb in 1973 as DeKalb General was opening new operating rooms and as the anesthesia group was beginning its anesthesia service at Decatur Hospital.

Keeton said he found DeKalb General an "incredible place to work."[8] The surgeons were performing exciting procedures, the doctors were smart and collegial, the nurses were outstanding, people knew and liked each other, and they liked working at the hospital. He also was impressed that Sessions, who had the sole anesthesia contract with the hospital, voluntarily shared equally with the partners the income generated by the service.

Opposite: William Keeton, MD (left), Mark Coppage, MD, and Donna Childers, RN in the DeKalb Medical Pain Center.

One of Keeton's special interests was pain management. He became interested in this area while a resident at Parkland. At the time, Burnell R. Brown, MD, PhD, was chief of the hospital's pain clinic, and Brown required each resident to attend his clinic one day a week. The residents dreaded going and would make any excuse to get out of it. One day, Brown asked Keeton to accompany him in the clinic to see an elderly woman who moved about with great difficulty because of excruciating lower back pain due to bone metastasis from cancer. Brown instructed Keeton to inject a "concoction" into the trigger point where the pain was most intense. After a few minutes, the woman stood up, exclaimed that her pain was gone, and danced around the room with Keeton. With that, Keeton said he was "hooked" on the value of managing pain.[9]

His interest and expertise in pain management were enhanced when he later met and became friends with Janet G. Travell, MD. Travell had been President John F. Kennedy's White House physician. Although it was not common knowledge at the time, the president suffered from chronic pain, and it was Travell's job to manage it.

Keeton established a pain clinic while in the Air Force and, once he came to DeKalb, he saw and also treated patients with chronic and acute pain, initially on his own time. Eventually, other members of the anesthesia group joined him, including Coppage, Nikola, Constantine Kokenes, MD, and Charles "Chip" Clifton, MD. His group established the Pain Center located first in the recovery room, later in the old Intermediate Intensive Care Unit, then on the 1700 wing of the hospital, and finally in the first Professional Office Building.

Keeton retired from the practice of general anesthesia in 1997 to devote himself full time to the Pain Center. Over the years, pain treatment modalities grew from the early practice of sympathetic

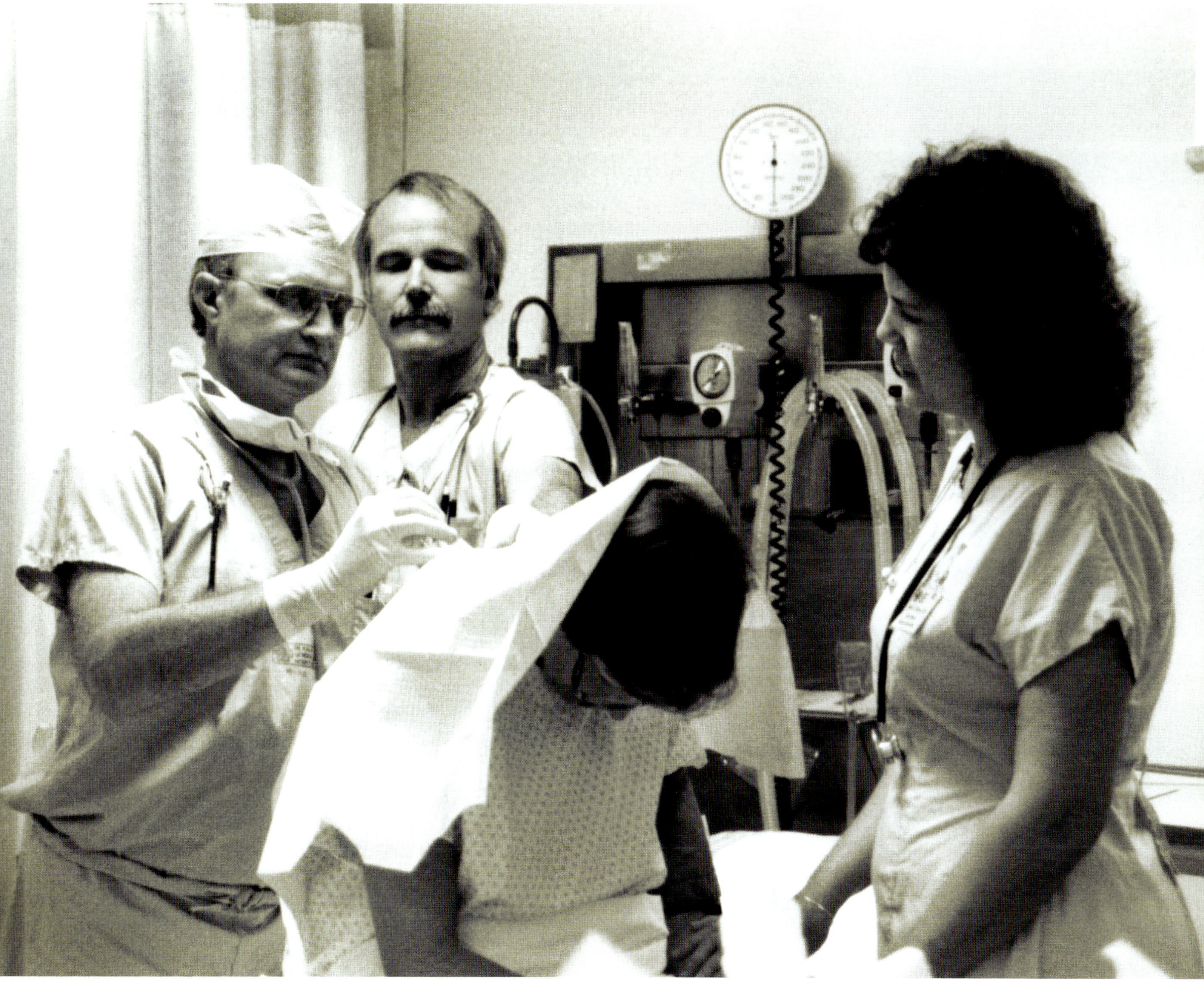

blocks and injecting trigger points to a variety of interventional techniques and the addition of medical management of pain. In August 2007 the Pain Center merged with Pain Consultants of Atlanta, headed by Rod Dularde, MD, and relocated to downtown Decatur.

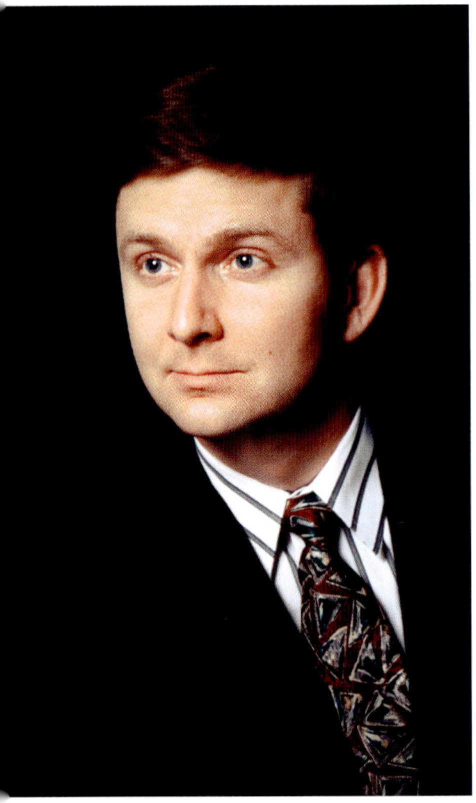

Charles "Chip" Clifton, MD, is the current chief of Anesthesia Services.

Nikola succeeded Keeton as chief of the Anesthesia Department for a brief period after which Keeton served a second term. Clifton became chief in 1996.

"Chip" Clifton joined DeKalb Anesthesia Associates in 1990. Having received his undergraduate and his medical degrees from Emory University, he returned to Emory for his anesthesia residency following four years of service as a flight surgeon. On the same night in 1990 he received phone calls with offers to join the Piedmont Hospital anesthesia group and the DeKalb Anesthesia Associates. He chose DeKalb and became the thirteenth physician in the group.

Keeton said that Clifton, as chief—with his intelligence, his business acumen, and his commitment to the service—elevated the anesthesia group to a new level.[10] Clifton acknowledged that as chief he had to deal with an entirely new set of challenges.[11] He had to recruit staffing. When several of the physicians and nurse anesthetists retired or left the group for other reasons he faced the need to recruit physicians and nurse anesthetists as well as practitioners from the newly created category of anesthesiology assistants. That meant, of course, that he and his associates had to monitor all recruits closely to ensure the quality of their competence and patient care.

DeKalb Anesthesia Associates during Clifton's tenure also faced major financial challenges. Sessions had established the group to be financially independent of the hospital; it billed and collected for all its own services. For many years, that system worked well. In 1992, however, Medicare began paying physicians a fixed amount, which was based on the procedure and a specified formula. That change resulted in a significant decrease in all physician reimbursements, including those made to anesthesiologists.[12] In addition, in 1997 when DeKalb Medical joined the PROMINA organization, DeKalb Anesthesia Associates was required to accept the reimbursement rates negotiated by PROMINA. At times these rates were less than the anesthesia group could have negotiated on its own. In addition, PROMINA experienced financial difficulties that made it unable to pay the DeKalb physicians all that they were owed.

In addition, surgical specialists increasingly established their own outpatient facilities. This meant the hospital lost many patients who had good insurance coverage or who were capable of paying out of pocket for services provided. The anesthesia group eventually found that more than 50 percent of the remaining patients were either underinsured or uninsured—people from whom little or nothing could be expected for services rendered.

While income declined, expenses increased. The cost of nurse anesthetists doubled in a decade. The addition of obstetrical and other surgically-related services at DeKalb Medical at Hillandale required the anesthesia group to provide in-house anesthesia coverage around the clock at two hospitals rather than one.

Those financial challenges created a new situation for the DeKalb Anesthesia Associates. Whereas George Sessions established the practice in 1961 with the firm determination that the group would be financially independent of the hospital, like 70 percent of anesthesia groups around the country, DeKalb Medical now supplements the group with a guaranteed income agreement.[13]

One of the original principles that remains, however, is "pride of ownership." DeKalb Anesthesia Associates still prides itself in maintaining a collegial relationship with physicians and hospital staff and in providing an uncompromising quality of competent patient care in a caring manner.[14]

Building Services and Materials Management

Most organizations have both visible and invisible heroes. DeKalb Medical is no exception. The visible heroes obviously are the doctors, nurses, and staff who take care of patients and provide patient care services, the team of executives who administer the affairs of the organization, the governing body that makes strategic decisions and ensures the financial stability of the institution, and the other leaders who are out front as the visible representatives of the organization.

The invisible heroes are there as well. They are on duty day and night, seven days a week, 365 days a year. They keep the facilities clean, safe, and operational. They are members of the Materials Management and Building Services teams.

Materials Management

Materials Management originally was known as the Purchasing Department, and Floyd "Mike" Mitchell was the director when DeKalb General opened in 1961. He remained in that position for only a year when he accepted the position as administrator of a hospital in Alabama.[1] As a means of economizing on expenses, the trustees elected not to name another director. Instead, they decentralized the responsibilities and named the head of Pharmacy as director of Pharmacy and Central Supply, asked the head of food services to order all dietary supplies and food, and asked the director of Building Services to purchase supplies for the laundry, housekeeping, and maintenance.

Several years later Sara Folger, who joined the Purchasing Department staff in 1961,[2] became the director.[3] At that time the department had only three or four personnel, one of whom was long-time em-

Below: Long-time employee Henry Elder, department head, Material Management. **Left:** Sara Folger, director of Purchasing with Roy Thomas, coordinator of Wages and Benefits.

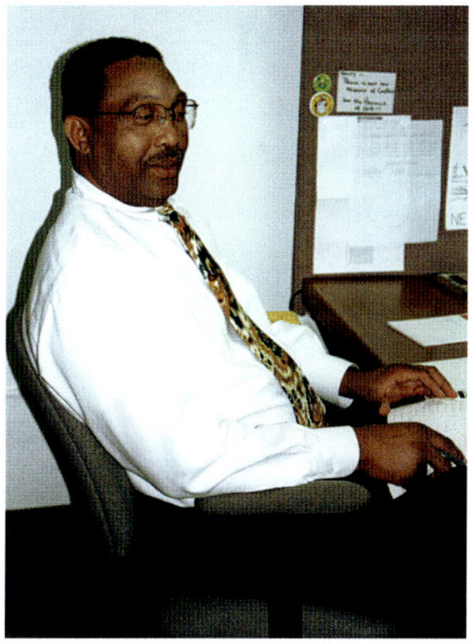

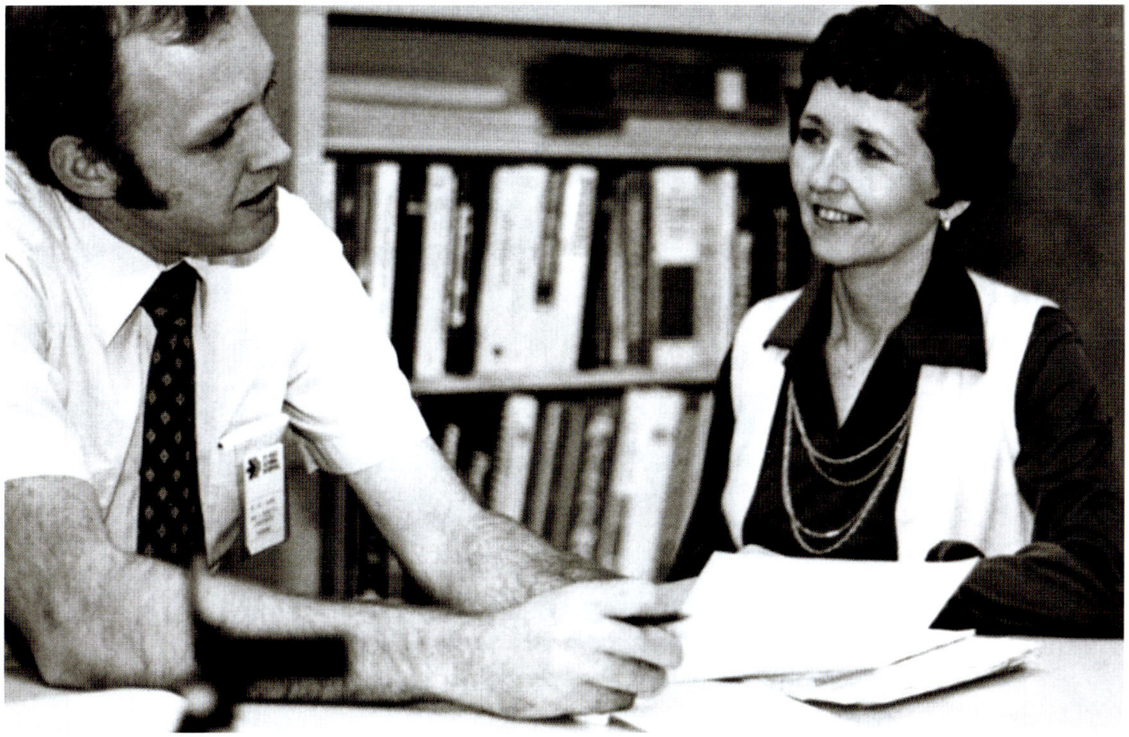

ployee Henry Elder.[4] Joe Hatchey succeeded Sarah Folger as director, and the name of the department was changed to Supply Purchasing and Distribution. Cynthia Perley replaced Joe Hatchey. John Washington and Dean Brown served as interim directors following Perley's resignation until Jack Sebree was appointed as the director in 2004.[5] Joe Jackson succeeded Sebree, and he remains the current director of Materials Management.

Materials Management now includes the Purchasing Department for which James Cistrunk is the coordinator, Distribution Services for which John Washington is the director, the Mail Room for which Maureen Dickson is the coordinator, and the Print Shop in which Richard "Rick" Carter and Claudell Johnson Jr., are the printers. Carter, originally a respiratory therapist in 1973, transferred to the Print Shop in 1985 and succeeded John Reagan, the hospital's first printer, when he retired in 1987.[6]

These services produce a staggering volume of work. The Mail Room processes and delivers nearly a half million pieces of mail each year. The Print Shop produces a million pieces of copy per month. Purchasing coordinates over 1,300 purchasing contracts and over 3,000 purchases, maintains 17,000 items in its database, and processes over $8.5 million in capital requests as well as $9 million in service contracts per year. Distribution Services daily receives and processes more than two hundred United Parcel Service (UPS) packages, fifty Federal Express packages, and fifteen overnight packages. It also handles between eight and fifteen pallets of supplies a day and keeps an average monthly inventory on hand valued at nearly $600,000. It restocks nearly one hundred areas and units in the hospital, delivers an average of thirty-five written requests to departments, and handles over 125 walk-up requests per day.[7] Materials Management truly "manages the supply chain" of DeKalb Medical.[8]

Below: Clayton Bailey, third director of Building Services who succeeded Dan Goolsbee in 1991. **Bottom:** Daniel "Dan" Goolsbee was the second director of Building Services who succeeded Rodney Sperry in 1969.

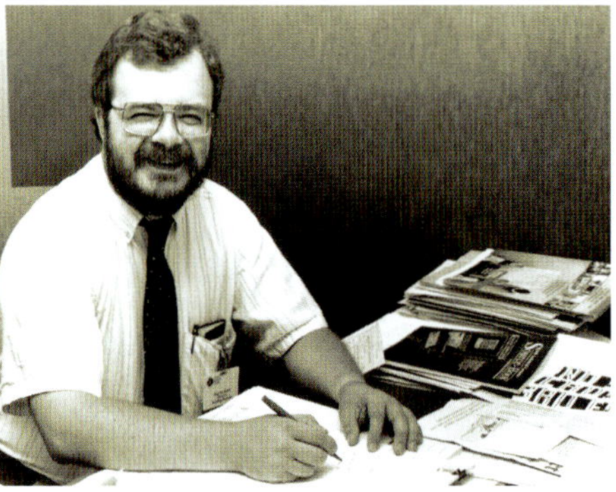

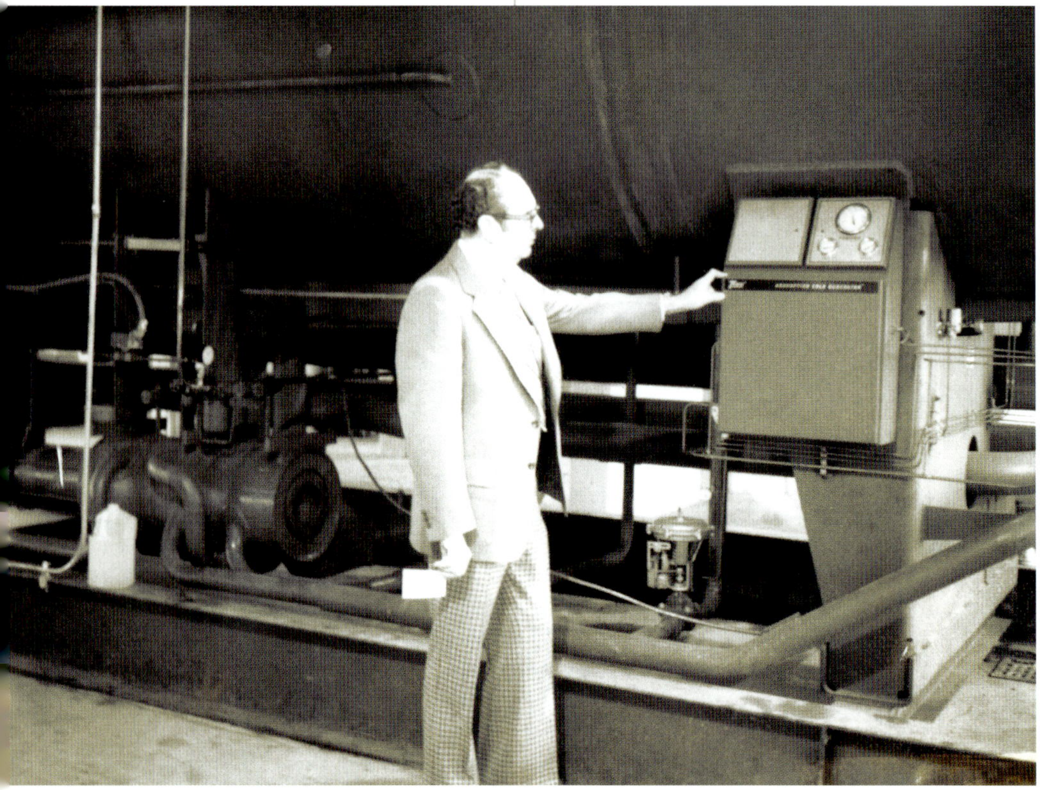

Building Services

Building Services originally included Maintenance, Housekeeping, and Laundry. Rodney Sperry was the director of Building Services, William Alexander was supervisor of Maintenance,[9] Cecil Hutchins was the first known manager of the Laundry,[10] and Mrs. Van Sickle was supervisor of Housekeeping.[11] Administrator William Thrasher reported to the trustees that Sperry resigned in 1969 for "a better salary, better advancement potential, and better location."[12] Dan Goolsbee succeeded Sperry and became the hospital's first full-time director of Building Services.[13] Goolsbee had recently retired from the U.S. Army with a strong background in hospital services, medical maintenance, and building construction. Clayton Bailey, who had served as Building Services' administrative engineering assistant, succeeded Goolsbee as director when Goolsbee retired in 1991.[14] Dan Callahan, who had joined the Building Service staff in 1994 and served as manager of the Engineering/Maintenance Department since 1995, became the fourth director in 1998 when Bailey resigned.[15]

Maintenance

The Maintenance Department in Building Services went through a series of reorganizations that reflected the increasing complexity of its responsibilities and the advancements in technology for which it was responsible.

In 1972 Joe Alexander was supervisor of the department. He began working at DeKalb General in 1961 as the hospital's only electrician.[16] As supervisor, he divided the department into four divisions: General Maintenance, Preventive Maintenance, Special Project, and Painting.[17] General Maintenance was responsible for general repairs, and William Ellis was lead foreman. Preventive Maintenance was responsible for servicing all equipment on a periodic basis, and Eugene Furey was the lead foreman. Special Projects handled all carpentry requests, including changes in the structure of the building, and Radus Ozburn was the lead foreman. Painting maintained the painting and wall repair needed in the hospital, and Otto Ransome was the lead foreman for this division.

Though the department was relatively small in size, things did not always go smoothly and required some effort at getting to a resolution. The 1971 employee newsletter carried the following notice of a "Dedication Ceremony."

> *A unique ceremony was held in the Maintenance Department this past week, dedicating a new comfort area. It was attended by top hospital officials. There was a ribbon cutting and an appropriate speech delivered by Thrasher, our Executive Director. A suitable gift was presented by another of our administrators. This culminates a seven-month effort to clear up a misunderstanding between Construction and Maintenance over installation problems in this area. The matter was climaxed to the satisfaction of all.*[18]

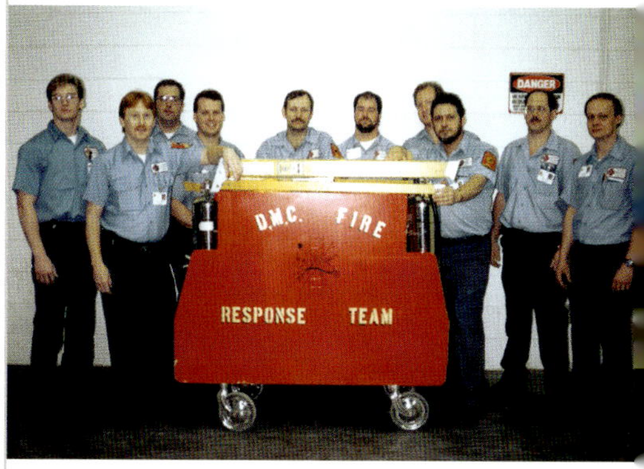

Members of the Building Services' Fire Response Team in 1988. Left to right: Robert Heard, James Tweedell, John Cates, Ladd Bancroft, Scott Hitt, Ken Boozer, Steve Tuthill, David Crowe, Randy Austin, and Michael Newberry.

Two decades later, in 1991, Building Services Director Clayton Bailey outlined another reorganization of the Maintenance Department into Mechanical Maintenance, General Maintenance, Technical Maintenance, and Paint Crew.[19] Eugene Furey had come to DeKalb in 1972 as lead foreman of Preventive Maintenance and had one technical equipment repairman in his department. In 1991, as supervisor of the new Technical Maintenance Department, he had a crew of seven people. They maintained and serviced everything from the microwave ovens all over the hospital to the defibrillators, ventilators, anesthesia machines, and laser equipment.[20]

By 1991 the new Energy Plant and Incinerator became operational, for which Building Services purchased all the major equipment. Mechanical Maintenance had responsibility for the plant's operation. While the incinerator offered the dual promise of disposing of the hospital's waste products and providing steam for the Energy Plant, increasingly stringent Environmental Protection Agency (EPA) requirements eventually led the hospital to shut it down.

While the incinerator was still in operation, the Federal Reserve Bank, the FBI, and the Secret Service occasionally used the Incinerator to destroy worn out bills, confiscated drugs, and contaminated or counterfeit money. One day Secret Service agents called to say they wanted to come out and review both the hospital's burning procedure and the personnel involved in the burning process. When they showed up at the hospital, they said some of the counterfeit money supposedly burned in the incinerator had been showing up in circulation. The Maintenance staff attending the meeting got uneasy, wondering if the finger of guilt was being pointed at them, until the authorities made it clear that they were concerned some of their own agents were holding out bills intended for the furnace.[21]

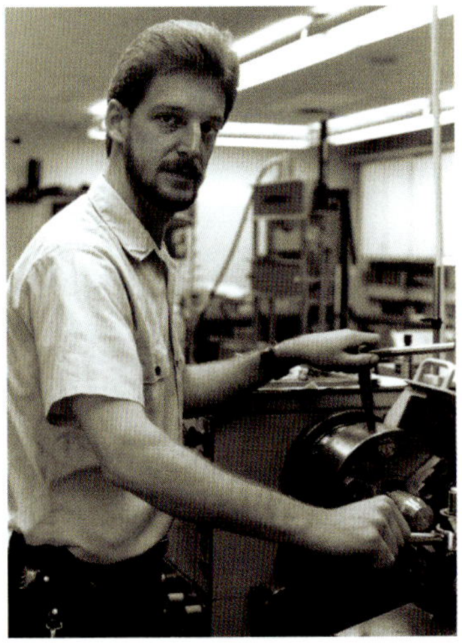

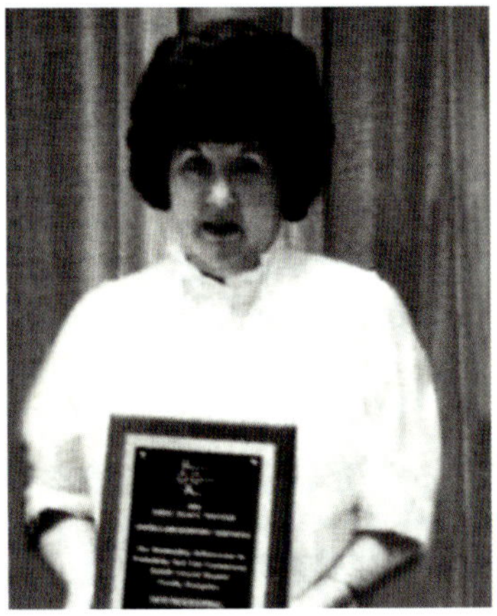

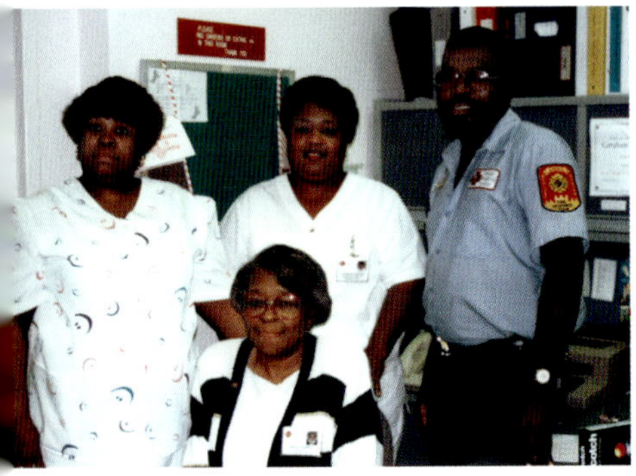

Top: Carl Lallerstedt, manager of the Engineering/Maintenance Department. **Center:** In 1986 Rae Easterling, DeKalb General's third executive housekeeper, was honored with an award for her cost-cutting measures. **Above:** The Anderson Family includes: Left to right standing; Carolyn G. Anderson, Juanquita Williams, Jackie Anderson, seated is their mother Carolyn Anderson. All are DeKalb Medical employees.

Currently the Maintenance Department's responsibilities include maintaining the facility and equipment in three hospitals, a series of primary care facilities, a Diagnostic Imaging Center, the professional buildings on two campuses and a Women's Center and Surgical Center. Such a great number of responsibilities called for even more creative structuring, operation, and leadership. The Technical Maintenance Department was restructured as the Biomedical Department, and those responsibilities were outsourced to General Electric Corporation, though still reporting to Building Services Director Dan Callahan. Many of the major pieces of technological equipment now are serviced by contracts with the manufacturers whose technicians are trained in the equipment. Mechanical Maintenance is now the Engineering/Maintenance Department for which Carl Lallerstedt is manager. It includes most of the duties previously assigned to the Mechanical and General Maintenance departments and the paint crew. The Facility Development Department, of which Ken Drury is project manager and Mike Paul coordinator, is responsible for renovation and construction projects.

In addition to keeping the facilities operational, Building Services has kept some of the institution's treasures safe. When DeKalb General Hospital was originally under construction, the trustees came up with an innovative idea to raise money. They mounted plaques on patient room doors in memory or in honor of a loved one in return for $1,000 donations. Later years brought more renovations and additional construction, and somewhere along the way many of the plaques were removed from their doors. For many years everyone thought the plaques had been lost. In 1990 an administrative resident discovered that, Jackie Anderson, Building Services' Parts and Tools Specialist who joined the staff in 1971, had been keeping and protecting the plaques in his personal locker through the years, waiting for someone to claim them.[22] Administration is planning to remount these treasures in a prominent display in the near future.

Environmental Services and Laundry Services

In addition to the various maintenance responsibilities, Building Services continues to retain oversight for Housekeeping/Environmental Services and Laundry Services.

Housekeeping/Environmental Services

When DeKalb General first opened, Mrs. Van Sickle was the Housekeeping supervisor and Frances Fannin her assistant. Van Sickle remained for a year, after which Fannin was named Housekeeping supervisor in 1962. When Fannin resigned in 1964, Rae Easterling became supervisor, a title that was later changed to executive housekeeper.[23]

Housekeeping had the following motto: "To radiate that 'clean look' to all who enter our doors."[24] The staff originally was known as maids and custodians.[25] All the staff was required to undergo a training class that dealt with personal hygiene and the required dress code, how to clean an occupied room and a vacated room, cleaning an isolation room, infection control, the use of chemicals, and other pertinent topics.[26]

James Solomon was one of the early stars on the Housekeeping staff. Coming to DeKalb General in April 1961 as custodian, he was rapidly promoted to group leader, training leader, floor supervisor, and assistant housekeeper.[27] He achieved the highest score of all those attending a national housekeeping seminar.[28] For three years he attended DeKalb Technical School, attended seminars, and took a correspondence course to become a Certified Housekeeper.[29] Many of the hospital staff still recall the daily rounds that Easterling and Solomon made together throughout the facility, Easterling calling out duties to be performed and Solomon making careful notes of instructions to pass on to the staff. When Easterling retired in 1991, Solomon was named manager, and the name of the department was changed from Housekeeping to Environmental Services.

Solomon retired in December 1996, and he was succeeded by David Jones. Shortly after Jones was appointed, DeKalb contracted the management of Environmental Services to a group known as First Management Services. Jones remained for a while as First Management's manager and was succeeded by Ray Darden in the fall of 1997.[30] In 2003 the hospital selected a new management company, Sodexho, for Environmental Services, and Regina Bradley became the director.[31] Even now, though the service is contracted to an outside source, the division continues to report to the director of Building Services.

Laundry Services

Like most things at DeKalb Medical, the workload in Laundry Services has continually increased. Six months after DeKalb General opened, the laundry was handling nearly seventeen pounds of laundry per patient per day for a total of nearly 57,000 pounds per month.[32] Following the hospital expansion in 1971, the division handled more than 184,000 pounds per month.[33] By 1985 the workload reached 270,000 pounds per month.[34] Currently Laundry Services processes more than 330,000 pounds per

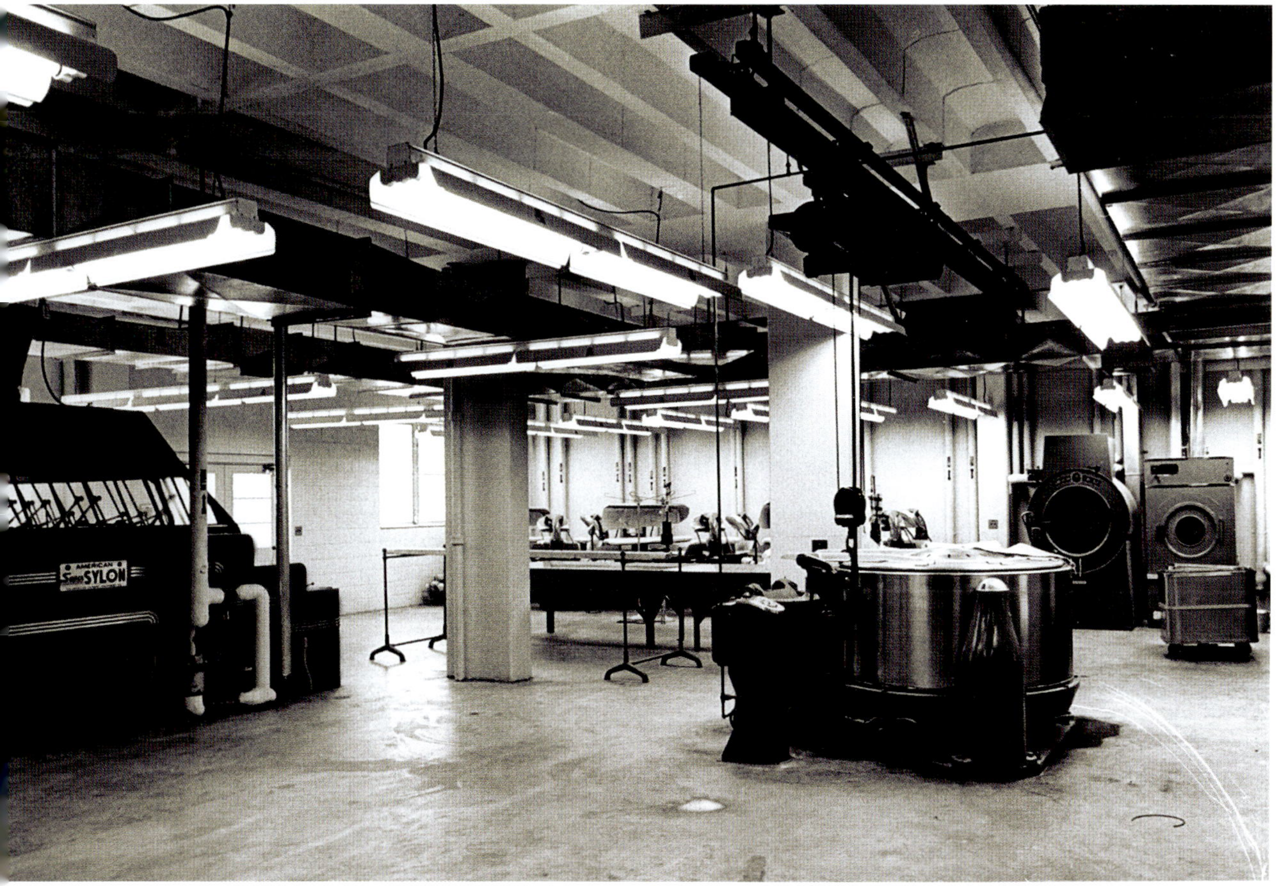

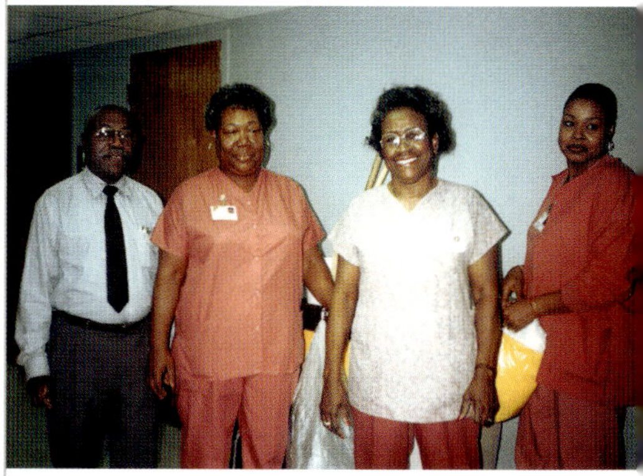

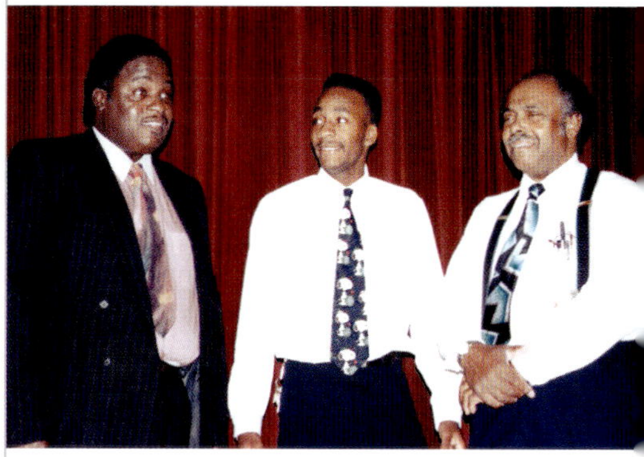

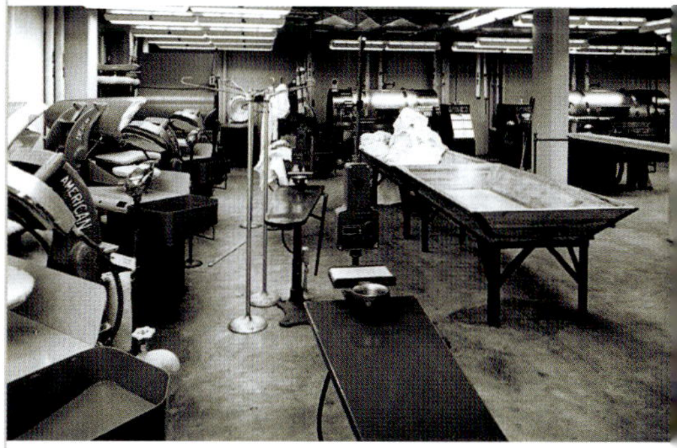

Top: Left to right; James Solomon was the third manager of Housekeeping/Environmental Services from 1991–1996. His coworkers are, left to right, Snow Weems, Annie Ruddison, and Patricia Williams. **Center:** Laundry Manager Grover Evans, center, with his colleagues and members of his singing trio Louis Coleman, left, and Claudell Johnson Sr., right. **Above and left:** The laundry areas as the hospital prepared for opening in 1961.

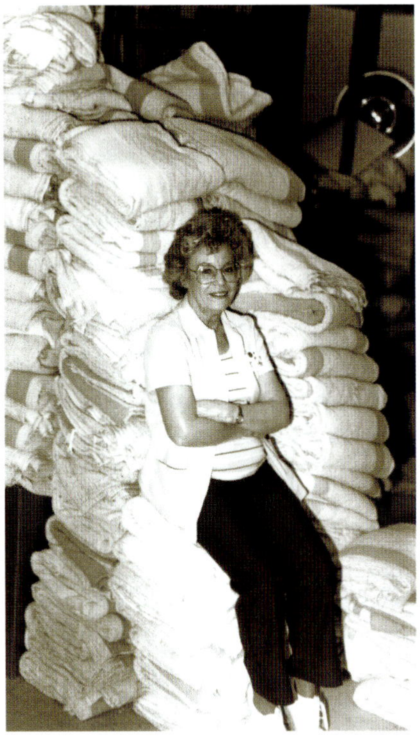

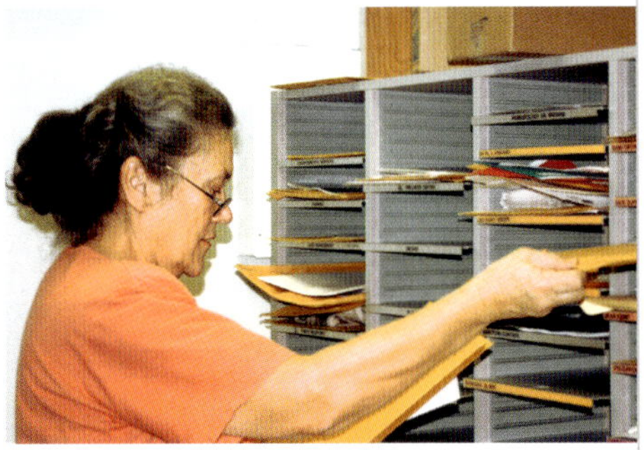

Top: Betty Bagwell takes a breather against a 1990 stack of torn blankets awaiting her repair. **Above:** Maureen Dickson hard at work in her "Mail Room."

month, or 4 million pounds annually.[35] It provides its services to all three of DeKalb Medical's hospitals, takes care of towels from the Wellness Center, and does a small amount of work from Emory University and Georgia State University. Yet it has done its work without increasing the size of its staff. In 1980 there were twenty-nine people on the staff.[36] Now there are only twenty-four.[37]

The work was always hard and, at times, hazardous. In 1962 the trustees added a cooling system to the laundry because fans were not doing the job, temperatures were rising to 105°, and employees were becoming ill. The workers even threatened a walkout.[38] The ceiling tiles were removed to allow the heat to rise, the exhaust fans elevated, and workers now are comfortable, sometimes wearing jackets.[39]

Protecting the staff not only from the excessive heat but also from infections has always been a top priority. All linens are considered contaminated and thus a potential source of infection. Those coming from patients on chemotherapy are considered "toxic" and are subject to an extra washing. All workers who collect, sort, or in any way handle soiled linens wear complete personal protective garments and equipment.

DeKalb Medical has had outstanding leadership in Laundry Services. Cecil Hutchins, who became manager of the Laundry in 1966, had thirty-five years of experience in the laundry business before coming to DeKalb General.[40] He was one of only 250 managers in the nation, and only the second in Georgia, to be named a Certified Institutional Laundry Manager by the American Institute of Laundering.[41] Grover Evans, who joined the Laundry staff in 1985 on the "ground floor" as a linen sorter, became manager of Laundry Services in 1996, was named Laundry Manager of the Year in 2000 and again in 2003 by the Georgia chapter of the National Association of Institutional Linen Management. He competed for the national title, only to be "beat out" by one manager from Massachussetts.[42] James Summey, who served as manager from 1978 to 1996 was recognized for maintaining high quality and productivity of laundry services.[43]

DeKalb has chosen to keep its Laundry Services in house rather than contracting it to outside agencies as many institutions have done. Keeping it in house enables the hospital to maintain control over the quality of its work and its customer service. The Laundry Services division at DeKalb continues to use a manual process for handling, washing, drying, ironing, and folding, rather than the automated systems in use in some institutions, yet it does so at a cost better than the national average.

When Grover Evans became manager, he established a task force to study DeKalb's laundry processes, and the team came up with ways to be efficient without sacrificing quality of service. The service developed a careful record of the linens actually utilized by each unit in the hospital so that the Laundry could provide each unit with just the amount needed. It also saved on the availability of scrub uniforms. Laundry Services now provides scrubs only for physicians, and it has ordered new scrubs for the doctors imprinted boldly and prominently with DeKalb Medical's logo. Evans contends that if DeKalb physicians choose to wear them outside the hospitals, at least they are advertising DeKalb Medical.

Laundry Services under Evans' leadership continues to focus on quality work, productivity, support for its workers, efficiency, customer service and safety for patients and staff. It is a service that directly affects patients and staff throughout DeKalb Medical, a service of heroic proportions.

Cancer Services

In 2007 DeKalb Medical's Charles B. Eberhart Cancer Center, having that year treated more than 2,000 new cases of cancer,[1] received the Outstanding Achievement Award with commendations from the American College of Surgeons' Commission on Cancer. Of the 453 hospitals surveyed, only 15 percent received this prestigious honor. It is reserved for those cancer centers that demonstrate high quality cancer care that not only meets but exceeds the commission's standards.[2] This was not the first time such an award was given. For example, in 2004 it was one of only thirty-nine programs nationwide to receive the Commission's Outstanding Achievement Award,[3] and the commission at that time declared the program to be "outstanding."[4]

Providing excellent care to patients with cancer has been one of DeKalb Medical's most notable achievements. From its inception, DeKalb has been committed to the prevention, diagnosis, and treatment of cancer and to the support of cancer patients and their families. It has given leadership, creativity, energy, and resources to the task so that Cancer Services has warranted DeKalb Medical's designation as a "center of excellence."

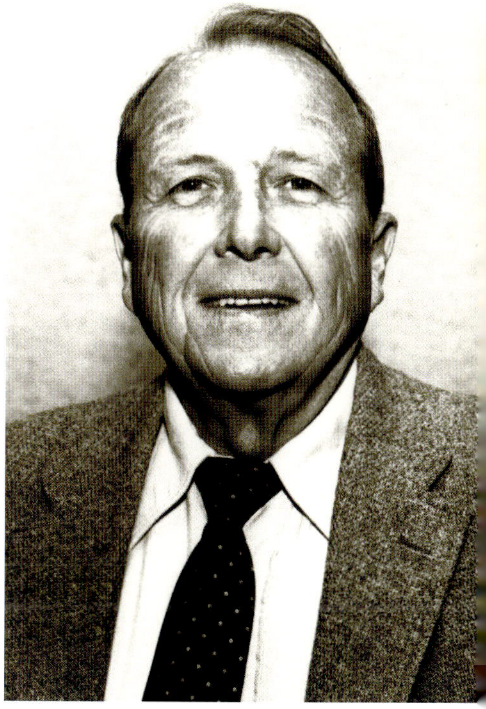

Angier Wills, MD, an original staff member from 1961, was a surgical oncologist who recommended establishing DeKalb General Hospital's Cancer Committee and Tumor Registry and served as the first chairman of the Cancer Committee.

Angier Wills, MD, a surgical oncologist, was a member of the original medical staff in 1961 and a leader in the early development and growth of the hospital's Cancer Services. In 1969 he recommended that the medical staff establish a Cancer Committee and that the hospital create a Tumor Registry to maintain records of patients diagnosed with cancer, the types of cancer diagnosed, treatments rendered, and the outcome of treatment.[5] The medical staff supported his recommendation for a Cancer Committee and, to no one's surprise, elected Wills as its chairman. The Cancer Committee instituted a Tumor Conference that met twice monthly to present lectures on cancer topics and to conduct multidisciplinary discussions of difficult cancer cases.[6] The hospital established a Tumor Registry in 1973,[7] and three years later the Commission on Cancer of the American College of Surgeons certified DeKalb General Hospital as a Cancer Treatment Center.[8]

That is not to say the hospital was expeditious in dealing with every cancer-related issue. Smoking was one such exception. In 1961 DeKalb General sold cigarettes in its vending machines and in the gift shop. Smoking was permitted throughout the hospital, including patient rooms. A cartoon in a 1961 employee newsletter was entitled "John Q. Patient—Be Nice to Him," and it pictured a nurse standing beside a patient's bed holding the patient's left hand while he dangled a lighted cigarette from his right hand.[9] A 1962 employee newsletter referred to a hospital staff member's relocation to another state and said, "We miss the smell of Mitchell's pipe in the snack bar and hope he is enjoying his new job in Alabama."[10]

In 1968 the medical staff, by a split vote of fifty-four to twenty-four (even closer in the Surgery Department where the vote was nine to seven), asked the DeKalb County Hospital Authority to remove cigarette vending machines from the hospital.[11] The Authority declined the request[12] but did attach a sign to each vending machine that read: "Members of our medical staff recognize that smoking is an extreme health hazard. The use of this machine is not recommended."[13]

In 1971 the Authority prohibited smoking in pediatric and semiprivate rooms,[14] and a year later ceased selling cigarettes in the hospital.[15] The trustees adopted a "no-smoking" policy in the hospital in

1977,[16] but as late as 1985 ashtrays were still in all patient rooms.[17] Finally, in 1990, the Authority banned smoking throughout the hospital and in its office buildings, and it established outdoor smoking areas.[18] In 2003 the DeKalb Medical Center Board of Directors strengthened that no-smoking policy by stating that in the fall of 2005, following the completion of DeKalb Medical at Hillandale, all DeKalb Medical facilities would be completely smoke free.[19]

DeKalb Medical also traveled a long and difficult course before it achieved a state-of-the-art radiation oncology service. The 1961 hospital opened with a cobalt unit for radiation therapy. In 1973 the Authority approved a plan to create a section of Radiotherapy as a division of the Radiology Department, replace the existing cobalt unit, and recruit a certified radiation oncologist.[20] A year later LaMar McGinnis, MD, chief of staff, expressed to the trustees his disappointment that the plan had not been implemented.[21] Instead of proceeding with the 1973 plan, the hospital had explored a "shared" radiation therapy service with Crawford Long Hospital, Georgia Baptist Hospital, and Emory University Clinic.[22] When that collaborative option was deemed unworkable, the Authority voted in 1976 to spend up to $1 million to replace the existing cobalt unit with a linear accelerator, and it once again endorsed recruiting one or more radiation oncologists.[23]

Frank Critz, MD, and John McLaren, MD, joined the medical staff as radiation oncologists, and the hospital created the Radiation Therapy Department separate from the Radiology Department. However, when it applied to the state for permission to replace its cobalt unit with a linear accelerator,[24] the state denied the hospital's request.[25] The hospital, therefore, replaced the existing cobalt unit with an improved Theratron 80 cobalt rotational unit[26] and hired a consultant to help develop a five-year master plan for radiation oncology.[27]

In the spring of 1988, the Authority once again budgeted for a linear accelerator[28] but put those plans on hold when it learned that Frank Critz was building a radiation therapy center with a linear accelerator only a short distance from the hospital. It would be another nine years before DeKalb Medical Center would reactivate plans for its own state-of-the-art radiation oncology program.

While slow to deal with the issue of smoking in the hospital and the enhancement of its radiation oncology service, DeKalb was attending steadily to other cancer service initiatives. It added two medical oncologists to the medical staff: John Manfredi, MD, joined in 1974 and Herbert Kann, MD, in 1979. In 1981 the hospital designated the 4200 nursing unit as the Medical Oncology Unit and dedicated twenty-two of the unit's sixty-six beds for cancer patients.[29] Sandra Yates, RN, was named 4200 department head. Linda Schievelhud, RN, was made cancer nurse coordinator to provide education to cancer patients, their families, and hospital staff, to counsel with cancer patients, and to collaborate with Social Services in its monthly cancer support group.[30] The hospital established an enterostomal therapy program in 1974 with Helen Simmons, RN, as one of only twelve enterostomal therapists in Georgia at that time.[31] The service assisted ostomy patients, many of whom had undergone surgery for cancer.[32] Prebble Mitchell (later Smith), RN, followed Simmons as director of enterostomal therapy. Long-time Authority member, Wash W. Lively, provided funds to renovate and furnish the solarium on 4200 as "The Lively Room" for cancer patients to watch TV, listen to music, and enjoy other entertainment sources.[33]

In October 1984 DeKalb General Hospital opened its Diagnostic Breast Center to offer mammography services.[34] Breast cancer was the most frequently seen cancer at DeKalb General. This new service made possible earlier detection of cancer and better cure rates, and, as the technology evolved, it offered the surgical option of segmental resection (lumpectomy) for appropriate patients in place of the tradi-

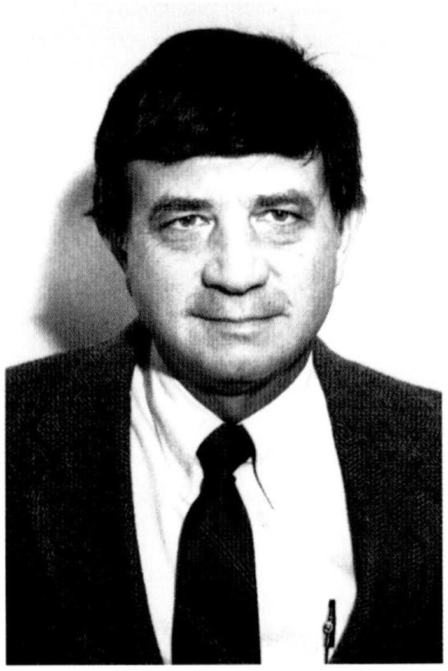

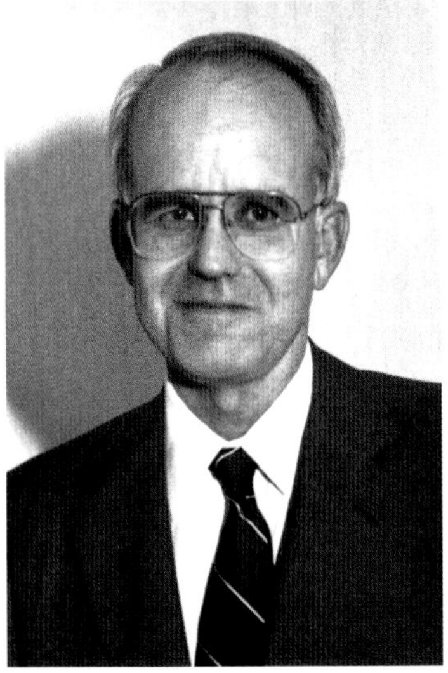

Top: John Manfredi, MD, was the hospital's first medical oncologist in 1974. **Above:** Herbert Kann, MD, was the second oncologist to join in 1979.

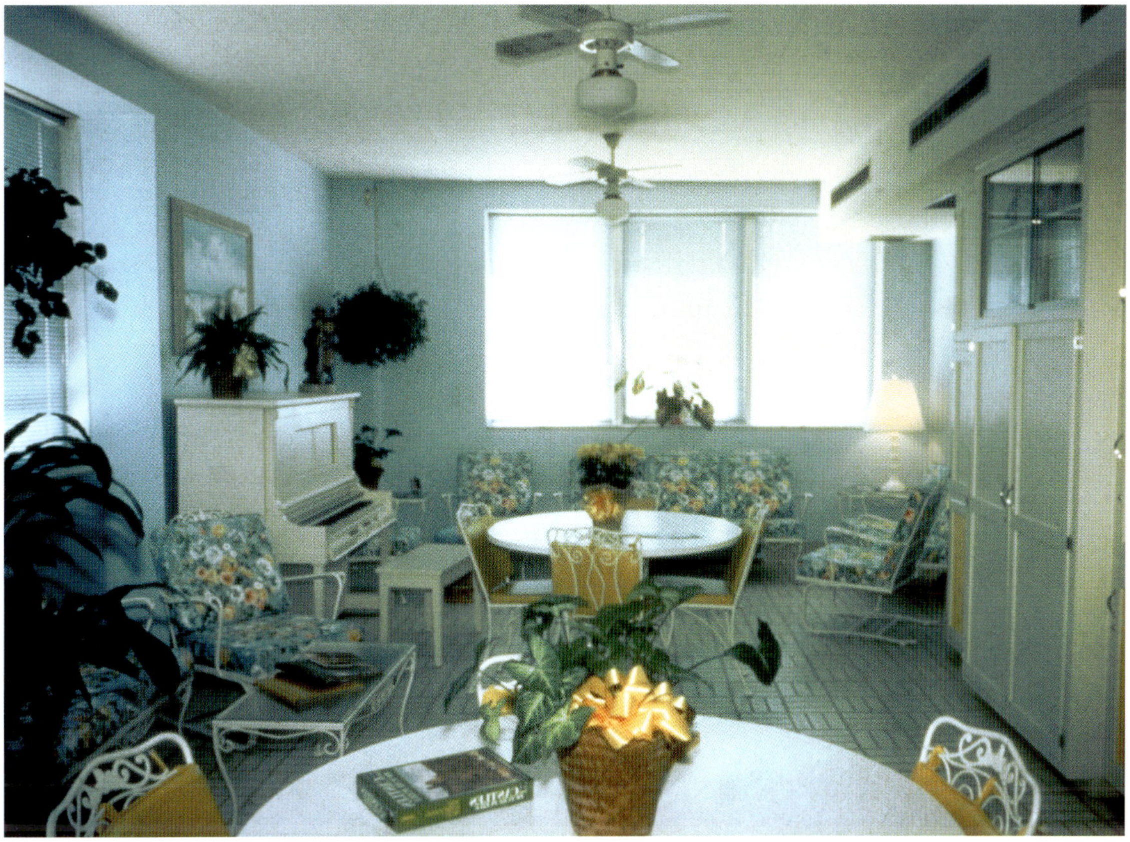

tional, more extensive, modified radical mastectomy.[35]

In 1988 Administrator Charles Eberhart engaged a consulting firm to study DeKalb General's Cancer Services and to make recommendations for its improvement. The consultants found that the hospital had most of the components of a cancer service, but saw them as fragmented, isolated, and lacking in the coordination necessary to present an integrated, unified image and an effective cancer program.

As a result of those findings, Eberhart created a Cancer Services Development Team composed of physicians, nurses, support staff, and administration.[36] He charged the team with identifying what it would take to elevate the existing cancer services to the level of a Cancer Center of Excellence. He named Betty Castellani, MDiv, associate hospital chaplain, as the director of the cancer center and LaMar McGinnis, MD, as its medical director;[37] and he charged the Cancer Services Development Team with providing the support that Castellani and McGinnis needed to create the new service.

Castellani envisioned a cancer center that was patient-centered unlike traditional services found even in prestigious academic settings. One of her first acts was to invite a group of cancer patients to meet with physicians who treat patients with cancer. She asked the patients to tell the physicians about their experience with cancer, how they had been treated, what they liked, what they did not like, what they wanted, and what they needed from a cancer center and from those who provided their care. They were articulate, insightful, and informative, and they helped create a roadmap for the future of DeKalb Medical's cancer center.

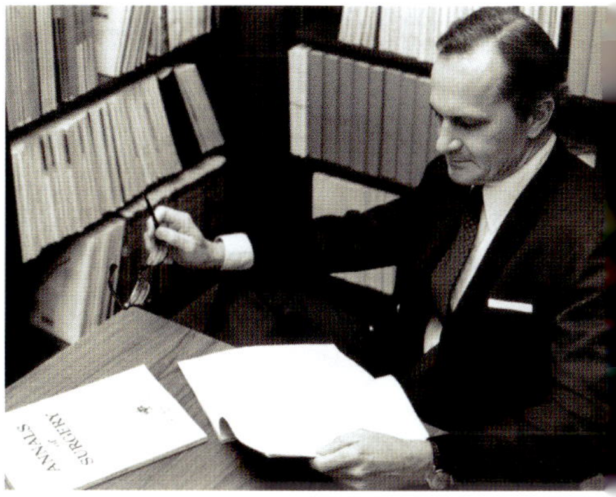

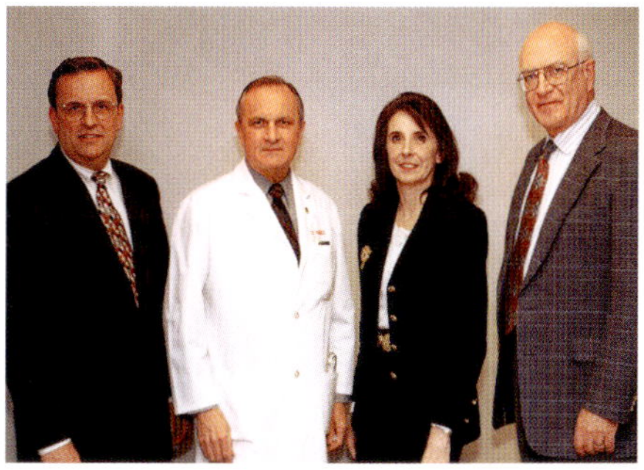

Above left: The Lively Room, a respite for cancer patients where they can watch TV, listen to music, and relax, was generously furnished by longtime Authority member Wash W. Lively. **Top right:** LaMar McGinnis, MD, a general surgeon, was the first medical director of the cancer center. **Above:** Cancer center leaders left to right; John Gerlach, LaMar McGinnis, MD, Betty Castellani, and Paul Crank, MD.

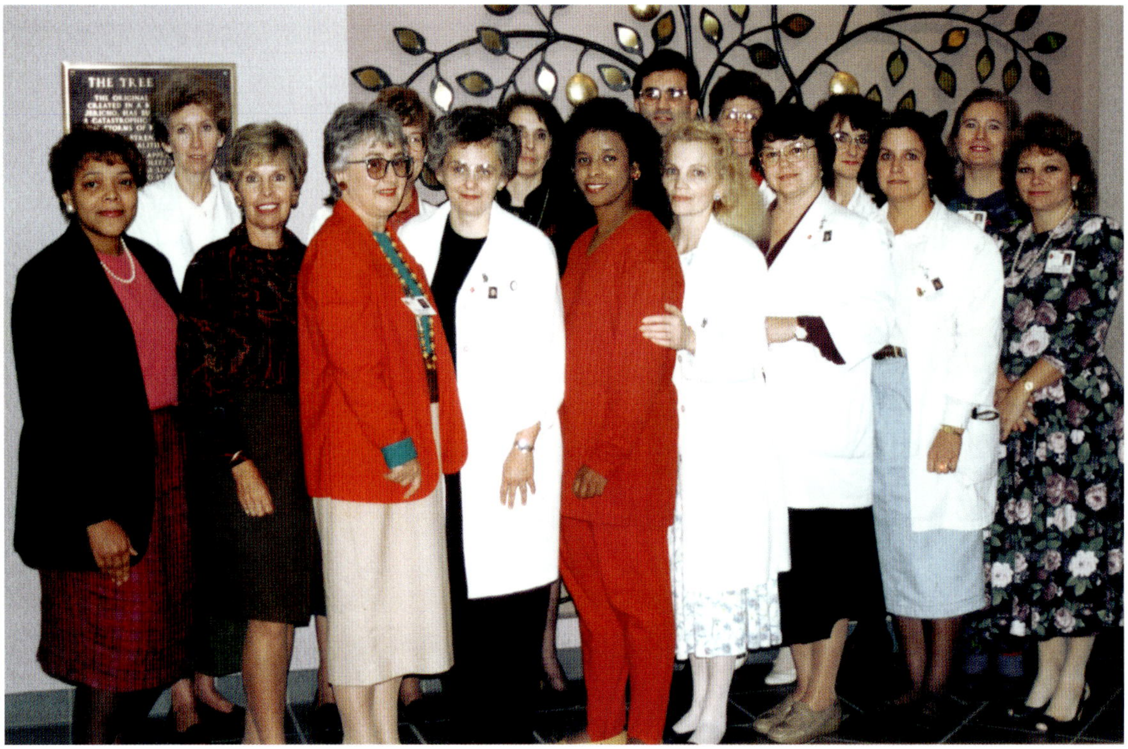

Right: Cancer center team. **Below:** Richard Leff, MD, medical oncologist who established the stem-cell transplant program.

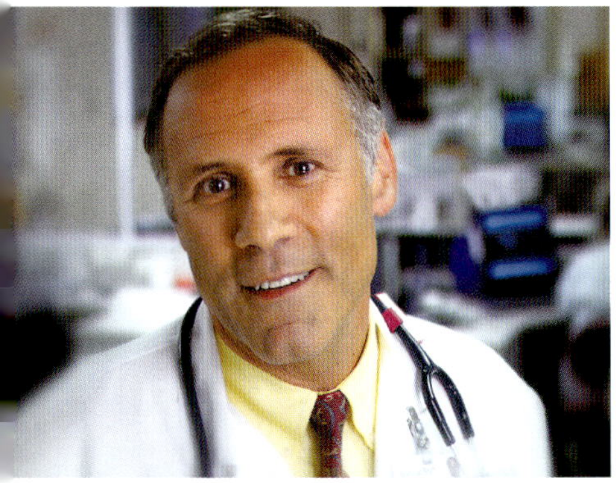

They wanted state-of-the-art cancer services comparable to the best that could be found anywhere. They wanted their physicians to communicate with each other and with them as patients so that they could understand their condition and their best options for its management. They wanted to be informed about cancer and to have an active role in decisions pertaining to their care. They wanted to be treated in a positive atmosphere that was permeated with hope, not handed a death sentence because of their cancer. They wanted care that recognized not only the vital role of the body, but also the mind and the spirit in coping with cancer.

Director Castellani, the physicians, and the cancer center team listened and developed an oncology program that met and exceeded the patients' expectations. It now provides the most advanced clinical care with state-of-the-art equipment, the latest medical technology, a well-trained and well-versed medical staff, a wide variety of treatment options, and unique support services for patients and their families. The center focuses on taking care of the patient, listening to the patient, and responding to the patient's needs.

In 1992 the cancer center established the first stem-cell transplant unit in Georgia, and one of the first in the southeast, under the medical direction of Richard Leff, MD.[38] Stem-cell transplantation offered an alternative to the more expensive, risky, and traumatic traditional bone-marrow transplantation for patients needing high dose chemotherapy. The procedure harvests embryonic cells from the patient's circulating blood, stores the cells, and reinfuses them to "rescue" the bone marrow's capacity to make blood cells following high-dose chemotherapy. The cancer center has performed over two hundred stem-cell transplants.[39] The procedure proved to be so safe and successful that, once offered only on an inpatient basis, it now is performed in the outpatient setting.[40] DeKalb Medical's stem-cell transplant program is accredited by the Foundation for Accreditation of Cellular Therapies,

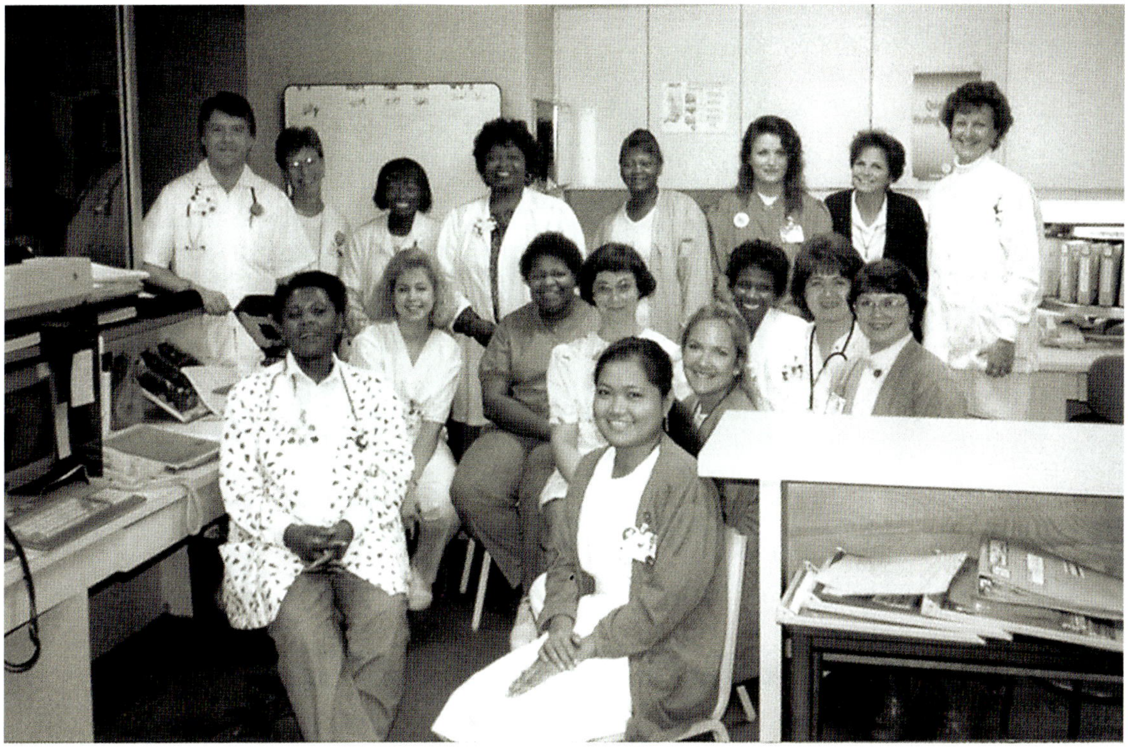

Left: 4200 unit nurses. **Below:** David Holladay, MD, the medical director of Radiation Oncology.

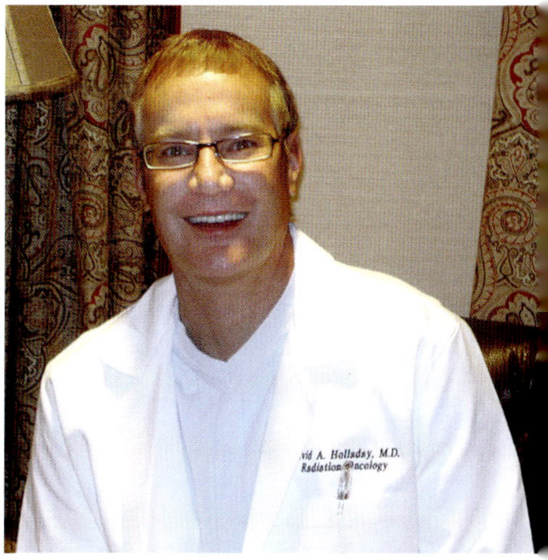

which sets quality standards for all blood- and marrow-transplant programs in the United States. The accreditation not only is a stamp of approval for the quality of DeKalb Medical's stem-cell program, but it provides the credentials necessary for the cancer center to participate in additional research studies affiliated with the National Cancer Institute.[41]

In 1997 the cancer center reestablished its radiation oncology service with a linear accelerator and the latest techniques in radiation therapy. In 2001 it added technology at a cost of $1.65 million that configures the radiation beam to conform specifically to the shape of the tumor, permitting higher doses of radiation, better outcomes, more protection to surrounding normal tissues, and the ability to treat sites previously considered too risky.[42] In 2007 David Holladay, MD, one of the nation's premier radiation oncologists, became the medical director of Radiation Oncology. In one year the center increased the number of patients receiving external beam radiation from approximately ten per day to fifty-five per day.[43] In addition Holladay performs high-dose radiation (HDR) implants for patients with gynecological cancer as well as MammoSite Radiation Therapy implants for patients with breast cancer who have undergone a segmental resection (lumpectomy) surgical procedure. In both procedures a radiation source is inserted near the surgical cancer site. Both have been highly effective, inflict less exposure on surrounding healthy tissues, and are completed in a much shorter period of time than is true with traditional radiation.[44] The DeKalb Medical Foundation provided funds to purchase the equipment needed for the Radiology Oncology Department to offer high-dose radiation.

Imaging Services (the new name for Radiology Services) has played a vital role in the cancer center's advances. It has the latest digital mammography equipment and conducts nearly 35,000 procedures annually.[45] It acquired the combined positron emission tomography (PET)/computerized tomography (CT) that enabled an assessment of body functions as well as anatomy. It established interventional radiology as an added diagnostic and treatment modality.

The cancer center established a genetic screening and risk-assessment program to identify individuals at increased risk of developing cancer of the breast, ovaries, colon, skin, and other sites.[46] Patients with breast cancer also can now participate in the Oncotype DX clinical trial. In that study patients with estrogen-positive, node-negative tumors can have their tumor tissue assessed to indicate whether they are at a high risk, intermediate risk, or low risk for recurrence. That determination helps patients and their physicians know how aggressive follow-up treatment should be to minimize the risk of recurrence.[47]

A DeKalb physician, oncology surgeon Michael Quinones, MD, was the first in Georgia to administer heated chemotherapy directly to abdominal cancer sites during surgery as a supplement to conventional chemotherapy.[48]

All of the cancer center nurses became certified in their specialty. William P. Tatum and his daughter Susan established a scholarship fund in memory of Mrs. Tatum to reward those nurses who successfully complete their certification.

Of the eight hospitals in the Atlanta Regional Community Clinical Oncology Program (CCOP), DeKalb's cancer center had 112 patients enrolled in 2007, the largest number in any participating hospital.[49]

There is a new, ten-bed Specialized Oncology Inpatient Unit on 4200 for the sickest medical and surgical cancer patients. The unit is staffed with oncology nurses who serve only that unit and who work with a staffing ratio of one nurse and one technician for no more than five patients. It is a model unit that has created great satisfaction on the part of patients, staff, and physicians.[50]

The Herbert E. Kann Outpatient Treatment Center, named in memory of DeKalb's second medical oncologist, was established to offer patients the convenience and efficiency of appropriate oncology care on an outpatient basis. Annually the Kann Center has over 10,000 patient visits, performs over 600 transfusions, administers over 1,800 chemotherapy treatments, and conducts more than a dozen stem-cell transplants.[51]

The cancer center offers education and information to patients and their families. It provides patient education programs, professional seminars, and community learning resources. The DeKalb Medical Health Sciences Library provides resources for patients and their families. In addition, the family of Rosemary Wilson made a major donation to establish a resource library in her name in the cancer center. The cancer center team has created more than six publications to inform and encourage patients. These include *The Cancer Hope Line*, a quarterly newsletter for patients; *The Cancer Challenge*, a book on nutrition, treatment options, spirituality, coping skills, patient stories, and recovery advice; *A Center for All Seasons*, a book containing the story of cancer survivors; *Easy Answers*, a booklet to help understand cancer diagnosis; and *Screening Guidelines*, a guide for appropriate cancer-screening practices.

The cancer center conducts a weekly Tumor Conference with an average attendance of over fifty individuals. The conference brings together physicians from various specialties to review patients with challenging diagnostic and treatment options to discuss the best options available.[52] If desired, a patient whose case is being presented can attend and ask questions. Physicians rate it as "one of the best conferences anywhere."

A multidisciplinary team of professionals provides a Second Opinion Panel to review patients' diagnosis and treatment plans. The cancer center also has an Easy Access Program with physicians available to evaluate within twenty-four hours patients who have signs or symptoms suggestive of cancer.

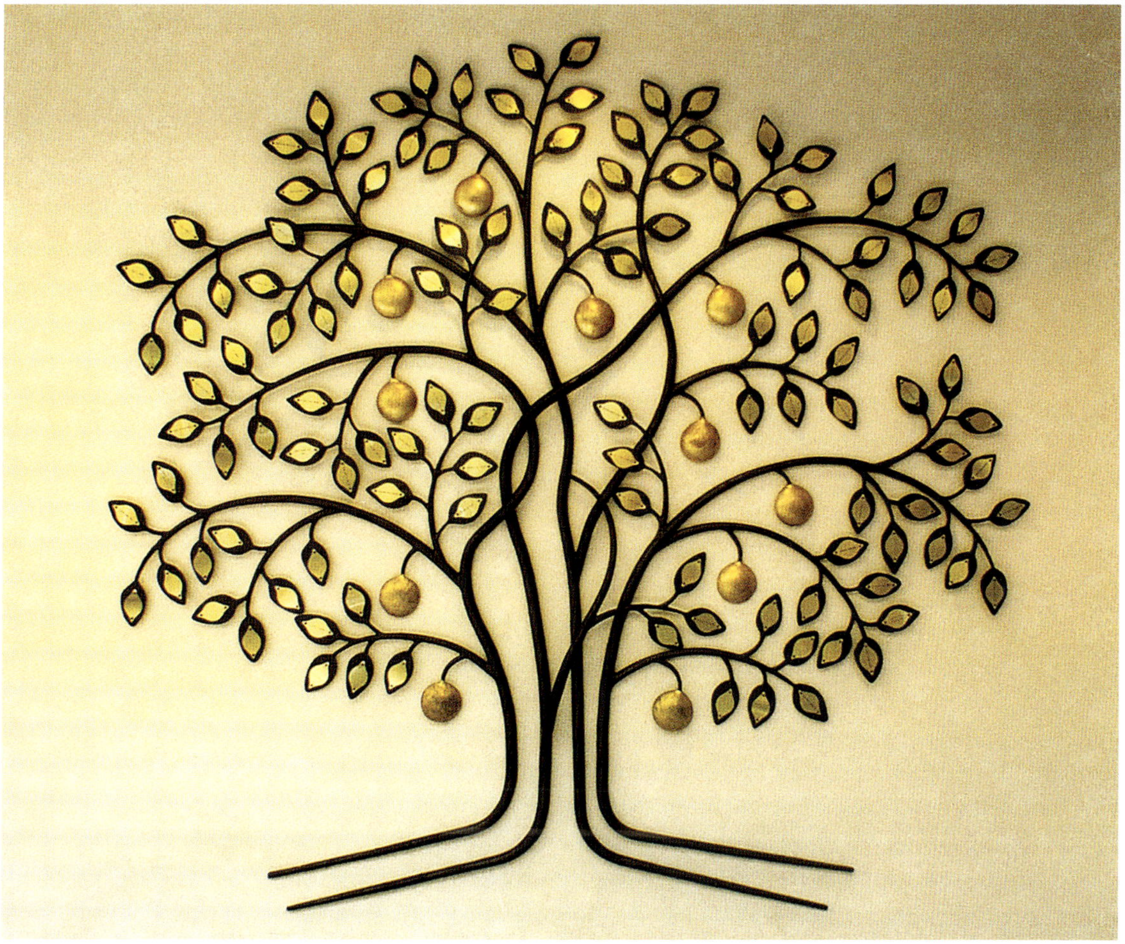

The "Tree of Life" is the powerful symbol for the cancer center representing the strength, endurance, and hope of all the cancer center patients.

Betty Castellani emphasizes that, while the cancer center offers the most advanced clinical care, the thing that sets the program apart is the uncompromising support it offers those experiencing cancer and its effects. She says, "Our patients are the soul of our institution and the motivation for all we do."[53] The center makes a commitment to the patients, pledging to be there for them in whatever way they need help, to teach them how to cope with cancer, and to make cancer a call for living with hope.[54]

The cancer center was one of the first centers to refer to its patients as "cancer survivors." It chose as its symbol the "Tree of Life," modeled after a mosaic that survived more than 1,200 years in the floor of a demolished palace in Jericho. The tree illustrates the strength, endurance, and hope of the center's patients. The center's motto is *carpe diem*, or "seize the day." Its publications tell the story of cancer survivors who epitomize the center's symbol and motto.

The center has adult patient "survivor groups" that have met weekly for more than twenty years, a support group for families of cancer patients, and a "Tree House Gang" for children who have a family member with cancer. As many as two hundred cancer survivors and their families may belong to one of the many groups at any one time. They celebrate successes, support those in distress, laugh together, share information, offer encouragement, develop coping skills, bond with one another, and provide a constant affirmation of hope.[55]

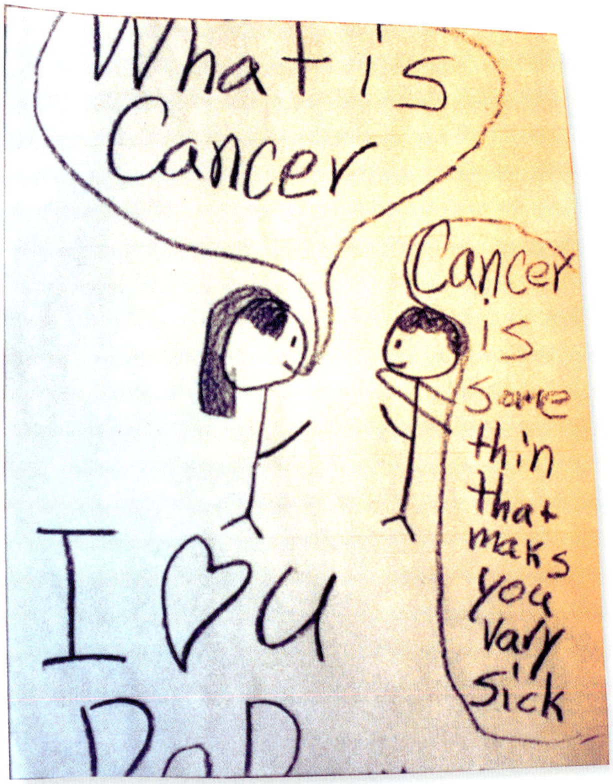

They teach one another how to survive, to overcome the fear associated with cancer, and to change each patient's perspective from that of a "victim" to a "survivor." They offer survival skills that include adjusting lifestyles to meet the physical challenges of cancer. They network with social workers, dieticians, physical therapists, occupational therapists, clinical nurses, and chaplains, all of whom offer their specialized support services. Patients learn about nutrition, stress reduction, relaxation, meditation, and spiritual growth. They are encouraged to keep a journal to which they commit their fears. They attend Return to Wellness classes to recover from their treatments and art therapy classes to heal through active expressions of the cancer experience. They learn to focus on hope, make each day count, and enhance relationships with their family and friends.[56]

The Tree House Gang, a suggestion of cancer patients with children and organized by Rose McKeever, LPN, was the first Atlanta support group for children of cancer patients. A new group is created quarterly for children between the ages of five and eighteen, and each group has three ninety-minute sessions that are led by a child therapist and an oncology nurse. The Tree House Gang deals with the unanswered questions, the new emotions, the fears, and the lifestyle changes that occur for children in a family where cancer is diagnosed. They are given the opportunity to talk, learn, and share their experiences. They learn about cancer and its treatment. They go to the laboratory and look at cancer cells through the microscope. They visit the Diagnostic Imaging Center and learn about the MRI, PET, and CT scans. They learn about radiation oncology, chemotherapy, and stem-cell transplantation. They learn that cancer does not necessarily mean death, that it is not contagious, and that it is not their fault that it occurred to a family member.[57]

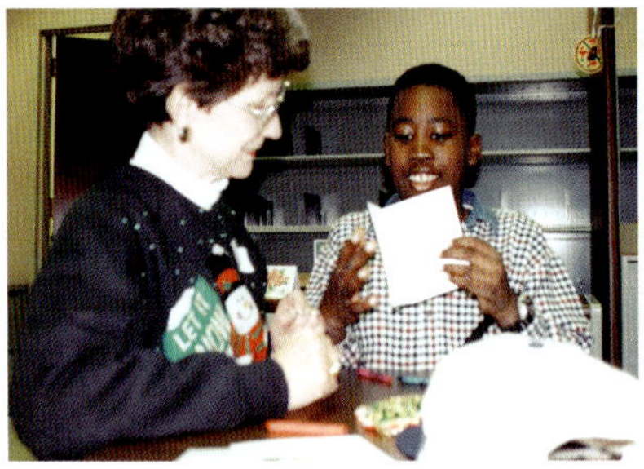

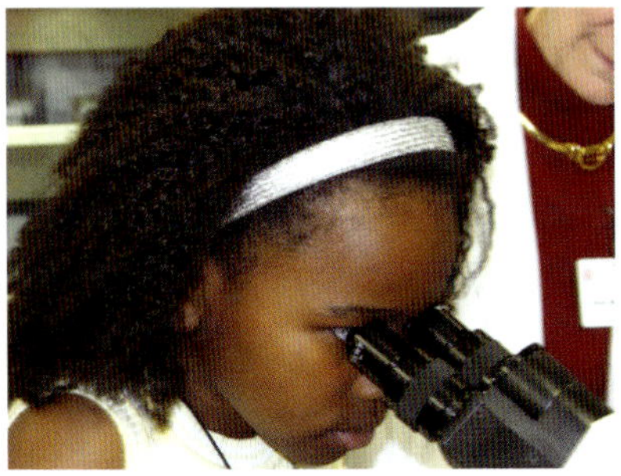

Top, center, and above: Rose McKeever, LPN, organized The Tree House Gang, the first Atlanta support group for children of cancer patients. Children learn about cancer, view cells through a microscope, and share their experiences through discussion and art.
Right: Allen Lawhead, MD, is a gynecological oncologist and medical director of the cancer center.

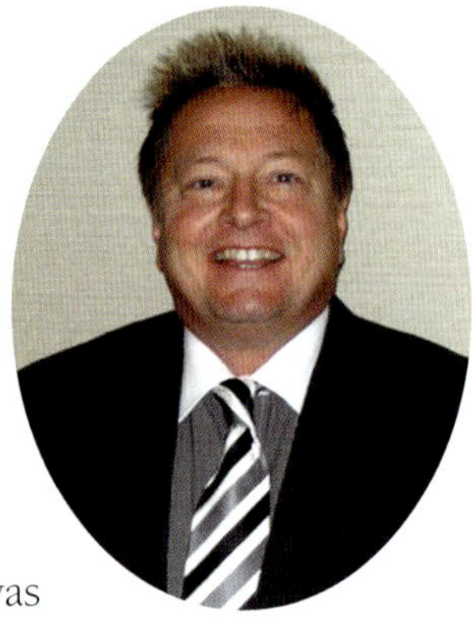

The cancer center recently created a cancer executive team under the direction of Betty Castellani and chaired by Allen Lawhead, MD, a gynecological oncologist. The team includes key physicians and administrative leaders. Its goal is to make DeKalb Medical a center of excellence in five areas of cancer: breast, gynecology, lung, prostate, and colon.[58] The team already has created a Comprehensive Breast Care program,[59] established the specialized inpatient oncology unit, worked with the leadership of the Radiology Department to enhance its services, and supported the cancer center team in its continued growth and development.

In August 1994 Charles Eberhart, CEO of DeKalb Medical Center, was diagnosed with a malignant brain tumor. Eberhart died in May 1995. During his illness, he lived each day to the fullest and demonstrated a courage, hope, compassion, and affection for others that amazed and inspired all who knew him. He personified the strength and attitudes that the center strived to help its patients discover. From its origin in 1990, the cancer center's leaders had been unable to choose an appropriate name for the center. After witnessing Eberhart's heroic journey with cancer, the cancer center team and the board of directors agreed that its proper name should be the Charles B. Eberhart Cancer Center.

The strength of the Charles B. Eberhart Cancer Center is due in large measure to the outstanding leadership of Betty Castellani, her team, the nurses and the physicians; the commitment

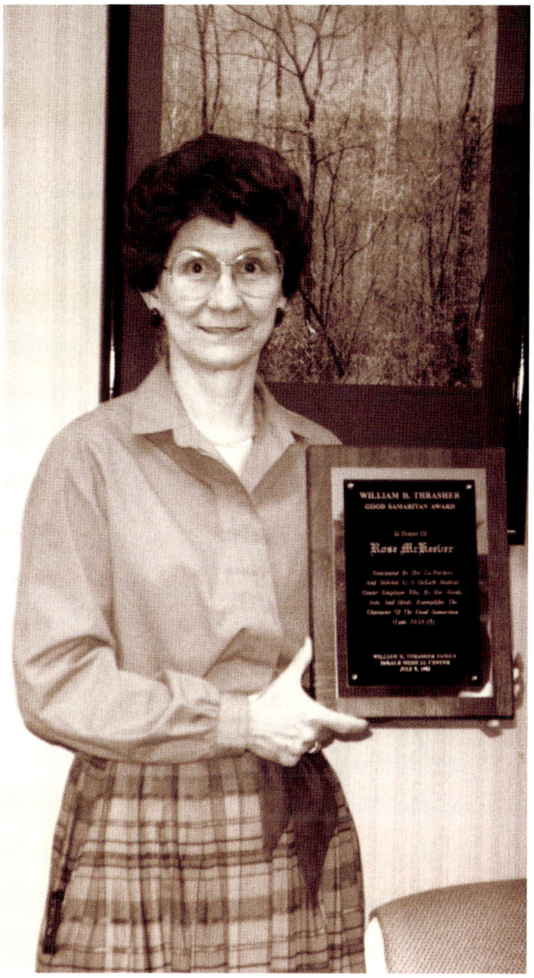

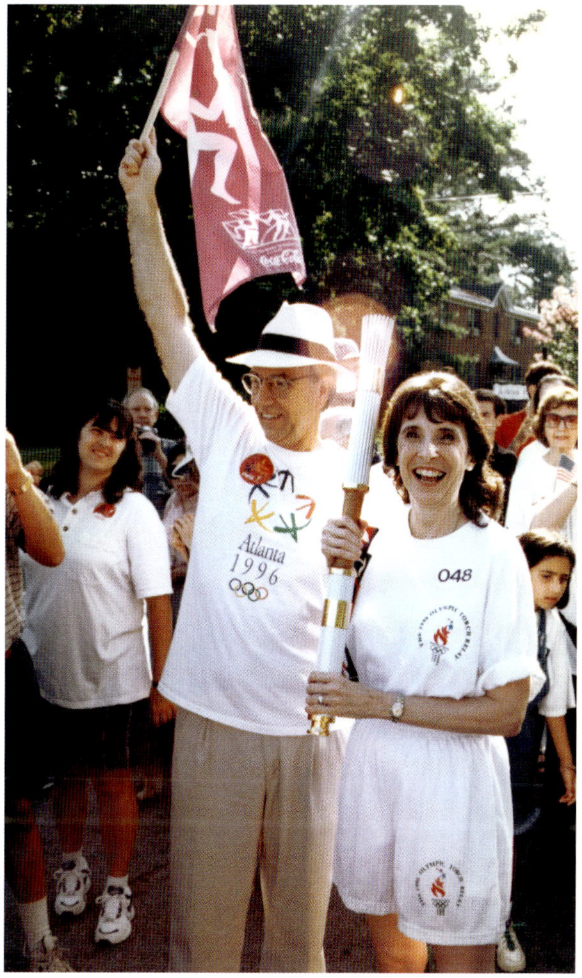

Far left: Rose McKeever, LPN, received the 1993 William H. Thrasher Good Samaritan Award. **Left:** Betty Castellani and her husband Robert as she carries the Olympic torch through Atlanta in 1996.

and support of the DeKalb Medical Foundation, administration, and governing bodies; and the participation of the patients it serves. As director, Betty Castellani took the early roadmap laid down by the cancer patients to a new level. She has created a vital, state-of-the-art organization imbued with a spirit of hope, love, and service that has made it unique among cancer centers. In 1996 her patients and staff nominated her to carry the Olympic Torch for the 1996 Olympics in Atlanta, and she was selected for the honor. She was recognized in 2001 as the recipient of the *Atlanta Business Chronicle's* Health Care Hero Award for her leadership in developing DeKalb Medical's cancer service.[60] In 2007 she was only the third nonphysician in thirty-four years to be awarded DeKalb Medical Society's prestigious Julius McCurdy Citizenship Award. It is not surprising that Rose McKeever, a member of the oncology team already caring for a disabled family member, took a cancer patient under her wing and into her home for the duration of the patient's care;[61] or that Donna Cannon, RN, another oncology team member, seeing a single mom with breast cancer and a ten-year old son, unemployed and broke, took the patient and her son into her home and helped the patient get both a job and back on her feet.[62] That, among other things, is what the cancer team does.

Cardiovascular Services

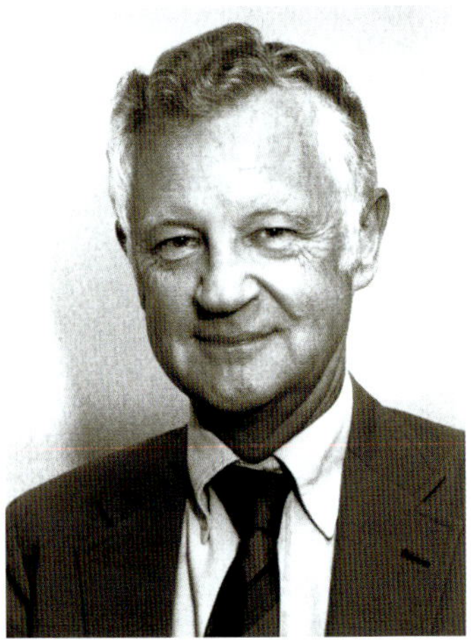

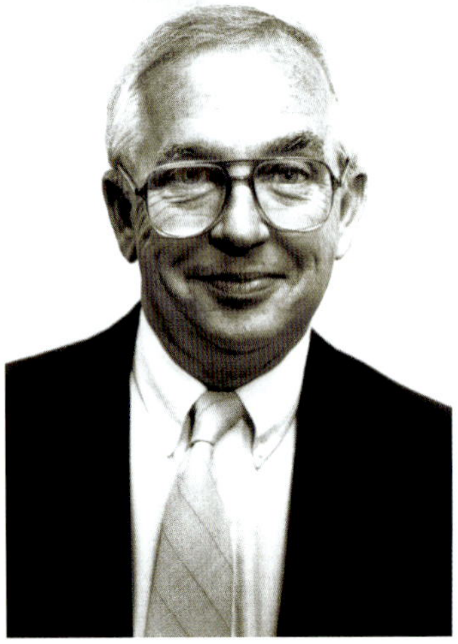

Above: In June 1965 two cardiologists, Benjamin Okel, MD (top) and Robert Hubbell, MD, (bottom) contracted with the hospital to supervise the EKG Department at DeKalb General Hospital. **Right:** Marie Schuster, RN, became the coordinator of the Coronary Rehabilitation Program (CRP) in 1988.

When DeKalb General Hospital opened in 1961, there was no separate medical staff section of cardiology, there was no separate coronary care unit, and there were no physicians specifically designated to read electrocardiograms (EKGs) or provide other cardiovascular studies. The twenty-four general practitioners and sixteen internists (including two cardiologists) provided the cardiovascular care for hospitalized patients. Daniel Jordan, MD, joined the medical staff in 1966 as the hospital's first specialist trained in vascular surgery.

In June 1965 DeKalb General's two cardiologists, Robert Hubbell, MD, and Benjamin Okel, MD, signed a contract with the hospital to supervise the EKG Department, to advise administration on matters pertaining to the department, and to read EKGs, rhythm strips, exercise tolerance test studies, and cardioversion tracings.[1] As more cardiologists joined the medical staff, those who were interested and qualified were added to the list of EKG readers.

In 1966 the hospital inaugurated the "Blue Alert" system. Whenever a patient experienced a cardiac or respiratory arrest, the hospital operator was immediately notified and announced "blue alert" over the loudspeaker, giving the patient's location. An emergency department physician and any other available physician in the hospital, along with a team from nursing, anesthesia, and respiratory therapy would immediately respond with an EKG machine, defibrillator, and Ambu hand-held ventilation bag. In the first eighteen months that the Blue Alert system was in effect, ninety-seven patients were resuscitated.[2] The system remains in effect today.

Acutely ill heart patients originally were admitted to the Intensive Care Unit (ICU) along with other surgical, seriously ill, or injured patients. In 1969 six beds in the ICU were designated as a Coronary Care Unit (CCU).[3] Administrator William Thrasher sent two nursing supervisors to Miami, Florida, to attend an institute on CCUs, and he and Nursing Director Opal Hopkins visited the Athens (Georgia) General Hospital CCU program.[4] The DeKalb County Hospital Authority approved a list of qualified physicians from the departments of internal medicine and general practice to have CCU privileges. The Medical Staff Executive Committee established a Coronary Care Committee to provide general oversight for the unit.[5] The hospital created a separate CCU in the 1971 expansion, and in 1974 the 4400 nursing unit was designated as an Intermediate Coronary Care Unit (ICCU) to monitor patients who no longer required CCU care.[6]

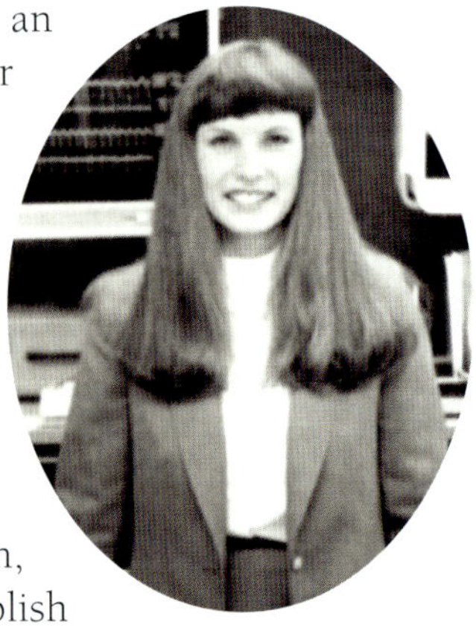

In 1973 DeKalb General initiated a Cardiac Rehabilitation Program (CRP) to which physicians could refer patients with angina or significant heart risks as well as those who had suffered a heart attack.[7] Initially started as an inpatient program, CRP later expanded to serve patients on an outpatient basis as well. In addition to the patient's physician, the CRP team was staffed by nurses, physical and occupational therapists, nutritionists, and social workers. In its first year, it enrolled 370 patients.[8] The program helped patients deal with the emotions that often accompany their condition, educated them and their families about heart disease, helped them establish positive health habits, improved physical strength and stamina with a prescribed exercise program, and assisted them to return to an optimal quality lifestyle. In the prescribed exercise program, patients were monitored by EKG while using exercise bikes, performing arm exercises, or walking on the treadmill.[9]

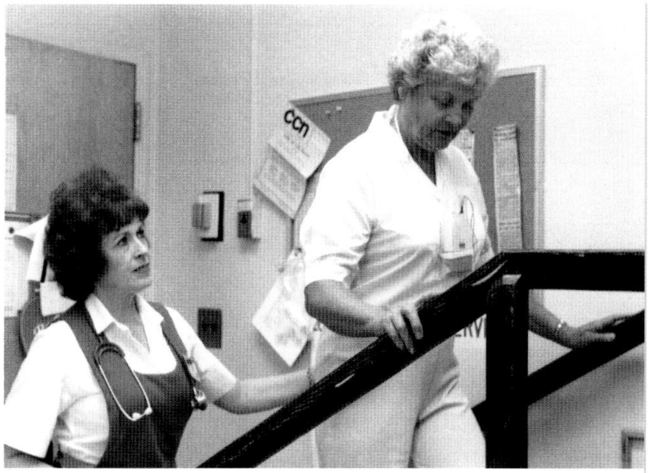

Left: Colleen Coffman, RN, and Betty Burns, RN, demonstrate the CRP equipment. **Below:** Bonnie Phipps, former CFO of DeKalb Medical, served as chairperson of the Cardiology Service Line Development Team that initiated the Catheterization Laboratory. **Bottom:** Paul Kirschbaum, MD, cardiologist is medical director of the Catheterization Laboratory.

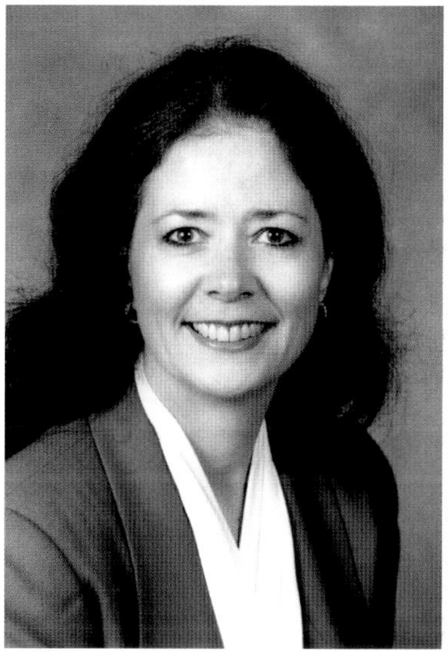

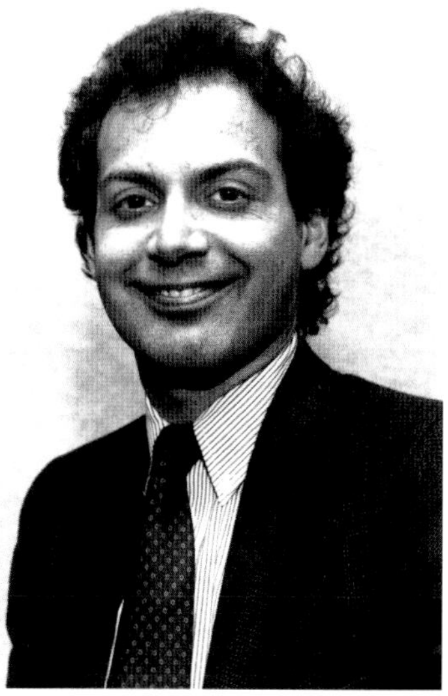

In 1984 the medical staff asked the hospital to file a certificate of need (CON) application with the state for a cardiac catheterization laboratory (cath lab).[10] Administration took no action on the request until 1988 when Administrator Eberhart appointed a Cardiology Services Development Team chaired by Chief Financial Officer Bonnie Phipps. The team included cardiologists, other physicians, administrators, nurses, and support personnel. Eberhart asked the team to study the feasibility of a cardiac cath lab and to recommend other cardiovascular services the hospital should provide.[11]

The team found that DeKalb had a significant number of patients who needed cardiac catheterization, that DeKalb physicians were referring those and their office patients to other facilities for the procedure, and that the hospital's medical staff now included physicians qualified to perform the procedure.[12] Emory University Hospital agreed to accept on an emergency basis any DeKalb General heart patients from the cath lab needing emergency cardiac surgery.[13] The team endorsed the concept of a cath lab, and the hospital filed a CON application in April 1989.[14] The state approved DeKalb's application the following fall, and the cath lab opened in January 1990. Sharon Evans was the first manager of the lab,[15] and the physicians initially credentialed to use the cath lab included B. J. Erb, MD, Spencer King, MD, Paul Kirschbaum, MD, Jerre Lutz, MD, and Naresh Parikh, MD.[16] Currently fifteen physicians are credentialed to use the lab, and Paul Kirschbaum is the medical director.

DeKalb physicians perform an average of more than 1,300 cardiac catheterization procedures per year.[17] In 2003 the hospital renovated the lab and installed digital imaging technology. This new technology was the first of its kind in Atlanta, and DeKalb was the fifth hospital in the nation to have it.[18] According to Medical Director Kirschbaum, it permitted higher-quality images, more precise detection of coronary artery lesions, the use of smaller catheters, less pain in the course of the procedure, lower doses of radiation, greater safety, and more information.[19]

In 1985 the hospital instituted a Congestive Heart Failure (CHF) program[20] available to all patients admitted to the hospital with heart failure, heart attack, or cardiomyopathy (inflammation and dysfunction of the heart muscle). Patients were enrolled prior to discharge and continued on an outpatient basis. It remains active today and provides CHF education, rehabilitation and wellness programs, and home health services. The CHF team includes physicians, nurses, pharmacists, nutritionists, and representatives from Care Management, Performance Improvement, and the Heart Mates support group. The program has contributed to a decrease in mortality for DeKalb's CHF patients, a decrease in the number of patients having to be readmitted to the hospital, and an improved quality of life.[21] In 2001 it received top honors among hospitals from Georgia and seven other states

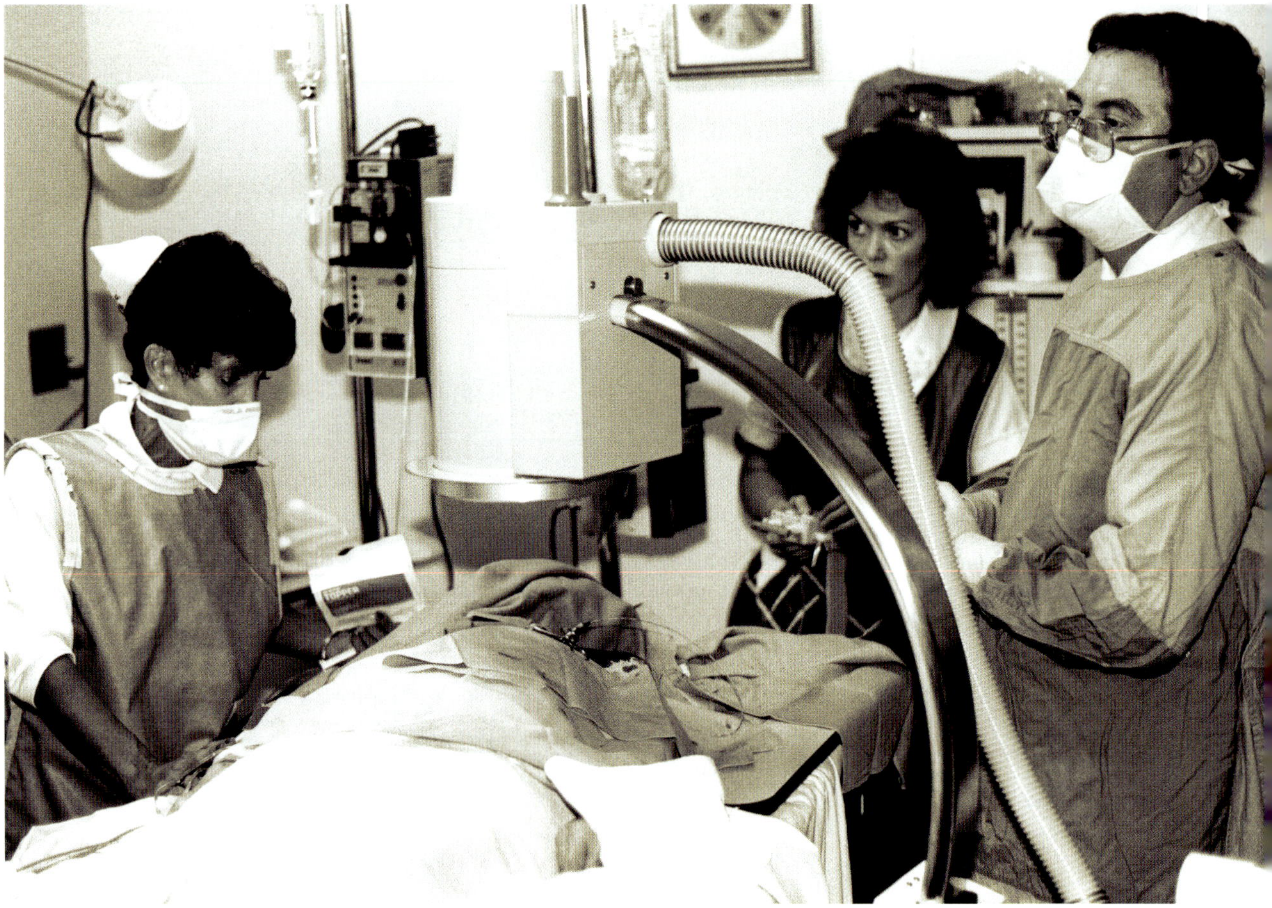

A cardiac catheterization procedure being performed

for its quality of care and its quantifiable, beneficial results.[22]

In 1991 DeKalb Medical's cardiologists helped create the Chest Pain Center in the Emergency Department as described in Emergency Services, which is located in this section of the book. DeKalb Medical Center, during one period, treated more heart attack patients than any hospital in Georgia and ranked fifth in the nation.

In 2001 DeKalb Medical established the Coumadin® Clinic to which physicians could refer their patients. Coumadin® is a "blood thinner" used to prevent the formation of blood clots.[23] Patients receive regularly scheduled appointments at the clinic to determine if they are taking the proper dosage of blood thinner. They also receive education regarding the purpose of their medication and the potential for interactions with certain foods and other medications.[24] The clinic is staffed by a clinical pharmacist and a nurse practitioner, and it is under the medical direction of a physician. More than one hundred physicians have referred patients to the clinic. In 2002 the clinic earned the Georgia Hospital Association's Quality and Patient Safety Award.[25]

The state denied DeKalb Medical permission to provide two cardiovascular services it sought to offer. The first was its request to perform open-heart surgery. The second was its request to be one of ten Georgia community hospitals without open-heart surgery in a research study to perform coronary angioplasty (dilating obstructed coronary arteries).

The denial to perform open heart surgery came in 1993. In December 1992, at the request of the medical staff and the Cardiology Services Development Team, the hospital filed a CON application with the state to provide open-heart surgery and coronary angioplasty. It presented a strong justification for its application. It was a leading provider of cardiovascular, emergency, trauma, and medical/surgical services to the citizens of the county and surrounding areas. Its services included its Chest Pain Emergency Center, cardiac catheterization laboratory, and general cardiac care. It was qualified to perform the service. In addition, without the ability to perform open-heart surgery, the hospital was limited in its ability to recruit cardiothoracic physician coverage for its trauma program and its existing cardiovascular services.[26] Despite DeKalb's strong petition, the state denied its application along with those from several other metropolitan Atlanta hospitals.[27]

The second denial came in 2005. DeKalb Medical applied unsuccessfully to be one of ten community hospitals in the state without open-heart surgery to participate in a research study conducted by Johns Hopkins University.[28] Studies suggested, but had not confirmed, that patients with heart attacks who underwent coronary angioplasty had better outcomes than those receiving intravenous medication to dissolve blood clots ("clot buster" therapy). Most of the heart-attack patients receiving angioplasty, however, were those admitted to hospitals with open-heart capabilities. A majority of heart-attack patients were managed in hospitals without open-heart surgery and angioplasty capabilities. The study focused on two issues. It wanted to study a larger number of heart-attack patients to confirm the conclusion that coronary angioplasty was more beneficial than intravenous clot-buster therapy. It also wanted to confirm the position that angioplasty could be offered safely in community hospitals without open heart capabilities.[29]

DeKalb Medical Center was one of twenty-five Georgia community hospitals that applied to be one of the ten community hospitals selected for the study.[30] DeKalb met all the requirements, including the recruiting of more interventional cardiologists and obtaining a transfer agreement with Emory University Hospital to be available should the need for cardiac surgery arise.[31] DeKalb Medical Center, however, was not selected.[32]

Despite these denials, Cardiovascular Services continue to be one of the system's major contributions to the community and one of its most important services. In its 2007 strategic plan, DeKalb Medical identified heart and vascular services as one of the principal programs it would support for further growth and development. It established a Comprehensive Heart and Vascular Institute and named Patrick Green as executive director.[33] As the first phase of the institute, DeKalb Medical filed a CON application to add a $3.7 million endovascular laboratory to be used by vascular surgeons, interventional radiologists, and cardiologists. The lab will combine diagnostic and interventional cardiac and vascular procedures using the latest Toshiba Infinix System[34] that is capable of performing all those procedures. The laboratory will serve more patients and provide more types of cardiac and vascular procedures than are currently available, including coronary angioplasty should regulations be modified. The institute also calls for establishing two specialized nursing units, one in the imaging area and one adjacent to the endovascular lab where patients are prepared for and recover from procedures and where some procedures may be performed.[35] The endovascular laboratory is in the planning stage subject to available capital funds.

Cardiovascular diseases remain major threats to the health and well being of the nation. DeKalb Medical has from its origins, provided education about these diseases as well as quality services for their prevention and treatment. They remain one of the institution's foremost priorities.

The Child Care Center

Providing a child care center for children of hospital employees proved to be an important but surprisingly daunting challenge for DeKalb General Hospital.

In 1963 Director of Nursing Opal Hopkins and the medical staff jointly expressed to the DeKalb County Hospital Authority their concern regarding the hospital's difficulty in recruiting and retaining nurses. The physicians asked the trustees to establish a nursery as at least one solution to the nursing shortage.[1] The Hospital Authority agreed that having a nursery, especially for employees on the three-to-eleven shift, might contribute as much to nurse retention and recruitment as increasing their salaries. It instructed administration to arrange for one of the local child care centers to accept children of DeKalb General employees.[2] None of the centers, however, were willing to add the staff needed to care for children until 11 PM or to assume the additional liability.[3]

Six years later DeKalb General Hospital still did not have a child care center, and its absence was one of several unresolved grievances that led to the resignation of one hundred of the hospital's nurses.[4]

In February 1969, following the mass resignation of nurses, the hospital created a temporary child care center on one wing of the hospital.[5] John Gerlach, assistant to the administrator, presented the Authority with five options for a more permanent solution: (1) purchase a home adjoining the hospital property, (2) try again to contract with an existing child care center to provide the service, (3) use a portable building, (4) construct a prefabricated building, or (5) construct a permanent building.[6] Gerlach recommended constructing a permanent, modular building that could accommodate up to sixty children.[7] He had discussed such a facility with a contractor who said he could build it and have it ready for use in two months.

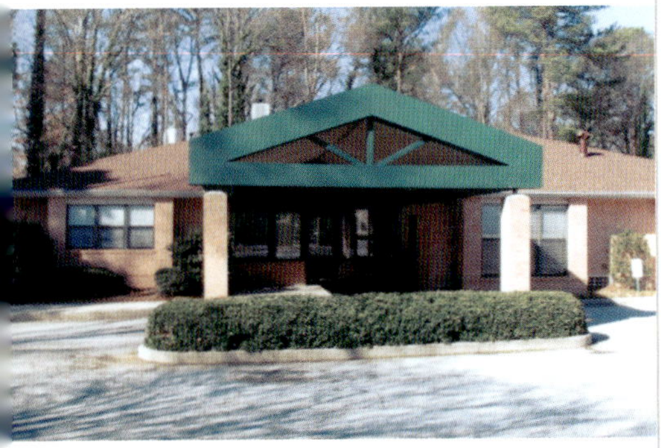

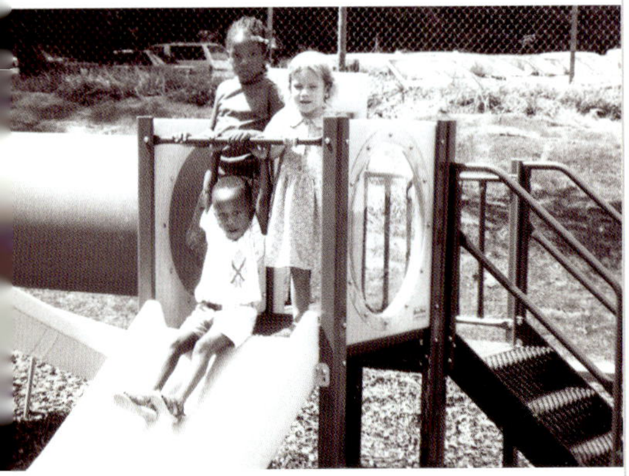

In July of 1970, the original Child Care Center opened its doors and could accommodate forty-five children. In 1993 a brand new facility opened its doors to 125 children.

The trustees agreed. They considered three possible locations: adjacent to the North Decatur Methodist Church, behind the new mental health unit, or on Winn Way at the hospital's southern boundary, adjacent to the DeKalb County Department of Public Health property. In May 1969 they decided on the last of these options and negotiated a contract with Richard Hodges of Modular Concepts Inc. He promised to have the facility ready by July 1969 at a cost of $41,000.[8] The hospital began using a portion of the facility in December 1969, but the building was not completed until July 1970.[9]

Once in operation the center was open from 6:30 AM until 11:30 PM, seven days a week except Christmas Day. Employees were charged $12.50 per child per week.[10] It accommodated up to forty-five children, and it was available to children from six weeks to five years of age.[11] In 1971 the center added a kindergarten for children four and five years of age for $10 per child per pay period (every two weeks).[12] Jane Dwyer was the first director.[13]

Because of the center's persistent financial deficit, the Authority announced plans in 1975 to close the operation on weekends and holidays.[14] That idea, however, met with such vocal employee resistance that the trustees quickly elected to look for some other way to reduce costs and increase revenue.[15]

By 1992 the twenty-two-year-old facility was in poor condition, space was inadequate, and the quality of care less than optimal. CEO Charles Eberhart appointed a team to study what needed

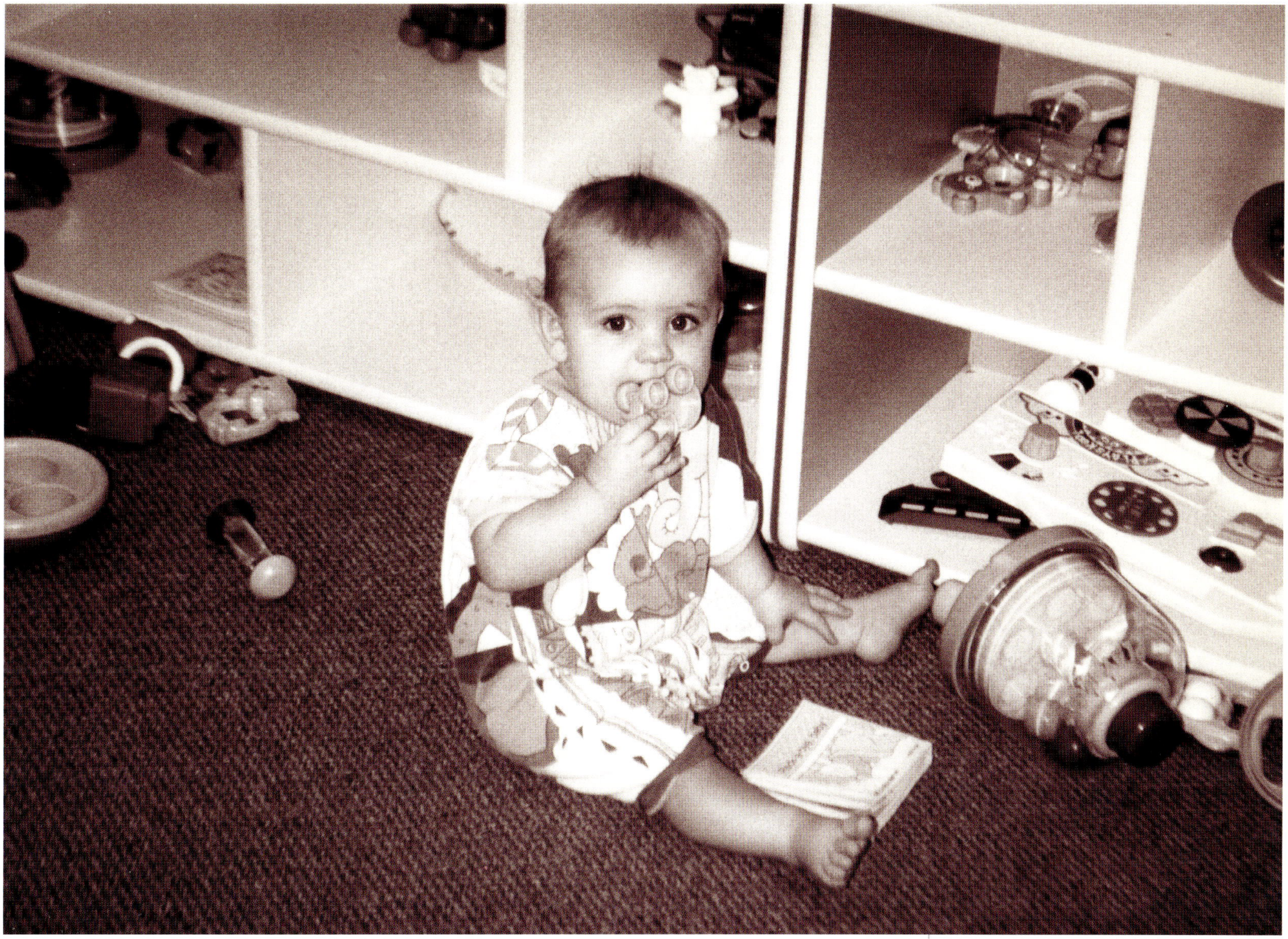

to be done. The team recommended the construction of a new facility,[16] and the DeKalb Medical Center Board of Directors approved $600,000 for its construction.[17] While the old building was being demolished and the new center constructed, the children were housed in the North Decatur Methodist Church educational building.[18]

The hospital elected to outsource the child care service and negotiated a contract with AmeriCare Early Learning Centers, a company specializing in day care centers, to plan, construct, and manage the new center. It was completed in the fall of 1993, had twelve new staff members and enrolled 125 children.[19] By the end of the year, 150 children were enrolled, 80 from employees, 32 from physicians and their office workers, and 38 from the community.[20] The facility, currently known as the Sunshine House, continues to serve the DeKalb Medical family.[21]

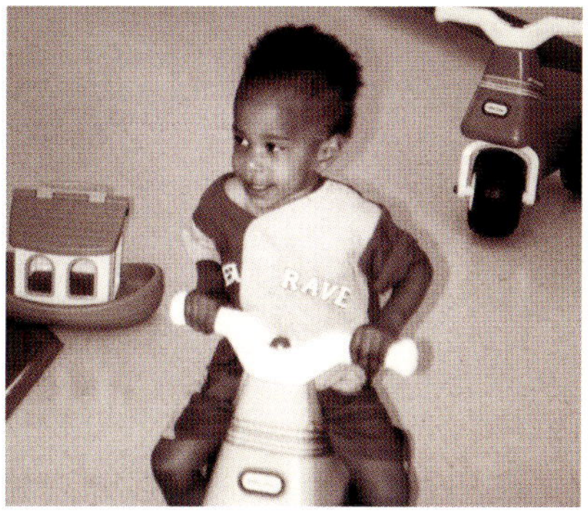

Communication: DeKalb Medical's Employee Newsletter

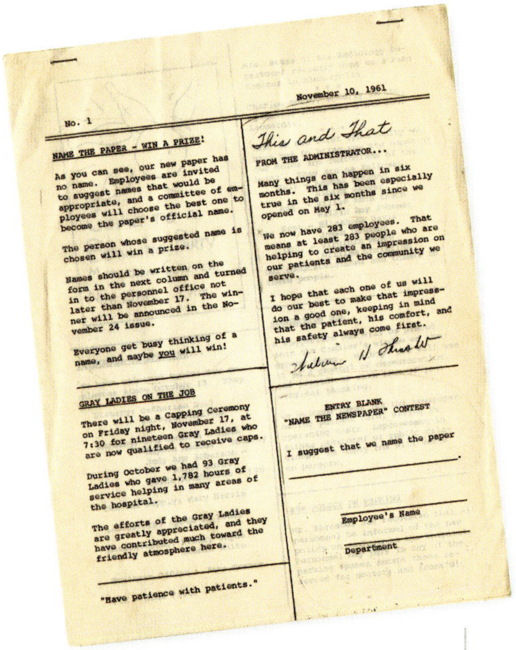

No. 1

November 10, 1961

NAME THE PAPER - WIN A PRIZE!

As you can see, our new paper has no name. Employees are invited to suggest names that would be appropriate, and a committee of employees will choose the best one to become the paper's official name.

The person whose suggested name is chosen will win a prize.

Names should be written on the form in the next column and turned in to the personnel office not later than November 17. The winner will be announced in the November 24 issue.

Everyone get busy thinking of a name, and maybe you will win!

GRAY LADIES ON THE JOB

There will be a Capping Ceremony on Friday night, November 17, at 7:30 for nineteen Gray Ladies who are now qualified to receive caps.

During October we had 93 Gray Ladies who gave 1,782 hours of service helping in many areas of the hospital.

The efforts of the Gray Ladies are greatly appreciated, and they have contributed much toward the friendly atmosphere here.

"Have patience with patients."

This and That

FROM THE ADMINISTRATOR...

Many things can happen in six months. This has been especially true in the six months since we opened on May 1.

We now have 283 employees. That means at least 283 people who are helping to create an impression on our patients and the community we serve.

I hope that each one of us will do our best to make that impression a good one, keeping in mind that the patient, his comfort, and his safety always come first.

ENTRY BLANK
"NAME THE NEWSPAPER" CONTEST

I suggest that we name the paper ________.

Employee's Name

Department

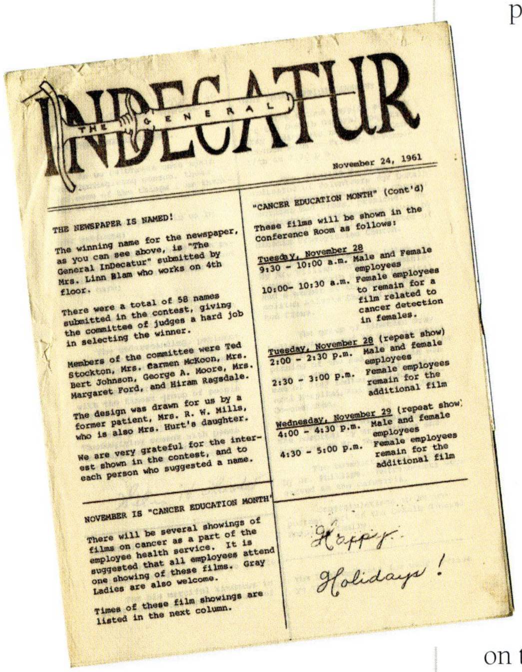

THE GENERAL INDECATUR

November 24, 1961

THE NEWSPAPER IS NAMED!

The winning name for the newspaper, as you can see above, is "The General InDecatur" submitted by Mrs. Linn Elam who works on 4th floor.

There were a total of 58 names submitted in the contest, giving the committee of judges a hard job in selecting the winner.

Members of the committee were Ted Stockton, Mrs. Carmen McKoon, Mrs. Bert Johnson, George A. Moore, Mrs. Margaret Ford, and Hiram Ragsdale.

The design was drawn for us by a former patient, Mrs. R. W. Mills, who is also Mrs. Hurt's daughter.

We are very grateful for the interest shown in the contest, and to each person who suggested a name.

NOVEMBER IS "CANCER EDUCATION MONTH"

There will be several showings of films on cancer as a part of the employee health service. It is suggested that all employees attend one showing of these films. Gray Ladies are also welcome.

Times of these film showings are listed in the next column.

"CANCER EDUCATION MONTH" (Cont'd)

These films will be shown in the Conference Room as follows:

Tuesday, November 28
9:30 - 10:00 a.m. Male and Female employees
10:00- 10:30 a.m. Female employees to remain for a film related to cancer detection in females.

Tuesday, November 28 (repeat show)
2:00 - 2:30 p.m. Male and female employees
2:30 - 3:00 p.m. Female employees remain for the additional film

Wednesday, November 29 (repeat show)
4:00 - 4:30 p.m. Male and female employees
4:30 - 5:00 p.m. Female employees remain for the additional film

Happy Holidays!

In November 1961, six months after DeKalb General Hospital opened, Helen Bush, secretary to Administrator William Thrasher, published the hospital's first employee newsletter. In it Thrasher announced that the hospital now had 283 employees and asked that all 283 work to make a good impression, "keeping in mind that the patient, his comfort, and his safety always come first." The newsletter also recognized the ninety-three Red Cross Gray Ladies who gave 1,782 hours of service in October, and Helen Bush announced in a lead article a contest to name the newsletter. She promised a prize to the winner.[1]

Out of fifty-eight names submitted, Linn Elam, RN, a fourth-floor nurse, had the winning entry: *The General InDecatur.* She received a flower arrangement as her winning prize. Mrs. R. W. Mills, a former patient and daughter of Personnel Director Mary Lou Hurt, submitted the winning design for the masthead. It depicted a loaded syringe imprinted with the words, "The General" overlying the background words, "InDecatur." There is no reference to Mills having received a prize for her winning design.[2]

Early editions of the newsletter contained numerous personal items, notices of lost items such as "the prized medical dictionary missing from the fourth floor nursing station," and congratulatory letters from patients praising the nurses, doctors, and DeKalb General for being "the best hospital, not only in Atlanta, but the best one you can find anywhere."[3] There also were personal items from nursing units and departments:

Third floor news: Miss Underwood is enjoying her new apartment, and who wouldn't with a swimming pool, air conditioning, etc. Mrs. Hardin's son, Ronnie, pitched for his Little League baseball game Tuesday. This was his first time, and his mother was about ready for the hospital when it was over.[4]

From Dietary: Harold Huston had bad luck on his vacation in Florida. First, his car washed out to sea and had to be towed in. Then it caught fire in Macon on his way home and burned up.[5]

Administrator Thrasher made it clear that the newsletter was for important employee information as well as entertainment. When 122 employees failed to vote for or against a proposed major medical insurance plan described in one newsletter, he wrote in the next issue:

You can be assured that if you read in the paper that each employee is expected to attend a meeting, or vote on a matter, etc., that is exactly what we mean. Employees who repeatedly disregard those instructions will be noted and kept in mind in the future.[6]

In addition to the newsletter, a DeKalb General Hospital Employees' News Center was located on the ground floor near the cafeteria, described in the employee newsletter as "the official medium of communication between all of us on matters of mutual interest. Bulletins, posters, letters, important notices, and instructions, announcements, and news flashes will be featured regularly. Give it a look every day."[7]

Helen Bush was referenced as editor of *The General InDecatur* from 1961 to 1965 and Mary Lou Hurt, director of Personnel, as editor from 1965 to 1970. There are, however, no available issues of the newsletter from October 1962 to January 1970. There is speculation that it was not published during that period. There was no response to public notices posted in 2007 requesting any issues from those dates. Monnie Mitchell, the first director of Public Relations, became editor in 1971 and continued in that role until 1981, with the title of managing editor, until her retirement in 1985.[8] Anne LeMasuier followed Monnie Mitchell and held the editor's position until 1988, when she was succeeded by Linda Abell Tierney who remained managing editor until her resignation in 2007.[9]

The newsletter went through a series of format and content changes. The original editions were handmade. Sara Folger in Purchasing printed the paper on a mimeograph machine using typed stencils, and Mary Lou Hurt, director of Personnel, assembled and stapled the copies.[10] In February 1962 the newsletter appeared with a preprinted masthead.[11] It took on a new look in 1975 when DeKalb General Hospital adopted its first logo that pictured an arrow piercing a red cross. The logo represented "a modern, progressive healthcare facility which is continually moving forward in a rapidly changing community and one that is willing to move forward to maintain a position of leadership."[12] The name of the newsletter was changed from *The General InDecatur* to *The InDecatur*, and the overlying loaded syringe was replaced with the new hospital logo. A new font was used, and the paper was printed on four pages of rich, brown paper.

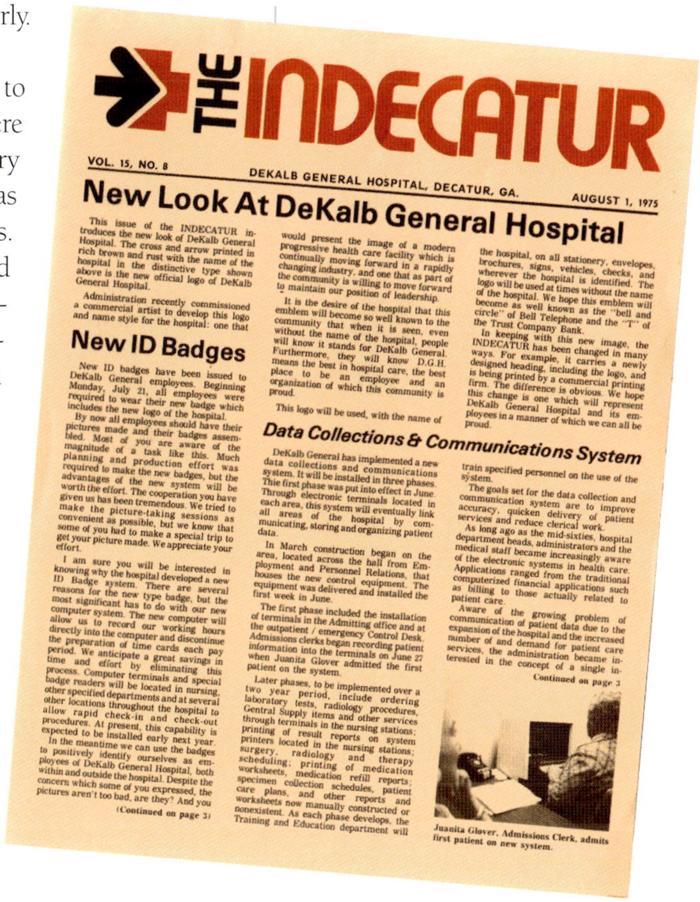

THE INDECATUR

VOL. 15, NO. 8 — DEKALB GENERAL HOSPITAL, DECATUR, GA. — AUGUST 1, 1975

New Look At DeKalb General Hospital

This issue of the INDECATUR introduces the new look of DeKalb General Hospital. The cross and arrow printed in rich brown and rust with the name of the hospital in the distinctive type shown above is the new official logo of DeKalb General Hospital.

Administration recently commissioned a commercial artist to develop this logo and name style for the hospital: one that would present the image of a modern progressive health care facility which is continually moving forward in a rapidly changing industry, and one that as part of the community is willing to move forward to maintain our position of leadership.

It is the desire of the hospital that this emblem will become so well known to the community that when it is seen, even without the name of the hospital, people will know it stands for DeKalb General. Furthermore, they will know D.G.H. means the best in hospital care, the best place to be an employee and an organization of which this community is proud.

This logo will be used, with the name of the hospital, on all stationery, envelopes, brochures, signs, vehicles, checks, and wherever the hospital is identified. The logo will be used at times without the name of the hospital. We hope this emblem will become as well known as the "bell and circle" of Bell Telephone and the "T" of the Trust Company Bank.

In keeping with this new image, the INDECATUR has been changed in many ways. For example, it carries a newly designed heading, including the logo, and is being printed by a commercial printing firm. The difference is obvious. We hope this change is one which will represent DeKalb General Hospital and its employees in a manner of which we can all be proud.

New ID Badges

New ID badges have been issued to DeKalb General employees. Beginning Monday, July 21, all employees were required to wear their new badge which includes the new logo of the hospital.

By now all employees should have their pictures made and their badges assembled. Most of you are aware of the magnitude of a task like this. Much planning and production effort was required to make the new badges, but the advantages of the new system will be worth the effort. The cooperation you have given us has been tremendous. We tried to make the picture-taking sessions as convenient as possible, but we know that some of you had to make a special trip to get your picture made. We appreciate your effort.

I am sure you will be interested in knowing why the hospital developed a new ID Badge system. There are several reasons for the new type badge, but the most significant has to do with our new computer system. The new computer will allow us to record our working hours directly into the computer and discontinue the preparation of time cards each pay period. We anticipate a great savings in time and effort by eliminating this process. Computer terminals and special badge readers will be located in nursing, other specified departments and at several other locations throughout the hospital to allow rapid check-in and check-out procedures. At present, this capability is expected to be installed early next year.

In the meantime we can use the badges to positively identify ourselves as employees of DeKalb General Hospital, both within and outside the hospital. Despite the concern which some of you expressed, the pictures aren't too bad, are they? And you

(Continued on page 3)

Data Collections & Communications System

DeKalb General has implemented a new data collections and communications system. It will be installed in three phases. Thie first phase was put into effect in June. Through electronic terminals located in each area, this system will eventually link all areas of the hospital by communicating, storing and organizing patient data.

In March construction began on the area, located across the hall from Employment and Personnel Relations, that houses the new control equipment. The equipment was delivered and installed the first week in June.

The first phase included the installation of terminals in the Admitting office and at the outpatient / emergency Control Desk. Admissions clerks began recording patient information into the terminals on June 27 when Juanita Glover admitted the first patient on the system.

Later phases, to be implemented over a two year period, include ordering laboratory tests, radiology procedures, Gentral Supply items and other services through terminals in the nursing stations; printing of result reports on system printers located in the nursing stations; surgery, radiology and therapy scheduling; printing of medication worksheets, medication refill reports; specimen collection schedules, patient care plans, and other reports and worksheets now manually constructed or nonexistent. As each phase develops, the Training and Education department will train specified personnel on the use of the system.

The goals set for the data collection and communication system are to improve accuracy, quicken delivery of patient services and reduce clerical work.

As long ago as the mid-sixties, hospital department heads, administrators and the medical staff became increasingly aware of the electronic systems in health care. Applications ranged from the traditional computerized financial applications such as billing to those actually related to patient care.

Aware of the growing problem of communication of patient data due to the expansion of the hospital and the increased number of and demand for patient care services, the administration became interested in the concept of a single in-

Continued on page 3

Juanita Glover, Admissions Clerk, admits first patient on new system.

In 1984, for an unknown reason, the masthead temporarily incorporated "DeKalb Medical Center" in the title, four years before the hospital changed its name, when the newsletter became *The DeKalb General Hospital/DeKalb Medical Center Indecatur*.[13] From 1987 to 1989 the heading was simply *indecatur* in script form. It became *INDECATUR* in 1988 when Linda Abell Tierney was named editor,[14] and several variations of the title followed.

The newsletter carried an inserted "Supplement" from 1978 to 1985 that provided detailed information about new employees, promotions, deaths, marriages, and work anniversaries. In the early 1980s, the *InDecatur* also began featuring the medical staff, highlighting medical staff officers, department chiefs with pictures and biographical sketches, and a list of new physicians joining the medical staff.[15]

In January 1999 the staff again modified the content of the newsletter with the stated goal of its serving as the news source for the entire health system, consolidating into one publication the many departmental newsletters, calendars, and memos currently in circulation.[16]

In December, 2005, *dateline DeKalb* replaced the *InDecatur* as the official employee newsletter. It included information from the three campuses in the health system. It was published twice each month in print form and electronically. Currently DeKalb Medical publishes a weekly electronic newsletter for employees and physicians entitled *datelineDeKalb E-Digest* and a daily news bulletin under the direction of Michael Tu.

Communicating effectively with staff, physicians, and community remains one of DeKalb Medical's commitments and one of its challenges.

The Credit Union

In January 1963 Administrator William Thrasher told the trustees that a few hospital employees had requested a credit union. He added that he had looked into the matter, and he did not think the time was right for one.[1] The trustees agreed. Four and a half years later, he reported that there now was considerable interest in a credit union, and he thought the time was right. He asked the Finance Committee to investigate what would be involved and to make a recommendation to the DeKalb County Hospital Authority.[2]

The Finance Committee studied the idea for two years. In June 1969, the committee recommended to the Authority that a credit union be formed and that it be open for loans and savings by February 1970.[3] The Authority agreed, named it the DeKalb Medical Employees' Federal Credit Union, and authorized a $10,000 loan to capitalize it.[4] Its organizational meeting was held on January 28, 1970.[5]

The credit union was an immediate success. Within two months it had 164 members and was making loans up to $200.[6] In its first year it realized sufficient revenue to pay a 3 percent annual dividend on savings deposits.[7] In its second year it was able to make $1,000-a-month repayments to the Authority for its capitalizing loan,[8] make loans of up to $800 to members,[9] and pay 5½ percent dividends on savings accounts.[10] By the third year it made new car loans of up to $3,000.[11]

In 1982 the credit union expanded its membership to include the medical staff, volunteers, and their immediate family members. A member bringing in a new member during the month of October received a silver dollar.[12]

While recommended by administration, authorized by the governing body, and supported by the hospital with space, personnel, and equipment,[13] the credit union was independent of DeKalb Medical's governance. As required by federal rules and regulations, a federal credit union is a not-for-profit, co-operative, financial institution owned and controlled by its members. Policies governing interest rates and other matters are set by a volunteer board of directors elected by and from the membership. Only members may deposit money with or borrow money from the credit union. Credit unions also must restrict their membership to a defined segment of the population as, for example, employees of the hospital. Credit unions typically pay higher dividends on deposits and charge lower interest rates on loans than commercial banks.[14]

The DeKalb credit union complied with all the federal rules and regulations, including having volunteer officers, a volunteer board of directors, and a volunteer supervisory committee that served as the credit union's watchdog.

It consistently demonstrated a healthy, stable financial status. In 1993 it was upgraded from a rating of "two" to the highest rating of "one" when surveyed by the National Credit Union Administration examiners.[15] Beginning in 1970 with a $10,000 capitalizing loan, in 1993 it had total assets of more than $6,500,000, including $5.5 million in outstanding loans, nearly $316,000 in cash, and $520,000 in investments.[16] In that same year it expanded its membership again to include employees of South Fulton Hospital, converted to a new in-house computer system and, while maintaining a branch office at DeKalb Medical Center, opened a new main office on Winn Way.[17] By 1994 it had a membership of 3,500 and assets of $7 million.[18]

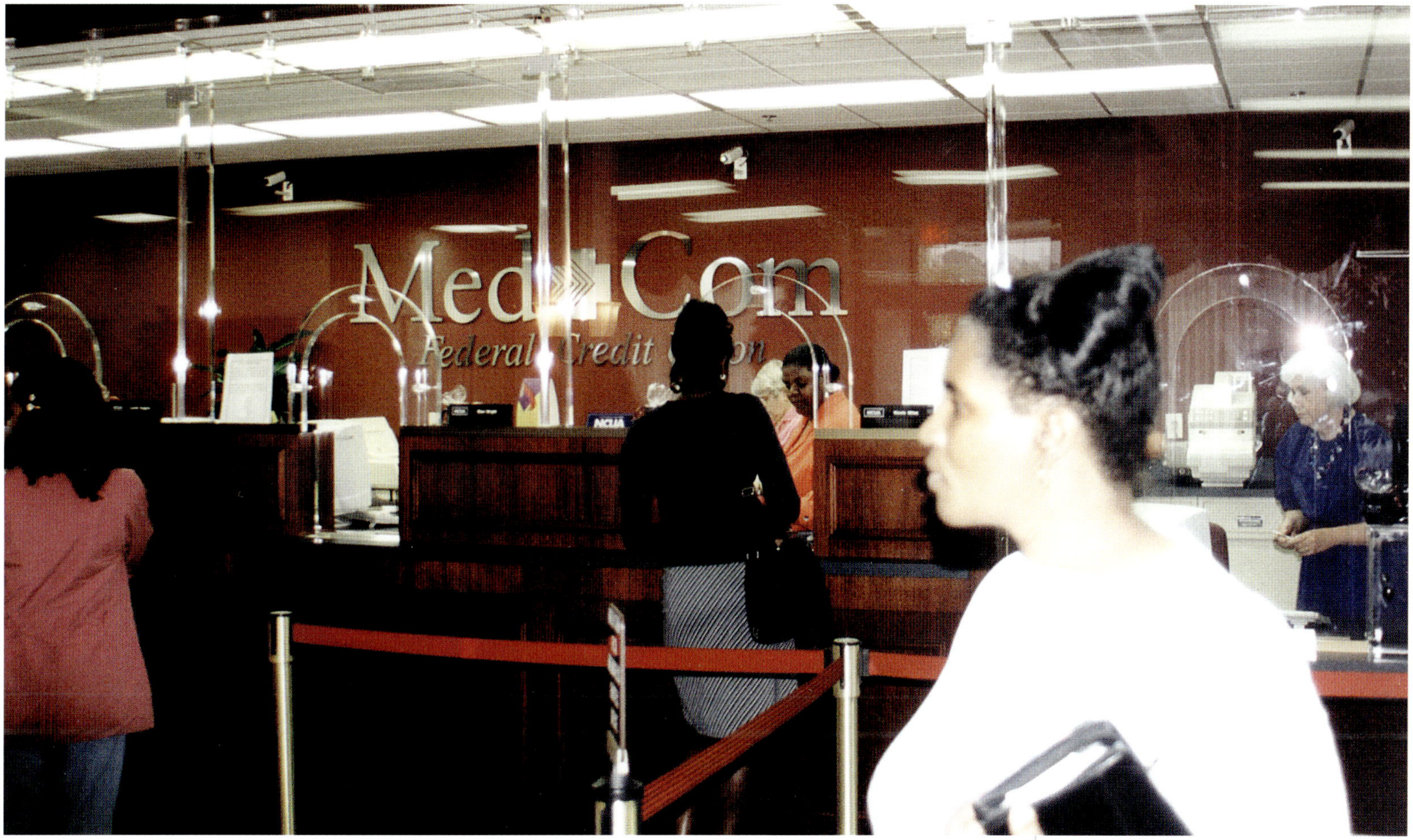

In 1995 the credit union board voted to change its name to "MedCom Federal Credit Union" to signify its expansion from being a healthcare–related institution to one serving a broader constituency. It formed a partnership with West Georgia Federal Credit Union that included employees of Paulding County Board of Education and Douglas County Board of Education. MedCom relocated its main office from Winn Way to a site on Lawrenceville Highway.

In December 2004 Wellstar Credit Union and MedCom Federal Credit Union formed a partnership, which the board of directors renamed "MembersFirst Federal Credit Union."[19] MembersFirst, in addition to serving DeKalb Medical, serves thirty-two other entities, including healthcare-related institutions, educational institutions, and a variety of businesses.[20] From its beginning in January 1970 as the DeKalb Medical Employees' Federal Credit Union with a share value of $5, MembersFirst Federal Credit Union has grown into a full-service financial institution with assets of over $56 million, 17,000 member-owners and seven branches throughout Georgia.[21]

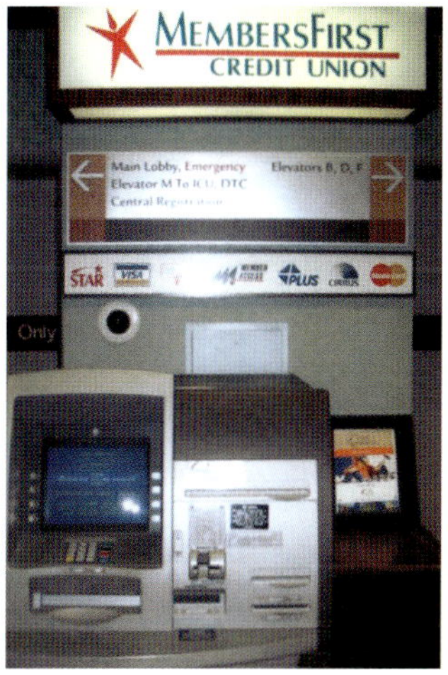

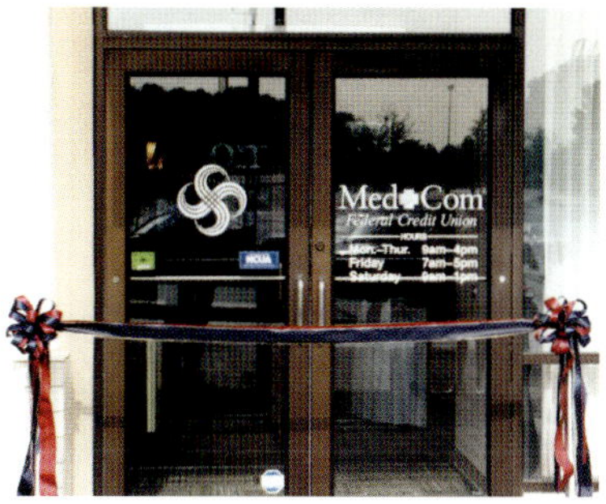

In 1995 the credit union's name was changed from DeKalb Medical Employees' Federal Credit Union to MedCom Federal Credit Union. In 2004 it partnered with Wellstar Credit Union and became MembersFirst Federal Credit Union. Since its birth in 1970, it has become a full-service financial resource with over $56 million in assets.

Demographic Changes with Rich Opportunities

"There are more than 150 different languages and dialects spoken here, making ours a truly international community. This diversity creates one of the rich, cultural fabrics with which we work...."

— Eric Norwood
President and CEO
DeKalb Medical

In the year 2000, CEO John Gerlach reflected on DeKalb Medical's values when he wrote:

> *Our four values are diversity, respect, healing, and service .... While all of our values are important, I believe diversity has a special place for us. We're located in DeKalb County, the most diverse county in Georgia. We experience this diversity in our workplace in terms of race, sexual orientation, gender, parental status, age, language, geographic origin, religion, and culture, just to name a few.... To value diversity, we must develop a sensitivity toward and appreciation of each other's differences. To demonstrate respect, we must show admiration for and consideration of others and ourselves, including our coworkers and our patients.*[1]

Four years later, President and CEO Eric Norwood added:

> *DeKalb County is the most diverse community in the southeastern [United States]. There are more than 150 different languages and dialects spoken here, making ours a truly international community. This diversity creates one of the rich, cultural fabrics with which we work.... The value that makes diversity a strength is respect.*[2]

The organization's leadership obviously appreciated the presence and value of DeKalb Medical's diversity and the rich opportunities presented by the community's dramatic demographic changes. The task remained daunting, however, to demonstrate in a convincing manner an appreciation for the value of the changes that emerged.

Chapter 3 described the issue of diversity as it arose in the hospital's first decade with the passage of the 1964 Civil Rights Act; the complaint filed with the Department of Health, Education, and Welfare (HEW) alleging discrimination at DeKalb General Hospital; the DeKalb County Hospital Authority's actions to abolish its segregated nursing unit and pass a resolution that "Patients will be assigned to hospital facilities according to their medical needs with no distinction to be made on grounds of race, color, religion, or national origin" and the pronouncement by HEW that it found no problems in terms of racial discrimination at DeKalb General.

The challenge of dealing positively and effectively with diversity, however, did not disappear with the hospital's 1965 resolution or HEW's pronouncement. In 1970 and again in 1975, blacks filed complaints with the Equal Employment Opportunity Commission (EEOC) against the hospital.[3] In each case the EEOC ruled in favor of the hospital, but the complaints demonstrated the difficulty of creating the perception of a fair and impartial environment.

In 1995 a physician and nurse manager acceded to a patient's request that the patient not be attended to or treated by a minority member of the staff.[4] The physician and nurse manager subsequently apologized to the staff, and the hospital issued a public apology. CEO John Gerlach declared, "DeKalb Medical Center does not tolerate or condone any acts of discrimination, and we value the diversity of our staff and the multicultural environment in which we work."[5] He appointed a Diversity Committee to identify and address key issues associated with diversity.[6]

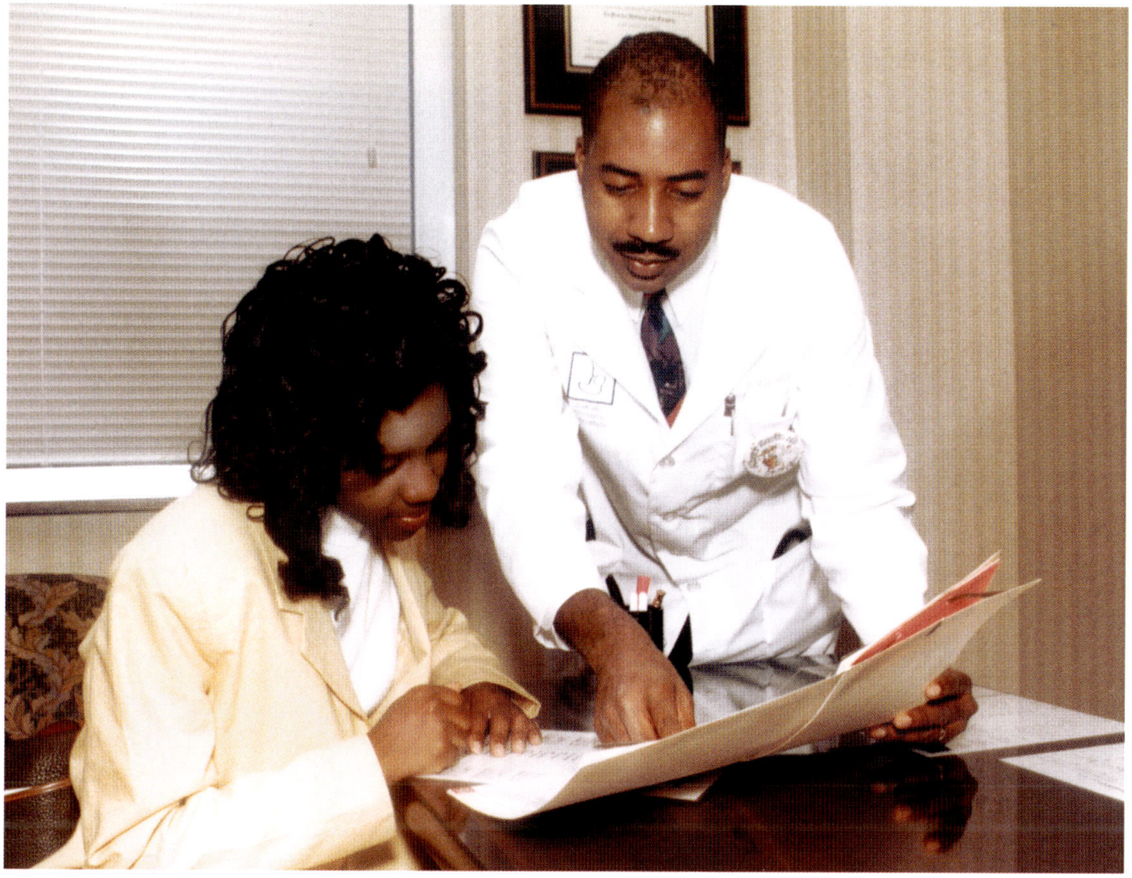

In 2005, Albert Scott, MD, became the first African American to be elected chief of staff at DeKalb Medical.

In 2005 CEO Eric Norwood engaged a consulting firm to help DeKalb Medical deal with the challenges and the opportunities presented by diversity.[7] That also was the year that Albert Scott, MD, became the first African American to be elected chief of staff at the North Decatur hospital; and that Cornelius Flowers, MD, also African American, was elected as the first chief of staff at the Hillandale hospital.[8]

By the mid-1970s diversity was no longer an issue of simply dealing fairly and appropriately with African Americans. Diversity encompassed race, nationality, language, culture, ethnicity, religion, and other differences, broad changes for which the hospital found itself only partially prepared. A 1975 issue of the employee newsletter reported the following incident that reflected the need to enhance its preparedness for the new elements of the community's diversity:

> *Recently we had need of an interpreter. The patient was a young Vietnamese mother who was not able to communicate with the nursing staff. . . .Social Services was contacted which called Personnel. Personnel knew of a Vietnamese [employment] applicant who also spoke English. He was called on the phone and brought to the hospital by Perry Stephens, assistant director of Personnel. Thanh Dai Nguyen was most helpful in interpreting essential words of their vocabulary for the hospital. A list was made in both languages that enabled the nursing staff and patient to understand each other. . . . [The newsletter added,] if you speak a language other than English, please complete the form below and return to Personnel.*[9]

DeKalb County rapidly experienced a dramatic influx of individuals of different nationalities, religions, and cultures. They became patients, members of the medical staff, and members of the hospital staff. By 1984 an employee survey produced a list of hospital employees who, in addition to English, were fluent in Chinese, French, German, Indian, Iranian, Korean, Lebanese, Portuguese, Spanish, Thai, Vietnamese, Yiddish, and sign language.[10]

In the year 2000 the county had six Baha'i, ten Buddhist, three Hindu, one Jain, four Muslim, and one Sikh religious congregations.[11] Approximately 13 percent, or 101,320, of the 665,865 people in DeKalb County were foreign born.[12] There was a 177 percent increase in foreign-born individuals between 1990 and 2000 as compared to an increase of 11 percent of native-born individuals. Nearly 65 percent of the county's foreign-born population entered the county after 1990.[13] The ten countries from which the largest number of immigrants came were Vietnam, Russia, Ethiopia, India, China, Somalia, Jamaica, Mexico, Yugoslavia, and Nigeria.[14]

From 2000 to 2007 the county's total population grew from 665,865 to 737,093, an increase of 71,228, almost an 11 percent gain.[15] Whites increased by 8,764 for a total of 228,499 (accounting for 31 percent of the county's population), blacks increased by 38,463 for a total of 398,030 (54 percent), Hispanics by 20,440 for a total of 73,709 (10 percent), and Asians by 3,562 for a total of 36,855 (5 percent).[16]

The changes in DeKalb County's demographics, however, involved not only more nationalities, religions, and cultures, but other population characteristics as well. Many of the newcomers moved into DeKalb Medical's neighborhood from outlying communities. The traffic congestion to be endured in commuting from outlying suburbs, the high cost of fuel, the attractive and available housing in DeKalb Medical's service area, and the employment opportunities inside the I-285 perimeter expressway led to a significant population growth in DeKalb Medical's immediate community. Younger, more-affluent families became DeKalb Medical's neighbors. Nearly 35 percent of the county's population was twenty-four years of age or younger, and another 35 percent was between the ages of twenty-five and forty-four years. A total of 92 percent were under the age of sixty-five years.[17]

More than 85 percent of those people twenty-five years of age or older were high school graduates, and more than 36 percent were college graduates.[18] The average household income in the county in 2000 was $60,098,[19] and DeKalb County became the second most affluent county with an African American majority in the United States after Prince George's County, Maryland.[20]

The changes have arrived. DeKalb Medical's responses have been extensive, creative, and effective. The opportunities remain rich, and the challenges remain great.

Diabetes Services

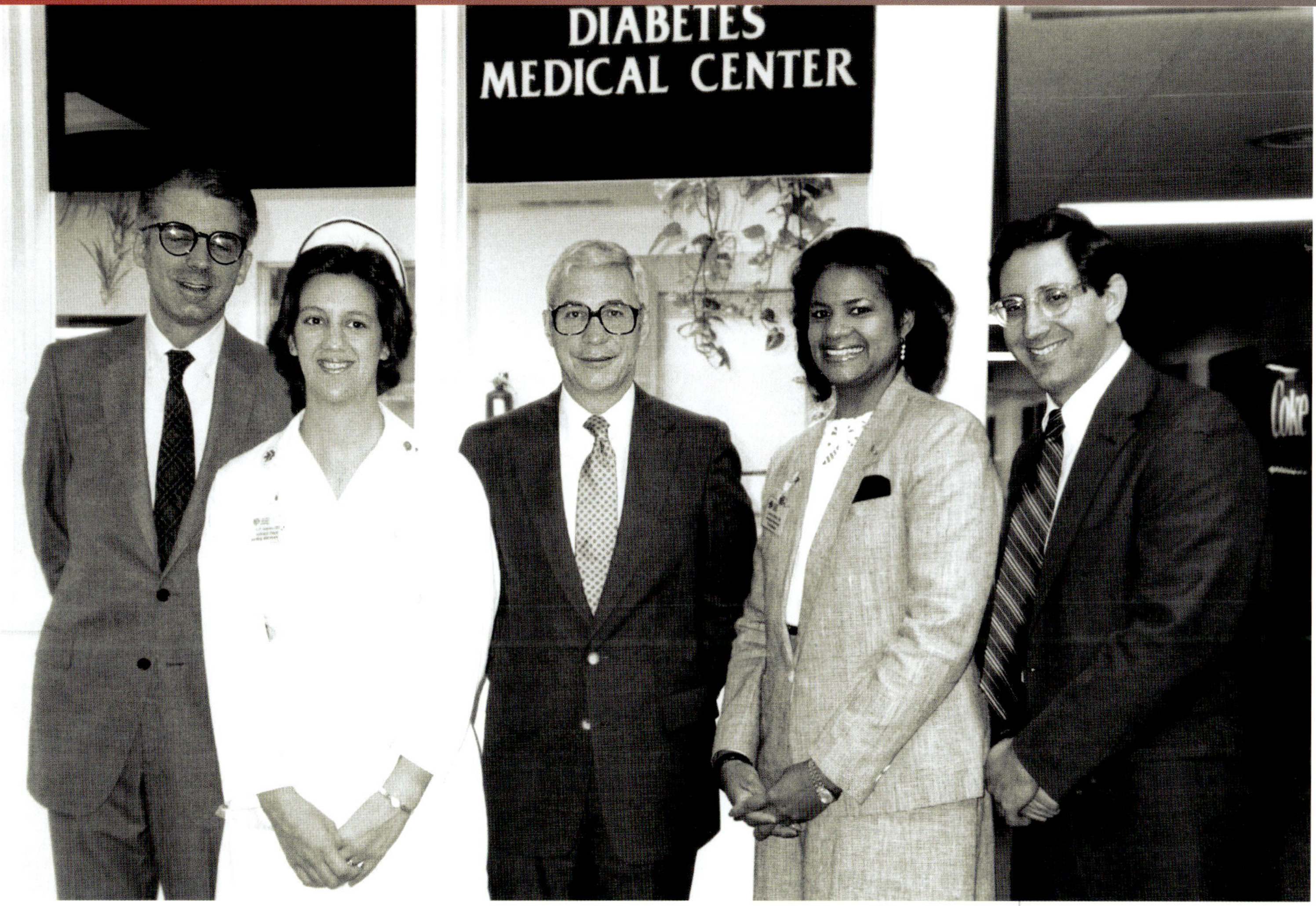

The Diabetes Medical Center, left to right: Donald DeBra, MD, endocrinologist; Peggy Jenkins, RN, department head; John Service, MD, guest speaker; Laura Hurt, RN, Patient Care Coordinator; and David Jacobson, MD, endocrinologist and medical director.

In 1985 endocrinologists David Jacobson, MD, Carol Teutsch, MD, and Donald DeBra, MD, proposed that DeKalb General Hospital establish a diabetes treatment center.[1] The trustees approved the concept and negotiated a contract with David Jacobson to serve as its medical director.[2]

The Diabetes Medical Center opened with twelve beds on the 1700 nursing unit in March 1986. It established a program for outpatient and inpatient services and for people of all ages.[3] Peggy Jenkins, RN, a certified diabetes educator, was the first department head; she led a staff of fifteen plus five part-time support personnel. When Jenkins became the hospital's diabetes education coordinator, she was succeeded by Donna McGehee, RN, as department head.[4]

In the first year, the Diabetes Medical Center admitted 292 patients to the 1700 nursing unit and provided educational services to 60 outpatients and their families. The center served not only patients admitted to the 1700 unit but also other patients with diabetes located throughout the hospital,

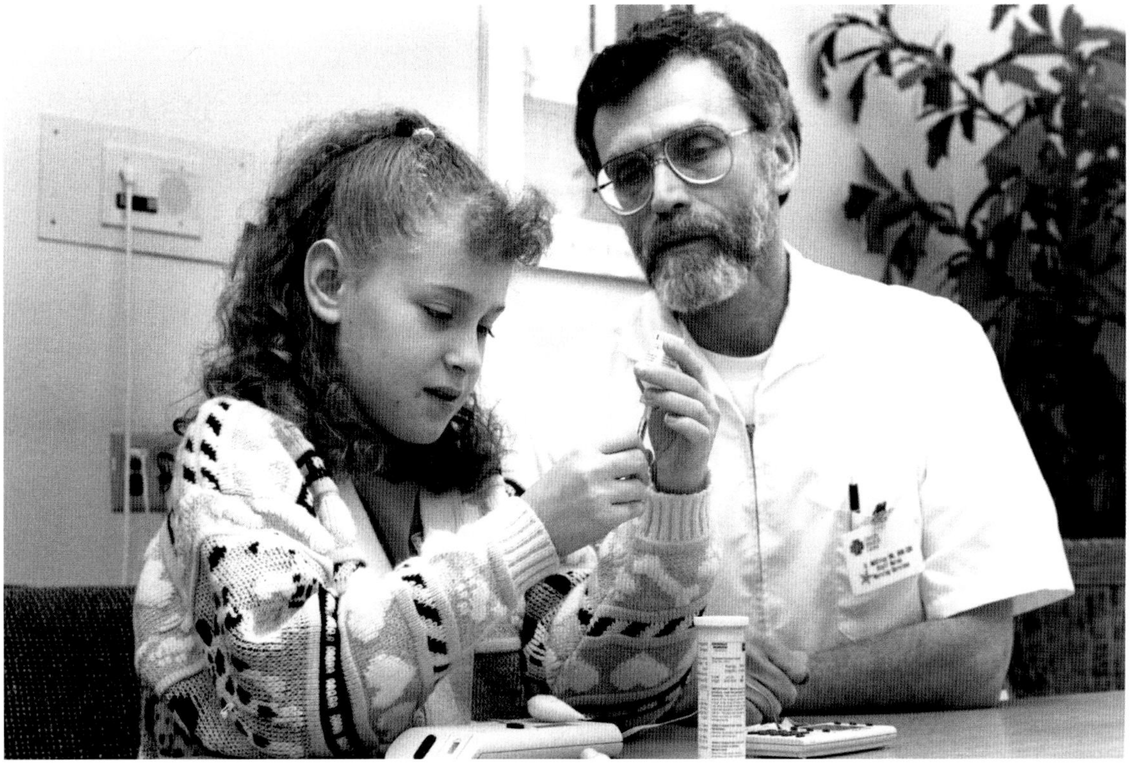

Karen McElroy learns how to prepare an insulin injection from her father Steve McElroy, RN, a certified diabetes educator.

numbering approximately forty on any given day.[5]

In 1991 the center expanded from twelve to sixteen beds and from fifteen to twenty-three staff members. In addition to physicians and nurses, the staff included an education coordinator, a dietician, an occupational therapist, a physical therapist, and a social worker. More than half of the nurses on the unit passed or qualified to take the diabetes educator certification examination. To sit for the examination a nurse must have had at least two years or two thousand hours of diabetes-care experience.[6]

In addition to its inpatient and outpatient services, the center offered screening and educational services to the community. In 1987 David Jacobson and the staff hosted more than six hundred people for a day of screenings, information, and cooking demonstrations at nearby Market Square shopping mall.[7]

The Diabetes Medical Center continued in operation until 1992 when it was replaced by the Center for Outpatient Diabetes Education.[8] The goal of the outpatient center is to offer educational services to the almost thirty thousand residents of DeKalb County with diabetes.[9] The outpatient center is one of the services supported by the DeKalb Medical Foundation's 2006–2009 campaign, "Building a Healthier Tomorrow."[10]

The outpatient center offers classes in the prevention, recognition, and management of type 1 and type 2 diabetes[11] as well as the recognition and management of gestational diabetes of pregnancy.[12] It provides group classes and one-on-one instruction.[13] The program has received high marks in customer satisfaction by its participants.[14] It also received certification by the American Diabetes Association and was recognized for its diversity initiatives, including diabetes education programs in Spanish and Chinese. The center's staff includes registered nurses, dieticians, and support staff who provided services to almost ten thousand diabetes patients in 2004.[15] The center's services now are provided at the North Decatur and the Hillandale campuses.

Education Services

A wise (and strict) high school mathematics teacher was fond of saying to her students, "It is not practice that makes perfect, but the right kind of practice that makes perfect."[1] Peter Senge wrote *The Fifth Discipline* in which he developed the theme that any vital organization must be a "learning organization."[2] DeKalb Medical's educational initiatives have been a keystone of its efforts to be a learning organization engaged in the right kind of practices.

Its early education activities were rudimentary when compared with today's scope of services. There was no medical library, no resource library for patients and their families, no community education programs, no established program of continuing professional education, and the in-service training program was in its infancy.

Over the years, DeKalb Medical established three stalwart pillars of education services: the Education Services Department, the Health Sciences Library, and a host of continuing professional education offerings.

It is not practice that makes perfect, but the right kind of practice that makes perfect.

Education Services Department

Margaret Ford, RN, was DeKalb General Hospital's first director of Employee Training and Health Service.[3] She alone constituted the in-service training section of Nursing.[4] The hospital required every new employee to attend only a "one-hour orientation program" under her direction. She also taught a twelve-week course in basic medical terminology and offered a class in hospital safety for all employees.[5] She apparently was an exceptional instructor because the employee newsletter reported that her students were "enthusiastic about their classes, even on test days."[6]

In 1962 Ford resigned to become director of Nursing at Aidmore Hospital, and Mary Hollis, RN, succeeded her with the title of supervisor of Employee Training and Health. Hollis trained nurses aides, orderlies, and diet clerks, and she provided continuing education classes for nurses.[7] The 1962 DeKalb County Hospital Authority minutes noted that "her primary responsibility will be to coordinate the training of nursing personnel with the medical staff's Nursing Committee," which also reflects the level of authority the medical staff had over nursing practices at DeKalb General at that time.[8]

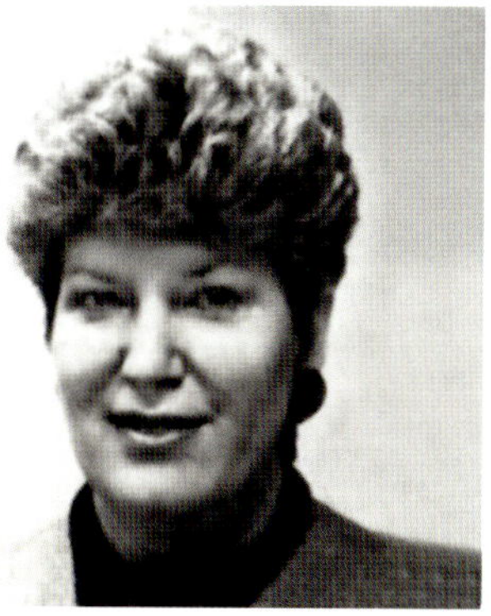

Barbara Lewis, RN, was director of Training and Continuing Education from 1976–1995.

Mary Hollis remained in the position until 1972 and was succeeded by Grace Morris, RN, (1972–1976), Barbara Lewis, RN, (1976–1995), Linda Stokes, (1995–1996), Jeff Curtis (1996–1999), and Anne Jones Fears (1999–present). Margaret Ford and Mary Hollis were responsible for employee health as well as training and education. Grace Morris was the first director solely assigned to Education Services. George Fischer was named the first Media Services coordinator,[9] and Karlton McIver succeeded him in 2003.[10]

In 1972 Bill Sublett, director of Human Resources, announced that Training and Continuing Education would become a new section in his department rather than a section in Nursing.[11] In 1980, during Barbara Lewis's tenure, Training and Education became a department rather than a section of Human Resources, but the department continued reporting to the director of Human Resources. In the 1990s the department briefly reported to the director of Hospital Relations[12] but subsequently reported again to the director of Human Resources. The name of the department also was changed from Training and Continuing Education to Education Services.

Education Services' responsibilities evolved over time. In the 1970s under Grace Morris' leadership it offered training and educational programs for nursing and non-nursing personnel as well as patients and their families, job-specific orientation for all new employees, medical terminology, cardio-pulmonary resuscitation (CPR) training, classes in breast-feeding for new mothers, diabetes education for the public, and a training program for all housekeeping employees.[13]

In 1972 Administrator Charles Eberhart, Bill Sublett, and Grace Morris created an eight-week Supervisory Management course[14] that inaugurated the concept of management and leadership training. The outgrowth of that course, the current Management Institute, remains an integral part of Education Services' program. The institute now has fourteen classes that include coaching, managing conflict, managing organizational transition, dealing with difficult people, employee satisfaction and retention, diversity as a strength, relationships with physicians, teamwork, and DeKalb Medical's image in the community.[15] Dannie Bell became Management Development coordinator in 1991 and was responsible for both top management and frontline management training. When Jeff Curtis joined the department, he was given responsibility for the top management program, and he developed a self-learning module that accommodated the specific learning needs of administrators.[16] According to Anne Fears, the program has been a "life-changing event" for managers.[17]

In 1973 Grace Morris established a three-month, advanced training course for the county's Emergency Medical Technicians (EMTs). Those who had completed a basic course in emergency training and who had become certified EMTs were enrolled. The program provided hands-on clinical experience relative to emergency care. Each class rotated through the Emergency Department, Intensive

In 1973 members of Education Services began conducting advanced training courses for members of DeKalb County's Emergency Medical Service.

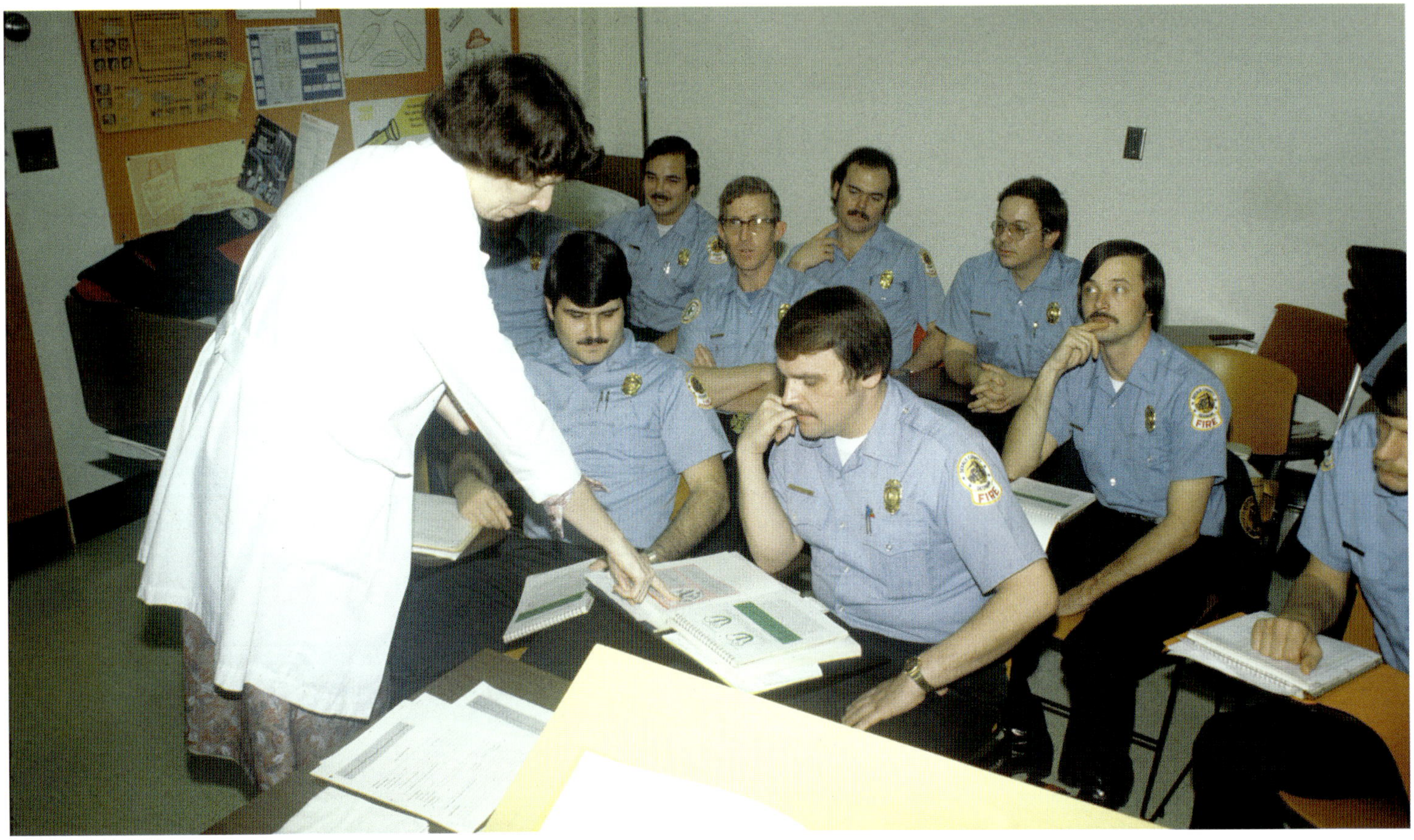

Care Unit, Coronary Care Unit, IV Team, and Laboratory.[18]

Barbara Lewis's early staff of educators focused on direct patient services and on education and support for patients and their families.[19] They provided general orientation and management development for all departments, clinical orientation for nurses, and a critical-care course. Personal instructors, known as preceptors, assisted employees with their specific areas of responsibilities after they began their work assignments.[20] The department also offered a variety of community education classes such as "how to be an effective babysitter" for teenagers, diabetes education for patients and their families, and coping with cancer—a service that currently is provided primarily by the Wellness Center in collaboration with the Cancer Center.[21]

In 1985 Barbara Lewis organized the department into three divisions: education services, health education, and media services. Amy Sabo, RN, and her team in education services coordinated educational and management development for nursing and non-nursing departments. Linda Schievelhud, RN, and her team in health education were responsible for community outreach programs and health education activities that included cancer, diabetes, and ostomy care. Jean Yates, RN, developed and produced media and coordinated the Learning Resource Center.[22]

The Learning Resource Center was established in 1985. It had study stations and audiovisual stations where hospital staff could access required in-service training materials.[23] It gave employees the option of classroom instruction or receiving individual training programs and information using interactive video technology.[24] The center also offered courses that were required by the Joint Commission on Accreditation of Healthcare Organizations (JCAHO), such as fire safety, back safety, electrical safety, and hazardous waste. The courses were available twenty-four hours a day, 365 days a year.

In a 1990s reorganization, most of nursing education was moved from Education Services to Nursing Services and placed in the hands of clinical nurse specialists and preceptors on the individual nursing units. Specialty education such as diabetes and oncology was conducted on the nursing unit where most of those patients were located. Education Services retained responsibility for general clinical orientation.[25]

While some services were removed from the department, others were added. During Linda Stokes' term as director, the department became known temporarily as the Education, Quality, and Performance Improvement Department.[26] Ann Rinaldi, RN, Crosby Turner and Martin Isganitis were responsible for Quality and Performance Improvement, including service excellence and customer satisfaction. As the Quality and Performance Improvement initiative focused increasingly on clinical issues, that function was moved into the newly formed Quality and Performance Improvement Council under the direction of Steve Mayfield.[27] Service excellence and customer satisfaction remained the responsibility of Education Services until the DeKalb Quality Institute was created and assumed that assignment. Education Services retained general orientation, management training, and a new responsibility—computer training.[28]

The widespread use of computers throughout the organization initiated a new training and education responsibility and a new opportunity. Computers required training in their use, and they provided a new method of learning. Training in the use of computers and the organization's software programs ranged from a basic introduction to the computer to the more advanced training in the use of the Sunrise Clinical Manager electronic medical record system.[29]

Computers also provided a new instrument for learning.[30] In 2001 DeKalb Medical implemented the Learning Management System that allows employees to obtain annual certification and training through Intranet-based learning programs. There are twenty-two JCAHO mandatory course modules. Employees can see what classes they need and the date by which they must be completed for their annual performance review. The courses may be taken on any computer that has Intranet-access twenty-four hours a day, seven days a week.[31]

Anne Fears estimates that approximately 50 percent of Education Services' activities currently involve orientation, computer training, and management training. One of her goals is to add more emphasis on improving skills in communication, dealing with conflict, and team-building. She also wants to increase the availability of open enrollment classes for the few individuals in each department who may need specific training without involving the entire department.[32] Education Services went through a recent transition with a turnover in personnel. Fears is pleased with her new team and the direction in which DeKalb Medical is going.[33]

Health Sciences Library

DeKalb General Hospital was open for only two years before the medical staff recognized the need for a medical library. Floyd Sanders, MD, chief of staff, appointed a Medical Library Committee, chaired by Baker Huff, MD. At the committee's request, the hospital bought a few textbooks for the physicians,[34] and Huff asked all active and courtesy members of the medical staff to contribute $3 a year to a library fund. By the end of 1963, the medical library subscribed to fourteen periodicals and owned sixty-seven books, eleven of which were reported missing.[35]

Frances Black, director of Medical Records, managed the library for a decade. It was located on the ground floor in a small space near her department. During the 1969–1971 renovation and expansion project, the small library shared its space with the EKG Department while a new EKG location was under construction.[36]

At the January 1972 Quarterly Medical Staff meeting, the chair of the Medical Library Committee asked the physicians what changes they would recommend in the current library. The doctors said to leave it like it was.[37] A year later, however, they complained that the library was too small.[38] In 1974 the hospital renovated a large storage space on the ground floor around the corner from Medical Records and relocated the library.[39] The medical staff agreed to increase its annual library assessment to $25 per member,[40] and physicians contributed $7,215 toward the purchase of a "core library" of reference books and periodicals.[41]

In September 1974 DeKalb General also hired Marilyn Gibbs (later Barry) as its part-time medical librarian, but she soon became full-time.[42] Barry is the daughter of internist and former chief of staff Robert Gibbs, MD. Earnest Atkins, MD, one of the original surgeons on the medical staff and former chief of staff, said in one of his speeches that "of the many contributions that Dr. Gibbs made to the hospital, Marilyn was the best."[43] Robert Gibbs, now retired, is a regular volunteer in the library where he works alongside his daughter.

Before coming to DeKalb General Hospital, Marilyn Barry received her undergraduate degree in English literature from Vanderbilt University, her master's degree in librarianship from Emory University, and she served on the staff of the Science Library at the University of Georgia.[44] In 1978 she was one of eleven librarians nationwide selected to participate in a National Library of Medicine conference to explore the needs of hospital libraries.[45] In 1994 she received the Recognition Award by the Southeastern Conference of Hospital Librarians; and in 1995 she was named Librarian of the Year by the Southern Chapter of the Medical Library Association.[46]

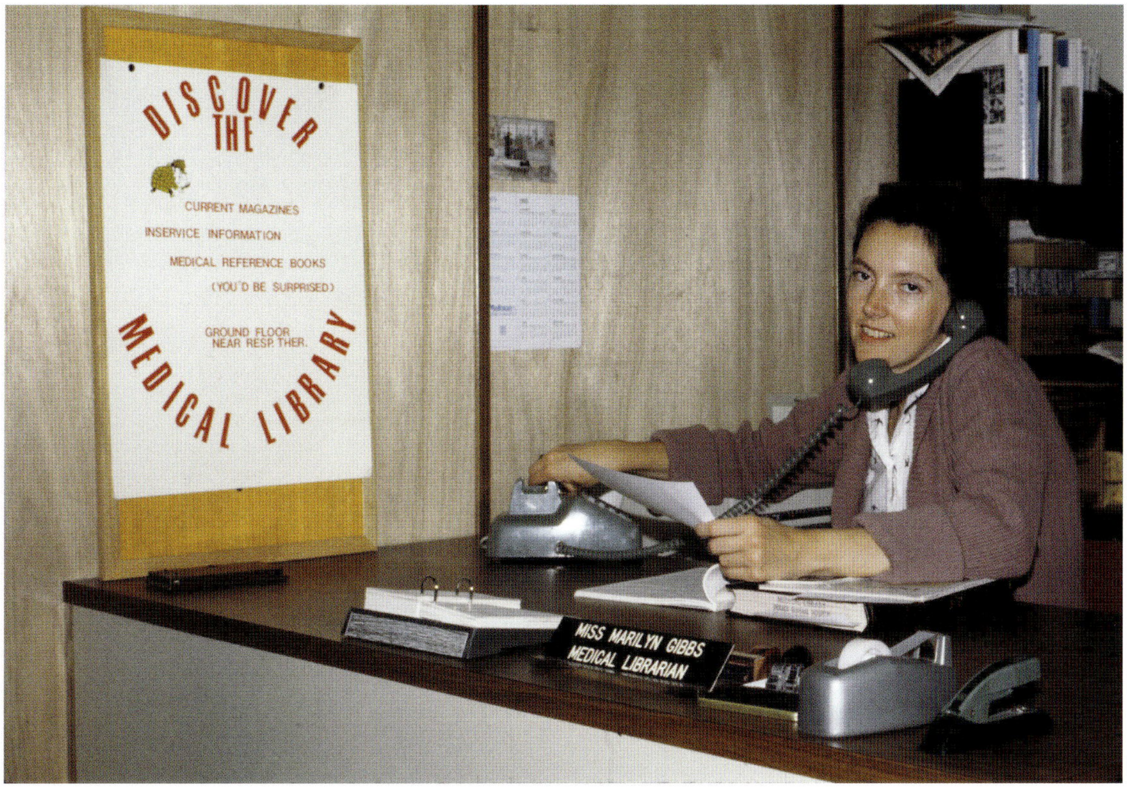

In 1974, Marilyn Gibbs (Barry) became director of the Health Sciences Library and remains in that position today.

Over the years, the library's capabilities and its collections have grown. In the 1970s it subscribed to Index Medicus that gave library users access to four million article citations if the user had good enough vision to read the small print and the fortitude to explore the exhaustive categories of the medical literature. Marilyn Barry observed that "despite its limitations, that now-prehistoric tool yielded evidence-based decision support for patient care."[47]

In the 1980s the library acquired MEDLINE, an online version of Index Medicus. The only "hitch" in the advancement was that the library user did not have direct access to MEDLINE. Requests for searches on topics of interest had to be channeled through the librarian who would print out voluminous paper reports. Still, according to Marilyn Barry, the system was a "thrill and boon."[48]

In 1988 the library acquired a MEDLINE CD-ROM that permitted the user direct access to article citations and abstracts in two hundred medical journals.[49] Along with this advancement, however, came a greater demand for library space to house journals in print.

In 1982 the library was relocated from the ground floor to the first floor near the physicians' entrance.[50] That location was convenient, but it included no room for expansion. Fortuitously, the space occupied by the library was needed for an expansion of the Outpatient Surgery Department. In 1994, to meet both needs, the library was relocated to the ground floor near the conference room and theater—the sites of most educational conferences—and it was expanded. The space was doubled, and a higher technical information delivery system was introduced in the form of a CD-ROM tower. MEDLINE discs also were networked so that as many as three users could search simultaneously.[51]

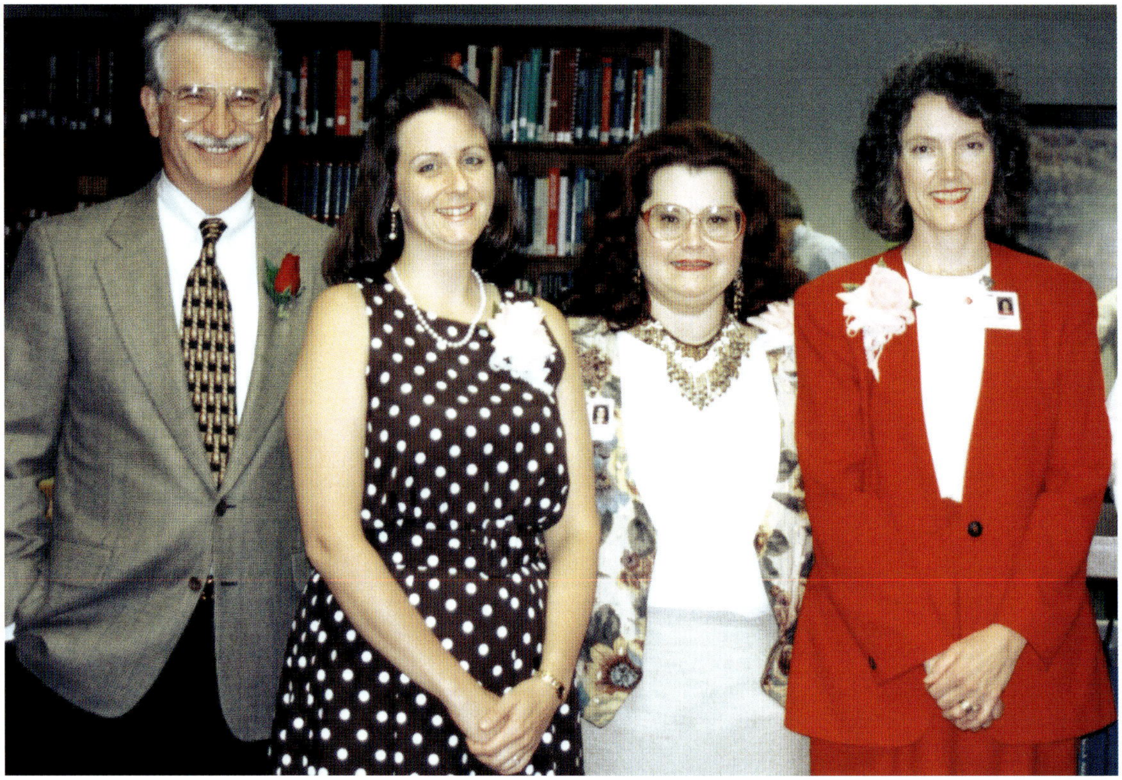

In 1994 a new library was celebrated with an open house. Left to right: Alex Parkinson, MD, chairman of the Medical Education Committee, Pat Herndon, assistant Librarian, Sharon Atkinson, information specialist, and Marilyn Barry, director of Health Sciences Library.

By 1994 the library's holdings had grown from the original sixty-seven books and fourteen periodicals to more than ten thousand books and journal volumes, more than three hundred periodicals (of which fifty were nursing journals), and 500 videotapes. The medical staff's annual library assessment was increased to $75 per member. Physicians had donated more than $275,000 during the previous twenty years in addition to the gifts of many books.[52]

Today the barriers are gone to direct access. Physicians and other library users can read books and articles from their offices, their homes, or wherever they may be with their computers. More than two-thousand journals and 160 books are available electronically, and the number is growing. While maintaining a core print collection of books and journals, the library has transferred some of its funds to enhance its electronic capabilities. Even the traditional services have taken on electronic features. The AutoAlert program automatically generates periodic updated references to users' topics of interest. Requests for articles from the core print collection are now scanned and emailed to users. The UpToDate program offers a regularly updated electronic database of 7,400 clinical reviews.[53] Library users currently may access electronically over 150 clinical texts, over two thousand periodicals, extensive patient resources, a library "card" catalog, and an array of additional links to key healthcare websites.[54]

In 1990 the Medical Library was renamed the Health Sciences Library to reflect its broader scope of materials and its services to all hospital professionals.[55] All electronic resources are available today at each of the three campuses and in DeKalb Medical's satellite primary care centers. In addition to the resources available in the North Decatur library, there are core clinical reference books and computer work stations in the libraries at the Downtown Decatur and the Hillandale hospitals.

In 1996 the Health Sciences Library teamed up with the Wellness Center and DeKalb Medical

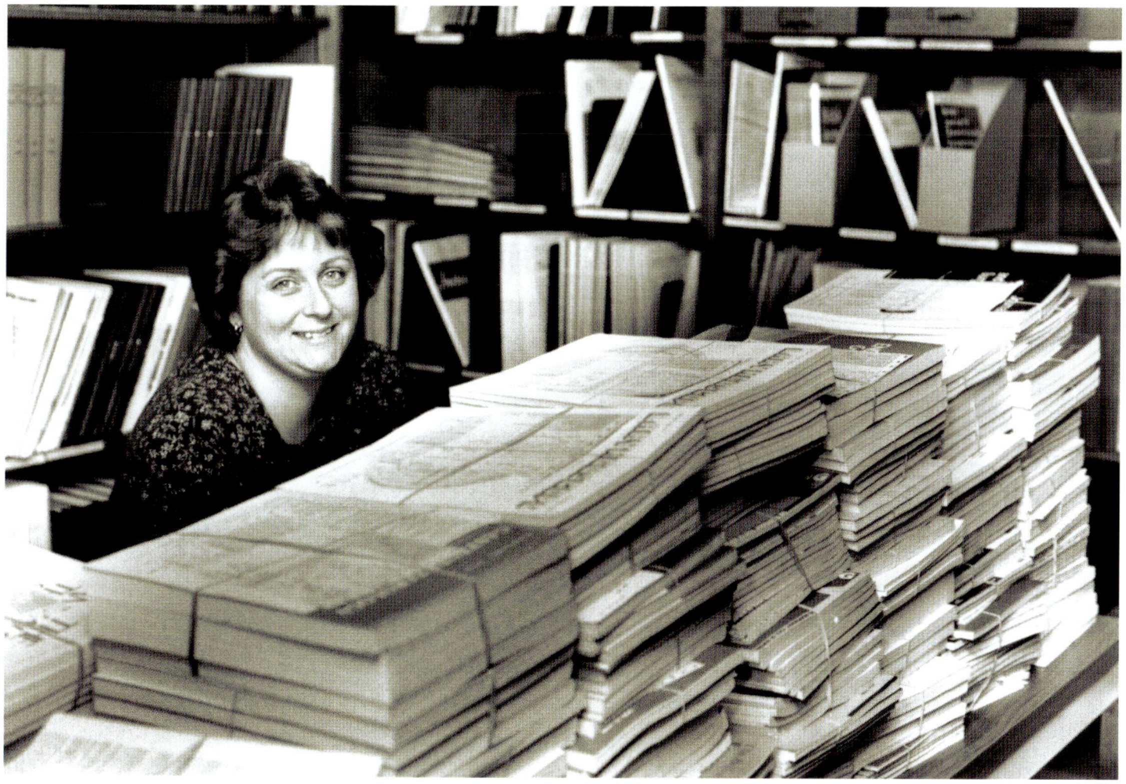

Pat Herndon, assistant librarian, processes a sea of newly arrived journals.

Center Auxiliary volunteers to create a Consumer Health Library, now known as the Family Resource Center. Originally located in the Wellness Center, it recently was moved to the new Women's Center and Surgery Center. The auxiliary has provided ongoing assistance to the facility including funding for special information resources. The Family Resource Center is free to patients, their families, and the public. The center contains a diverse selection of magazines, pamphlets, books, and videos, and its printouts of health information are available at no charge.[56] It provides information on health, wellness, illnesses, and other medical conditions.

In addition to its traditional information services, the staff of the Health Sciences Library has assumed two additional responsibilities. It now is in charge of the medical staff's continuing medical education (CME) program; and it has volunteered to offer a leadership role in archiving, managing, and making available documents that pertain to DeKalb Medical's history. The current staff of the Health Sciences Library and Continuing Medical Education include Marilyn G. Barry, director, Sharon Atkinson, information specialist, and Timothy Lammers, librarian.

Continuing Education

Continuing Medical Education

DeKalb Medical provides a wide variety of educational programs to its staff and physicians that include not only required assessment of their knowledge and skills but also enrichment opportunities to advance their knowledge and skills and to open new career opportunities.

In the hospital's early days, voluntary, service-specific educational opportunities occasionally were offered. In 1967 Benjamin Okel, MD, announced that DeKalb General's cardiologists were offering a course in coronary intensive care open to nurses and doctors every Wednesday night.[57] Stansell's O2 Service held an Inhalation Therapy Technical Conference every other Monday morning to which it invited interested employees and physicians.[58]

In 1970 the medical staff's Cancer Committee, chaired by Angier Wills, MD, established the first formal CME program for physicians and other health professionals when it instituted a tumor conference. The conference met twice a month, offered lectures on various cancer-related subjects, and presented complex and interesting cancer cases for discussion.[59]

In 1973 Chief of Staff LaMar McGinnis, MD, reported to the trustees that the medical staff wanted more CME.[60] John Harrel, MD, newly appointed director of Medical Affairs, subsequently established the Tuesday morning CME conference for physicians and other health professionals.[61] The Cancer Committee was responsible for the first Tuesday of each month, Emory School of Medicine professors presented lectures on the second and third Tuesdays, and a DeKalb General physician presented Ground Rounds every fourth Tuesday.[62] J. Willis Hurst, MD, chairman of Emory's Department of Medicine, was the first Emory speaker to present a lecture at DeKalb General's new Tuesday morning conference.[63]

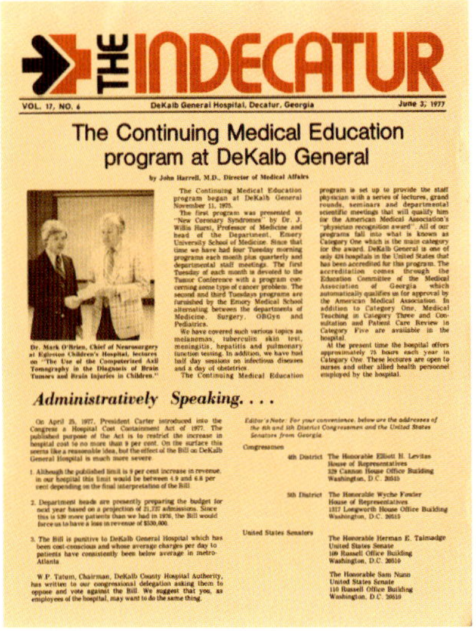
THE INDECATUR

VOL. 17, NO. 6 — DeKalb General Hospital, Decatur, Georgia — June 3, 1977

The Continuing Medical Education program at DeKalb General

by John Harrell, M.D., Director of Medical Affairs

Dr. Mark O'Brien, Chief of Neurosurgery at Egleston Children's Hospital, lectures on "The Use of the Computerized Axil Tomography in the Diagnosis of Brain Tumors and Brain Injuries in Children."

The Continuing Medical Education program began at DeKalb General November 11, 1975.

The first program was presented on "New Coronary Syndromes" by Dr. J. Willis Hurst, Professor of Medicine and head of the Department, Emory University School of Medicine. Since that time we have had four Tuesday morning programs each month plus quarterly and departmental staff meetings. The first Tuesday of each month is devoted to the Tumor Conference with a program concerning some type of cancer problem. The second and third Tuesdays programs are furnished by the Emory Medical School alternating between the departments of Medicine, Surgery, OBGyn and Pediatrics.

We have covered such various topics as melanomas, tuberculin skin test, meningitis, hepatitis and pulmonary function testing. In addition, we have had half day sessions on infectious diseases and a day of obstetrics.

The Continuing Medical Education program is set up to provide the staff physician with a series of lectures, grand rounds, seminars and departmental scientific meetings that will qualify him for the American Medical Association's "physician recognition award". All of our programs fall into what is known as Category One which is the main category for the award. DeKalb General is one of only 424 hospitals in the United States that has been accredited for this program. The accreditation comes through the Education Committee of the Medical Association of Georgia which automatically qualifies us for approval by the American Medical Association. In addition to Category One, Medical Teaching in Category Three and Consultation and Patient Care Review in Category Five are available in the hospital.

At the present time the hospital offers approximately 75 hours each year in Category One. These lectures are open to nurses and other allied health personnel employed by the hospital.

Administratively Speaking. . . .

On April 25, 1977, President Carter introduced into the Congress a Hospital Cost Containment Act of 1977. The published purpose of the Act is to restrict the increase in hospital cost to no more than 9 per cent. On the surface this seems like a reasonable idea, but the effect of the Bill on DeKalb General Hospital is much more severe.

1. Although the published limit is 9 per cent increase in revenue, in our hospital this limit would be between 4.9 and 6.8 per cent depending on the final interpretation of the Bill.

2. Department heads are presently preparing the budget for next year based on a projection of 21,737 admissions. Since this is 539 more patients than we had in 1976, the Bill would force us to have a loss in revenue of $530,000.

3. The Bill is punitive to DeKalb General Hospital which has been cost-conscious and whose average charges per day to patients have consistently been below average in metro-Atlanta.

W.P. Tatum, Chairman, DeKalb County Hospital Authority, has written to our congressional delegation asking them to oppose and vote against the Bill. We suggest that you, as employees of the hospital, may want to do the same thing.

Editor's Note: For your convenience, below are the addresses of the 4th and 5th District Congressmen and the United States Senators from Georgia.

Congressmen

4th District — The Honorable Elliott H. Levitas, House of Representatives, 329 Cannon House Office Building, Washington, D.C. 20515

5th District — The Honorable Wyche Fowler, House of Representatives, 1317 Longworth House Office Building, Washington, D.C. 20515

United States Senators

The Honorable Herman E. Talmadge, United States Senate, 109 Russell Office Building, Washington, D.C. 20510

The Honorable Sam Nunn, United States Senate, 110 Russell Office Building, Washington, D.C. 20510

In 1977, the *InDecatur* reports on the creation of a new Continuing Medical Education program at DeKalb General.

That format remained in place for fifteen years. Harrel's staff arranged for speakers. By the late 1980s, however, the DeKalb medical staff had grown not only in numbers but in expertise. Many highly trained physicians had joined the medical staff. The Medical Education Committee, chaired by Alex Parkinson, MD, decided it was time to take a new approach to the Tuesday conference. The Cancer Committee would continue being responsible for the first Tuesday morning, but members of the Medical Education Committee assumed responsibility for the remaining sessions. The committee as a whole agreed on a range of topics to be presented, and members of the committee invited DeKalb physicians to present topics in their area of expertise or special interest. The response was overwhelming. Attendance grew so that frequently there was standing room only in the auditorium. Parkinson's committee not only provided substantive information, but it also introduced the medical community to the competence and expertise of the physician presenters.

In addition to the Tuesday morning conferences, a number of monthly, lunchtime specialty conferences emerged, such as endocrinology, cardiology, dermatology, and neurology. Currently fifteen specialty conferences are held each month.[64] In addition, physicians now can participate in individualized, practice-based learning experiences that are accredited by the American Medical Association. One such format is Performance Improvement CME, through which a physician may demonstrate improvements in selected practice processes involving the physician's own practice.[65]

Marilyn Barry, Health Sciences Library director, currently has responsibility for the administration of DeKalb Medical's CME program. Since its inception, it has received successive three-year accreditations by the Education Committee of the Medical Association of Georgia, including "accreditation with commendation" on its most recent survey.[66]

Other Continuing Education Opportunities

In addition to its continuing medical education activities, DeKalb Medical has made available to its staff and physicians a number of other educational opportunities. Among these, in the early 1970s, DeKalb General joined Emory University Hospital, Northside Hospital, and DeKalb Community College in providing a nine-month course in Operating Room Technology to prepare students for service in the operating room.[67]

DeKalb Medical's Education Assistance Program encourages staff to pursue educational opportunities that improve their job-related skills and competence. Qualifying programs may include hospital business or healthcare–related diploma or degree programs offered by an accredited university, college, or vocational/technical schools. In 1976 the hospital reimbursed up to $250 in educational expenditures per year to those who had been employed at least six months and who successfully completed an approved course of study.[68] In 1978 that amount was increased to $400 per year, and in 2001 it was increased to $2,400 per year for full-time employees and $1,200 per year for part-time employees.[69]

Beginning in the early 1980s, many DeKalb staff members received a bachelor of science and health degree from the College of St. Francis located in Joliet, Illinois, through classes offered on-campus at the hospital.[70] In 1991 St. Francis expanded its program to offer a nine-semester master of science degree in healthcare administration.[71]

In 1997 DeKalb Medical Center contracted with Mercer University to offer an on-campus master's degree in business administration. DeKalb paid a portion of the tuition for any physician or staff member who successfully completed the program. In May 1999 fifteen DeKalb Medical staff members and four physicians received their master's degree. One of the recipients, Chief of Staff Sanford Hartman, MD, wrote the following farewell poem for his classmates:

Things looked extremely hopeful as we began this trek,
They told us there'd be lots of work, but we said, "What the heck!"
They told us "You'll spend hours in class then more hours at home;
There'll be no time for sports or fun, there'll be no time to roam.
For every hour you spend in class, you spend twice that outside;
The homework will at times give you the thought you wish you'd died.

Accounting, Econ, Ethics and Management they taught,
Statistics, Finance, Marketing gave knowledge that we sought.
Decision Theory, Info Systems, Managed Care, and Law,
International Management and Capstone we saw.
We learned, we wrote, we met in groups, we all became adept.
We spoke and we computed, and some in the class they slept.

I thank you for everything, it's almost sad to part.
I thank you from my inner depths, I thank you from my heart.[72]

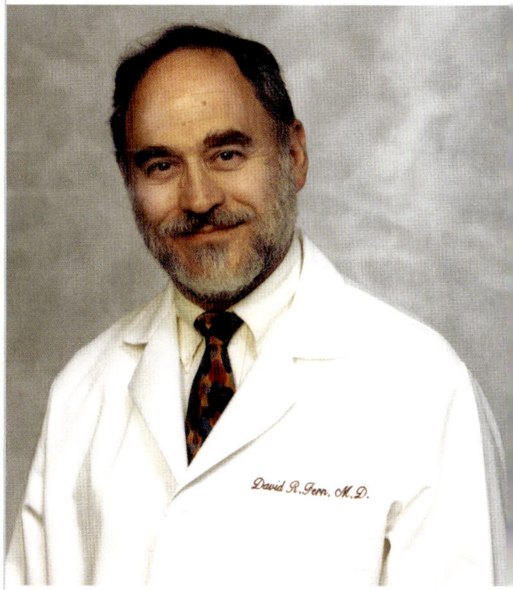

In 1999, Chief of Staff Sanford Hartman, MD, wrote a farewell poem to his classmates upon completing an on-campus master's degree in business administration.

Conclusion

The evolution and growth of DeKalb Medical's education services reflect the acknowledgment and commitment of governance and management to Peter Senge's thesis that a vital organization must be a learning organization. The demands on staff, physicians, and the institution imposed by increasingly complex technology; the increasing demands of regulatory agencies, third-party payers, and the public; the ever-changing understanding of disease, its prevention, and its treatment; and the need to discover better ways to achieve health and wellness all call for a continued dynamic, informed, and integrated emphasis on continuing education to which DeKalb Medical is committed.

Emergency Services

The rapid growth of the Emergency Department, the surprisingly major role of its services, and the need to establish full-time physician coverage with the DeKalb Emergency Group (DEG) was described in chapter 3, "A Decade of Growth and Challenges." Providing adequate physician staffing proved to be a continuing challenge. Initially the patient volume required only one DEG physician per shift. Even then, the lone physician on the night shift often was free to retire to the "sleep room" for two or three hours' rest. That privilege, however, was short-lived. Soon each physician shift required doubling, and then tripling, the number of doctors on duty. By the mid-1990s, the department included fourteen full-time physicians, six part-time physicians, and six physician assistants, plus a growing number of nurses, clerical staff, and volunteers.

A contributing factor to DeKalb's expanding load of emergency patients was Emory Hospital's decision to close its emergency department in 1972.[1] Most of Emory's emergency patients came to DeKalb General. One of those patients happened to be the dean of the Emory School of Medicine who sustained a dog bite and, to his chagrin at having to go elsewhere for his care, resorted to being treated at DeKalb's Emergency Department.

Freeman Simmons, MD, served as chief of the DEG and medical director of the Emergency Room from 1965 to 1973. He was followed by Tom Lowry, MD, (1973–1979), Patrick O'Neal, MD, (1979–

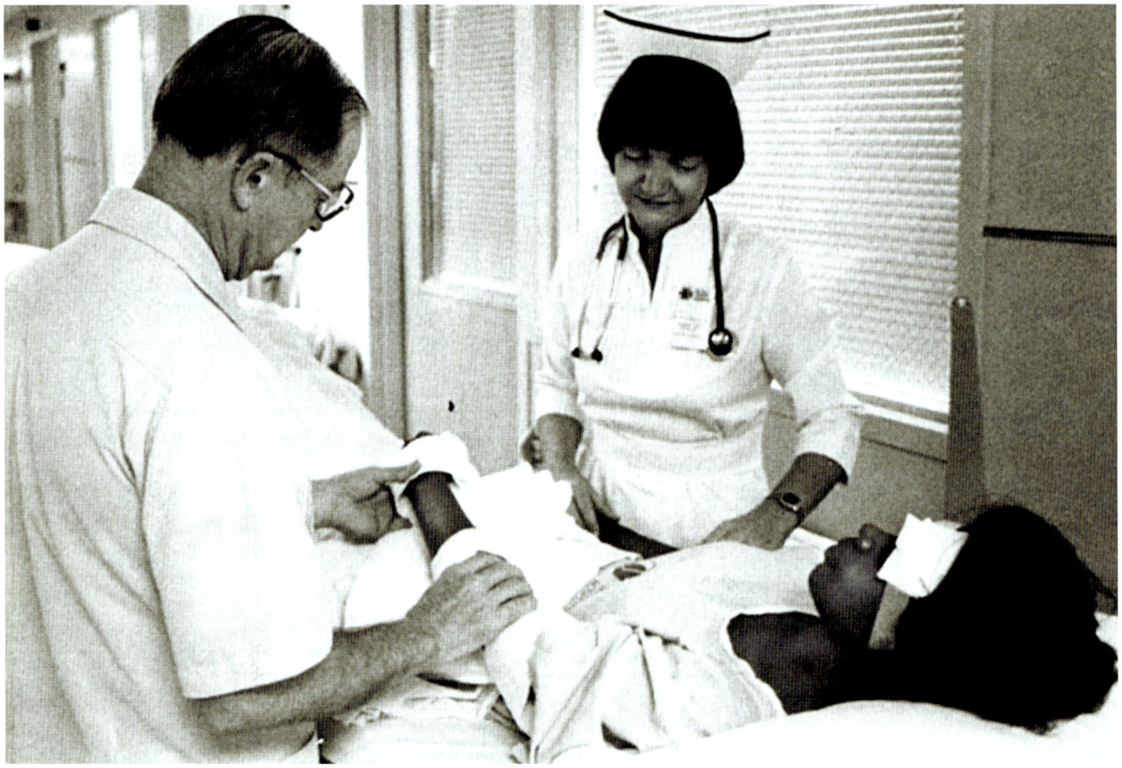

Freeman Simmons, MD, chief of DeKalb Emergency Group and medical director of the Emergency Department, assesses a patient in the emergency room with Donna Lewellyn, RN, emergency room manager.

1983 and 1986–2002),[2] David Carson, MD, (1983–1986),[3] and Steve Holbrook, MD, (2002–2006).[4] In 2006 Paschal Crosby, MD, was named medical director of the Emergency Department at the North Decatur campus and Gail Matthews, MD, became medical director of the department at Hillandale.[5]

In the nursing leadership, Mary Hollis, RN, was named director of Emergency Services in 1969,[6] and she was followed by Deborah Whelchel, RN, in 1991.[7] Frankie Jackson, RN, became the director of the department in 1990,[8] and Patricia Horton was named administrative director of Critical Care and Emergency Services in 1995.[9]

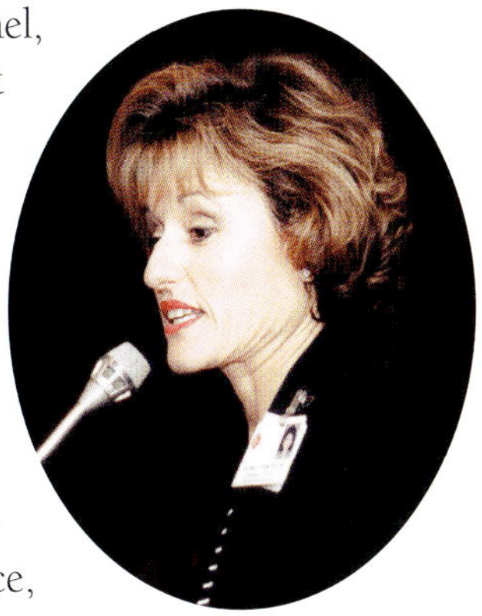

Patrick O'Neal took a leave of absence in 1983 as chief of DEG and medical director of the department to explore the need and opportunities for American physicians in Saudi Arabia. He was consultant to the first Saudi Trauma Center at King Fahd Hospital in Rizadh, Saudi Arabia.[10] He quickly decided he was needed back in Georgia, however, when an American obstetrician from Chicago and a British surgeon were apprehended with alcohol by the Mutaween religious police, severely beaten, and thrown in jail before being shipped back to their respective countries.[11]

The DEG worked as contract physicians for thirty years. In 1995 DeKalb Medical Center made Emergency Department physicians hospital employees.[12] In 2005, however, the hospital resumed a contract relationship[13] and selected California Emergency Physicians Medical Group to provide medical management for the emergency departments at the North Decatur and Hillandale hospitals.[14]

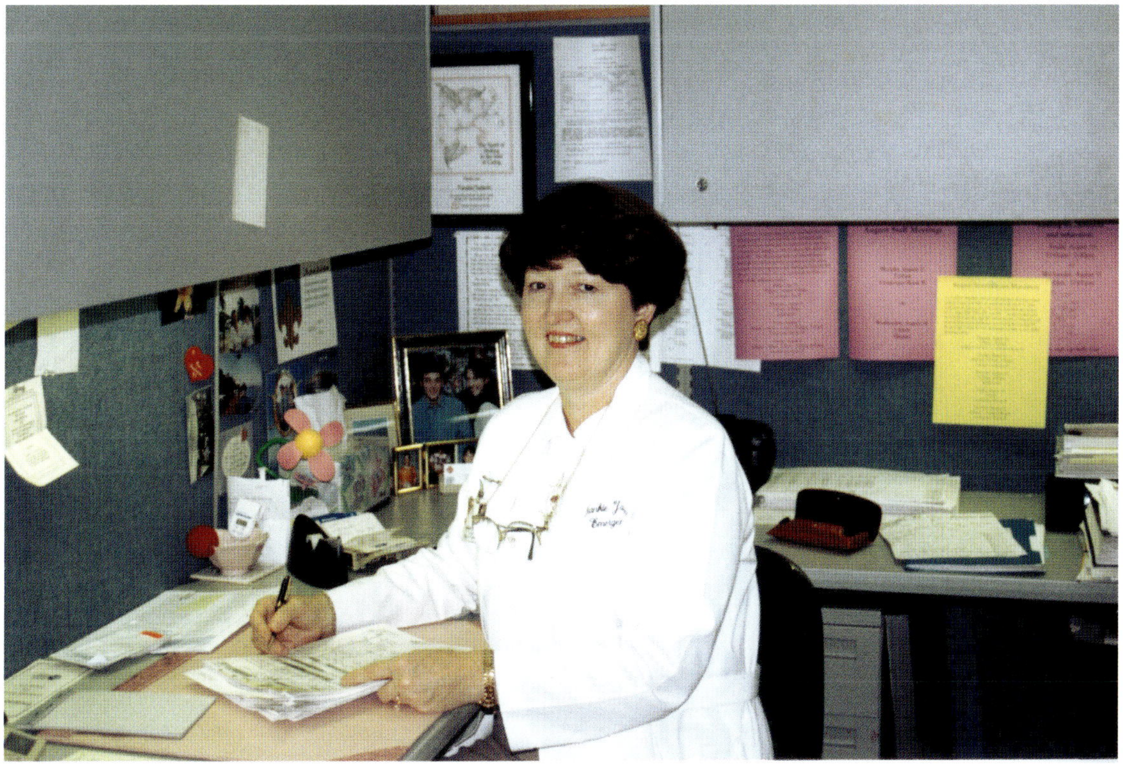

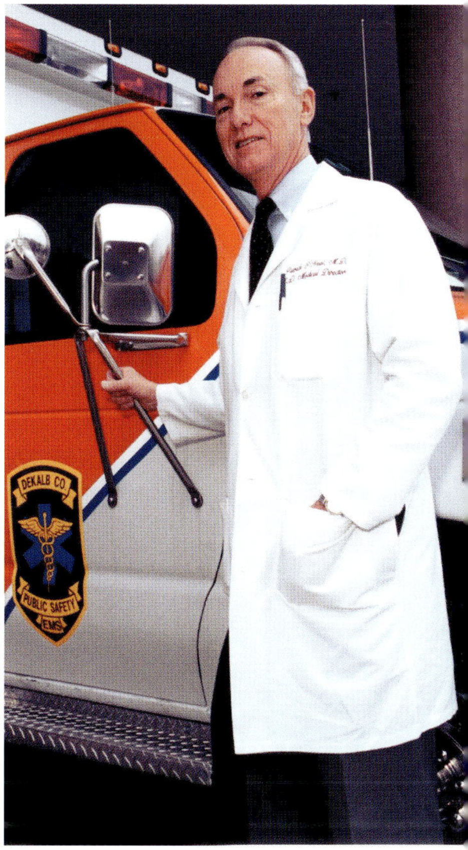

Above: Patrick O'Neal, MD, was the third chief of the DeKalb Emergency Group and medical director of the Emergency Department. **Above left:** Patricia Horton, RN, was named administrative director of Critical Care and Emergency Services in 1995. **Left:** In 1990 Frankie Jackson, RN, became director of the Emergency Department.

In addition to needing a larger staff to handle the growing patient volume, the Emergency Department needed more space. In its first decade, the department saw more than four thousand patients a month,[15] and the hospital doubled the department's space with the major expansion of 1971. Given its expanded space and enlarged scope of services, in 1973 its name was officially changed from "Emergency Room" to "Emergency Department."

In 1975 the hospital enlarged the entrance to the Emergency Department with a new ramp and a canopy that accommodated as many as eight vehicles at a time. The enlarged entrance was used to discharge inpatients and to facilitate a more efficient entrance and exit for emergency patients.[16]

The enlarged facility soon proved inadequate once again. By the early 1990s, the annual emergency patient volume grew to 55,000,[17] and within another five years it reached 74,000.[18] The medical severity of patients also increased. Critical emergency patients who presented for care increased from a ratio of one in ten to one in every five patients.[19]

In 1975 the hospital added a new canopy and ramp to the entrance of the Emergency Department to more easily accommodate patients arriving and leaving.

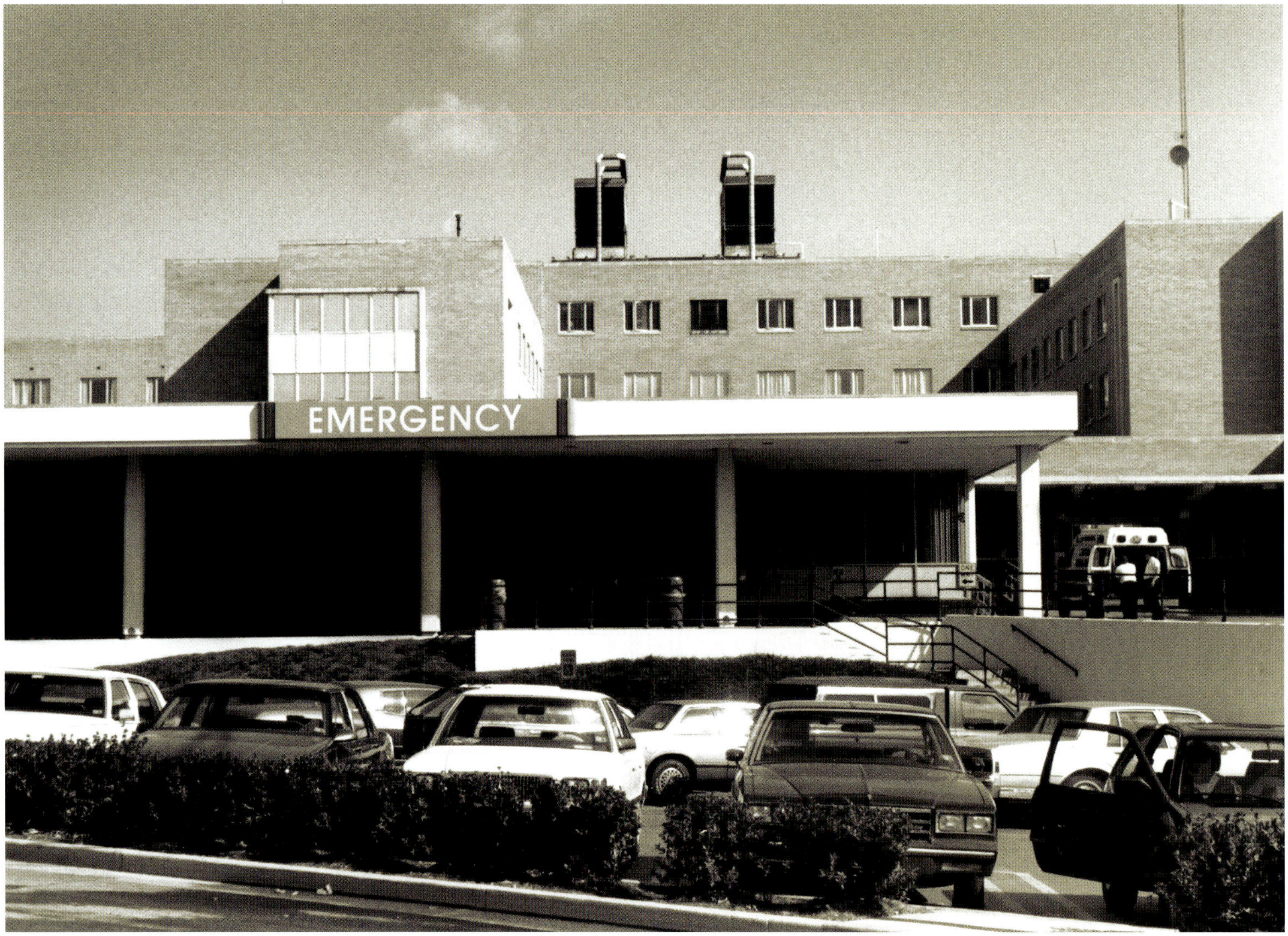

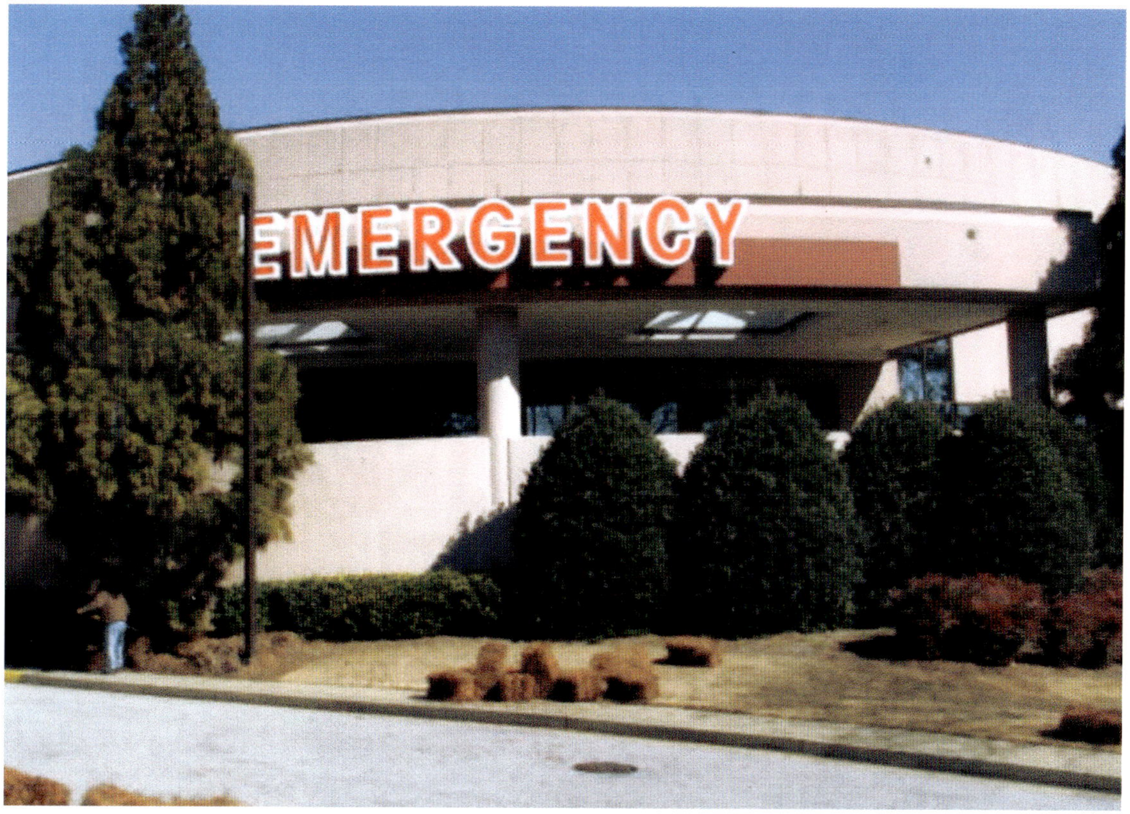

In 1995, the hospital enlarged its Emergency Department to 22,000 square feet, tripling its size. The addition also included an on-site laboratory and radiology rooms.

In 1995 the hospital began a 70,000-square-foot, $11.5 million project that included additions to the Emergency Department, the combined Intensive Care Unit (ICU) and Coronary Care Unit (CCU), and the Diagnostic and Treatment Center (DTC). It gave the Emergency Department 22,000 square feet of new space and 6,000 square feet of renovated space to triple its size. The enlarged department contained thirty-two patient rooms, eleven of which were for the more serious trauma and chest pain patients, three rooms for pediatric patients, three specially equipped for sexual assault patients, and seven for patients with minor emergencies and illnesses.[20] It also had an on-site laboratory and radiology rooms. The new Emergency Department opened in the fall of 1996.

Despite the enlarged staff and facility, long waiting times and a backlog of patients to be seen or admitted to the hospital were still common. There were three underlying causes. First, the Emergency Department was often crowded with nonemergency patients. Second, many patients came to the Emergency Department to meet with their private physicians, especially after physician office hours. Finally there were patients who needed to be hospitalized but had no doctor or none that was on the hospital's medical staff. In these cases, doctors had to be located to assume management—including admission—of these patients. Emergency physicians were not permitted to admit patients to the hospital.

The hospital and Emergency Department initiated three solutions to address those crowded conditions. First, the hospital constructed and equipped the Diagnostic and Treatment Center (DTC), where private physicians and emergency physicians could see, evaluate, and manage nonemergent patients without utilizing Emergency Department space and resources.[21] Next, it established a Fast Track program (later known as the Care Center) for nonurgent patients with minor medical problems.

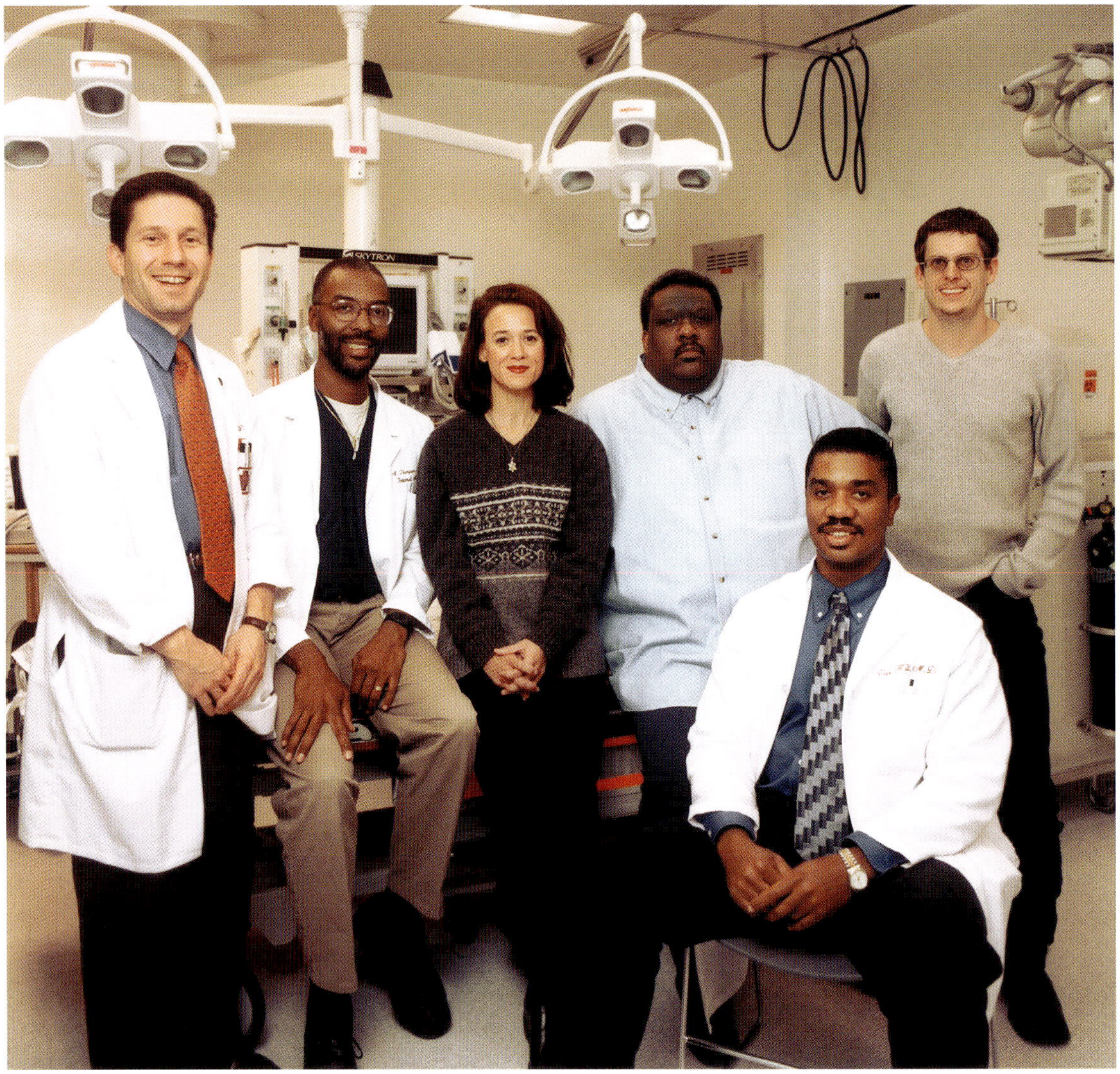

DeKalb Medical Center's Medical Emergency Associates (MEAs), the first hospitalists in the state of Georgia. Left to right: Robert Holloway, MD, Michael Thompson, MD, Stacy Goldsholl, MD, Kirk Brown, MD, Van Hill, MD, and Scott Steinbach, MD.

The department designated rooms for the Fast Track and assigned staff nurses and physician assistants under the supervision of emergency physicians to see and manage those patients. The Fast Track staff endeavored to see, treat, and discharge patients within sixty minutes.[22] Finally, the hospital contracted with four board-certified internists to be the Medical Emergency Associates (MEAs), later known as "hospitalists," to see, admit, and manage patients who had no physician or none on the medical staff.[23] Robert Holloway, MD, was chief of the MEAs.[24] Those three initiatives significantly improved the Emergency Department's ability to see patients with urgent and emergency conditions in a more timely and efficient manner.

In addition to improving the timeliness and efficiency of care, the Emergency Department undertook three other initiatives to enhance the scope and quality of its service. Those three initiatives included the establishment of the DeKalb Rape Crisis Center, creation of the Chest Pain Center, and designation of the department as a Level 3 Trauma Center.

The DeKalb Rape Crisis Center

Of all the patients who came to the Emergency Department, none were more challenging than the victims of sexual assault. They came with critical physical, medical, emotional, and legal needs, all of which required simultaneous attention and skilled care. Each patient also presented a public safety concern, requiring the proper collection, preservation, and transmittal of criminal evidence associated with the assault. They needed physicians and nurses with special interest, sensitivity, training, skill, and experience, and they needed a support staff capable of participating appropriately in their care.

Traditionally most DeKalb County sexual assault victims went to Grady Memorial Hospital's emergency department. In 1987 Sue Ellen Mears, chairman of the DeKalb County Rape Crisis Task Force, asked DeKalb General Hospital to participate in discussions as to how the community's rape victims could be served more appropriately.[25] The DeKalb Junior League, the Decatur Cooperative Ministry, the DeKalb Medical Society, and the local press all endorsed the need to provide better local service to those individuals.[26]

The Task Force struggled for three years with the complexities of establishing a workable program. Finally, in 1990, in spite of objections, concerns, and resistance from various quarters, the DeKalb County Hospital Authority approved Administrator Charles Eberhart's recommendation that DeKalb Medical Center's Emergency Department serve as the site for the DeKalb County Rape Crisis Center.

The DeKalb Junior League recruited and trained volunteers to counsel and support victims of sexual assault. The DeKalb County Rape Crisis Task Force contracted with obstetricians, family physicians, and internists to be trained in the proper care of these patients. The DeKalb Medical Center Auxiliary donated $50,000 to help establish the service.[27] The DeKalb Rape Crisis Center at DeKalb General Hospital officially opened on July 1, 1990.[28]

The DeKalb County Rape Crisis Task Force gradually expanded its services not only to include the care of those presenting with sexual assault but also to be a crisis counseling service with a hotline, individual and group therapy, follow-up care, and community education.[29]

The Rape Crisis Center attended to nearly six thousand sexual assault survivors in its first fifteen years.[30] Its success was the result of volunteers and a staff that was committed to this important service. The center honored physician assistant Jo Stearns for her service and dedication that included volunteering as an expert witness; training more than eight hundred volunteer crisis advocates, physicians, and nurses; and providing her own care and support to sexual-assault survivors.[31]

The Chest Pain Center

While the victims of rape and sexual assault were among the most challenging patients presenting to the Emergency Department, those presenting with chest pain were among the most critical. The proper diagnosis and management often meant the difference between life and death. And the patients are many. DeKalb's Emergency Department sees more than 2,500 chest pain patients each year.[32]

In 1991 emergency physicians, cardiologists, other physicians, hospital staff, and administration formed a task force to assess the current management of chest pain patients, look at existing best practices, and devise a plan to make the Emergency Department's management equal to or better than the best currently available anywhere. The task force identified five requirements: (1) establish a Chest Pain Center in the Emergency Department with space, equipment, and trained personnel to provide appropriate care;[33] (2) devise protocols (care maps) based on the best-known practices for optimal care; (3) educate the public on proper response to chest pain; (4) involve Emergency Medical Service (EMS) in the development of protocols and their role in them; and (5) enroll the Chest Pain Center in a major clinical trial program to assess the effectiveness of the center's chest pain management.

The task force created management protocols that focused on two significant aspects of caring for confirmed heart attacks. The first was to provide appropriate patients with thrombolytic ("clot buster") medication capable of dissolving the blockage in the heart's blood vessels. The second was to provide those drugs early when they were indicated. It had been demonstrated that the first hour after a heart attack occurs was "the golden hour" when best results are achieved.

To assess the effectiveness of DeKalb's management of chest pain patients, the task force enrolled in a prominent international study that was evaluating the use of thrombolytic agents. During one period of time, DeKalb's Chest Pain Center treated more heart attack patients than any hospital in Georgia and ranked fifth in the nation.[34] The Chest Pain Center not only enhanced the Emergency Department's prestige and its quality and scope of services, but also enhanced one of its most vital services to the community.

A Level 3 Trauma Center

DeKalb Medical's third initiative to enhance the scope and quality of its emergency services was to enroll in the Georgia Trauma Network as a Level 3 Trauma Center.

Trauma centers are assigned a numerical level according to their ability to provide prescribed resources as required by the American College of Surgeons. Level 1 trauma centers are at the highest level of trauma care and must have the ability to perform open-heart cardiac surgery; must have in-house emergency, anesthesia, and general surgery services; and must have immediately available a wide variety of major surgical and nonsurgical specialists. Level 2 trauma centers must have in-house emergency, anesthesia services, and a general surgery trauma team; and must have on-call other major surgical specialties available to respond within a short time to a trauma alert. Level 3 trauma centers must have a dedicated team of trauma surgeons capable of being at the injured patient's bedside within twenty minutes; in-house anesthesia services and emergency physicians capable of managing the injured patient until the trauma surgeon arrives; and specialists such as orthopedists, neurosurgeons, thoracic surgeons, and plastic surgeons on call as needed.

In 1969 the Fulton County Medical Society asked DeKalb General Hospital if it wished to be listed in a directory as a hospital willing to handle multiple trauma cases. DeKalb replied that, even though its volume of trauma cases was second only to Grady Memorial Hospital, it had to decline because it was in the midst of a major expansion project and recovering from a mass resignation of nurses. It was not in a position at that time to solicit more trauma cases.[35]

In 1974 Congress passed the Emergency Medical Services Act and the Georgia General Assembly established the state's Office of Emergency Medicine/Trauma.[36] In 1985 DeKalb General considered becoming a trauma center.[37] Administration was in favor,[38] but the Department of Surgery and the Medical Staff Executive Committee said the time was not right.[39] The Authority agreed with the doctors.[40]

In 1988 the state's trauma network was in jeopardy and nearing collapse.[41] Like DeKalb, other hospitals around the state had declined to become trauma centers. The state put out a call for hospitals to reconsider and come to the trauma network's rescue. Despite persistant reluctance on the part of many members of the medical staff, DeKalb decided to join.[42] Providing enhanced trauma care clearly was a needed community service, and the hospital was at risk of losing patients and revenue if it did not become a part of the state's trauma network.

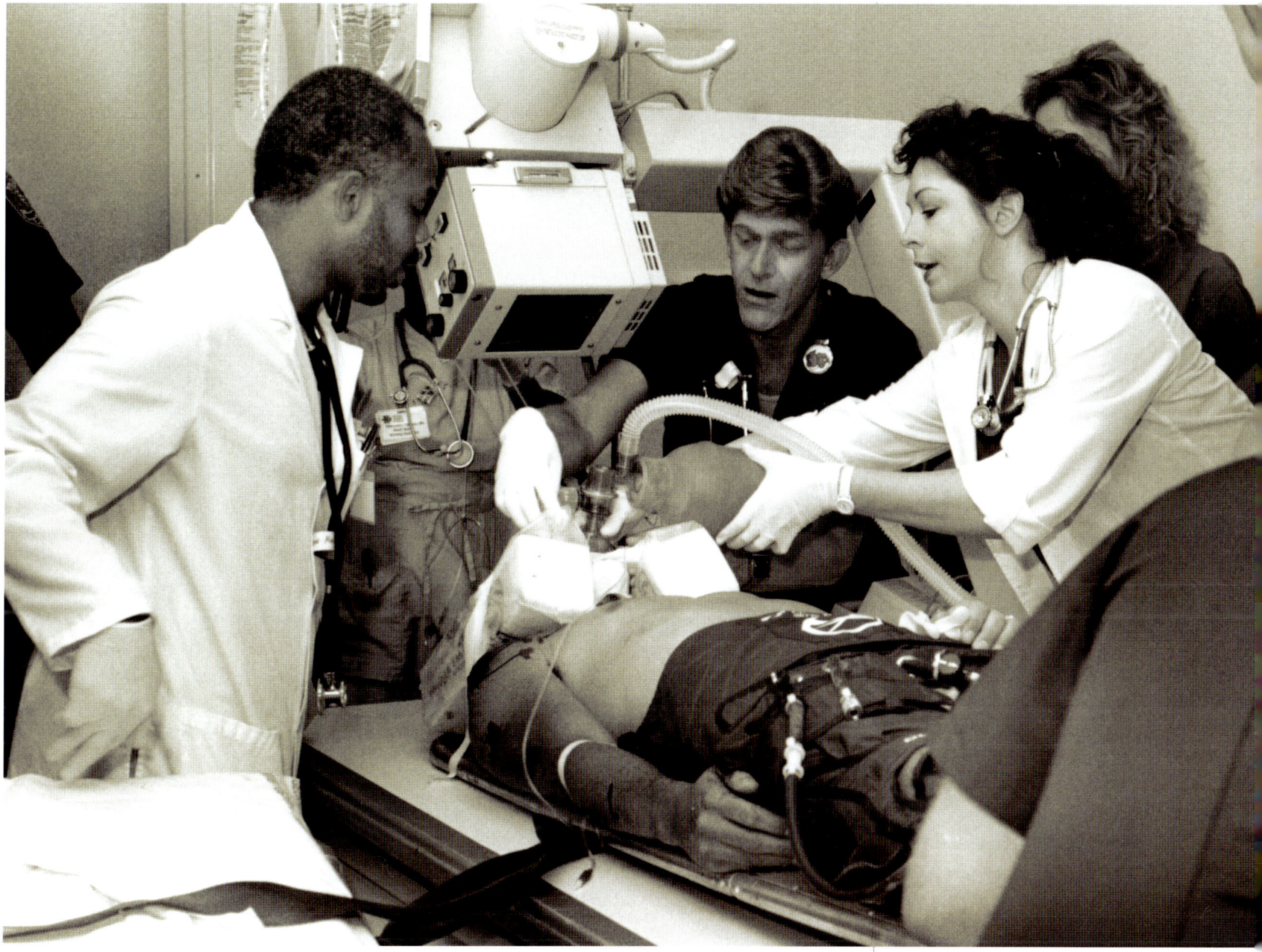

Emergency staff attending to a trauma patient, left to right: Leon Martin, MD, Rick Tillman, RT, and June Shephard, CRT.

Approximately one third of all the patients admitted to the hospital entered through the Emergency Department. Most were transported by the DeKalb Emergency Medical Service (EMS). In fact, DeKalb General Hospital received a majority of EMS-transported patients because the hospital was both the county's triage center and the medical control center for EMS.[43] If another hospital became the area's designated trauma center, DeKalb General stood to lose both of those ties with the DeKalb EMS and subsequently could lose many of the patients the EMS traditionally brought to the hospital.[44] Those patients were an important source of revenue not only for the hospital but for its physicians.

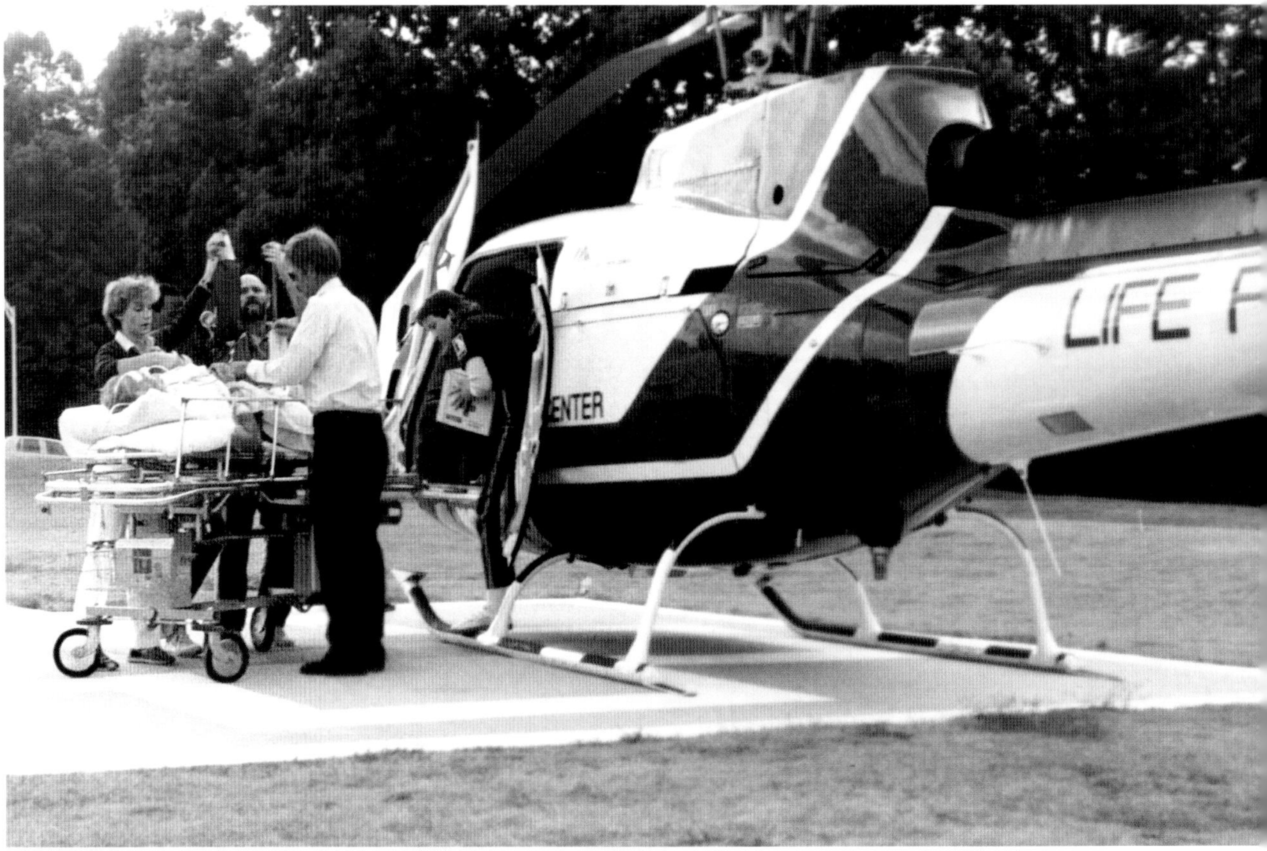

An emergency patient arrives by helicopter.

In November 1989 DeKalb Medical Center (the hospital now having a new name) signed a contract with the state trauma network to become a Level 3 Trauma Center.[45] The hospital enlisted seven of its general surgeons to form a trauma team.[46] The surgeons agreed not to schedule elective surgery the day they were on call so that they could be immediately available to see and manage trauma patients. William Hardcastle, MD, was named medical director and Kelly Nadeau, RN, coordinator of the Trauma Center.[47]

DeKalb Medical Center became one of fourteen trauma centers in the state. There were four Level 1 centers (Grady Memorial Hospital in Atlanta, Medical Center of Central Georgia in Macon, Medical College of Georgia in Augusta, and Memorial Health University Medical Center in Savannah), nine Level 2 centers (Atlanta Medical Center, Gwinnett Medical Center, and North Fulton Regional Hospital in the metropolitan Atlanta area and six others across the state), two pediatric centers (Children's Healthcare of Atlanta at Egleston and Scottish Rite), and one Level 3 center (DeKalb Medical Center).[48] On several occasions DeKalb considered applying for Level 2 status but elected to remain at a Level 3.[49]

Out of 75,000 emergency department patients in 2003, 1,135 were injured patients and 448 of those were serious enough to be classified as trauma patients.[50] Most were brought to the hospital by the DeKalb EMS,[51] and a fifth of the trauma patients required immediate surgery.[52] Nearly half of the patients required an orthopedist, 32 percent needed a neurosurgeon, 10 percent saw a plastic surgeon, and 12 percent were in need of other subspecialists.[53]

DeKalb's trauma center provided excellent care, but it faced numerous problems. Specialists contended they experienced significant financial losses in providing care to trauma patients because of the large number without insurance or the ability to pay for their care.[54] The hospital struggled with an equitable way to reimburse participating physicians, but it was difficult to reach an acceptable solution, especially with the neurosurgeons. A neurosurgical group that had been on the medical staff since 1963 elected to change its medical staff status from the "active" to "courtesy" category, a change in category that exempted it from emergency duty. The group eventually resigned from the staff.[55] Efforts to recruit replacement neurosurgeons or to work out neurosurgical coverage with other hospitals proved difficult.[56] Other specialists also withdrew from providing emergency coverage.

The hospital was frequently on trauma diversion, which meant the DeKalb EMS had to transport trauma patients to other hospitals. When appropriate specialty coverage was not available, or when necessary facilities such as ICU beds were not available, diversion was activated. The situation reached the point that at times the hospital was on trauma diversion as much as twenty-two days out of the month.[57]

DeKalb's trauma service, as well as that at most other hospitals, experienced steadily climbing financial losses. Nearly 35 percent of DeKalb's trauma patients had no insurance, and many of them lacked the financial resources to pay out-of-pocket for their care.[58] Already experiencing millions in a net operating loss in fiscal year 2006 and the possibility of a greater loss in fiscal year 2007, DeKalb Medical faced the difficult decision of how it could best allocate its resources to meet its commitment to provide health services to the community.[59] Georgia's Governor Perdue and the state legislature promised to deliver substantial financial support to the hospitals in the state's trauma network. Those promises, however, were subject to many contingencies and uncertainties. Even if the promise was honored, as only a Level 3 center, DeKalb stood to receive only a small share of the funds.

The board of directors considered several options,[60] appointed a committee to evaluate these and other options,[61] and engaged consultants to report back to the board with its recommendations. The board voted in March 2007 not to renew the hospital's contract with the state trauma network after June 30.[62] It negotiated a revised compensation agreement with a team of general surgeons to take first call for future trauma cases coming to the Emergency Department.

The state's remaining trauma centers awaited with great concern to see if the state's lawmakers would deliver on their promise to rescue the state's trauma network from possible collapse. To withdraw from the network was a difficult decision that DeKalb Medical felt it had to make.

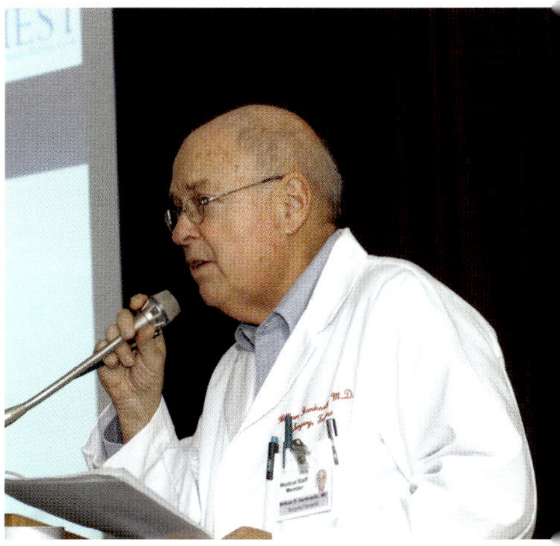

William Hardcastle, MD, medical director of the Trauma Center and chief of staff 2002–2004.

Conclusion

It was anticipated that DeKalb General Hospital's "Emergency Room" would play a peripheral, minor role in DeKalb's services when the hospital opened in 1961. But the Emergency Department rapidly emerged as one of the most identifiable capstones of the institution. It has been one of the main gates through which the community has entered DeKalb Medical. It has become one of the institution's most important facilities and services. Providing emergency services has not been simple or easy. It has been a complex task that carried with it enormous challenges of staffing, space, technology, competency, efficiency, liability, cost, and public relations. It has demanded unlimited attention, energy, creativity, commitment, and resources. It has received just that from volunteers, staff, physicians, management, and governing bodies. It has been a team effort of the highest order and has produced care of the highest quality. But "the beat goes on," and the challenges and demands remain present and unrelenting.

Home Health Services

In 1967 the DeKalb County Hospital Authority's long-range plan stated that "home health services should be developed."[1] It was not until 1985, however, that the hospital negotiated an affiliation agreement with DeKalb Home Health Agency and with Community Nurses' Service to provide home health services for the hospital's discharged patients who needed follow-up home care.[2] That arrangement soon ran into difficulties. The Home Health Agency was to share a portion of its profits with the hospital. The agency failed to pay DeKalb General anything for more than a year and asked the hospital to change the terms of the contract. The Authority said the agency had to pay the $62,000 it owed before there would be any discussions about modifying the contract.[3] The two parties reached an impasse, and that home health service arrangement ended in 1988.

In 1993 the DeKalb Regional Healthcare System (DRHS) Board of Directors discussed acquiring its own home health service.[4] In 1997 it purchased the Atlanta-based CareSouth and the Macon-based CareSouth Home Health Services.[5] The Atlanta-based company was a Medicare-certified home health agency, and the Macon-based company was a specialty ancillary home health agency licensed to provide infusion therapy, private-duty nursing, respiratory care, hospice services, and medical equipment.[6]

DRHS established the new agency as a for-profit subsidiary, named it the DeKalb Medical Home Care Services, and contracted with CareSouth to manage it.[7] In 1998 DRHS sold half interest in the agency to Southern Regional Healthcare System and changed the name to Atlanta Home Care Services.[8]

DRHS expected the agency to provide patients with a high level of home care and provide the system with revenue.[9] DeKalb Medical Center had referred approximately one thousand discharged patients to other home health agencies during the previous year. The new DRHS agency could serve those patients and accept referrals from other sources. It was projected to make more than fifty thousand patient visits during the first year.[10]

Its financial performance, however, was disappointing. In the first nine months, the gross revenue was more than 50 percent below budget and the net operating income 225 percent below budget.[11] DRHS also was dissatisfied with the quality of CareSouth's management service.[12] In August 2000 the DRHS Board of Directors voted to close Atlanta Health Care Services,[13] sold the equipment and pharmacy components, and terminated the business in December 2000.[14]

DeKalb Medical Center subsequently established its own home health department, and Joyce Osborne, RN, was named director and clinical manager.[15] It had a staff of thirty-eight employees that included registered nurses, physical therapists, occupational therapists, speech therapists, medical social workers, certified home health aides, and a certified wound/ostomy/continence nurse. Physicians could order home services that included wound care, cognitive skills training, diabetes monitoring and management, diet and nutritional education, enteral nutrition, rehabilitation services, and infusion therapy. The program had an average daily census of 145 patients.[16]

In October 2007 DRHS signed a preferred-provider agreement with Visiting Nurse Health Systems of Atlanta (VNHS) that served twenty-six counties.[17] DRHS retained its home health service

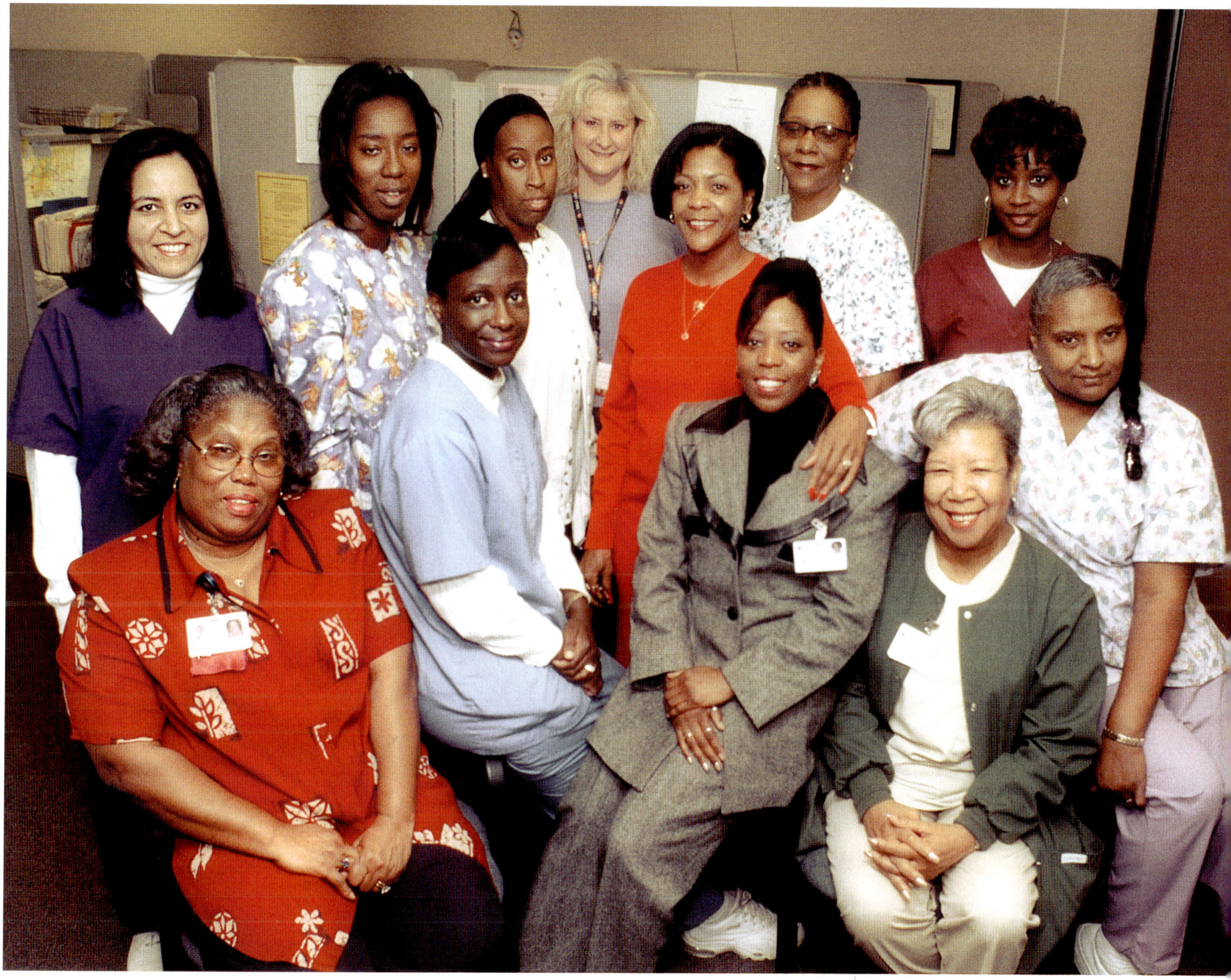

certificate of need (CON) but outsourced management of the home health service and staff to VNHS. VNHS named Joyce Osborne to be its full-time manager to facilitate discharge planning for those patients. VNHS agreed to accept referral of all patients, regardless of payer class, who had no other preference or who were not required by their insurer to use another service.[18] This arrangement appears to be working well for the hospital system and the community.

The Home Health staff in 2002.

INFORMATION TECHNOLOGY

DeKalb General Hospital opened in 1961 more technologically advanced than most hospitals in the area—-it had an IBM data processing system in the business office with hole-punched cards. Within a year, however, processing and storing nonclinical information became a challenge, and the business office looked to microfilming as a solution. Microfilming equipment was purchased after the DeKalb County Hospital Authority Finance Committee in its 1965–1966 annual report stated:

> *The matter of storage is becoming more critical every day . . . . The initial investment in [microfilming] equipment to move into this area would probably be $2,000. . . . If we do not begin microfilming, the storage space needed for records will cost considerably more than microfilming equipment.*[1]

A few months later the hospital took another technological step forward when Administrator William Thrasher announced that he was buying a small computer for the business office.[2] He "asked for physician patience while the bugs were being worked out."[3] The business office computer, however, did not perform as Thrasher expected, and he returned it. Pathologist Frank Matthews, MD, said "his

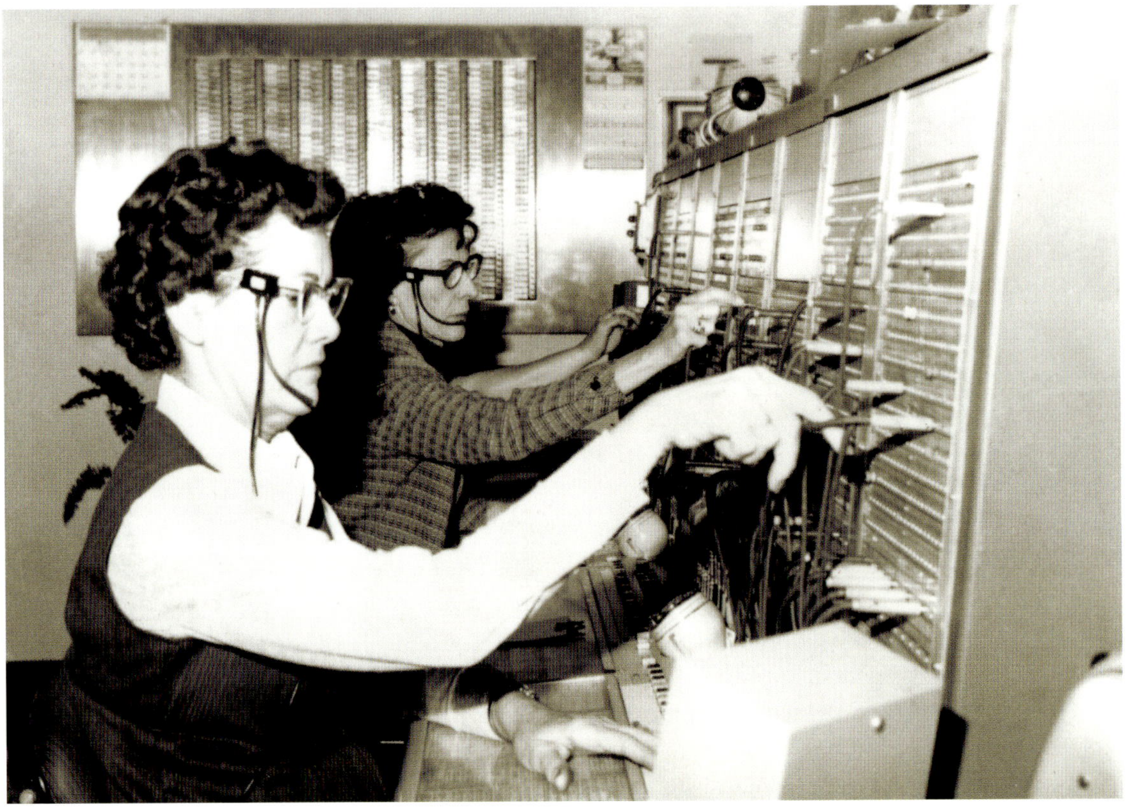

Margie Conoly and Eileen Ensor connect calls on an early switchboard system at the hospital.

department [the Laboratory] regretted that the hospital had given up its computer." He said that the Laboratory would utilize a computer if the hospital would finance the $3,000 cost.[4]

Disappointed in its first computer, DeKalb General participated in a "shared computer system among hospitals in Georgia."[5] In 1971 it joined the Georgia Hospitals Computer Group that included hospitals in Atlanta and others around the state as far away as Statesboro and Valdosta in south Georgia. The hospitals shared an IBM 360 Model 40 that printed paychecks, performed inpatient daily billing, recorded average daily census, and kept other statistics.[6] The need for DeKalb General to have its own computer prevailed, however, and later in 1971 the hospital purchased another computer for the business office for $70,250.[7]

Within two years DeKalb General began looking for a major system, separate from the financial system, to handle admissions and transfer data. It needed a system to improve the speed and efficiency of admitting patients, communicating doctors' orders, generating accurate charges, keeping track of patient transfers, and dismissing patients.[8] In 1974 it selected a system offered by Diversified Numerical Applications (DNA), a division of Avnet Inc.[9] The hospital purchased three initial phases of the Avnet/DNA system with an option to purchase two more. Avnet said all three phases would be installed and operational no later than October 1976.[10]

Avnet/DNA still had installed only phase one by the end of 1977, and phase one was functioning poorly. Avnet asked for more time and an additional $100,000 to install phase two. In the meantime, administration learned that Avnet was divesting itself of its DNA division.[11]

Avnet would not give the hospital assurance that it would abide by the terms of the contract or support the system. All efforts at negotiating a settlement failed.[12] DeKalb General filed suit, and in 1980 the courts ordered Avnet to repay the hospital more than $500,000.[13]

In the meantime, the business office had shut down the Avnet/DNA system and reverted to a laborious manual process while it looked for a new data collection and communication system.[14] This time it selected the Huff, Barrington, and Owns (HBO) Medpro product. HBO's Medpro was installed and in use by July 1979, and it worked well.[15] The system handled admissions, discharge, and transfer information. It also allowed nurses to enter orders on a computer terminal, send those orders to a printer in the appropriate department, review orders entered for a patient, review patient schedules, send maintenance requests, and place orders to the store room.[16] Patient billing, accounting, and other financial data functions were handled separately by a service company for a monthly fee of $20,000.[17]

Despite optimistic, long-term expectations for HBO's Medpro system, hospital needs exceeded the system's capacity within five years. Bob Brown, director of Information Technology, once again looked for a new system. In 1986 DeKalb General purchased the INVISION software program from Shared Medical Services Inc. (SMS) and an IBM Model 4381 computer to run the system. INVISION not only replaced the HBO Medpro data collection and communication system for admissions, discharge, and transfers, but brought in-house the financial functions that were provided by the service company for a monthly fee, and it handled materials management and other customized functions.[18] The new IBM computer was touted to have the capacity to store the equivalent of five million typed pages, amounting to a stack of paper more than 160 stories high.[19]

In 2001 the hospital invested $2 million in a document imaging system (SOVERA) to scan, store, and make patient records available electronically to the Medical Records Department and to the business office.[20] The system later was upgraded to an Internet-based version, making patient records also available to authorized physicians and other users.[21]

In the meantime, Siemens Inc. purchased SMS Inc. and its INVISION system. Siemens worked with DeKalb's Information Technology staff to "tweak" and customize the INVISION system to meet the hospital's changing and growing needs. By 2003 the 1986 system could no longer be updated. The board of directors allocated $8.5 million to convert the old version of INVISION to a new, two-part, browser-based system. It was rolled out in 2004 and known as FOCUS (Financial and Organizational Changes Underway for Success).[22] Part one was FOCUS Lawson, and part two was FOCUS INVISION.[23] The system not only performed the old system's tasks, but it also automated Materials Management processes, and it interfaced and shared information with the new clinical information system that was being installed.[24]

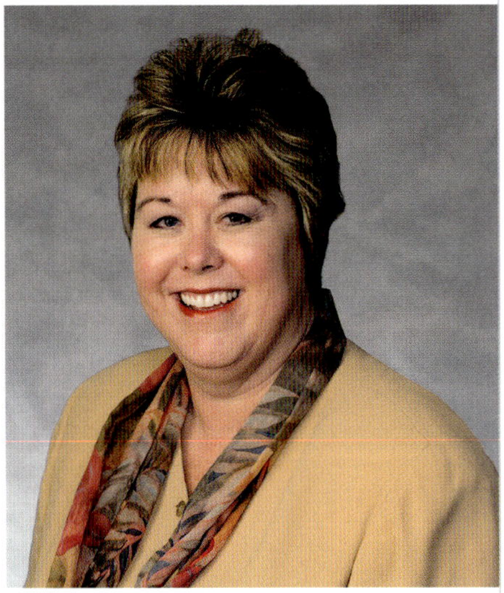

Cynthia Adgate Davis was named vice president of Information Technology and chief information officer in 2002.

A clinical information system was the big piece missing in the DeKalb Medical's information armamentarium. In 2000 DeKalb Medical Center implemented a Patient Care Delivery Model on nursing units 3400 and 4400. It featured a wireless telephone system, a new nurse call system, a physician-order interface, and specialized chart wall desks that housed patient charts outside each patient room.[25] That model, however, did not approach the need for an integrated system that linked the users and providers of patient care with clinical information.

That level of a clinical information system had its origin in the PROMINA organization of which DeKalb Medical was a member. Business coalitions and organizations such as The Leapfrog Group pressured hospitals and physicians to document and publish a record of the safety, efficiency, and quality of their care. PROMINA elected to establish QUEST (Quality, Uniformity, Efficiency, and Safety through Technology) in response to that demand. DeKalb Medical, Piedmont Hospital, Gwinnett Medical Center, and Southern Regional Medical Center agreed to invest $40 million to establish a clinical information system and to start QUEST together. The hardware and core technology staff was to be located at the PROMINA corporate headquarters.[26]

Gwinnett Medical Center, however, decided not to use the centralized hardware located at PROMINA headquarters. Southern Regional deferred its participation.[27] DeKalb Medical Center and Piedmont Hospital, therefore, decided to establish QUEST on their own. In 2002 the DMC board of directors allotted $8 million to the project,[28] and in 2004 they budgeted an additional $1 million to upgrade the existing infrastructure.[29] DeKalb's goal was to make patient care safer, more effective, and more efficient.

In the spring of 2002 DeKalb Medical Center named Jeff O'Neil director of its QUEST project. O'Neil assembled a strong team composed of clinical and support staff and physicians who got the project underway. In November 2002 DeKalb Medical named Cynthia Adgate (later Davis) as its first vice president of Information Technology and chief information officer (CIO).[30] Davis assembled an Information Technology Executive Governance Group to establish an information technology strategic plan and an Information Technology Steering Committee to evaluate and implement the plan.[31]

QUEST required the installation of a core information technology system and a series of interconnected building blocks. DeKalb purchased the Sunrise Clinical Manager's (SCM) clinical information system from Eclipsys Corporation as the foundation and linchpin for QUEST. It was the heart of the system, for it tied the other building blocks together. The other building blocks included Picture Archival Communication System (PACS) and STAR in Radiology, Softlab in the Laboratory, McKesson's Horizon Meds Manager in the Pharmacy, Computrition in Dietary, and Mediscribe in Medical Records.

In April 2004 DeKalb Medical contracted with Healthvision, a healthcare Internet company, to make DeKalb Medical's clinical information available to physicians via the Internet. By entering an ID and password, physicians and other authorized users anytime, anywhere, could access DeKalb Medical's website and view laboratory results, radiology images and reports, medical records, pharmacy orders, fetal tracings, labor and delivery monitors, access a secure email site, view consults, and get demographic and financial data pertaining to their patients.[32]

A key ingredient in the entire enterprise was physician leadership and participation. Norman Jacobs, MD, Mark Pollock, MD, and Albert Scott, MD, served as chief medical information officers.[33] These three leaders early on envisioned the need for a more effective way to enhance, measure, document, and demonstrate quality of patient care.[34] They were surprised and gratified that administration and the governing body were ready and willing to commit to such a long-term, resource-heavy, ahead-of-the-curve initiative.[35] These three leaders were instrumental in developing the concept, but they also participated in the hard work of deciphering existing work processes, configuring the clinical information system that would meet the needs and goals envisioned, recruiting other physician champions and "super users," learning the system, teaching others how to use the system, and being ambassadors and cheerleaders for the system and its value for patients, physicians, staff, and the organization.

In July 2004, after twelve thousand hours of staff and physician training and a mock "go-live" event, DeKalb Medical went live with SCM.[36] When DeKalb Medical at Hillandale opened its doors in July 2005, SCM's CPOE (computerized physician order entry) component and its computerized clinical documentation were operational. The electronic medical record was up and running.

With CPOE, physicians enter orders into a computer rather than on paper, thereby reducing potential errors of handwritten orders, integrating orders with patient information, and improving communication between the entire healthcare team. Orders include standardized order sets found to be most effective and efficient in diagnosing or treating specific conditions.[37] The order sets were developed by physicians and had the approval of the DeKalb Physician-Hospital Organization (DPHO) and the Medical Staff Executive Committee. The process of modifying existing order sets and developing new ones is ongoing.

In September 2007 CPOE and clinical documentation went live throughout the North Decatur hospital. In the first week, 60 percent of the physicians who admitted patients entered their orders via CPOE, accounting for 50 percent or all orders processed.[38]

When DeKalb Medical at Hillandale opened in 2005 with its remote internet-based physician viewing system in place and CPOE and computerized clinical documentation in operation, *Hospitals & Health Networks* magazine, the official journal of the American Hospital Association, ranked DeKalb Medical as one of the "Most Wired" hospitals and health systems in the nation. It cited DeKalb Medical at Hillandale as the first planned digital hospital in Georgia and one of only 2 percent of U. S. hospitals to successfully implement CPOE and computerized clinical documentation.[39] In 2006 the same magazine named DeKalb Medical as one of the nation's twenty-five "Most Wireless" hospitals.[40]

Along with all the pride, respect, and gratitude for the Information Technology team and the host of those who labored long and hard to bring about the significant achievements of QUEST, CEO Eric Norwood reminded everyone that "a transition like this isn't an 'Event,' it's a 'Process' that will evolve over the days and weeks to come."[41] With information technology and information systems, the challenges and opportunities never end.

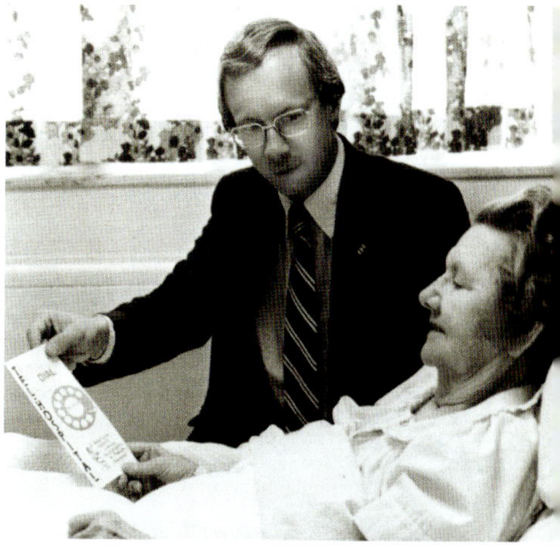

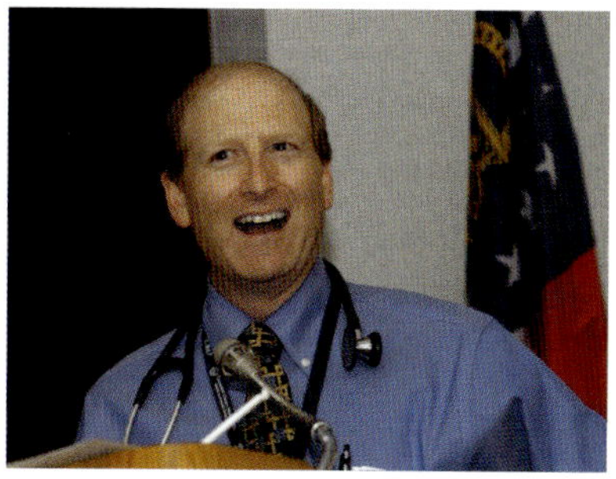

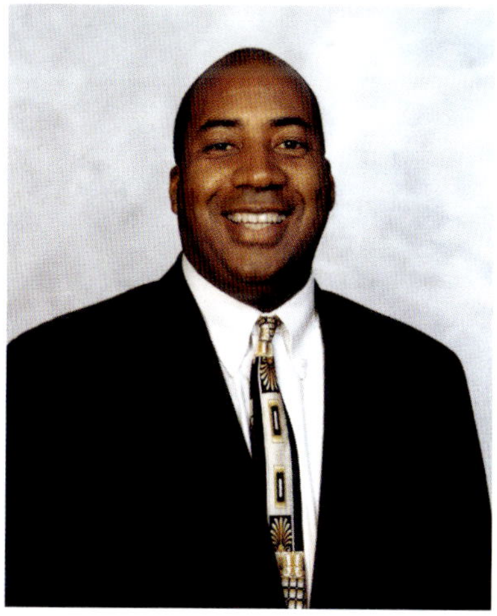

Three key leaders were chief medical information officers who championed and trained others in the new electronic medical record project at DeKalb Medical. Top to bottom: Norman Jacobs, MD, Mark Pollock, MD, and Albert Scott, MD.

Laboratory Services

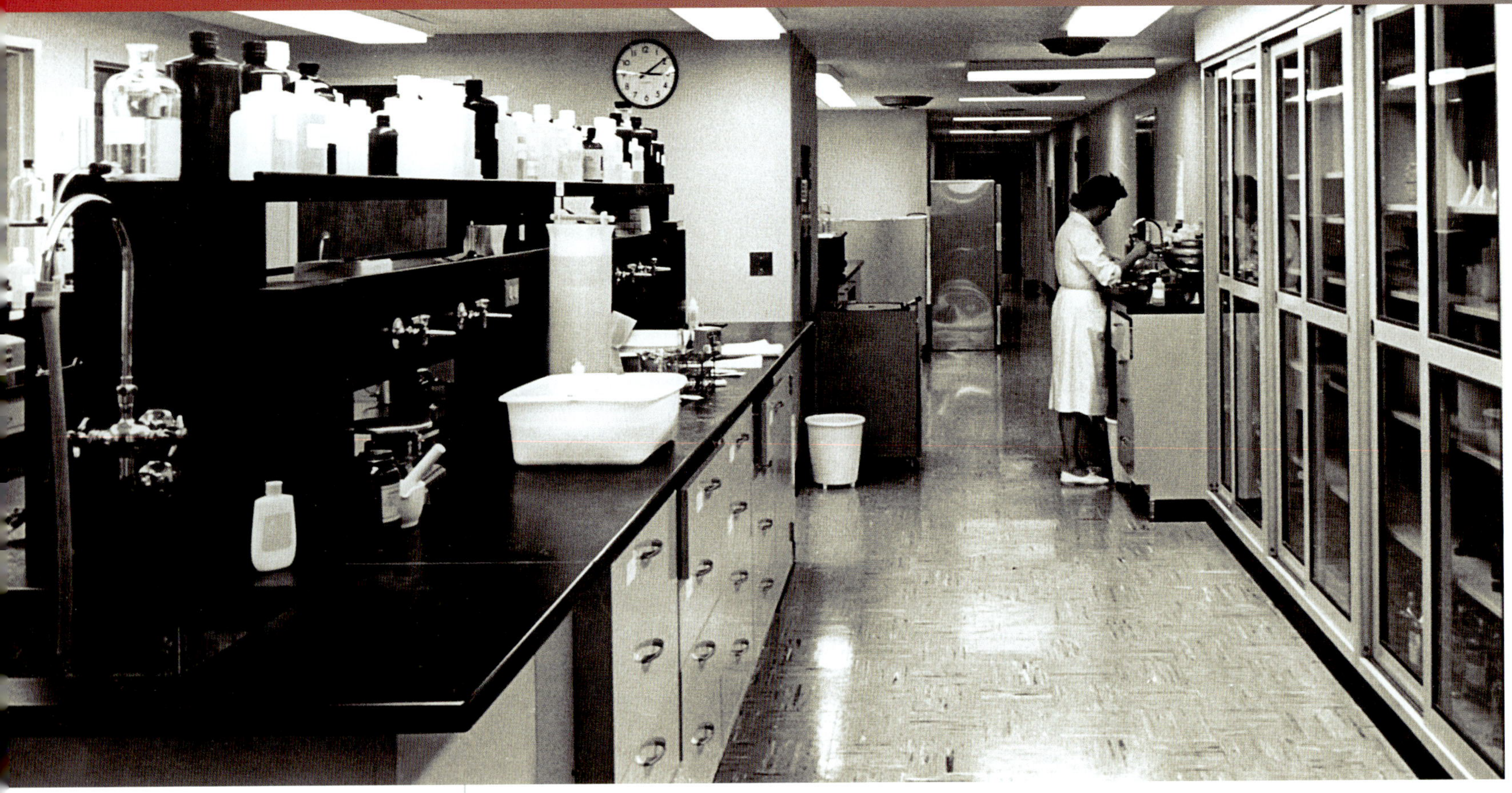

In 1961, the 2,500-square-foot laboratory at DeKalb General Hospital was state-of-the-art with all the latest technology.

In February 1960 the DeKalb County Hospital Authority selected Frank Matthews, MD, as DeKalb General's first chief pathologist and medical director of the Laboratory. However, he was not released from military service until nearly two months after the hospital opened in May 1961. Webster "Buck" Sherrer, MD, a pathologist at Frank Matthews's father's Kennestone Hospital laboratory, served as interim chief until Matthews arrived.[1] Matthews remained chief pathologist and medical director of the Laboratory for thirty-six years until his retirement in 1997.[2] Gee Aldridge, MT, wife of cardiologist Stanley Aldridge, MD, was the first administrative technologist. The nine other technical staff members on opening day included Frankie Murphy (later Pearce), MT, who would succeed Aldridge in 1967 and remain chief medical technologist until her retirement in 1996.[3]

Frankie Pearce had the reputation of being ready for any challenge. When, in 1970, the vice president of the United States paid a visit to Stone Mountain, the Secret Service put DeKalb General on standby for possible medical problems and provided the Laboratory with the vice president's blood type. Pearce knew that her husband had the same blood type, so she kept him close at hand just in case his blood was needed.[4]

Matthews's contract with the hospital stipulated that he would perform laboratory work on hospital personnel at no fee, that he would perform autopsies on hospital-related deaths at no fee, that he would pay any associates needed, and that he would receive 25 percent of laboratory charges after deducting his professional interpretation fees.[5]

DeKalb General's 1961 Laboratory was considered modern and state-of-the-art. It occupied 2,500 square feet of space, including the morgue, and was equipped with the latest available technology.[6] Though antiquated by today's standards, the studies available, the procedures by which they were performed, and the charges for those procedures were advanced for 1961. A urinalysis was performed in five parts, including boiling the specimen over a flame to measure its albumin content. Electrolyte tests had been available for only the previous five years, and each sample was passed laboriously through a flame photometer twice to measure sodium and potassium. Carbon dioxide was measured using a technique that involved mercury spills, which seemed to concern no one at the time. Calcium, phosphorus, uric acid, and cholesterol were performed with the vastly improved Coleman spectrophotometer. Enzyme determinations from the liver, adrenal gland, brain, pancreas, liver and other organs were performed only in highly specialized reference laboratories, and a technique for measuring blood gases had not been developed.[7]

A small oven capable of reaching several hundred degrees centigrade made possible the new protein binding iodine (PBI) test for thyroid function; this test was a replacement for the less-accurate basal metabolic rate (BMR) test. Pregnancy was detected by injecting a woman's urine into frogs and subsequently examining the frog's urine for spermatozoa. This "frog test" was used at DeKalb General in lieu of the traditional "rabbit test" in which a woman's urine was injected into a female rabbit, a few days after which the rabbit was sacrificed and its ovaries examined for tell-tale changes caused by increased levels of human chorionic gonadotropin that occur in pregnancy.[8]

In 1961 blood collected for transfusions was screened only for adequate hemoglobin and evidence of syphilis. The discovery of the Australia antigen in 1963 in patients with acute and chronic hepatitis led to radical changes in the screening process. The AIDS epidemic led to additional screening in 1985, and the Federal Drug Administration (FDA) eventually mandated that all blood for transfusion be screened for hepatitis B, hepatitis C, the t-lymphotropic virus, the West Nile virus, and the AIDS virus.[9]

The 1961 charge for a complete blood count (CBC) was $5, urinalysis $3, blood glucose $3, Pap smear $5, and examining a surgical specimen $8. The gross laboratory billings for the month of October 1961, including EKGs that were a part of the Laboratory, were $13,153.[10] By 2007 the charge for a CBC was $72, urinalysis $55, blood glucose $20, basic surgical specimen $29, and billings for 107,000 tests in a peak month totaled $6,201,019.[11] As Matthews observed, however, since Medicare, managed-care companies, and other insurers "pay pretty much what they want to, laboratory charges now are often only a nominal fiction" and essentially meaningless.[12]

The Laboratory rapidly moved toward automation for many of its studies. In 1967 Matthews spent $10,000 of his $51,000 equipment budget for a Coulter Counter to count blood cells and an AutoAnalyzer to measure blood glucose and blood urea nitrogen (BUN), a kidney-function test.[13] In 1974 the Laboratory began performing arterial blood gases, which revolutionized the management of critically ill patients. In the late 1970s electrolyte determinations were automated and the biochemical profile (BCP) with twelve standard tests became available.

Microbiology studies were automated in the mid-1980s so that positive blood cultures could be reported in six hours rather than in the traditional eighteen hours. Tuberculosis could be identified in

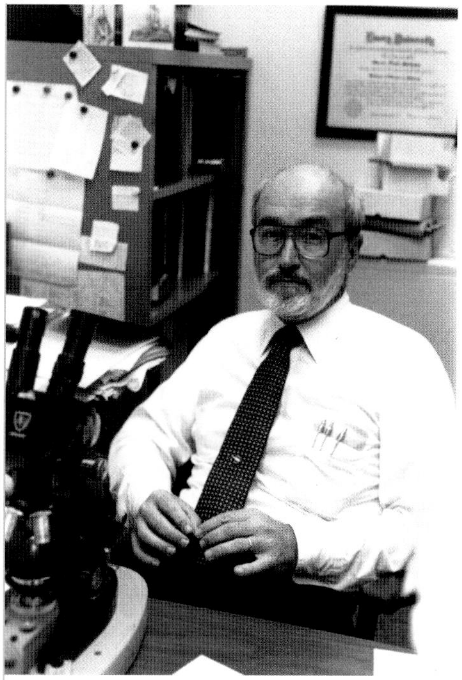

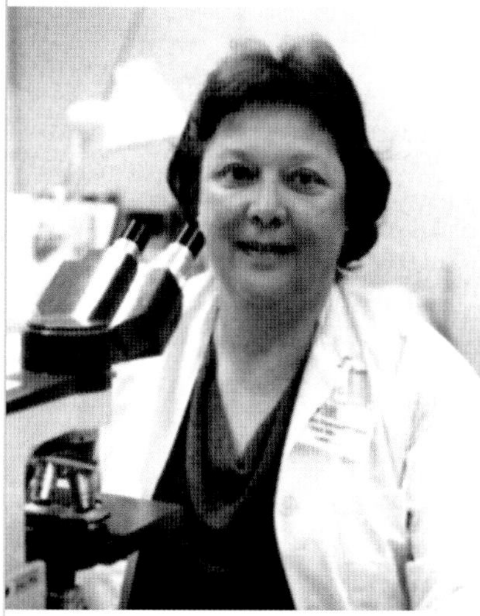

Top: Frank Matthews, MD, was DeKalb General's first chief pathologist and medical director at the Laboratory from 1961–1997. **Above:** Frankie Murphy Pearce, MT, was chief medical technologist from 1967–1996.

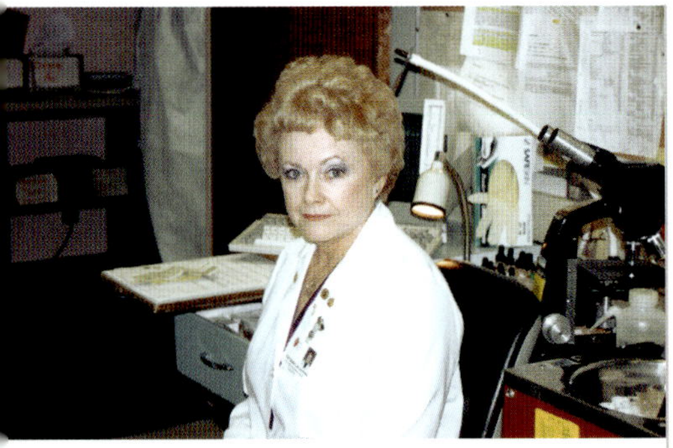

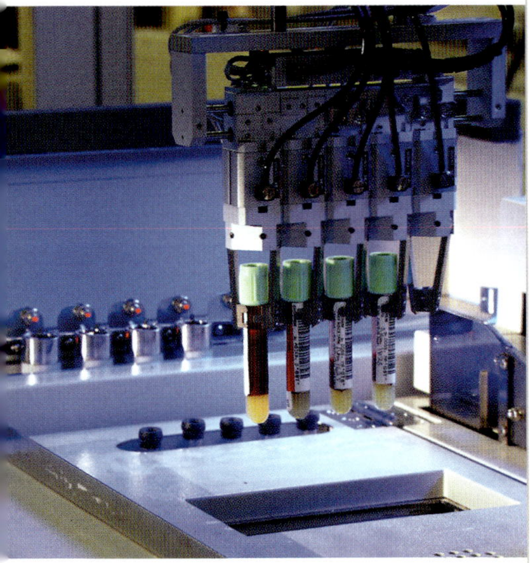

Top: Mary Murray, MT, manager of the laboratory's Blood Bank. **Above:** The hospital Laboratory quickly embraced automated technology.

days rather than weeks.

The Laboratory recently acquired an automated hematology analyzer that makes its own blood-smear slides for examination; differentiates and counts six different types of white blood cells including those in early, primitive formation; performs auto-verification of normal results; and displays cells for the Laboratory technician's review on a screen with amazing detail and clarity.[14]

DeKalb General found it practical and economical in the early days to send some of its chemistry studies to outside laboratories. In 1966 a group of Atlanta pathologists created a cooperative central laboratory known as Pathologists' Services, PA (PSPA). For the next fifteen years, PSPA provided clinical chemistry services to most, if not all, hospitals in Atlanta and other parts of north Georgia. Laboratory results were returned to each hospital by Teletype. This outside service saved DeKalb General and other users the cost of equipment and personnel since biochemistry machines, of which there were only three in Atlanta, cost approximately $150,000 each and required a large, trained staff. In 1981 PSPA sold its equipment and services to Smith Kline Beecham (SKB) Clinical Laboratories, and Quest Diagnostics Inc. subsequently bought the service from SKB.[15] By 1990 DeKalb Medical Center began performing more of its own biochemical studies due to its large volume and the need for rapid turnaround on reports. Currently 98 percent of its studies are performed in-house on automated equipment provided by a vendor to whom the hospital pays a fee for each specimen performed.[16]

Tom Raaen, MD, who had served as chief pathologist at Grady Memorial Hospital, joined Matthews in 1963 as DeKalb General's second pathologist. Earl Barton, MD, the third pathologist followed in 1969; James David Stacy, MD, joined in 1972; and Rene Tapia, MD, joined in 1974 when Barton relocated to the Veterans' Administration (VA) Hospital. Alex Parkinson, MD, became a member of the staff in 1980, followed by Hilary Hargreaves, MD, in 1982 when Raaen retired. William McNeill, MD, and Edwin Nunnery, MD, joined in the late 1980s, Gail Walker, MD, arrived in 1991 and Aileen O'Neill, MD, came in 1993. The full-time Pathology staff in 2007 includes Hargreaves, McNeill, Nunnery, and Walker, Diane Jarrett, MD, Jan Kennedy, MD, Cynthia Lambert, MD, and Vida Gowda, MD. "Retired" Matthews and Steven Covington, MD, are part-time pathologists. DeKalb's pathologists service, in addition to the three DeKalb Medical campuses, Eastside Hospital, Henry Medical Center, and Georgia Urology Prostate Laboratory.[17]

Philip Carlquist, PhD, came to DeKalb General in 1965 as clinical microbiologist, possibly the first doctoral-level microbiologist in a nonuniversity hospital in Georgia.[18] Robert C. Jerris, PhD, succeeded Carlquist in 1985 and established professional microbiology consultation as a valued laboratory service. Following Jerris's resignation to take a position with Children's Healthcare of Atlanta, Adam Bressler, MD, an infectious disease specialist, became DeKalb Medical's microbiologist.[19]

Earnest Ochoa, PhD, was DeKalb General's first clinical chemist in 1968, followed by Joe Stabile, PhD, in 1969, and Jerry McHan, PhD, in 1996.[20] McHan established the forensic toxicology laboratory in 2000 to provide workplace drug testing, legally defensible forensic toxicology testing, and drug testing for commonly abused drugs and prescription medications.[21] The legal proceedings for which many of the laboratory's test results were used requires both elaborate steps to ensure accuracy of results and meticulous "chain of custody" documentation to verify who had custody of the specimen at all times and all actions taken with each specimen. Most forensic toxicology work now is performed by Quest laboratories.[22]

Hiram Ragsdale, one of DeKalb General's earliest employees, was hired in February 1961 as a member of the Housekeeping staff to get the hospital ready for occupancy. He joined the Pathology

Department later in 1961 and was trained as a denier, the morgue attendant who is responsible for handling and cleaning the bodies of the deceased and, in some cases, assisting in autopsies. He became senior denier and also was recognized as a leading citizen of the hospital staff. The employee newsletter recognized Ragsdale for his nine years of service as chairman of the Good Neighbor Fund committee and for "the many contributions [he] has made to DeKalb General Hospital and its employees."[23] Ragsdale was succeeded by Norman Saunders who remains DeKalb's senior denier.[24]

The Laboratory was certified following its first inspection by the College of American Pathologists in 1967 and has maintained uninterrupted accreditation ever since. In 2007 it was inspected by four accrediting bodies with twenty inspectors and "all went well."[25]

In addition to meeting the requirements of inspecting agencies, however, the Laboratory has been diligent in eliminating errors, whether technical or caused by miscommunication. The advent of computer systems significantly reduced such communication errors as wrong test request, wrong patient's name, or misfiling laboratory reports. Each laboratory specimen now is bar-coded for accuracy and ease of tracking.[26]

In 1984 the Laboratory purchased a Meditech System with a 55-megabyte (MB) hard drive to store and transmit laboratory information.[27] While that system had a meager capacity compared to today's computers, it reduced communication errors at least ten-fold.[28] In 1999 the Laboratory replaced the Meditech computer with Softlab Computer Company's laboratory program that was capable of receiving orders from the hospital system's new Sunrise Clinical Manager and sending results to Sunrise Clinical Manager to make them available to physicians, nurses, pharmacists, and others responsible for a given patient's care.

The Laboratory grew in size as well as in functions. While the 1961 Laboratory occupied 2,500 square feet, including the morgue, in 1971 the Laboratory was awarded 10,000 square feet, the space being divided between two floors, with the hospital's first major expansion project. In 1997, in addition to the Outpatient Laboratory located in Professional Office Building II, the Laboratory moved into new quarters that doubled its space to 18,000 square feet.[29] A pneumatic tube system was installed in critical care areas to facilitate a rapid transport system for those patients and to reduce the need for satellite laboratories. Hematology, microbiology and chemistry occupied the core area of the Laboratory. Flow cytometry, pathology, histology, oncology, and blood-bank functions were performed in a separate area.

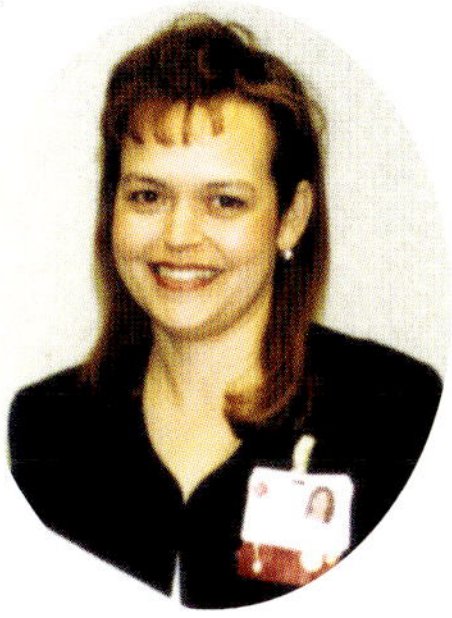

In 1996, with the new Laboratory under construction with its expanded services, the position of chief medical technologist was replaced with a director of Laboratory Administrative Services. James Craft, MT, was the first director. He held the position until 2000 when he was succeeded by the current director, Roslyn "Roz" Heath, MT.[30]

Alex Parkinson assumed the post of chief pathologist and medical director of the Laboratory when Matthews retired in May 1997.[31] When Parkinson retired in December 2006, Hargreaves became chief of overall operations, and McNeill became chief of Pathology and medical director of the Laboratory at the North Decatur campus.[32]

Since DeKalb Medical's beginning, the Laboratory has served a vital role in the diagnosis and management of nearly every patient whether admitted to one of the three hospitals or served on an outpatient basis. The commitment and competence of the staff and the quality of the service they have rendered have been and remain vital to the mission and reputation of the institution.

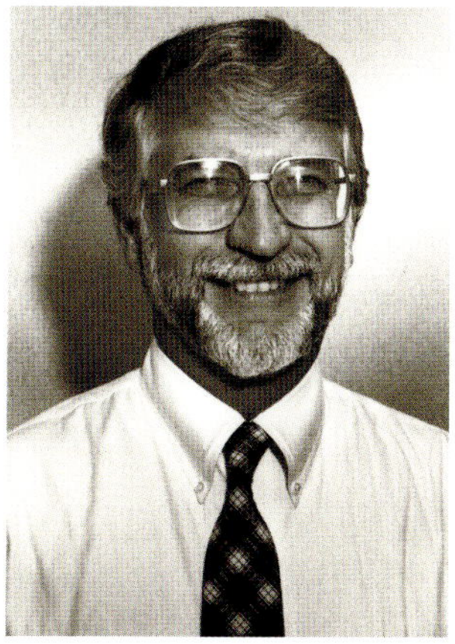

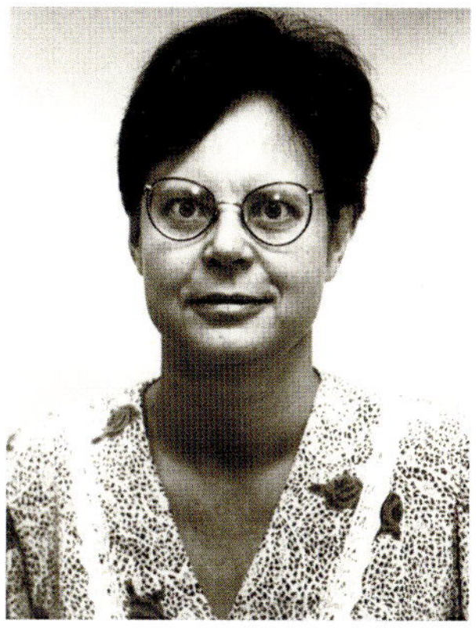

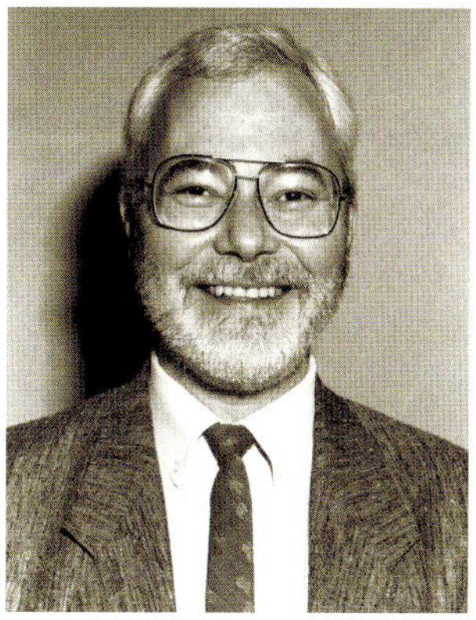

Above: When Frank Matthews retired in 1997, Alex Parkinson, MD, (top) became chief pathologist and medical director, followed by Hilary Hargreaves, MD (center), and William McNeill, MD (bottom).
Left inset: Roslyn "Roz" Heath, MT, is the current director of Laboratory Administrative Services.

Medical Records

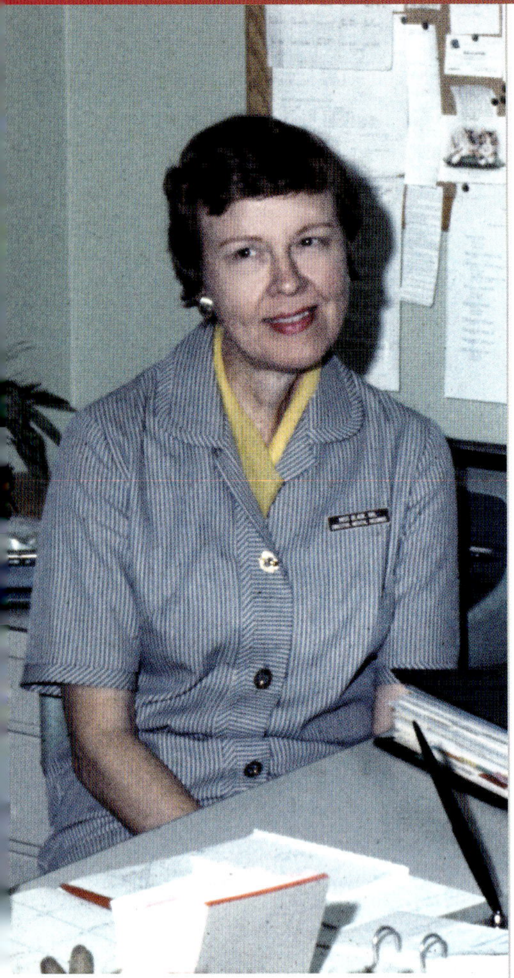

Frances Black, RRA, was hired by William Thrasher as the first director of Medical Records. She retired in 1984.

Administrator William Thrasher chose his neighbor, Frances Black, RRA, from among several applicants to be DeKalb General Hospital's first director of Medical Records. Black once was a writer and the editor of a trade magazine. She later decided to make medical records her career and earned her degree in health records administration at Emory University. She once said of her job at DeKalb General, "Mr. Thrasher gave me a chance to see what I could do."

Initially her department was located in two areas. Transcriptionists were housed on the first floor of the hospital while the remainder of the department was on the ground floor. Medical Records was united and moved to its present location on the ground floor when the renovation and expansion was completed in 1971.

For eleven years, until Marilyn Gibbs Barry was named librarian in 1974, Frances Black was in charge of the medical library as well as medical records.

Doctors were convinced that Frances Black had been a student of President Teddy Roosevelt, for she knew how to "speak softly and carry a big stick." She ran the department with a firm but fair hand, with pride and devotion. She also saw to it that her department "kept up with the changes." She purchased equipment for physicians to dictate their discharge summaries. In 1970 she acquired several of the newly released IBM Magnetic Tape Selective Typewriters for transcribing dictated discharge summaries.[1] She devised improved ways to audit patient records for completeness and relevance.[2] She recruited a staff of people who provided continuity, creativity, and leadership to the department. Susan Hill, Laverne Neighbours, and Hilda Jackson are among the people Black hired who have remained with the department for more than thirty years.[3]

On the occasion of her retirement in 1984, Black admitted a twinge of guilt for "getting a paycheck for doing something you love."[4] Though retired for nearly a quarter of a century, she continued checking on how things were going in "her" department with occasional phone calls and personal visits.[5]

One of the people Black hired as a coding analyst in 1975 was Faye Sophy, RRA. She quickly recognized Sophy's competence and named her assistant director of the department. When Black retired in 1984 Faye Sophy was a "natural" to succeed her as director.[6] Sophy served in that position for nineteen years until she retired in 1999.[7]

The world of technology exploded during Faye Sophy's administration, and she took advantage of it by incorporating it effectively into Medical Records. She initiated computerization of medical records in the early 1980s. She instituted bar codes to track the location and current use being made of patient charts. She established an interface system with the Business Office so that diagnostic codes that were applied to patient records in her department were automatically available in Finance for billing purposes and filing insurance claims. She established a system in which her transcriptionists could work from home to access, transcribe, and transmit back to the hospital physicians' dictated charts. She envisioned and initiated the document imaging project that was completed after her retirement.[8]

Like Frances Black before her, Faye Sophy continued to build a team of loyal, dedicated staff members, many of whom remain today, including Virginia "Ginna" Evans, current manager of Medical Records. Another gift that Sophy shared with others was the spirit of courage and strength with which she dealt with ovarian cancer. She died from her cancer in July 2000, six years after being diagnosed and eight months after retiring.

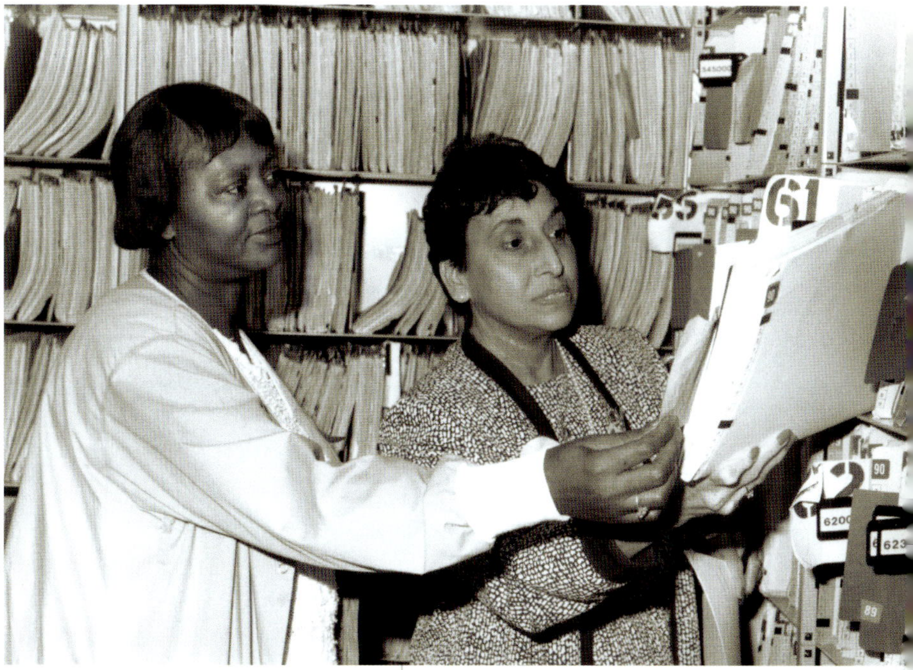

Ron McCranie, RRA, joined the Medical Records staff in 1969. The June 1970 issue of the employee newsletter announced that "Ron McCranie, who has been with the department of medical records since last November, is being promoted to the position of Clerk-General."[9] McCranie was considering a career in medicine, but Black recognized his propensity for medical records and encouraged him to reexamine his career options. But a medical records career was not the only thing McCranie found in the department; he also found his wife.[10]

In 1974 McCranie enrolled in the Health Records Administration program at Emory University. With his degree in hand, he worked for a while at Emory and then at Clayton General Hospital (later named Southern Regional Medical Center). He returned to DeKalb Medical Center in 1999 and succeeded Faye Sophy as director of Medical Records.

As director, McCranie completed the revolutionary SOVERA document-imaging project that Faye Sophy had envisioned and initiated. DeKalb Medical Center spent $2 million to purchase the system.[11] Now, patient orders, progress notes, and other data entered into the electronic medical record are automatically entered into the patient's SOVERA record. Following discharge, the patient's remaining paper record is indexed and scanned into the SOVERA electronic record. The paper chart is stored offsite for two years after which it is destroyed, and the electronic record is backed up in multiple sites. It is immediately available by computer to the Business Office, to physicians, and to other authorized individuals from anywhere via the physician portal system. Physicians can, from anywhere at any time, review, complete, and sign their patient records electronically.

As for future projects in Medical Records, McCranie's primary short-term focus is to fine-tune the electronic medical record. Voice recognition documentation is another technology that is receiving increasing interest in the medical records world. It has undergone exponential improvements, making it increasingly attractive and potentially applicable as a future tool. Finally, computer-automated coding is evolving in which the computer extracts data from the electronic medical record and generates diagnostic codes for billing purposes. Human coders become the editors to confirm or alter the computer-designated codes.[12]

The department has come a long way from the days of all-paper charts, manual entry and extraction of information, sending someone to Medical Records to retrieve an old chart when a patient presented to the hospital, and the IBM Magnetic Tape Selective Typewriter. Today there is document imaging and the electronic medical record, available instantly anywhere, any time. Medical Records has been at the forefront of utilizing the best people, the best available tools, and the best services to ensure optimal accuracy, usefulness, and timeliness of information that is essential to quality patient care.

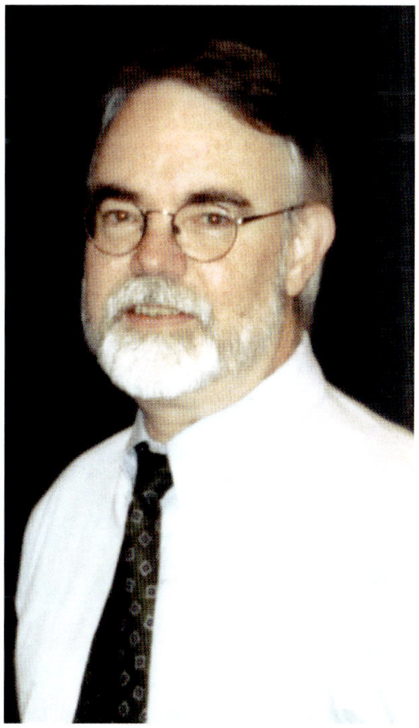

Top: Faye Sophy, RRA, (right) became DeKalb Medical's second director of Medical Records in 1984. She is seen here with Myrtle Favors, NA.
Above: Ron McCranie, RRA, became director of Medical Records in 1999.

The Medical Staff

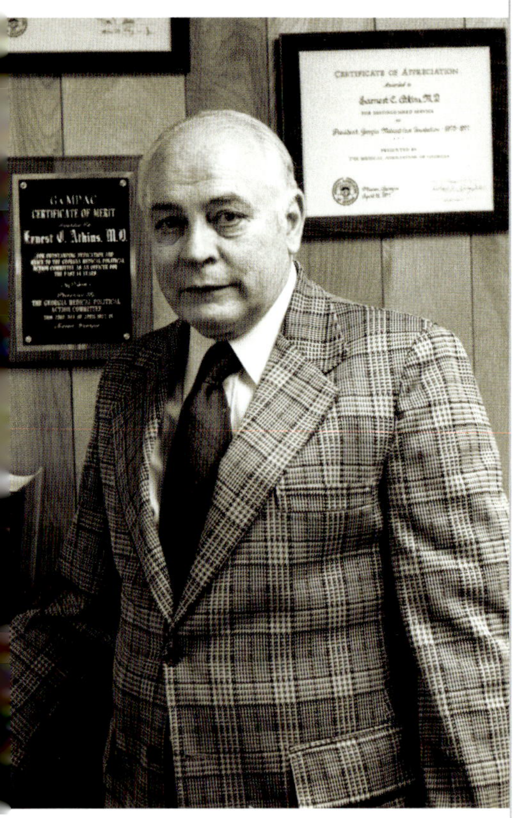

Earnest Atkins, MD, was a general surgeon and former chief of staff. He was also former president of the DeKalb Medical Society, former president of the Medical Association of Georgia, and the 1984 recipient of the Julius A. McCurdy Citizenship Award.

DeKalb Medical's relationship with its physicians has been close and evolving through the years. The original trustees had strong ties with the medical community and the medical staff. J. Rufus Evans, MD, a physician, was instrumental in creating the hospital and served as chairman of the DeKalb County Hospital Authority for more than a decade. He and the other trustees regularly sought physician counsel and were attentive to physician concerns and recommendations.

The trustees called on the DeKalb Medical Society to frame and implement the initial medical staff bylaws, rules and regulations, credentialing process, and organizational structure until such time as there were a sufficient number of physicians on staff to assume responsibility for their own organization. The hospital and medical society maintained such close ties that, for the first several years, a physician had to be a member of the DeKalb Medical Society to qualify for membership on the medical staff.

When the hospital opened in May 1961, there were sixty-six physicians in eight departments: Anesthesia, General Practice, Internal Medicine, Obstetrics and Gynecology, Pathology, Pediatrics, Radiology, and Surgery. The Department of Psychiatry became a section of the Department of Medicine in 1969[1] and a separate department in 1971. In 1973 the Department of Emergency Medicine was created,[2] and the General Practice Department was renamed the Department of Family Practice.[3]

As more physicians joined the medical staff, departments established specialty sections. The Department of Surgery, in addition to general surgery, created sections of oral and maxillofacial surgery, urology, ophthalmology, orthopedics, plastic surgery, colon and rectal surgery, otolaryngology, neurosurgery, thoracic surgery, vascular surgery, and podiatry. In addition to internal medicine, the Department of Medicine established sections of cardiology, dermatology, gastroenterology, hematology and oncology, neurology, pulmonary medicine, infectious disease, nephrology, endocrinology, rheumatology, hospitalists, and pain and rehabilitation medicine.

There were seven original medical staff committees: Executive, Credentials, Infections, Interns and Residents, Medical Records, Pharmacy and Therapeutics, and Tissue. Tissue investigated inconsistencies in preoperative and postoperative diagnoses. The Committee on Interns and Residents was eliminated when the hospital decided it would not have a postgraduate training program. The number of other committees grew steadily. By 1990 there were forty-two medical staff committees. The Medical Staff Executive Committee appointed one more, the "Committee on Committees," to recommend those that could be eliminated or combined. As a result of its work, the number was reduced from forty-two to nineteen.

In 1961 technology was basic and minimal, the cost of healthcare reasonable, the doctor-doctor relationship collegial, the doctor-nurse relationship respectful, and the doctor-patient relationship paramount. Earnest Atkins, MD, once observed that Lawrence P. Matthews, MD, former chief of the Department of Obstetrics and Gynecology, "was one of the finest men I ever knew. His fees were very low, and he never sent any patient a bill when he saw that patient in consultation at the request of another doctor. Matthews saw that as an opportunity to render a favor to the referring physician."[4]

Floyd Sanders, MD, DeKalb General's second chief of staff from 1962 to 1964, recalls that his fee for a routine office visit was $3, a house call $4, and a night visit to the Emergency Department $5.[5]

Greg Hinesley, RN, said that he saw a live demonstration of what the doctor-patient relationship looked like when Earnest Atkins, MD, asked Hinesley to accompany him to see a patient scheduled for surgery the next day. Atkins sat on the edge of the bed, held the patient's hand, and explained everything about the surgery. When he finished, he asked the patient if she had any more questions. He assured her that if other questions came to mind after he left, she should feel free to ask the nurse or call him at home. Then he left his home telephone number with her.[6]

Physicians and the hospital were committed to protecting patient safety. They went to great lengths to verify that physicians were competent to perform the services for which they were granted privileges. Surgeons were monitored by a colleague on every surgical procedure performed for their first two years on the medical staff. If a surgeon's performance was not up to standard, that physician might be required to undergo additional training, have certain privileges limited, or have privileges revoked. Physicians who did not use the hospital enough to have their competency assessed were removed from the staff.

Originally physicians were admitted to either the active or the courtesy staff. The medical staff soon required that all physicians be admitted first to the "provisional" staff for a period of two years. During those two years, their performance was observed and their medical records evaluated to determine if they were qualified to be placed on the active or courtesy staff. The courtesy staff was accorded to those who admitted a limited number of patients or performed a limited number of procedures and services.

Occasionally an applicant's past performance in other hospitals disqualified the physician from becoming a member of the medical staff. At times, an existing member of the medical staff's performance called for the physician's removal. Whenever those situations arose, the governing body carefully followed fair procedures and the legally required due process of law, but consistently supported the medical staff's recommendation. That support at times came at the cost of much time, effort, and legal expense and the potential for legal suits filed by the physician in question. The medical staff leadership and the governing body laid such a solid foundation for their decisions, however, that there was never a case where the final decision of the governing body was not upheld by the courts.

The trustees were consistently responsive to the concerns and recommendations of the medical staff. Shortly after the hospital opened, L. C. Buchanan, MD, the first chief of staff, presented the Authority with the recommendation that there be a formal system by which the Authority and the medical staff might communicate.[7] The trustees created the Joint Conference Committee, composed of the officers of the medical staff and the officers of the Authority, and the committee met monthly to hear and consider physician concerns and recommendations. The trustees further stated that there would be physician input on all questions pertaining to the clinical aspects of running the hospital.[8] In 1969 the Professional Service Committee, chaired by W. P. Tatum, replaced the Joint Conference Committee to provide "in-depth discussions with representatives of the medical staff regarding various medical problems that might arise in the hospital."[9] In the most recent DeKalb Medical reorganization, the duties of the Professional Service Committee and other responsibilities were transferred to the board of directors' Quality Committee chaired by Roy Vandiver, MD.

In 1964 Sanders, the second chief of staff, was invited to attend meetings of the Authority on a regular basis for consultation, but he was not allowed a vote.[10] The current chiefs of staff are now

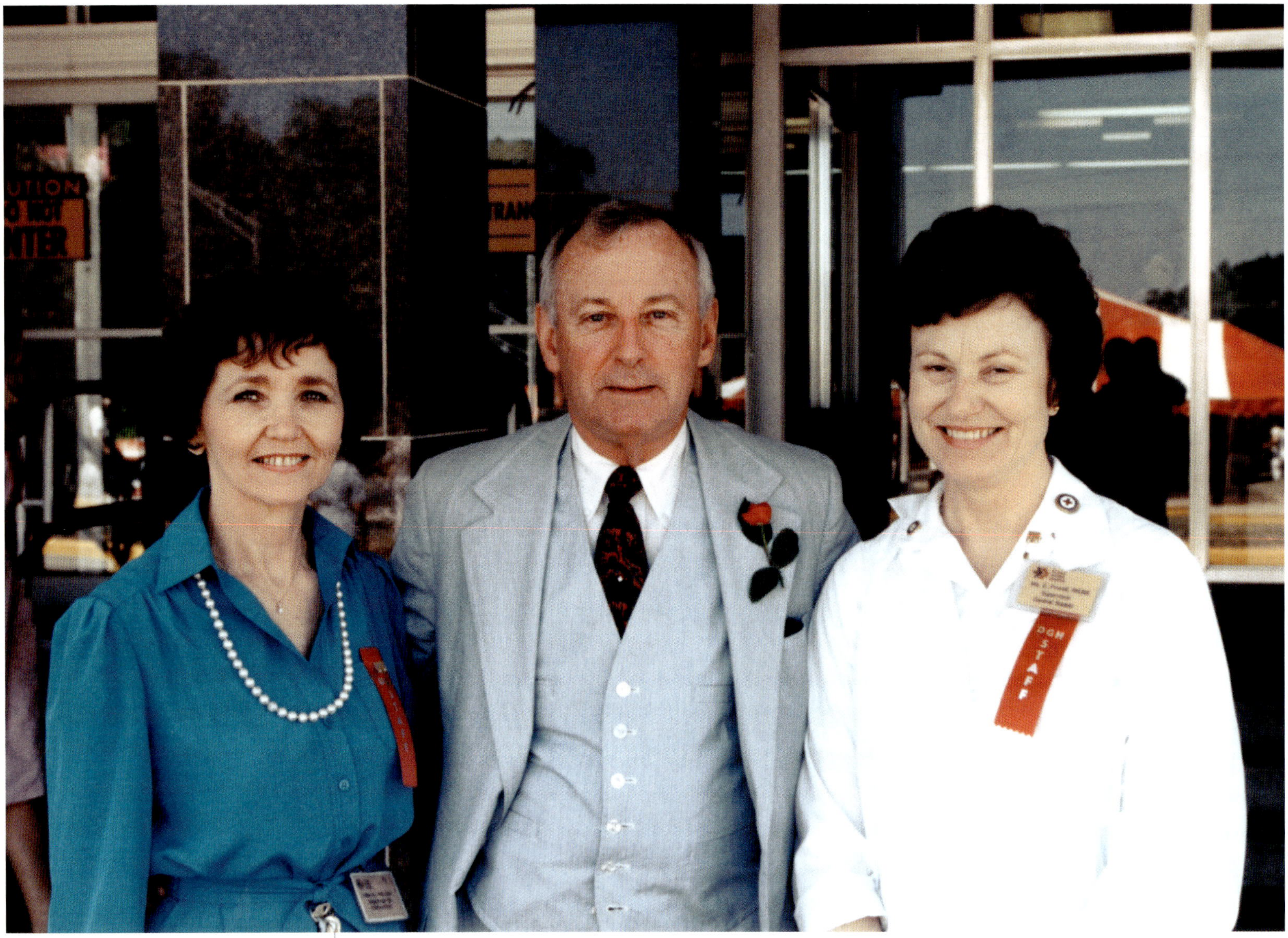

John Harrel, MD, (center) was appointed first director of Medical Affairs in 1974. He is pictured here with Sara Folger, director of Purchasing (left) and Libby Powell, RN, Supervisor Sterile Processing and Distribution (right).

a voting member of the governing body. In 1965 Sanders was elected a trustee to replace the late Ross McCain, and in 1973 L. C. Buchanan became the third physician to be elected to the Authority.

Physicians were not only members, but assumed positions of leadership on the governing body. Rufus Evans, Floyd Sanders, and Duane Blair, MD, each served as chairman of the Authority. Blair also was elected as chairman of the DeKalb Medical Center (DMC) Board of Directors and the DeKalb Regional Healthcare System (DRHS) Board of Directors. Physicians serving on the DRHS Board in 2007 include Roy Vandiver, MD, Peter Gordon, MD, Gulshan Harjee, MD, Michael Quinones, MD, and Charles "Chip" Clifton, MD, (ex officio as chief of staff).

One of the recommendations of the one hundred nurses who resigned in 1969 was for the hospital to have a director of Medical Affairs to serve as a liaison between the medical staff and the administration.[11] Fincher Powell, MD, chief of staff, recommended that the Authority appoint a committee to investigate the position.[12] The committee developed a job description[13] that Administrator

Charles Eberhart refined into a position paper that he submitted to the medical staff in 1973.[14] The Medical Staff Executive Committee voted eight in favor of hiring a director, one opposed, and six abstaining.[15] The principal concern of those abstaining or objecting was the question of how loyal a director could be to the medical staff if paid by the hospital. The physicians' concern did not, however, go as far as to recommend that the medical staff pay the director's salary. In May 1974 the Authority approved the position with one dissenting vote.[16] Thirty applicants responded to the advertised position,[17] and John Harrel, MD, a pediatrician from Arkansas, was selected as DeKalb General's first director of Medical Affairs.[18] Harrel remained in that position for fourteen years until he retired in 1988. He was succeeded by Wytch Stubbs, MD, (1988–1996),[19] Paul Crank, MD, (1996–2001),[20] and Nancy Rampell, MD, (2002–2004).[21] The position was discontinued in 2004 following Rampell's retirement, and its responsibilities were divided among the elected medical staff officers, Primary Care Division Director Duane Barclay, DO, and other administrative leaders.

One of the vexing decisions the medical staff and the governing body faced pertained to applications for membership and privileges from practitioners who did not have a doctor of medicine (MD) degree. The first such application came from oral surgeon, Thomas Conner, DDS, in 1962. There was a recognized need for the services of his specialty, particularly for patients presenting to the Emergency Room. The medical staff and Authority readily agreed to amend the medical staff bylaws to include dentists with advanced degrees in oral surgery,[22] establish a section of Oral Surgery in the Department of Surgery, and admit Thomas Conner to the medical staff.[23] Perry Brickman, DDS, was subsequently admitted in January 1965,[24] and Edward Green, DDS, joined in March 1966.[25]

The next two categories of non-MD applicants involved more deliberation. In January 1972 Gordon Dugger, a doctor of podiatric medicine (DPM), applied for membership and privileges in podiatry; and in March 1972 Darrel Dean, a doctor of osteopathy (DO), made application for membership and privileges in the Department of General Practice.[26] The Medical Staff Executive Committee recommended that, since the bylaws did not recognize either of these two degrees, both applications should be denied.[27]

The Authority deferred taking action on the medical staff's osteopathy recommendation in light of recent court rulings, pending rulings by the state's attorney general, and a pending Cobb County court case soon to be heard.[28] When the Cobb County court ruled in favor of admitting osteopathic physicians, the Authority asked the medical staff to reconsider its position. The medical staff Bylaws Committee convened and recommended at the May 1974 quarterly medical staff meeting that the bylaws be amended to permit the admission of osteopathic physicians. By a narrow margin of two votes, thirty-nine to thirty-seven, the physicians defeated the proposed amendment. In light of established state and federal law and the Cobb County court ruling, in a rare move the Authority exercised its prerogative and overrode the action of the medical staff. It adopted the recommended amendment of the Bylaws Committee to permit qualified osteopathic physicians to join the medical staff.[29]

At that time the Authority supported the medical staff's recommendation regarding podiatrists.[30] Podiatrists were accepted on the medical staff at the private Decatur Hospital when it opened in 1973, and the DeKalb Medical Center (DMC) Board of Directors recognized their membership at Decatur Hospital when it acquired the operation of the hospital in 1994. In 1996 James Bouchard, DPM, chairman of the Department of Podiatry at Decatur Hospital, petitioned DeKalb Medical Center to reconsider its position.[31] In 1998 Chief of Staff Sanford Hartman, MD, asked the department chiefs to take a poll of their members regarding allowing podiatrists to join DeKalb Medical Center's medical staff.[32] The consensus was that the time was right to admit podiatrists. The bylaws were amended, and in May 1999 the DMC Board of Directors approved a section of Podiatry in the Department of Surgery.[33] Bouchard was named the section's first chief.[34] The North Decatur and the Downtown Decatur hospitals jointly established a podiatry residency program in January 2007.[35]

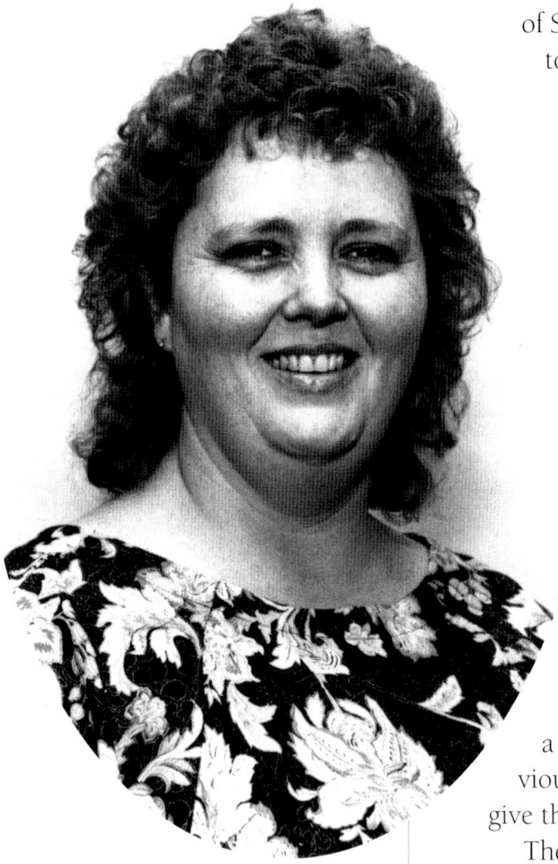

Catherine Huggins, MD, a family physician, was the first and only female physician to serve as chief of staff.

For the first three decades, the growing size of the medical staff was not a concern to the hospital's leadership. Shortly after DeKalb General opened in 1961 with sixty-six doctors, physicians from across metropolitan Atlanta applied for and were granted membership and privileges. Some became very active on the medical staff while others made little use of the facility and eventually resigned or were removed from the membership roster for lack of utilization. DeKalb General was seen as a reputable institution, the population of DeKalb County continued to grow, and physicians in all the specialties joined the medical staff. And they were welcomed. In the late 1980s and early 1990s, the hospital actively supported existing practices with such initiatives as placing computers in physician offices and in assisting the practices to recruit physicians and expand. Pam Richardson was named director of Medical Staff Recruitment and Development to support practices and assist them to recruit physicians.[36]

In the mid-1990s, however, there was a virtual explosion in the size of the medical staff. Within a short period of time, the number of physicians increased from less than five hundred to nearly one thousand. The growth was due not only to the good reputation of the hospital but also to the attractive contracts that DeKalb Medical Center secured with managed-care organizations and other third-party payers. Chief Financial Officer Bonnie Phipps was a skillful and effective contract negotiator, and DeKalb Medical Center enjoyed a good reputation among the insurers. Physicians across the city, many of whom had no previous interest in DeKalb Medical Center, wanted to be identified with the hospital that might give them leverage in negotiating their own contracts.

The rapid increase in the size of the medical staff posed a new challenge for the governing body. Governance recognized its responsibility to provide for the needs of the community, to support its existing physician practices, and to provide adequate facilities and services for its physicians and the patients they served. But it also recognized that there was a limit to the number of physicians for whom it could provide adequate support, facilities, and services.

In February 1998 the board of directors approved a Medical Staff Development Plan.[37] Based on the plan, DeKalb Medical Center would continue accepting applications in the primary care specialties of family practice, general internal medicine, pediatrics, obstetrics/gynecology, and the hospital-based specialties such as anesthesiology, emergency medicine, pathology, and radiology. It would not, however, accept additional applications from physicians in seventeen specialties that included cardiology, colon and rectal surgery, otolaryngology, gastroenterology, general surgery, gynecologic oncology, hematology/oncology, infectious disease, nephrology, neurosurgery, orthopedic surgery, perinatology, pulmonary medicine, radiation oncology, rheumatology, urology, and vascular surgery unless the applicant was replacing an active medical staff member who was retiring or leaving the medical staff for other reasons.[38]

The plan achieved the goal of curbing the rapid growth of the medical staff. However, in a relatively short period of time, it created a major problem—the need for more physicians. Several factors created a need to recruit more physicians. Many key physicians were getting older. Those more than fifty years of age accounted for nearly 20 percent of the medical staff. They admitted many of the hospital's patients, and many were approaching retirement. There was a 41 percent decrease in general surgeons, and a precipitous decline in the number of procedures performed by all surgeons. Surgical specialists were retiring or relocating their practices to other facilities. In addition to DeKalb Medical Center's need for more doctors, the anticipated construction of a new hospital in the growing South DeKalb area created an urgent need to expand the medical staff to serve the growing population of that community and the new hospital.[39]

In June 2003 the DMC Board of Directors rescinded the 1998 Medical Staff Development Plan[40] and retained the services of Steve Bible as director of Physician Recruitment and Retention[41] to build the medical staff's primary care physicians and the specialists who would utilize the services and the facilities of the three hospitals.

In addition to rebuilding the medical staff, DeKalb Medical reorganized the staff. With the completion of DeKalb Medical at Hillandale in 2005, the DRHS Board of Directors unified the three medical staffs with shared governance. The chiefs and representatives from each hospital now form the DeKalb Medical Executive Committee. The new structure provides that each hospital will have its own distinct medical staff privilege requirements, but the three hospitals will have a common set of bylaws, the same clinical department structure, one credentialing process, and a uniform peer review process.[42]

Today DeKalb Medical physicians have, more than ever, a strategic role in the organization. The relationship between physician and hospital was in early years essentially one of laissez-faire. Medical staff leaders volunteered their services and counsel. Today theirs is an integrated relationship in which physician leaders not only sit on the governing boards, but they have become partners in the business aspects of the organization. Members of the DeKalb Physician-Hospital Organization (DPHO) have, since the establishment of the DPHO in the late 1990s, played a vital role in negotiating and managing contracts with insurers. More recently they have become vital partners with DeKalb Medical in a clinical integration initiative.

DeKalb Medical's latest strategic plan identified key services to be developed and promoted, and it has asked physicians to be leaders of development teams to build and enhance those services. DeKalb Medical has entered into joint ventures with physicians in selected service ventures where physicians and hospital share risks and benefits.

The physician's relationship with the hospital has evolved from laissez-faire to that of a true partnership.[43] The unprecedented challenges that confront all healthcare organizations confirm the need for that partnership.

Mental (Behavioral) Health Services

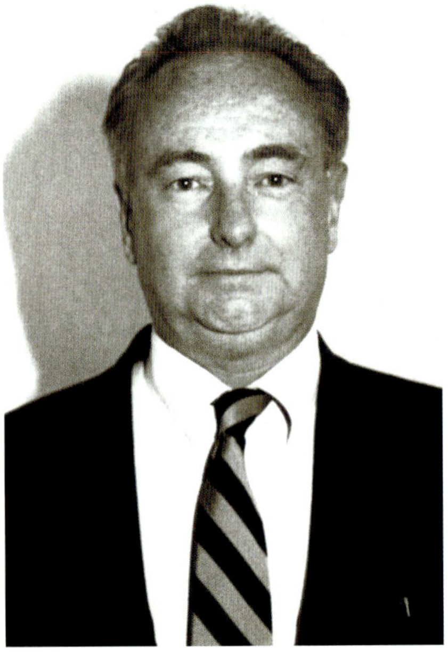

Clyde Rountree, MD, psychiatrist, helped establish the Mental Health unit and was the first chief of the Department of Psychiatry and medical director of Mental (Behavioral) Health Services.

In 1958, while DeKalb General Hospital was in the early planning stages, the president of the Greater Atlanta Mental Health Association (GAMHA) asked the DeKalb County Hospital Authority to include an eighteen or twenty-bed psychiatric unit in the new hospital for the treatment of the mentally ill. The trustees declined to include a dedicated unit, but stipulated that mentally ill patients could be housed temporarily in the four isolation rooms planned for the hospital. They also agreed to consider a psychiatric unit in any future expansion.[1]

GAMHA was not the only group looking to DeKalb General to address the needs of the county's mentally ill, and the need was real. DeKalb County patients with mental illness awaiting transfer to the state psychiatric hospital in Milledgeville, Georgia, were placed in jail with criminals until they could be transferred. There was no other place to house them. In 1959 the DeKalb County Junior Chamber of Commerce (Jaycees) said that securing beds for mental patients in the new hospital was its number one priority. A committee of the chamber met with the Hospital Authority and asked for at least two rooms in the hospital to accommodate patients awaiting transfer to Milledgeville.[2]

The local press joined in the campaign. A 1959 *Decatur-DeKalb News* editorial exclaimed that the lack of plans to provide space in the new hospital for those patients was "not only surprising but shocking."[3] The editorial went on to say, "A hospital is for the ill. Mental disorder is a form of illness. . . . *The Decatur-DeKalb News* joins with the DeKalb County Jaycees in begging the DeKalb County Hospital Authority to reconsider its decision not to have a place at least to temporarily house mental patients awaiting treatment."[4] A week later the same newspaper reported with satisfaction that "DeKalb General Hospital will have four isolation rooms that can be used by mentally ill patients from DeKalb County. . . .."[5] That promise, of course, was essentially the same offer the trustees had made to the Greater Atlanta Mental Health Association a year earlier.

In 1968, when it became known that the Authority planned to expand the hospital, GAMHA once again petitioned the Authority to include a psychiatric unit.[6] The Medical Staff Executive Committee supported the concept.[7] The Georgia Department of Public Health approved the hospital's proposal to build a mental health unit with up to fifty beds.[8] Clyde Rountree, MD, who had a private psychiatric practice and who worked part-time with the Georgia Mental Health Institute, offered to help DeKalb General develop a Department of Psychiatry and staff the proposed mental health unit.[9]

The hospital and the DeKalb County Department of Public Health jointly submitted a construction grant application to the National Institute of Mental Health for $743,000 to build a forty-four-bed mental health unit to serve a twofold purpose.[10] First, it would provide an inpatient facility to which DeKalb General's private psychiatrists could admit their patients. In addition, it would accommodate the DeKalb County Community Mental Health Program.

The proposed community mental health program consisted of six services: inpatient care, partial care, emergency care, aftercare, outpatient care, and psychiatric education and consultation services. The community program anticipated that DeKalb General's private psychiatrists would provide the first three services for the county for a fee, and the county would provide the last three services.[11] The National Institute of Mental Health granted the construction funds requested.

The joint venture quickly encountered problems. The first problem related to the care of the county's indigent inpatients. DeKalb General psychiatrists agreed to see and treat indigent patients, but they wanted to know how many the county expected them to see and who would pay for their care. The county health department said it wanted the psychiatrists to care for all of the county's indigent mental health patients. The county commissioners, however, said they had no money to pay for their care, and the hospital would have to work out that issue with the county health department.[12] The hospital, therefore, submitted a ten-point working agreement to the county health department in February 1970, including the stipulation that the health department would pay for the care of all indigent patients not covered by any other form of insurance.[13]

The medical staff proceeded to create a Department of Psychiatry and elected Rountree as its chief.[14] The hospital opened twenty mental health beds for private patients ages fourteen years and older in March 1971.[15] Edna Lang, RN, who had helped plan the facility, was named department head. The unit included two recreational rooms—one for teenagers and one for adults—a television room, a dining room, and a laundry room. In addition to individual therapy sessions, patients' daily schedules consisted of exercise sessions, occupational therapy, rest, and meals. Patients and staff wore street clothes.[16]

The county health department, however, delayed beginning its program. It would not agree to the terms of the ten-point agreement that the hospital had submitted in February 1970. The Authority called a special meeting of mental health representatives from the federal, state, and local levels to discuss the agreement. Everyone said the terms were reasonable, and T. O. Vinson, MD, director of the county health department, said his department would finance indigent inpatient care.[17]

Despite Vinson's verbal commitment, the county health department did not sign the agreement until April 1972.[18] As a result of the delay, the hospital was severely criticized for failing to provide the mental health services envisioned by the community even though it was the county that delayed for twenty-six months signing the agreement. Jim Fleming, vice president of the DeKalb chapter of the Metropolitan Atlanta Mental Health Association, said "the hospital is not living up to a contract." DeKalb Police Chief Fred D. Hand said that emergency mental patients present "a very serious problem" to his officers and that "We don't get too much help" from DeKalb General.[19]

The county health department finally signed the agreement, but then it ran into financial problems. It anticipated receiving a $600,000 federal grant to fund its staffing for its first year's program,[20] but those federal funds never came. The state granted only $75,000 for start-up expenses. The county health department had to abbreviate its plans.[21] It opened a unit on the ground floor in January 1973, but could afford only a partial staff and a limited outpatient program.[22]

The county never received the funds needed to carry out its plans. It also experienced a rapid turnover of its leadership.[23] It began a drug and alcohol program under the medical direction of Douglas Talbott, MD,[24] but transferred that program to its Briarcliff Road facility in 1976.[25] Finally, in the fall of 1981, the county announced that it would cease completely using DeKalb General's mental health facility due to a lack of funds and would relocate its program to a Scott Boulevard address in September 1982.[26]

Shortly after the county moved out of the facility, the National Institute of Mental Health demanded that DeKalb General Hospital reimburse it the $743,000 grant made to construct the facility, plus interest, for a total of $1.3 million. And it demanded payment within thirty days. When the Authority attempted to negotiate with the institute, it added additional interest to their demand. Fortunately, U.S. Senator Sam Nunn intervened, and the institute finally agreed to let the hospital purchase the

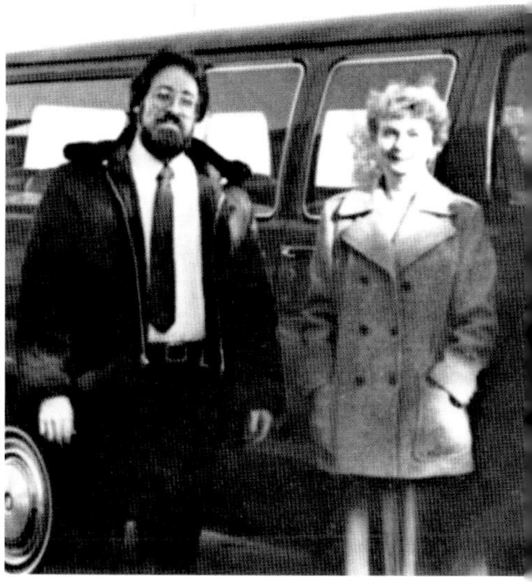

Edna Lang, RN, (right) helped plan DGH's mental health facility and served as its department head from its beginning in 1971 until her retirement in 1990. Richard Gerson, (left) was program coordinator.

mental health facility at a price that was even less than that of an appraisal.[27]

As sole occupant and owner of the facility, the hospital negotiated a contract with Clyde Rountree to serve as the medical director of DeKalb General's mental health program.[28] Edna Lang remained as department head until her retirement in 1990.[29] The unit established a substance abuse program under the direction of Ralph Alexander, MD,[30] that later expanded into a "New Day Recovery Substance Abuse" program in collaboration with an outside partner.[31] The DeKalb General Auxiliary donated a van to be used for patient outings.[32] In 1992, when Lee Woods was director of the department, it added a sixteen-bed medical/psychiatric service under the medical direction of Rob Riesenberg, MD, for patients with coexisting medical and psychiatric illnesses.[33]

In the mid-1990s DeKalb Medical Center and the newly acquired Decatur Hospital consolidated the mental health and addiction recovery programs of the two hospitals into a single department called DeKalb Behavioral Health Services located at DeKalb Medical Center. It included an eighteen-bed medical/psychiatric unit, an eighteen-bed general psychiatry unit, and an outpatient substance-abuse and eating-disorders programs. Following Lee Woods' resignation, Dorinda McCauley, PhD, who had served as director of Decatur Hospital's substance-abuse and eating-disorders program, was named director of DeKalb Behavioral Health Services.[34]

With the advent of managed care in the 1990s, DeKalb Regional Healthcare System (DRHS) entered into a joint venture with Strategic Decision Systems Inc. (SDS) to manage its mental health services and to create a managed-care mental health product to compete with other programs in the area. DRHS also entered into a joint venture with Behavioral Health Partners, another managed-care program created by Gary Lang who also was affiliated with Strategic Decision Systems. DRHS soon purchased a majority interest in Strategic Decision Systems and a 94 percent share of Behavioral Health Partners stocks.[35] The Behavioral Health Partners Board of Directors named Bill Sublett, director of DeKalb Medical Center Administrative Services, as chairman of the board and Gary Lang as president. DRHS then merged the two companies into one corporation, Behavioral Health Partners Inc. (BPH) to provide managed-care consulting, management, and other mental health services.[36] With a $500,000 loan from DRHS, BHP purchased a software program, Connex, to handle its managed-care initiatives.[37]

BHP negotiated a contract with the PROMINA Health Plan to manage its behavioral health benefits. It also negotiated contracts with other mental health organizations throughout the state to provide four types of services: to serve as a managed-care organization for behavioral health, to provide behavioral health consulting services, to provide behavioral health management, and to provide a behavioral health information system.[38]

Gary Lang predicted that by the end of the 1998 fiscal year BHP would show a profit of at least $300,000.[39] Those optimistic financial projections, however, were never realized. In the first eleven months of 1998, BHP sustained a loss of more than $1 million.[40] The following year showed more losses.[41] Not only had DRHS invested heavily in acquiring BPH and the Connex software, it had made substantial loans to cover the company's payroll and other operating expenses. DRHS served notice that it would not continue supporting BHP financially.[42] The BHP Board of Directors instructed Gary Lang to reconfigure BHP's operations, sell the Connex software, and curb ongoing losses. Otherwise, the board said, it would cease operating the company.[43]

Gary Lang sold the Connex software program,[44] but the operating losses continued. An audit also revealed inadequate management of expenses and of collecting fees for services rendered.[45] DRHS offered to sell its ownership shares in BHP to Gary Lang, but he would not agree to the terms of the sale.[46]

In April 2000 Gary Lang resigned as president of the company.[47] Employees offered to form a new company and take over servicing the contracts BHP had signed; but they could not honor BHP's debts and financial obligations, and the BHP Board of Directors could not accept their offer.[48] Ultimately the BHP board voted to "close the BHP doors" and go out of business on May 3, 2000. Bill Sublett, chairman of the BHP Board of Directors, sent the following notice to those organizations with which BHP had contracts:

> *As you know, Behavioral Health Partners Inc. has a contract with you to provide certain behavioral health services.*
>
> *It is necessary for me to advise you that the Board of Directors of Behavioral Health Partners Inc. has determined that the company no longer has the financial resources to continue in business. It has therefore closed its doors effective May 3, 2000, subject to retaining one representative who will wind down the business for a short time.*[49]

The BHP Board of Directors used the money on hand, what it received for previous services rendered, and financial assistance from DRHS to negotiate settlements with the BHP employees for payroll and benefits due them and to reimburse organizations that had made advanced payments to BHP for services they never received. Once all loose ends were resolved, the board members submitted their resignations, and BHP ceased to exist.[50]

With that management venture behind it, DeKalb Medical Center turned its attention to managing its own mental health services. Dorinda McCauley remained as director until she retired in 2001.[51] At that time, DeKalb Behavioral Health Services offered three kinds of service: a general psychiatric unit for adults, a medical-psychiatric unit mostly for older patients with psychiatric and medical conditions, and an outpatient group counseling service for those who could function with that level of service.[52]

Paul Olander, LCSW, succeeded Dorinda McCauley as director in 2001.[53] Shortly thereafter the hospital engaged consultants who recommended that Behavioral Health Services be "right sized."[54] The department subsequently reduced its inpatient capacity from thirty-four to eighteen beds and discontinued its medical-psychiatric program. Only general psychiatric patients and/or those with substance-dependency impairment qualified for inpatient admission. Outpatient services remained unchanged at that time.

In 2006 DeKalb Medical engaged another consulting firm that recommended additional staff reductions and the closing of outpatient services. Closing outpatient services involved the painful termination of staff members who had worked in the department for more than twenty-five years.

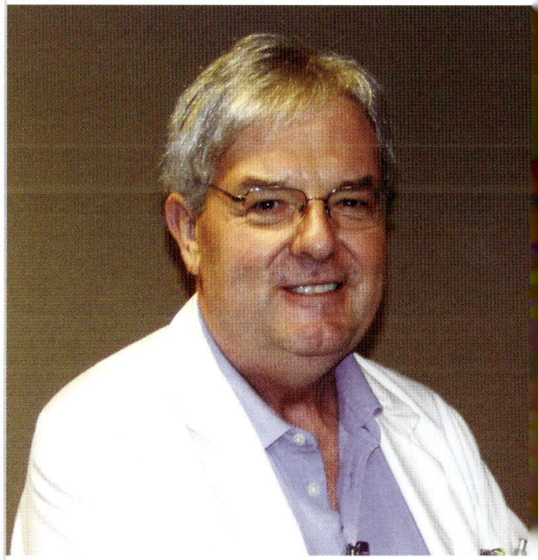
Paul Olander, LCSW, became director of Behavioral Health in 2001.

Behavioral Health Services now operates fourteen inpatient beds. It admits and stabilizes patients in crisis, whether they be psychotic, homicidal, suicidal, or in need of alcohol or drug detoxification. Once stabilized, they may be discharged or transferred to another facility. Most patients come from the Emergency Department, but some come from psychiatrists' offices and a few come from other hospitals. Whereas thirty-one psychiatrists used the mental health unit twenty years ago,[55] today there are only four. Todd Antin, MD, is the medical director, and Neil Kahn, MD, is chief of the Psychiatry Department.[56]

Though small in the size of its hospital and physician staffs and in the scope of its current services, Behavioral Health Services continues to meet an important community need. It also stands ready once again to enlarge its staff and services should the need and opportunity arise.

The Nursing Home
(Also known as Skilled Nursing Facility or Extended Care Facility)

The DeKalb County Hospital Authority acknowledged the need for a facility for "the elderly and the infirm" in some of its earliest deliberations. In 1958 the trustees discussed building a home for the aged on campus, but a legal review of the bond documents revealed that the county's bond money could be used only for "hospital facilities for the sick."[1] That restriction precluded using the money for a home for the aged.

In April 1960, a year before DeKalb General Hospital opened, the county and state public health representatives asked that any hospital plans for a future addition include a "facility for convalescents."[2] W. E. Uzzell of the Georgia Department of Public Health added that the state would partner with DeKalb General to build a model nursing home at DeKalb General if the hospital was interested.[3] The Authority responded in the affirmative.[4]

The Authority appointed a committee to develop a description of the facility, obtain architectural drawings, and provide cost estimates.[5] In January 1961 the committee proposed that the hospital construct a 100-to-150-bed "convalescent and rehabilitation unit" if the county would provide $1 million in the next bond election as its share of the cost.[6] A site plan for the hospital's forty acres was prepared in 1962 and showed an "Old Age Nursing Center" facing Winn Way, located on the southernmost part of the hospital's property at approximately the site of the present Child Care Center.[7]

In 1963 the county voted a bond referendum for the project. The county commissioners then passed a resolution "that the building of a facility of care for the aged be placed on the property . . . owned by the DeKalb County Hospital Authority, and that the DeKalb County Hospital Authority, the county administration, and the [state] public health department work together on the construction of the facility, and upon its completion, the DeKalb County Hospital Authority will assume the operation and supervision of the same."[8]

The county's plan, however, presented two problems. First, the bond that passed allocated only $200,000 to the project rather than the proposed $1 million.[9] The Authority told the county commissioners that $200,000 would build only a forty-bed free-standing facility that could not be operated economically.[10] In addition, the Authority said that the county should provide operating funds for the facility on a "permanent basis," which neither the bond referendum nor the county commissioners' resolution had addressed.[11] The Authority recommended that the commissioners put the plans on hold until another bond issue could be passed that provided enough money to construct and operate a larger free-standing facility.[12] The commissioners agreed and planned to have a bond election in early 1965 for enough money to build a "first-class one-hundred-bed" facility.[13]

Not everyone was happy with that decision. Consumer advocates were impatient with both the county and the hospital for the delay. At the April 1965 meeting of the Hospital Authority, Mrs. William Kamerer of the League of Women Voters and Mrs. Frank Brenner of the United Church Women appeared before the Authority and "grilled" Chairman Evans with ten lengthy questions as to the status of a home for "the chronically ill and infirm" and how the hospital was working with the county on that issue.[14] Chairman Evans answered as well as he could, given the unknown actions the county would take.

Because of the delay and the existing need to provide convalescent care for some of its discharged patients, the Authority negotiated contracts with three private nursing homes to accept its convalescent patients. DeKalb Convalescent Center, Fountainview Convalescent Center, and Moody Nursing Home all agreed to receive patients, and the hospital agreed to accept any of their patients needing hospitalization.[15]

By 1968 the Hospital Authority developed plans to renovate and expand the hospital. The trustees thought it logical to include a fifty-bed long-term care unit in the expanded hospital rather than build a separate free-standing facility. A fifty-bed unit as part of the hospital would be more economical to build and more efficient to operate.

The county and the state approved the hospital's proposal, agreed to its construction budget of more than $2 million, and authorized the hospital to advertise for construction bids.[16] The Hill-Burton Agency approved more than $1 million in federal funds for the project, and the county transferred to the Authority the 1963 bond funds of $200,000. The Authority paid the remaining $800,000 out of accumulated reserves and part of a 1968 revenue anticipation certificate.[17] The state provided no money. Groundbreaking for the renovation and expansion took place in July 1968, and the project was completed three years later in July 1971.

But red tape and bureaucratic delays over the unit's license prevented the hospital from opening the nursing home as a long-term care, skilled nursing facility for four and a half years. In April 1970—even before the renovation was complete—Administrator Thrasher reported a problem to the hospital Authority.[18] Since the unit was a part of the hospital building and under the direct control of the Authority, the trustees had asked the state to include the nursing home under the hospital's license. The state, however, contended that it had to be licensed separately as a nursing home.

Despite the fact that Medicare, the Metropolitan Council on Health, and the state board of health supported the hospital's request to operate the unit under a single hospital license,[19] the Georgia Department of Public Health stood its ground and would not alter its demand for a separate license. The hospital deferred opening the unit for more than four years while it continued requesting a single license and the Georgia Department of Public Health continued refusing it.[20] Finally, in November 1975, Administrator Thrasher's successor, Charles Eberhart, announced that the unit would open as a skilled nursing facility nursing home under a separate license as the state had demanded all along.

Director of Nursing Naomi Harman, RN, already licensed as a nursing home executive, was named administrator of the facility.[21] She retired in 1992 to be followed by Nell Adams, RN, Paul Barnes, Marie Gaspard, RN, Kathy LaPorte, RN and Kappa Strickland, RN.[22]

As a fifty-bed unit, twenty-six of the rooms were private. The first fifteen patients moved in on September 17, 1975. The patients could choose from available framed pictures to hang in their rooms. The unit included a "sun room" and a barber shop/beauty salon ("Granny's Parlor"). It provided rehabilitative nursing care with access to social services, physical therapy, occupational therapy, speech therapy, and recreational therapy.[23]

The staff provided good nursing care and entertainment for the residents. They went on picnics and riverboat rides at Stone Mountain Park.[24] They visited DeKalb General's adopted Stone Mountain High School where they attended classes in physics and calculus and had lunch with the students.[25]

They went on picnics and riverboat rides at Stone Mountain Park. They visited DeKalb General's adopted Stone Mountain High School where they attended classes in physics and calculus and had lunch with the students.

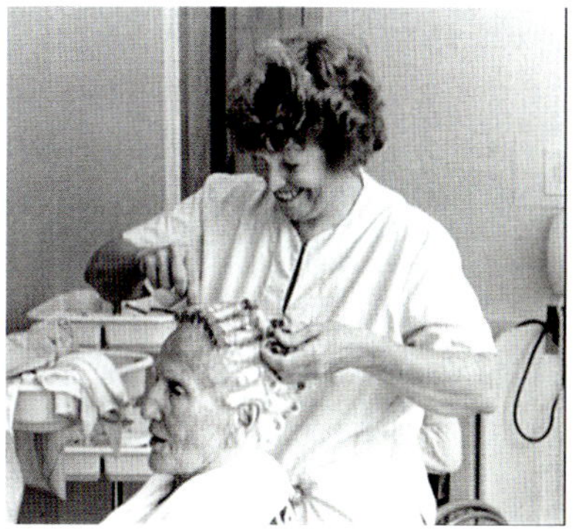

Granny's Parlor was operated by Ruth Kuester, and every Wednesday she and an assistant would wash, cut, set, perm, color, and style hair for DeKalb Medical Center patients and employees. Here she is setting the hair of Betty Pelton..

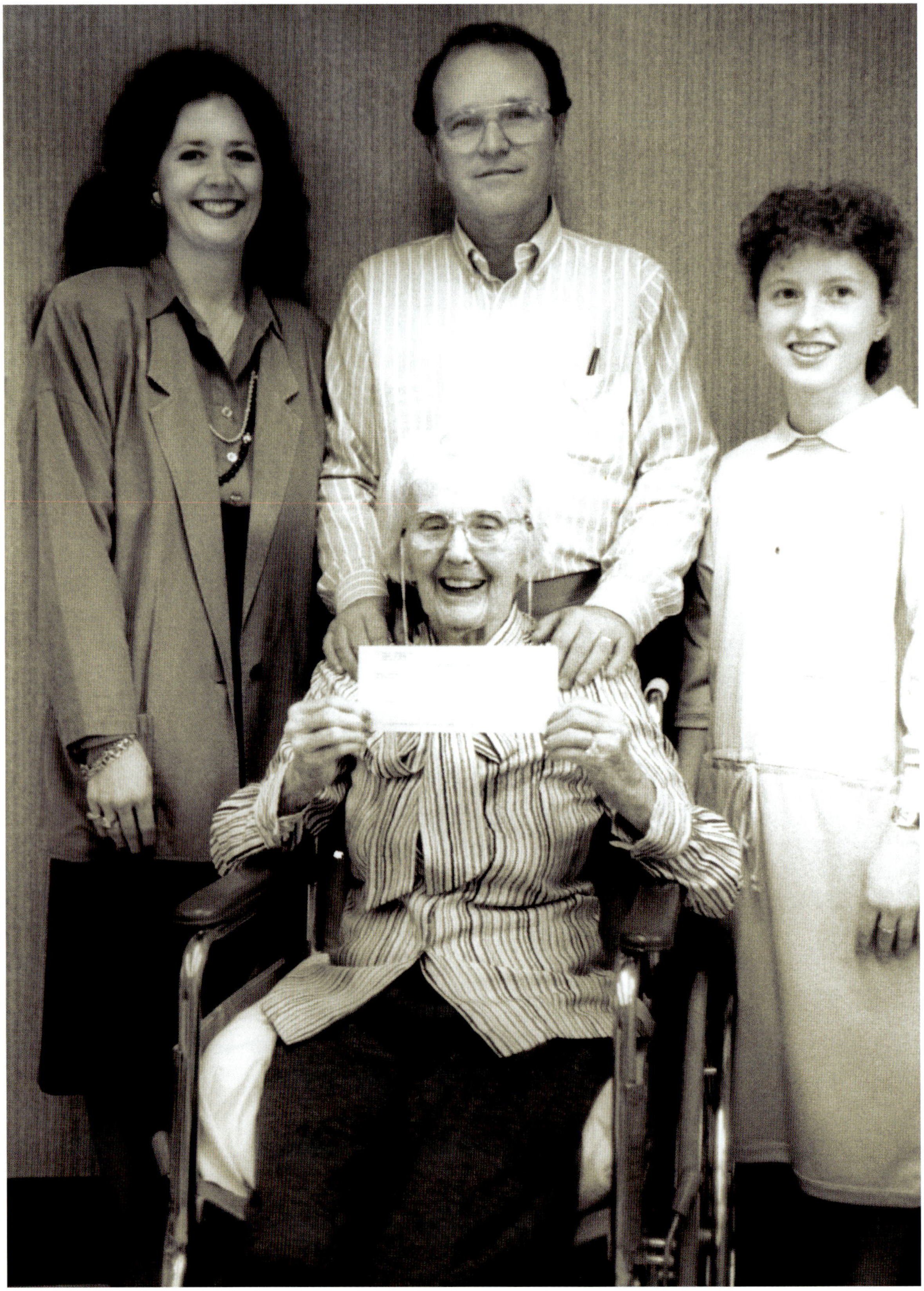

Betty Sumner (right) was voted Candy Striper of the Year and named Metro Atlanta's "Volunteer of the Year" for which she won a $1,500 cash award. She had spent many hours teaching art classes to the hospital residents and performing other volunteer duties. Rather than put her cash award toward her prenursing studies, she chose to donate the money back to the hospital to be used for the residents' outings, parties, craft supplies, and other activities. Accepting the donation is resident Johnnie McAnulty and with them are Bonnie Phipps, Fiscal Services Director, and Ben Harbour, Nursing Home Activities Coordinator.

There was an annual crowning of "Ms. DeKalb General Nursing Home."[26]

Once open, the unit ran smoothly and filled rapidly. The state approved it for Medicare and Medicaid patients, it was accredited with commendations by the Joint Commission on Accreditation of Healthcare Organizations, and within a month forty-four members of the medical staff had admitted patients to the unit. The unit had a lot to recommend it: it was close to the Emergency Department in case of emergencies, it was convenient to physicians seeing other patients in the hospital, other hospital nurses were available to provide nursing backup, and the rates were reasonable. A private room initially cost $870 per month, and a semiprivate room $780 per month.[27]

Eventually the unit experienced a growing financial challenge. It was increasingly expensive to operate, increasingly difficult to comply with expanding regulatory requirements, and increasingly difficult to realize a positive net income or break even. While expenses rose, reimbursements declined. Medicare payments became restrictive and limited, and Medicaid repeatedly reduced its rate of reimbursement. To reduce staff as a means of cutting expenses meant putting the quality of patient care at risk. The annual net operating loss reached more than $1 million and increased every year.[28] The board of directors finally made the difficult decision to close the facility.

Patricia Walker was hired as administrator to close the unit. She met personally with the residents' families to notify them of the decision and to help them make appropriate transfers for those residents who needed continued care. Many of the residents were transferred to the same facility, which made their adjustment to a new environment easier.[29] When the last resident was transferred, the nursing home closed on June 30, 2003.[30] The patient rooms were converted into an antepartum nursing unit.[31]

Nursing Services

A vast array of people are essential to provide quality care to hospital patients. That task requires competent and committed members of the governing body and administrative staff, physicians, technicians, and a host of others in all of the support services. Without any of these, there is a glaring gap in the kind of patient care for which the hospital exists and to which it is committed.

Few people are more important to quality care than the hospital's nurses. They are the very face of the hospital in patients' eyes: those who touch patients throughout the day, who administer their care, who witness their moment-to-moment changes for good or ill, who intervene and solicit assistance when urgent attention is needed, and who provide comfort for their pain, concerns, and anxieties.

The important task of securing nurses, training them, guiding them, supporting them, and empowering them is the primary responsibility of the hospital's nursing leadership. As of 2007 DeKalb Medical has had six leaders who have brought their unique gifts to that task and made special contributions to Nursing Services. The contributions of each reflect not only their leadership abilities but also their responses to the healthcare environment that evolved during their tenures and to the philosophy of nursing that emerged during their administrations.

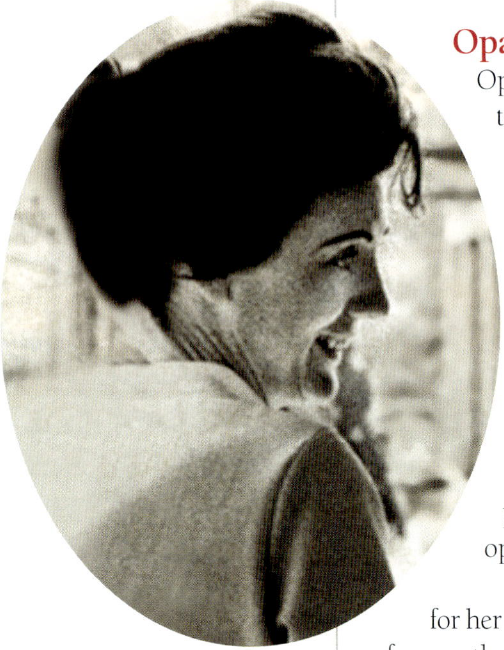

Opal Hopkins, (Fyffe), RN, was the first director of Nursing at DeKalb General Hospital.

Opal Hopkins (Fyffe)

Opal Hopkins (Fyffe), RN, was DeKalb General Hospital's first director of Nursing from 1960 to 1965. A member of the nursing staff at Georgia Baptist Hospital, Administrator William Thrasher selected her as his nursing leader because he liked her, felt he and she could work well together, agreed with her ideas about organizing the nursing service, and appreciated her background as an instructor in nursing education.

Despite a nationwide nursing shortage, Opal Hopkins was successful in recruiting 120 nurses by the time the hospital opened. Many of her recruits came from Georgia Baptist where she was known and where she knew the nurses. She filled all head nursing positions except one with nurses from Georgia Baptist. The majority of her nurses were graduates of three-year hospital diploma programs, as was she, and all were females.[1] Diploma programs were, in fact, the dominant type of nursing education at that time.[2] She and her staff did a remarkable job of developing policies, organizing the nursing units, preparing the hospital for opening day, and creating a nursing environment of collegiality, optimism, and even excitement at being in a progressive, new hospital.

Hopkins had a "hands-on" leadership style and created a supportive, intimate environment for her nurses. She knew the nurses personally, stayed in close touch with them and their units, and frequently made nursing rounds on all three shifts. She helped them change bed linens and perform other tasks to demonstrate her acknowledgement of and appreciation for even their most routine duties. She fought their battles. When she began losing nurses to other hospitals that caught up with and surpassed DeKalb General's salaries, she offered her resignation in protest and rescinded it only when administration and the governing body made a commitment to increase the nursing pay scale and improve benefits.[3]

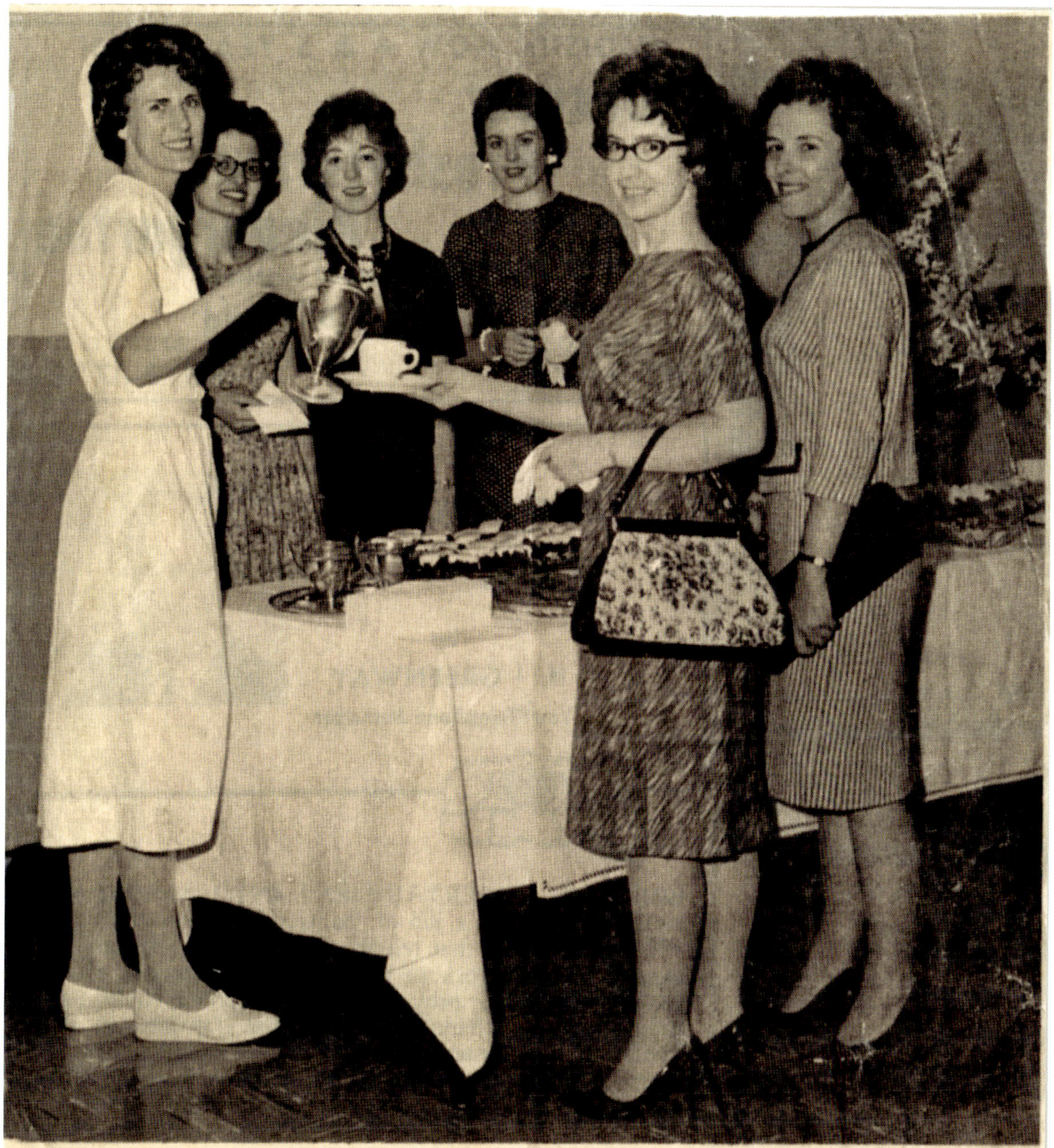

STUDENT NURSES HONORED—Students graduating in June from the nursing schools in Atlanta hospitals were guests of honor at a tea given by DeKalb General Hospital during National Hospital Week on May 14. Left to right are: Mrs. Opal Hopkins, Director of Nursing at DeKalb General; Emily Hendry; Lynn Walsh; Armenia Williams; Anita Lynes; and Portia Keller. Mrs. Hopkins was assisted in serving by the DeKalb General Hospital nursing supervisors, together with Mrs. Mary Lou Hurt, personnel director, and Mrs. Helen Bush, administrative assistant.

Opal Hopkins had a "hands-on" leadership style and created a supportive, intimate environment for her nurses.

The trustees did not invite Hopkins to attend their meetings as they did with subsequent nursing leaders. She depended on the administrator to report nursing's needs and concerns to the DeKalb County Hospital Authority. She also had to accept the authority that physicians had over nurses in that era at DeKalb General as well as at other hospitals around the nation. The hospital Authority said that in all matters of patient care, nursing procedures and treatment, the director of Nursing would be responsible to the medical staff. It also said that the medical staff's Nursing Committee would have ultimate responsibility for dealing with all unresolved deficiencies in the patient care provided by nurses.[4]

Despite those constraints, Hopkins brought an enthusiasm to DeKalb General's Nursing Services that permeated the staff and created a pleasant, familylike environment. The nurses felt valued and supported. Even with the authoritative role of the physicians, the medical and nursing professions showed a mutual appreciation and respect for one another. As Hopkins reflected in later years, "It was the best job I ever had; the best of all worlds. I would have done it for free."[5]

Margaret Ford

After her husband died in 1963, Hopkins remarried and retired in 1965 to attend to responsibilities at home. The trustees directed Administrator Thrasher to select a "degree nurse," someone who received her nursing degree from an academic institution, as Hopkins's successor. He chose Margaret Ford, RN, as the second director of Nursing. Ford received a bachelor of nursing education degree from the University of Georgia and a master's degree in nursing from Emory University.[6] She already was known at DeKalb General because she had served as the hospital's first director of Training and Health Services from 1961 to 1962 before taking a director of nursing position elsewhere.

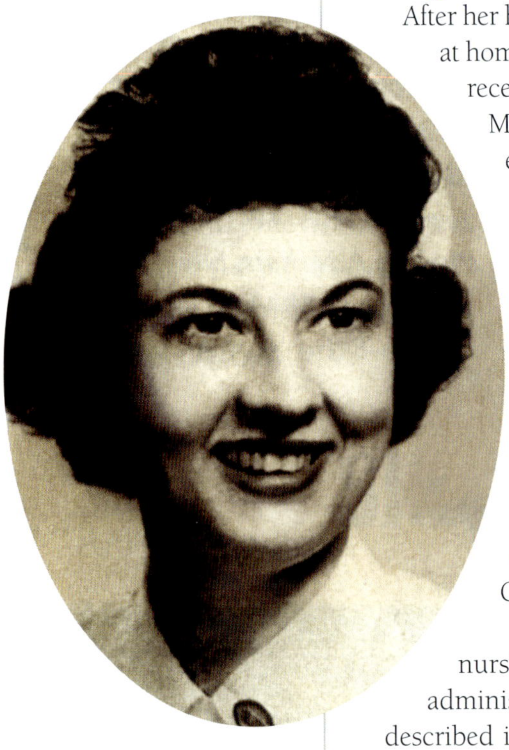

Margaret Ford, RN, second director of Nursing, was fired due to the hospital administration's perception that her loyalty was not with them, but with the nurses who decided to resign.

Margaret Ford had solid credentials and experience: she had a master's degree in nursing, she had been in the military, she was a former director of nursing education, and a former director of nursing. Ford brought an element of professionalism to DeKalb General's Nursing Services that differed from Fyffe's leadership style.[7] Ford preferred to hire nurses with bachelor of science in nursing (BSN) degrees from academic institutions, and she encouraged the diploma nurses to pursue a baccalaureate degree.[8] While she was liked by those who knew her well,[9] many described her as "cold, aloof, and private."[10] She did not enjoy the close relationship with the nursing staff that was a notable feature of Opal Hopkins Fyffe's administration.

Ford's tenure also was impacted overwhelmingly by an emerging philosophy of nursing that conflicted with the views of many nurses, most physicians, the trustees, and administration. It placed her in the middle of the growing crisis in Nursing at DeKalb General described in chapter 4. During her administration, the Georgia State Nurses Association (GSNA) adopted a statement of philosophy advocated by the American Nurses Association. That philosophy declared that the welfare of nurses was inseparable from the welfare of patients and that to insure optimum patient care, nurses had to have a voice in establishing their employment conditions. GSNA also said that nurses had a right to participate in planning and administering the nursing service, and they had a right to organize and choose a representative to engage in collective bargaining on their behalf as the most effective means of securing their rights.[11]

GSNA asked directors of Nursing to take a neutral position if they could not actively support their nurses' attempts to organize, and it said they should not interfere with organizing efforts even if they did not approve of them.[12] Ford tried to remain neutral when DeKalb General's nurses organized, but she would not be perceived by administration and trustees as being neutral.

DeKalb's nurses felt that administration and the Authority were not responsive to their need for improved salaries and benefits. A large number of DeKalb General's nurses asked GSNA to be their representative to engage in collective bargaining with the hospital to achieve their demands. Administration and the trustees refused to recognize the GSNA as their bargaining representative, and they fired Ford because they questioned her loyalty to the hospital. As a result of the impasse and being angered by Ford's dismissal, one hundred of the hospital's 130 nurses resigned in mass on January 22, 1969.

Despite enhancing the professional status and competence of the hospital's nurses, Ford's achievements regrettably remain overshadowed by the nurses' loss of confidence in DeKalb General's leadership, by the confrontational environment that ensued, and by the loss of the many valuable nurses who resigned.

Naomi Harman

Naomi Harman, RN, was called on to be the third director of Nursing and to re-build the decimated Nursing Services. She also was no stranger to DeKalb General; she had been the first night supervisor when the hospital opened in 1961. Opal Hopkins selected her as assistant director of Nursing when Hopkins had to reduce her responsibilities to attend to her terminally ill husband. When Opal Hopkins married David Fyffe and retired in 1965, Harman resigned to assist her husband in his new furniture business. She subsequently became night supervisor at Emory University Hospital and later was serving as director of Nursing at Fountainview Convalescent Center when Administrator Thrasher asked her to return to DeKalb General.[13]

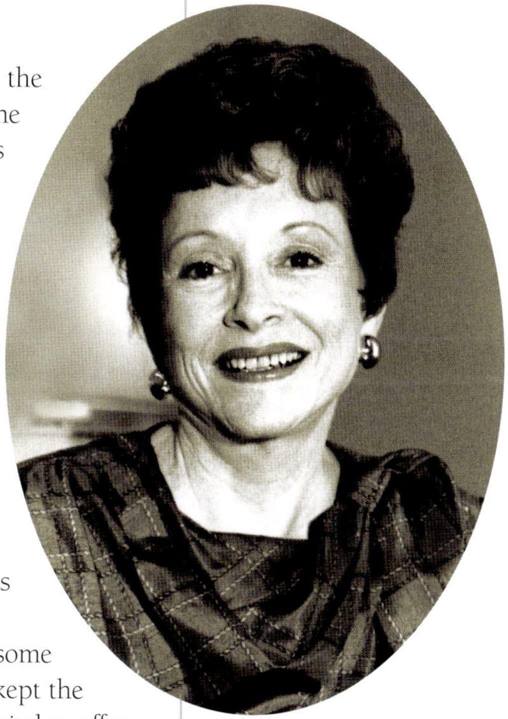

Naomi Harman, RN, succeeded Margaret Ford, becoming the third director of Nursing, and rebuilt the nursing staff.

Coming back to the hospital, Harman faced a monumental task, possibly one unparalleled in the annals of nursing services. She immediately had to provide nursing care for 220 patients with less than 25 percent of the usual nursing staff. In the aftermath of the hospital-nurse dispute noted above, very few of the nursing leaders remained. Harman had to rebuild Nursing Services almost "from scratch." And she also had to achieve that task in the midst of a major renovation and building project that added inconveniences for patients, staff, and physicians.

Former retired nurses, doctors, doctors' wives with a current nursing license, and some resigning nurses who rescinded their resignations answered her call. Harman not only kept the hospital running; within two months she had rebuilt a nursing staff that enabled the hospital to offer full services again. Within six months hospital life was essentially "back to normal."[14] As she rebuilt her staff, Harman personally interviewed all nursing applicants. She looked for competence in her recruits, knowing that uneasy physicians, the media, the community, and the Joint Commission on Accreditation of Healthcare Organizations (JCAHO) were watching closely to see if she could "pull it off."[15] She measured up to their standards and passed a JCAHO survey with "flying colors." It was truly a remarkable achievement in nursing leadership. That, however, was only the beginning of Harman's contributions in her twenty-three-year tenure as director of Nursing.

She created a more diverse nursing staff in terms of training and education than had her predecessors. She began with a staff still composed of mostly diploma nurses and a few baccalaureate nurses. But times were changing rapidly. Diploma training was being phased out in favor of collegiate education for

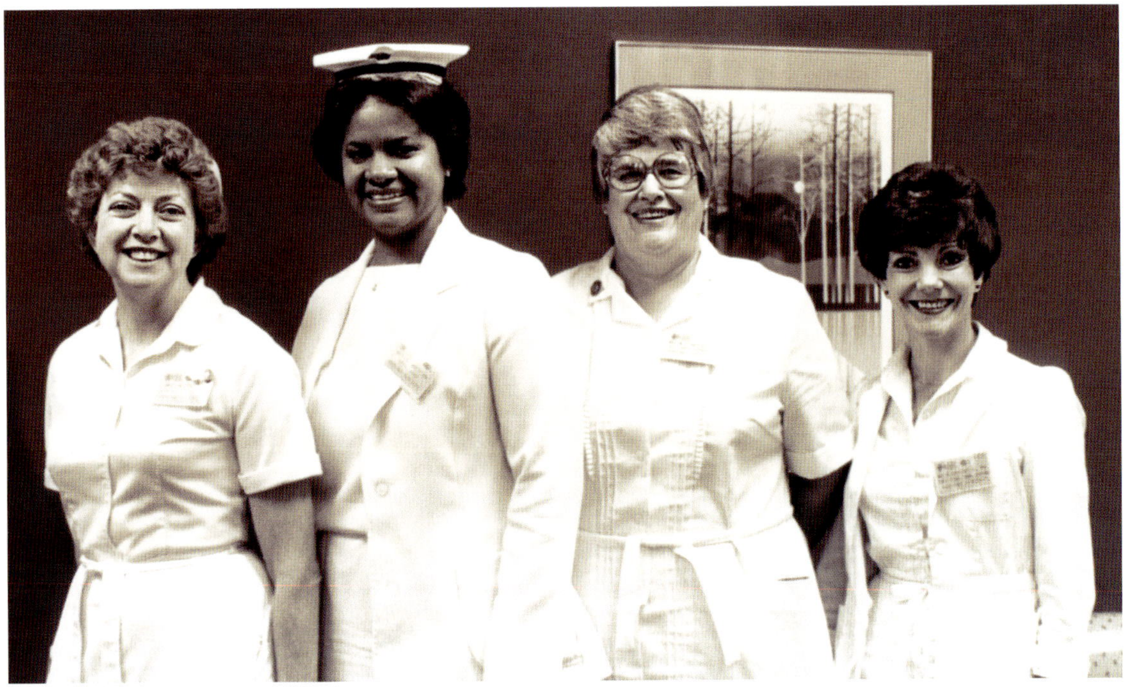

Naomi Harman's first Patient Care Coordinators, left to right: Mary Hollis, RN, Laura Hurt, RN, Mary Chambers, RN, and Melba Cantrell, RN.

nurses. Four-year colleges were granting bachelor of science in nursing degrees, and community colleges were granting associate degrees.[16] Technical schools offered a licensed practical nurse (LPN) certificate that prepared LPNs to work under the supervision of RNs or a physician and perform certain tasks previously performed only by RNs.[17]

Harman created refresher courses for former RNs and hired many of the graduates.[18] She encouraged further education for the nursing staff, appreciating its value for them as well as for the organization. With that in mind, she helped bring the College of St. Francis to the hospital from which she and many of her nurses received their baccalaureate or master's degrees.[19]

Harman created a new set of leaders that would fill the gap created by the leaders lost in the mass resignation. Once Harman identified and chose her leaders, she and the Personnel Department designed and conducted management training.[20] That creative initiative laid the groundwork for the significant emphasis on leadership development that the hospital has continued to pursue.

Harman also enhanced professionalism among the nurses. Once she identified and trained her lead nurses, she was one of the first in the city to elevate those nurses to new positions of professional responsibility. She made each of her head nurses a department head, giving each authority to manage the nursing unit in budgeting, staffing, employment issues, and general administration. That change achieved two goals. It enhanced the efficiency with which Nursing Services operated. It also enhanced the nurses' sense of worth and professional pride when empowered with new and appropriate leadership responsibilities.

Harman subsequently divided responsibility for the oversight of the nursing units among four Patient Care coordinators and appointed assistant directors of Nursing. Her first coordinators were Mary Chambers, RN, Melba Cantrell, RN, Laura Hurt, RN, and Mary Hollis, RN.[21] She then appointed Mary Hollis as her first assistant director of Nursing and later added Martha Cook (Nodal, Kalember), RN.[22]

In 1976, when Mary Hollis was promoted to another position, Charlotte Davis (Courtois), RN, succeeded her.[23]

In addition to developing nursing leadership, Naomi Harman oversaw the establishment of a "clinical ladders" program to acknowledge and reward nurses who chose to remain at the bedside. Clinical ladders gave the bedside nurse the opportunity to advance professionally and financially. The Program consisted of three levels that nurses could attain according to their ability to meet standards: clinical nursing practice, education and professional development, and leadership and institutional development.[24] As many as sixty-two nurses participated in the clinical ladders program.[25]

The status of Nursing Services was elevated during Harman's tenure. She became a member of the senior executive administrative team and represented Nursing Services at its weekly meetings. She attended the monthly meetings of the governing body. She attended the Medical Staff Executive Committee and interacted with the physician leaders. Harman and John Harrel, MD, director of Medical Affairs, made regular rounds together. They visited every nursing unit to inquire about the unit's needs and to share relevant information. Nurses to this day recall with delight their meaningful visits.[26] The presence of Harman and Harrel making rounds together was a visible symbol of the linkage between nursing and the medical staff as well as nursing and administration.

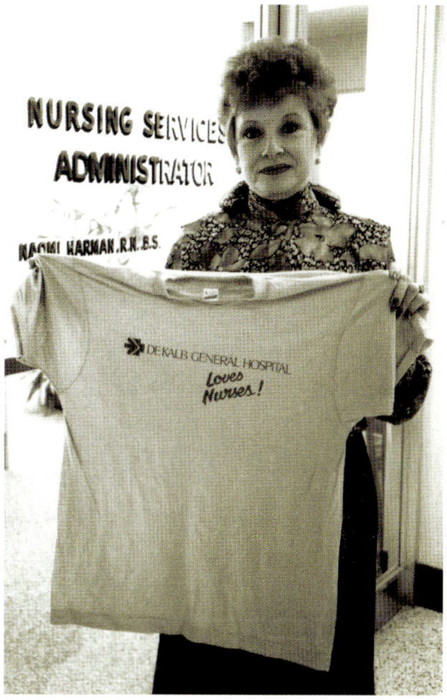

Naomi Harman displays a T-shirt presented to the nurses during Nurses Week, that says, "DeKalb General Hospital Loves Nurses!"

In the 1970s and 1980s, increasing specialization resulted in a growing complexity of patient management. The IV (intravenous) Team was organized, Mental Health (later known as Behavioral Health) Services was established, the Skilled Nursing Facility was opened, a Cardiac Rehabilitation Program was created, the Critical Care Unit was expanded to add an Intermediate Intensive Care Unit;[27] and the general medical units began to have such specialty designations as oncology, cardiology, and neurology. Each was staffed with nurses with interest and training in the specialty area. Nurses were encouraged to pursue advanced training and become certified in their specialty. Physicians utilized standing orders on some units as a reflection of their trust and confidence in the nurse's judgment and skills. Harman increasingly hired nurses with bachelor of science and master's degrees in nursing. She introduced clinical nurse specialists to the hospital to share their advanced training, knowledge, and skills with the patients, the nursing staff, and physicians.[28]

In her twenty-three years as director of Nursing, Naomi Harman helped reestablish a collegial atmosphere at DeKalb General. The hospital once again was considered a great place to work and a place with a warm, friendly, safe, supportive, familylike environment. Even though she still encouraged the nurses to stand and offer their chairs when a physician entered the nursing unit, the nurse-physician relationship was good. The focus was on the patient's well-being and good patient care. The nursing staff was confident that administration and the trustees were aware, concerned, involved, and supportive of that focus and of the importance of nursing in its achievement.[29]

There were emerging challenges that would become increasingly threatening in the decades to come. Nursing shortages were a growing problem, requiring the establishment of an in-house pool of PRN (from the Latin, *pro re nata*, "as needed") nurses and the expensive use of agency nurses. The growing emphasis on customer service led to what seemed to be a never-ending string of "service excellence" programs, often perceived by the nurses as artificial. The emerging focus on cost containment imposed by Medicare, Medicaid, managed care, and other third-party payers brought to the fore for the first time the challenge to "do more with less." The business model was arising for the first time to challenge the coveted primacy of the patient-care model that gave healthcare professionals a special pride in their practice.[30]

Ninfa Saunders

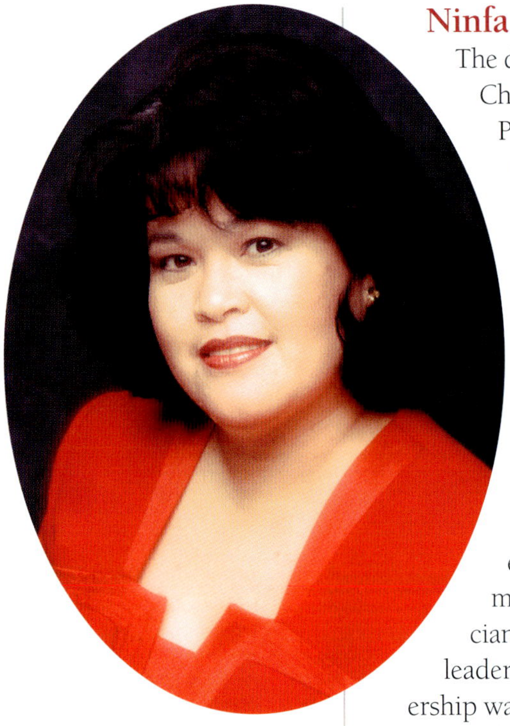

Ninfa Saunders, RN, was hired in 1992 upon the retirement of Naomi Harman. She was given the title of administrator of Patient Care Services.

The decade of the 1990s was one of rapid change. When Harman retired in 1992, Administrator Charles Eberhart named Ninfa Saunders, RN, as her successor with the title of administrator of Patient Care Services.[31] Saunders was a "true professional" of the times and considered by many to be ahead of her time. She held a bachelor's degree and a master's degree in nursing and a master's degree in business administration. She had attended the healthcare executive program at the Wharton School of Business and the international business program at the London (England) School of Business, and was pursuing a doctoral degree in healthcare administration at the Medical University of South Carolina.[32] She came to DeKalb from the position of director of nursing resources at the Emory University Hospital.

She was young, energetic, and inspiring. She immediately became a powerful and respected presence not only in nursing but throughout the hospital and in the wider community. She hired a number of new staff members with special expertise, especially clinical nurse specialists. Her leadership style was empowering and supportive. She encouraged creativity and the use of one's talents and interests. She placed a strong emphasis on education, including business and financial skills. She helped bring Mercer's masters in business administration (MBA) program onto campus to provide staff and physicians with the opportunity to obtain graduate business degrees.[33] She encouraged the nursing leaders to be exposed to the world outside DeKalb Medical Center. The culture under her leadership was one of enthusiasm and activity. Nursing had a new sense of authority in patient care and pride in the elevated level of nursing practice and knowledge.

Saunders implemented many changes in nursing practice and organization. She brought two important existing groups of nurses into the nursing division. One was the IV (intravenous) Team that she transitioned from Pharmacy to Nursing Services.[34] The other was the function of clinical nursing education that she transferred from Education Services to the individual nursing units as the responsibility of clinical nurse specialists and preceptors.[35]

She supported the successful critical care shared governance model of leadership established during Harman's tenure. She initiated multidisciplinary outcome-based care conferences with case reviews. She initiated "H Works" in collaboration with the Health Care Advisory Board Company to address the challenge of nursing recruitment and retention. DeKalb Medical Center was one of only five hospitals in the nation using the H Works program to deal with this problem.[36] The program surveyed eight hundred registered nurses and identified areas that needed attention to improve nursing satisfaction, retention, and recruitment.

She also introduced a new model of patient care. Spearheaded by Barbara Kleynen, department manager of Telemetry, patient charts were moved from the central nursing station to the wall directly outside the patient's room. The new chart racks held patients' charts as well as their daily medications and supplies. Kleynen facilitated the implementation of the new model throughout the medical-surgical areas. State-of-the-art Hill-Rom Composer system beds were purchased to replace the traditional call-light system with a wireless telephone system. All nurses carried portable phones to give them direct access to physicians, other caregivers, patients, and each other.[37]

Saunders also helped bring an inpatient hospice to the DeKalb Medical Center, and she supported the creation of the Chest Pain Center in the Emergency Department and the Acute Care of the Elderly (ACE) unit. She supported the development of the Congestive Heart Failure program, the first outpatient

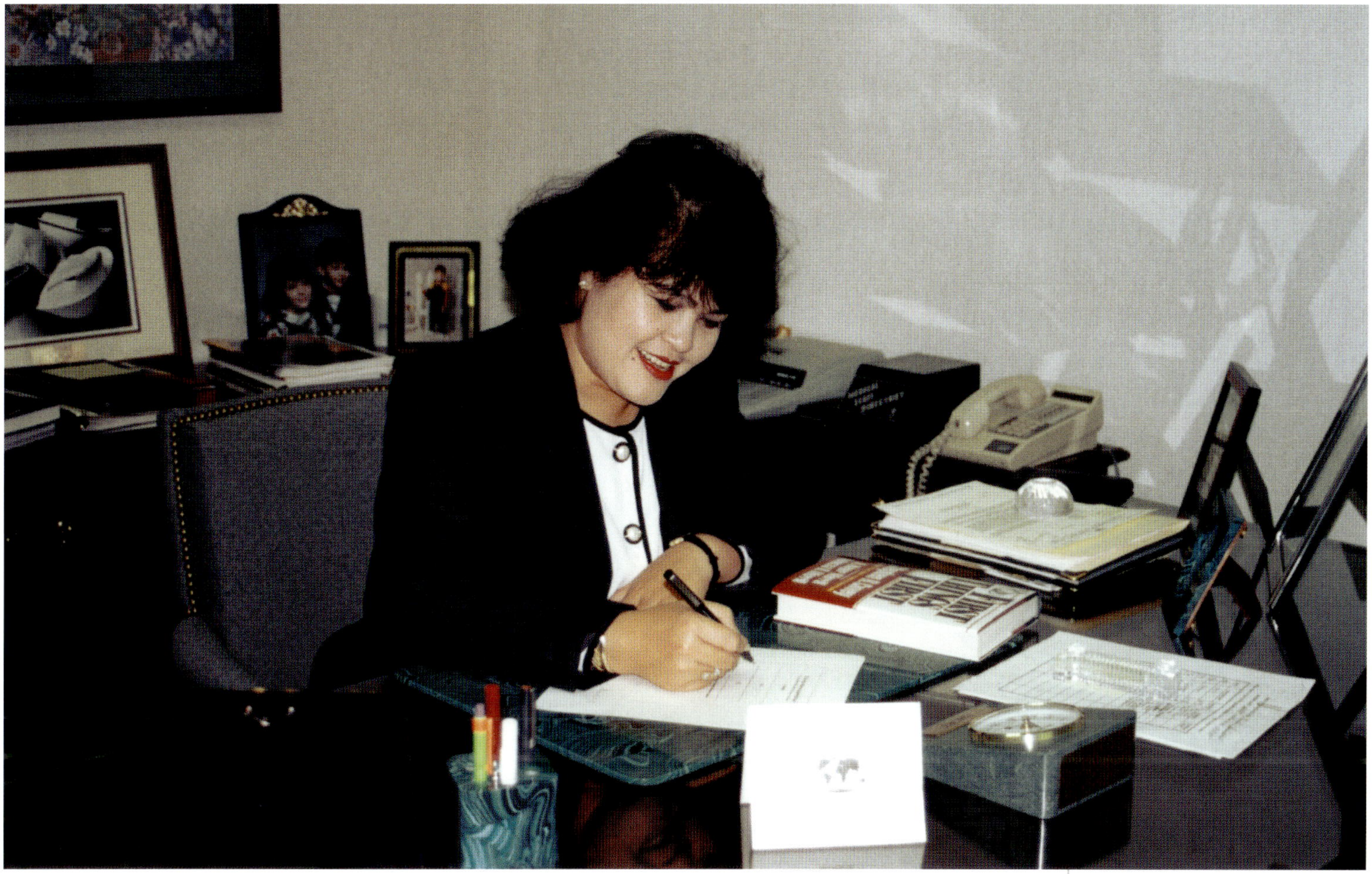

service run by a hospital-employed nurse practitioner, Nancy King (Curdy). Saunders initiated problem-oriented charting for nurses at DeKalb, a patient-acuity staffing model, and the use of quality scorecards.[38] Ninfa Saunders revolutionized the concept of nursing leadership at DeKalb Medical.

During Saunders's tenure DeKalb Medical Center was impacted by many of the growing challenges that first appeared in the 1980s. There was a growing diversity of patients, nursing staff, and physicians. There was an acute nursing shortage nationwide, and DeKalb felt it as well. The demand for documented and demonstrated quality patient care at less cost exploded in the decade of the 1990s. DeKalb Medical Center's entry into PROMINA offered the promise of many benefits but resulted in a great deal of difficult financial and leadership demands.

None impacted life at DeKalb Medical Center more than the financial environment. Saunders was named Chief Operating Officer (COO) in addition to retaining her Patient Care Services responsibilities. In that dual role, she assumed responsibility not only for Nursing Services but for all hospital departments. She had to manage and balance the growing tension between the emerging business model for fiscal survival—a challenge that stressed all members of administration—and the treasured traditional patient-care model championed by the medical and nursing professions.[39] Saunders was the last nursing leader asked to serve in that dual role.

Susan Parry

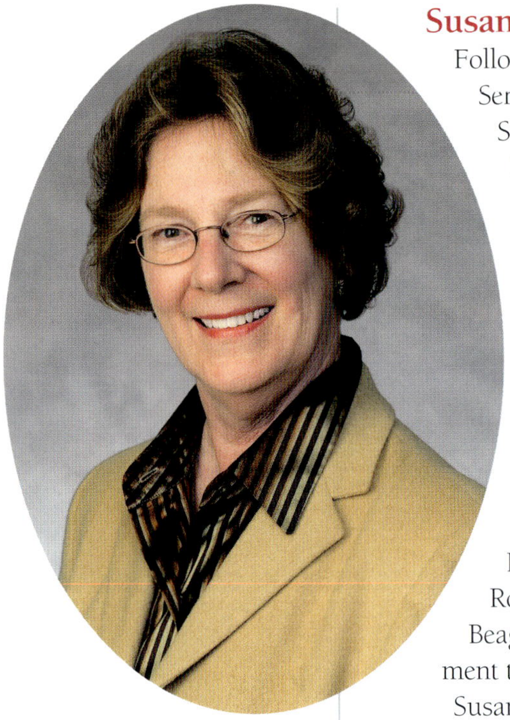

Susan Parry retired in 1998 after serving as a department head and a clinical nurse specialist. Then in 2001, John Gerlach asked her to return as director of Nursing Services and Patient Care Services.

Following Saunders' resignation in 2001, Jean Kemp, RN, served as interim director of Nursing Services until CEO John Gerlach called on Susan Parry, RN, to become the director of Nursing Services and Patient Care Services. Parry was well known by nurses and physicians and highly respected. She had come to DeKalb General in 1982 as a medical-surgical staff nurse, having a bachelor of science degree and a master's degree in nursing. She served as a department head and as a clinical nurse specialist before her first retirement in 1998. News of her return and acceptance of the position was received enthusiastically throughout the hospital.

She inherited a strong nursing leadership team, including four nursing directors with whom she had worked in the past: Susan Bales (Harris), RN, Patricia Horton, RN, Jean Kemp, RN, and Kathy LaPorte, RN. Kelly Arnold, RN, a systems analyst, was also there to support the team in matters of data management and budgeting.

Parry also recruited new members to her team of nursing directors. She named Margie Hunter, RN, as director for Women's and Infants' Services and promoted Carole Fortenberry, RN, to the newly created position of director for Nursing Resources. Brent Robinson, RN, replaced retiring Jean Kemp as director of Medical-Surgical Services. Becky Beagle, RN, assistant director of Critical Care Services, showcased the strength of the management team when she received the first systemwide Leader of the Year Award.

Susan Parry spent a great deal of time with the staff in the clinical areas, making rounds and attending staff meetings and informal get-togethers. She focused on saving and nourishing the many good things from Saunders's administration and the warm, safe, familylike culture that had characterized the Harman and Fyffe administrations.

When the administrative team underwent changes in membership, titles, and responsibilities, Parry's title became vice president for Patient Care Services and chief Nursing Officer (CNO) for the hospital system.

There were many challenges during her tenure, but one of the biggest was that of maintaining appropriate nursing staff to provide quality patient care while remaining within budget. Carole Fortenberry, in managing the use of agency nurses and the hospital's own PRN (as needed) nursing pool, played a key role in helping preserve adequate nurse-patient ratios within the constraints of tight budget controls. The nursing staff offered their own ideas. Ellen Hargett, RN, and Beth Singleton, RN, suggested a "Booster Nurse" program in which highly qualified nurses in nonclinical, salaried positions worked in support roles on clinical units particularly struggling with staffing. The first five Boosters possessed collectively more than eighty years of bedside nursing. In the Critical Care areas, their positive impact on patient care and staff morale was immeasurable. One of the participants said that being a Booster Nurse was one of the most rewarding experiences of her nursing career.[40]

While Parry faced numerous challenges, she achieved many notable accomplishments. Nursing Services received a perfect score on a JCAHO survey. Two other significant initiatives involved establishing the "Throughput" process and laying a foundation for the implementation of the QUEST (Quality, Uniformity, Efficiency, and Safety Through Technology) electronic medical record initiative.

The "Throughput" project dealt with finding ways to move patients through the system efficiently, appropriately, and safely without unnecessary delays at any point along the way. Every department was challenged to examine and streamline its processes where indicated. Nursing Services created the

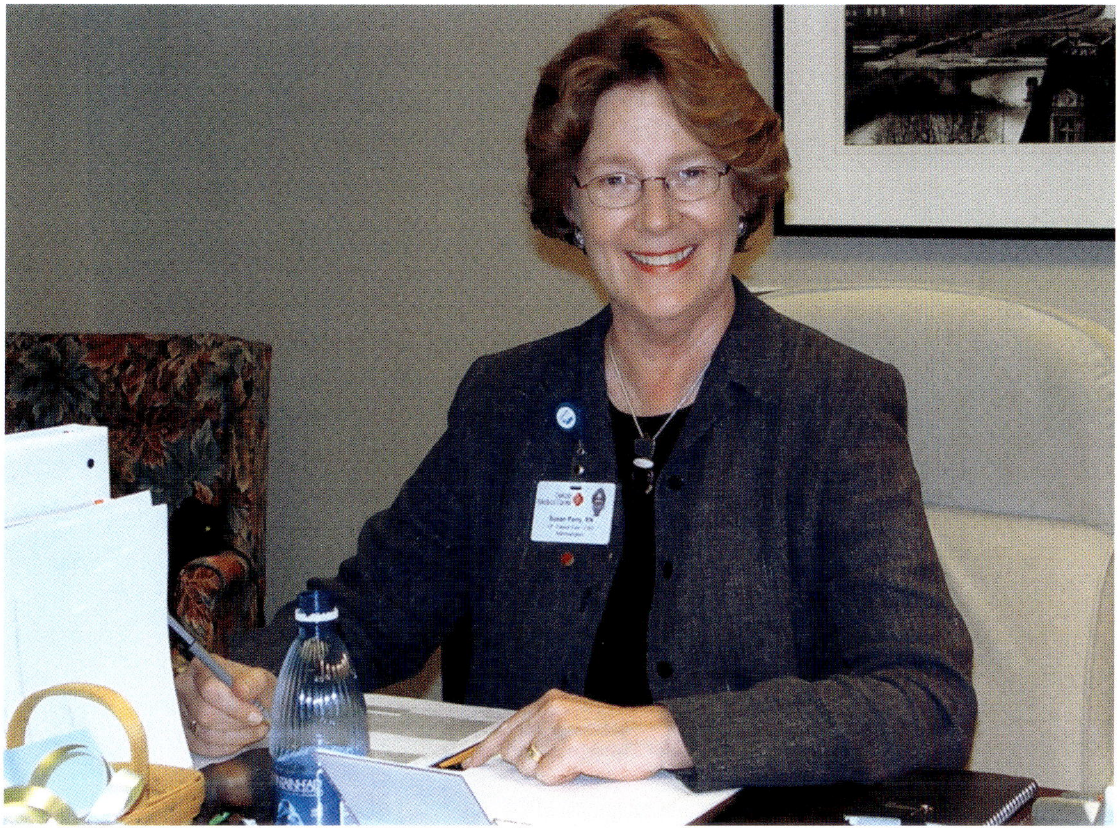

position of Bed Coordinator and assigned one nurse for each day and evening shift to monitor and facilitate the movement of patients housewide. Critical Care Services reestablished an Intermediate Intensive Care Unit to which appropriate patients might be transferred from the Intensive Care Unit. The Emergency Department created a Clinical Decision Unit for patients for whom the need for hospitalization remained to be determined. The Throughput project was the beginning of an ongoing process that continues today.

The QUEST initiative involved establishing the electronic medical record throughout the system. It consisted of a computerized system that handled ordering, communicating, and documenting a patient's care while in the hospital and maintaining the record for ease of access in the future. Parry's team undertook a successful program of intensive training for nurses and unit secretaries for phase one of the initiative, which training was completed with much relief and celebration when all went smoothly on the "Go Live" weekend.

When a gathering of nurses were asked to characterize Susan Parry's term as vice president for Patient Care Services and chief nursing officer, they said she enjoyed her nurses, she listened to them, she valued them, she supported them, and she inspired them. They also said she brought healing, health, and fun to Nursing Services.[41] When Parry was asked to characterize her tenure, she described it as one in which an already existing strong staff welcomed back and supported an old friend, and together they accomplished much. She believed she was leaving a strong situation upon which her successor could build.

When a gathering of nurses were asked to characterize Susan Parry's term . . . , they said she enjoyed her nurses, she listened to them, she valued them, she supported them, and she inspired them. They also said she brought healing, health, and fun to Nursing Services.

Brent Robinson

CEO Eric Norwood named DeKalb Medical's own Director of Medical-Surgical Services Brent Robinson, RN, as Parry's successor. Robinson was a certified family nurse practitioner and was board certified in medical-surgical nursing, adult critical care nursing, and cardiac rehabilitation nursing. He initially served as clinical manager of the 4400 Telemetry Nursing Unit after which he was made department head of the unit.[42]

During his 2004–2007 term as director of Patient Care Services and chief nursing officer, Robinson oversaw the development of three councils—the Patient Care Services Executive Council, the Oversight Council, and the unit-based Partnership Councils—in all of which staff members participated.[43] He reestablished participation in the Center for Frontline Nursing Leadership, a year-long course for those interested in frontline supervision.[44] He also standardized the dress code so that staff, physicians, and patients could more easily identify nurses.

Of all DeKalb Medical's nursing leaders, however, his tenure was impacted most heavily by the healthcare environment, including the system's financial losses. The financial challenge required deep reductions in staffing. Good people from many departments were released and morale declined. Physicians expressed great concerns that on some units the nurse-to-patient ratio might not be adequate to ensure quality patient care.[45] The administrative team of which Robinson was a part was under stress from all directions and was perceived as less visible to the staff. Those financial challenges, staffing reductions, sense of remote leadership, and diminished morale unfortunately overshadowed the goals Robinson set for his administration and the value of his accomplishments. He resigned at the end of 2007 to accept a position in another Atlanta hospital, and DeKalb Medical began the process of looking for his successor (See Timeline 2008).

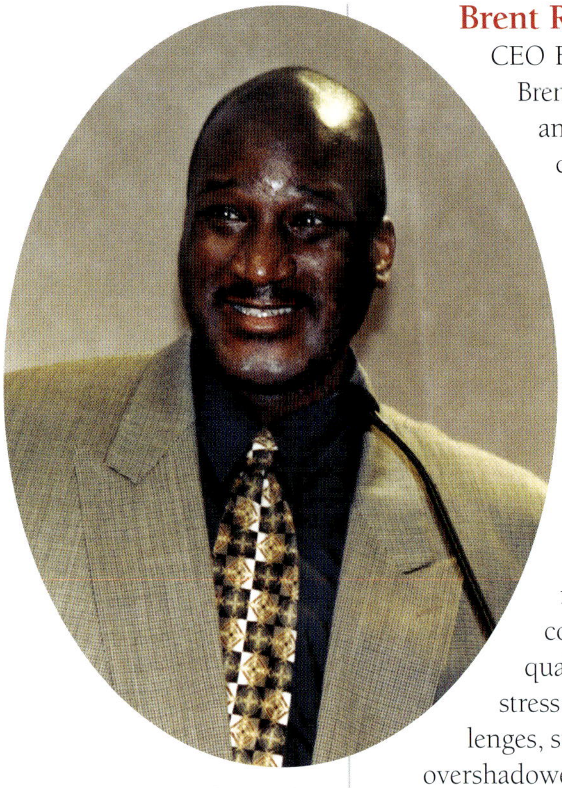

Brent Robinson, RN, was vice president of Patient Care Services and chief nursing officer from 2004–2007.

The Future

Like other hospitals nationwide, DeKalb Medical faces the challenge of maintaining quality patient care by its nurses in the face of financial constraints and a growing shortage of nurses. Yet, there is unqualified confidence that the new vice president for Patient Care Services and chief nursing officer, and the nurses with whom he or she will work, with the support of administration and the governing body will meet those challenges and elevate DeKalb Medical's Nursing Services to an even higher level of leadership and service in the days to come.

Nutrition Services

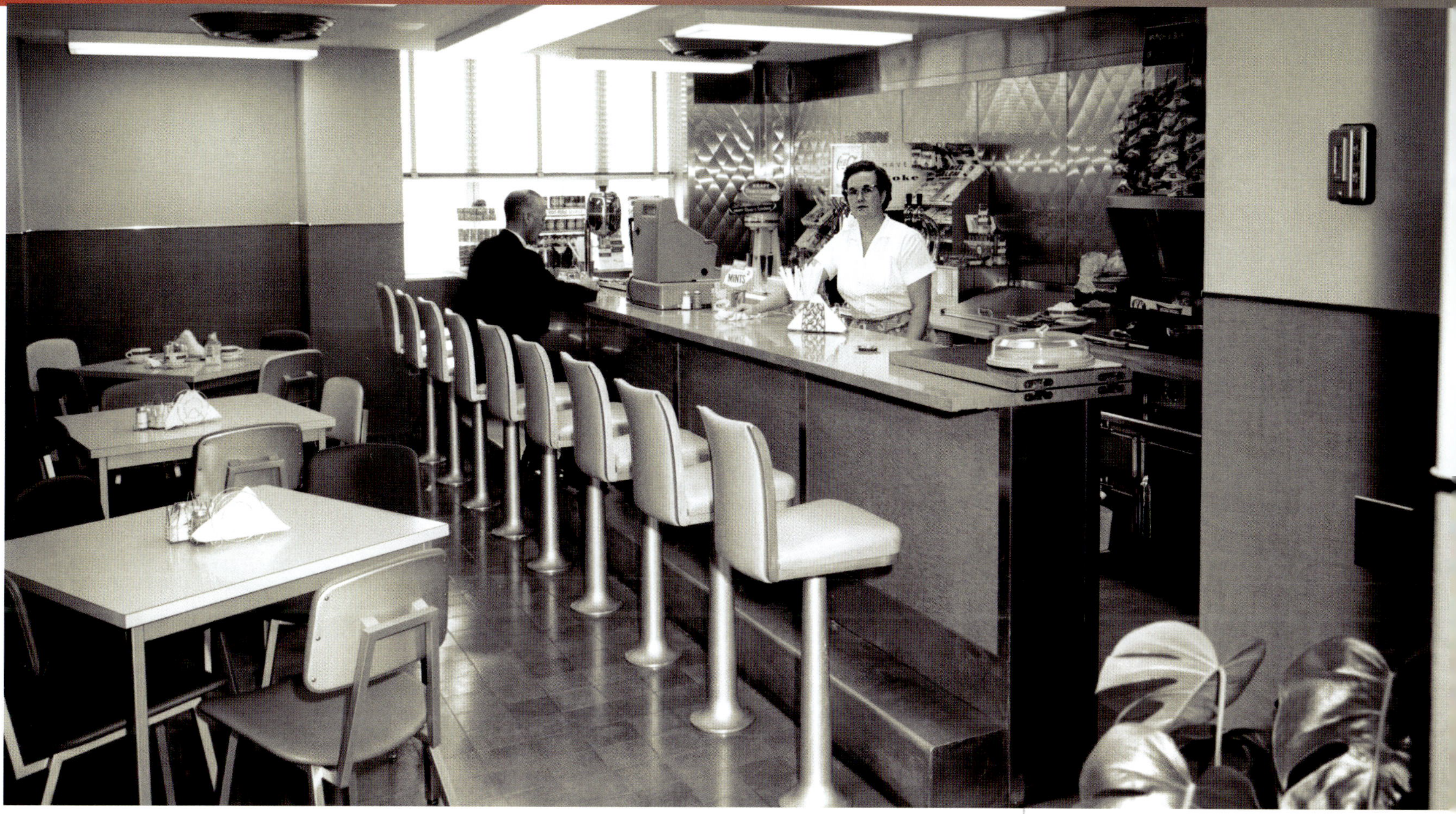

Jeanette Mayfield, manager of the Snack Bar, DeKalb General's first food service, was open even before the hospital itself opened its doors on May 1, 1961.

November 21, 1961
To Administrator William Thrasher
Dear Sir:
Recently . . . I was a patient in the DeKalb General Hospital. . . . I could not close this letter without commenting on the delicious food served by DeKalb General. A pet gripe of every hospital patient I've ever known has been the food in hospitals. Not so, in this case. The tasty food and the wholesome preparation of it would appeal to a gourmet. I still haven't recovered from the pleasant surprise of being able to select from a menu.[1]

The "tasty food and the wholesome preparation" was the handiwork of Mattie Lou Meadows, DeKalb General's director of the Dietary Department for fifteen years, from 1961 until she retired in 1975.[2] Administrator Thrasher recruited Meadows from Athens (Georgia) General where he had been administrator before coming to DeKalb General. She helped the architect design the cafeteria and kitchen

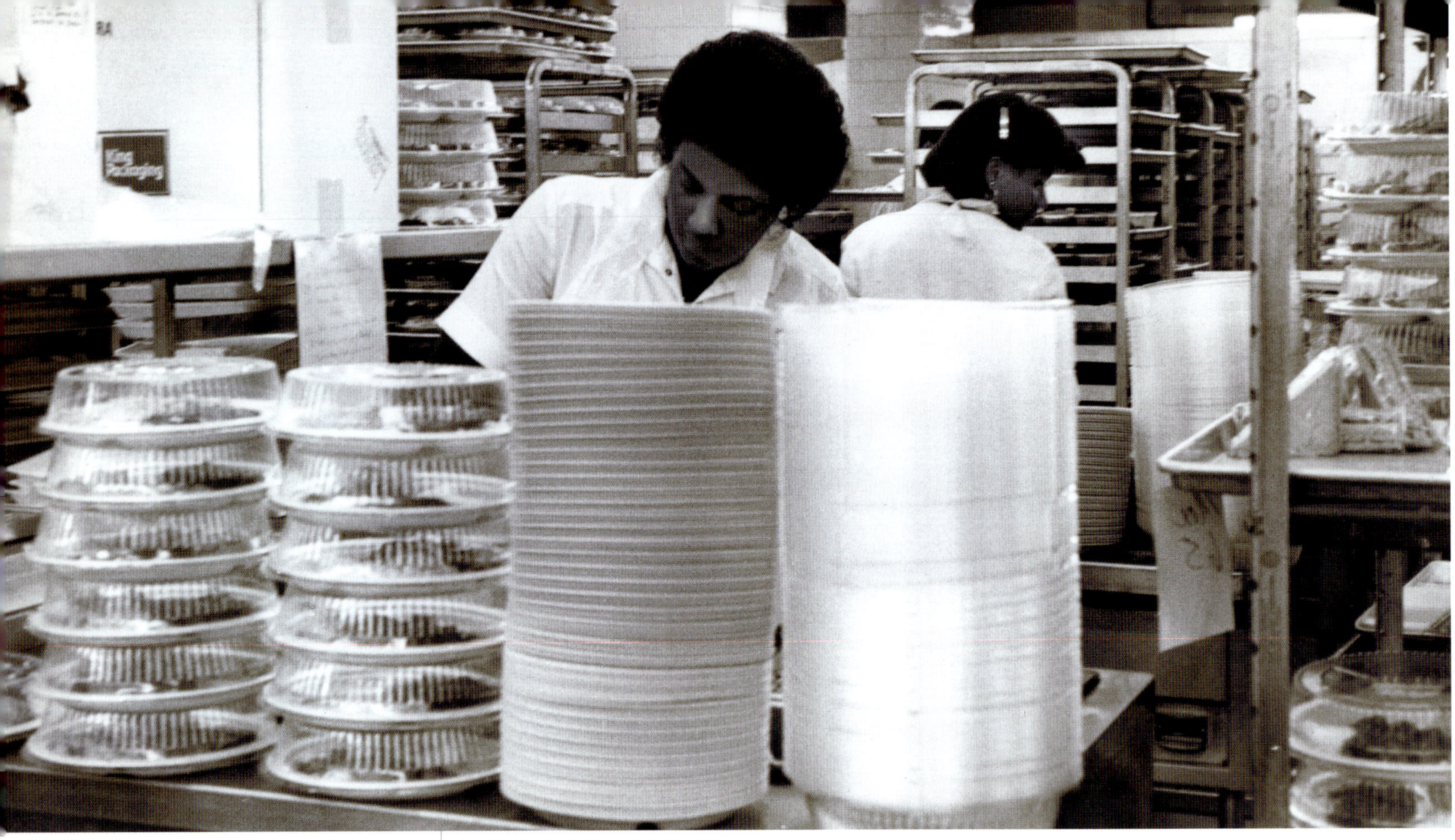

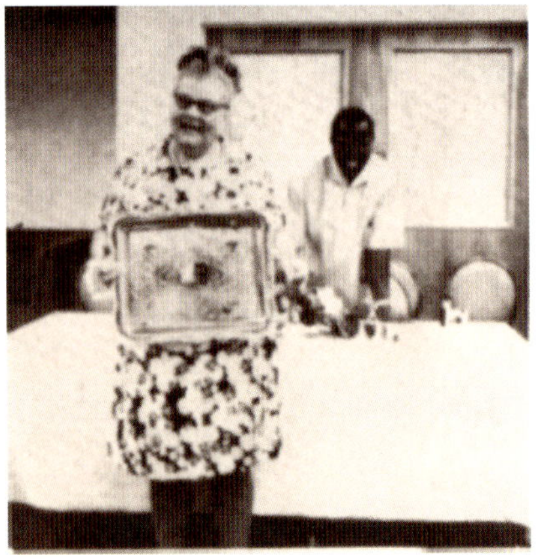

Top: Patient trays are prepared by Nutrition staff, Powell and McDavid. **Above:** Mattie Meadows was director of the Dietary Department for fifteen years from 1961 until she retired in 1975. The hospital here awards her many years of service with a silver tray.

and she decorated the doctors' dining room with ornate, red-velvet curtains.[3]

Meadows inaugurated DeKalb General Hospital's food service in three phases. First, in the spring of 1961 before the hospital was completed, she opened a snack bar that fed hungry employees, workmen finishing the hospital construction, and visitors. Jeanette Mayfield was the snack bar supervisor, and various food suppliers donated Mayfield's initial stock of food. The early "menus of the day" were whatever salesmen had brought in as free samples.[4]

Meadows' second food service was started in May, and it was for patients. She had seventeen inpatients to feed on opening day. When she retired, she was preparing meals for an average of 378 patients a day.[5]

She began the third phase shortly after May 1 when she opened the cafeteria for staff and visitors. She had only a few employees in the department, and part of their salary consisted of free meals.[6] She used mostly fresh produce, and she said she thoroughly enjoyed shelling peas or shucking corn.[7]

Meadows initiated several new food service ideas during her tenure. One popular innovation, to which the letter above referred, was the use of menus from which patients could select their diet. She also established the five-meal-a-day plan for patients (coffee and juice on waking, a large breakfast, a snack at noon, a large dinner in the late afternoon, and a snack at bedtime[8]) that pleased patients, staff, and physicians.[9]

Rather than discussing grams of meat and vegetables that patients were prescribed when they went home, Meadows asked Mary Towne to design a special food cart with wax food models to show patients what their home diet should look like. The models illustrated the size of servings prescribed by their doctor and what could be done to make the diet more appetizing.[10]

During the 1969–1971 hospital renovation and expansion, the Dietary staff had to relocate to temporary quarters. They prepared and set up six hundred patient trays a day in an area only 27' x 34'. The kitchen was moved to an old conference room that had two closets, which Meadows used as pantries. The pantries held a week's supply of food items except for bread, milk, sweet rolls, and pies that were delivered daily. Entrée items were ordered once a week and stored in the freezer. Meadows's equipment consisted of two home-type ranges, two upright freezers, one meat slicer, and one mixer. There was a cook's table, a salad table, a steam table, and forty tall racks. The makeshift kitchen had one cold-water faucet, but no sink. Housekeeping relinquished a mop closet in which maintenance installed a sink and drain board for washing pots and pans. Meadows used disposable paper and plastic products whenever possible to avoid the need for washing dishes. During the construction period, Dietary served two meals and three snacks a day.[11]

Before the major construction project was started, trays were placed on carts and taken to the floors where nurses' aides delivered them to patients. When construction was completed, Meadows instituted a new "quick-food" preparation system and a new work schedule for her employees. They worked eight, ten-hour days after which they were off six days. The staff did most of the cooking for patient meals on Thursday and those meals were frozen for the coming week. She began using "convenience foods" instead of fresh produce for most of the food items in that system. Trays were prepared and placed in a cooler on the floors, then heated in microwave ovens located on each patient floor and distributed hot to patients.[12]

Helen Scherer, RD, was DeKalb General's first registered dietitian. She remained on the staff for twenty-one years, from 1961 until she retired in 1982.[13] She wrote the hospital's first diet manual, prepared the daily menus and menus for special diets, and oversaw the preparation of patient food trays.[14] Doris Trail, RD, was the hospital's second dietitian,[15] and Gail Shackelford, RD, became the third in 1971.[16]

While the role of registered dietitian originally involved duties in the food preparation area, Gail Shackelford worked primarily with patients, assessing their nutritional needs and offering nutritional education.[17] She created a program of outpatient nutrition education that also was available to patients referred from physicians' offices. Her program included instruction in the special diets for the management of obesity, diabetes, cardiac rehabilitation, and other medical requirements.[18]

Dennis Ryan succeeded Mattie Lou Meadows in 1975 as director of Dietary. He had received an associate degree in hotel management from the University of New York and had served as president of the Chattanooga District American Hospital Food Administration before coming to DeKalb General.[19]

Ryan made several changes in food services. He added a fourth registered dietitian and named Gail Shackelford chief dietitian with responsibilities for dietary education for patients and the food services staff. He combined the cafeteria kitchen and the patient kitchen into one main kitchen; and he named Bertha Johnson to the new position of manager of Production, Alice Giles as manager of the main kitchen, and Johnny Tyus as manager of the cafeteria.[20]

Ryan inaugurated a restaurant-style patient menu with daily specials and a hostess program. A hostess visited each patient daily during the patient's stay in the hospital to introduce the menu and

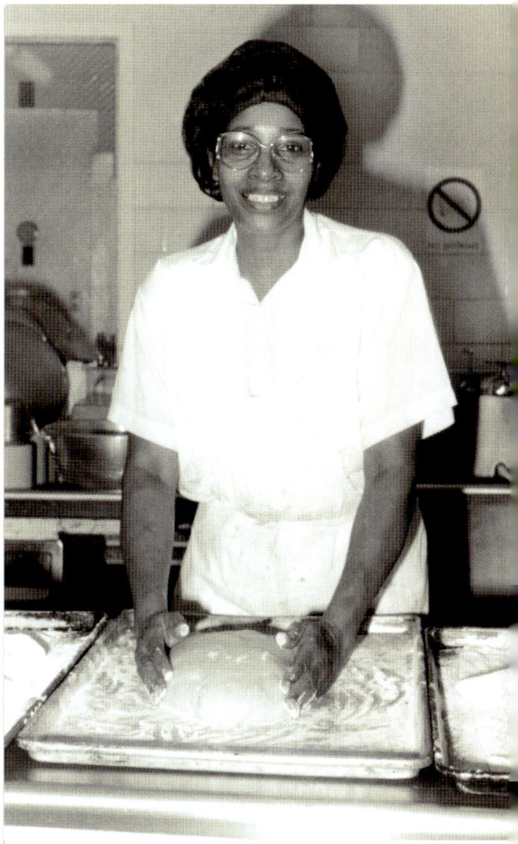

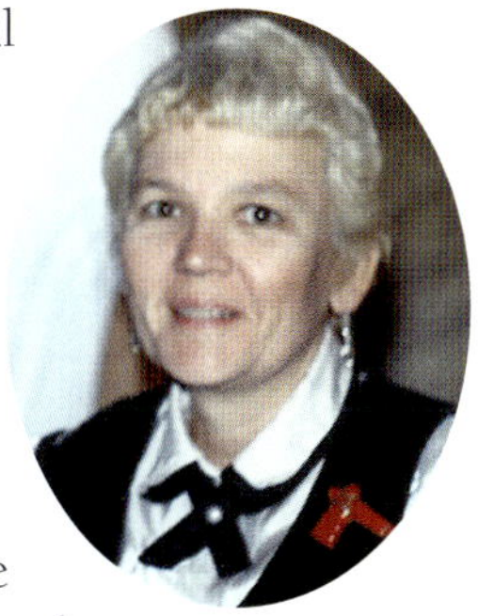

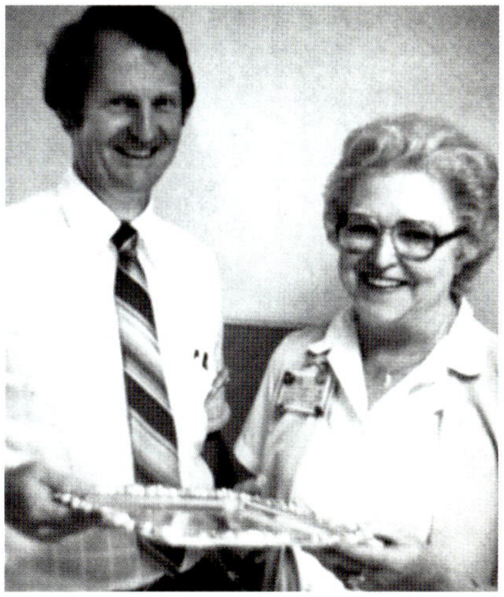

Top: Shirley Butler, head baker, prepares dough for all the pastries that will be made that day. **Left:** Gail Shackelford, RD, became the hospital's third registered dietician in 1971. **Above:** Director of Food Services, Dennis Ryan awards Helen Scherer, RD, with a silver tray upon retiring from dietary in 1981.

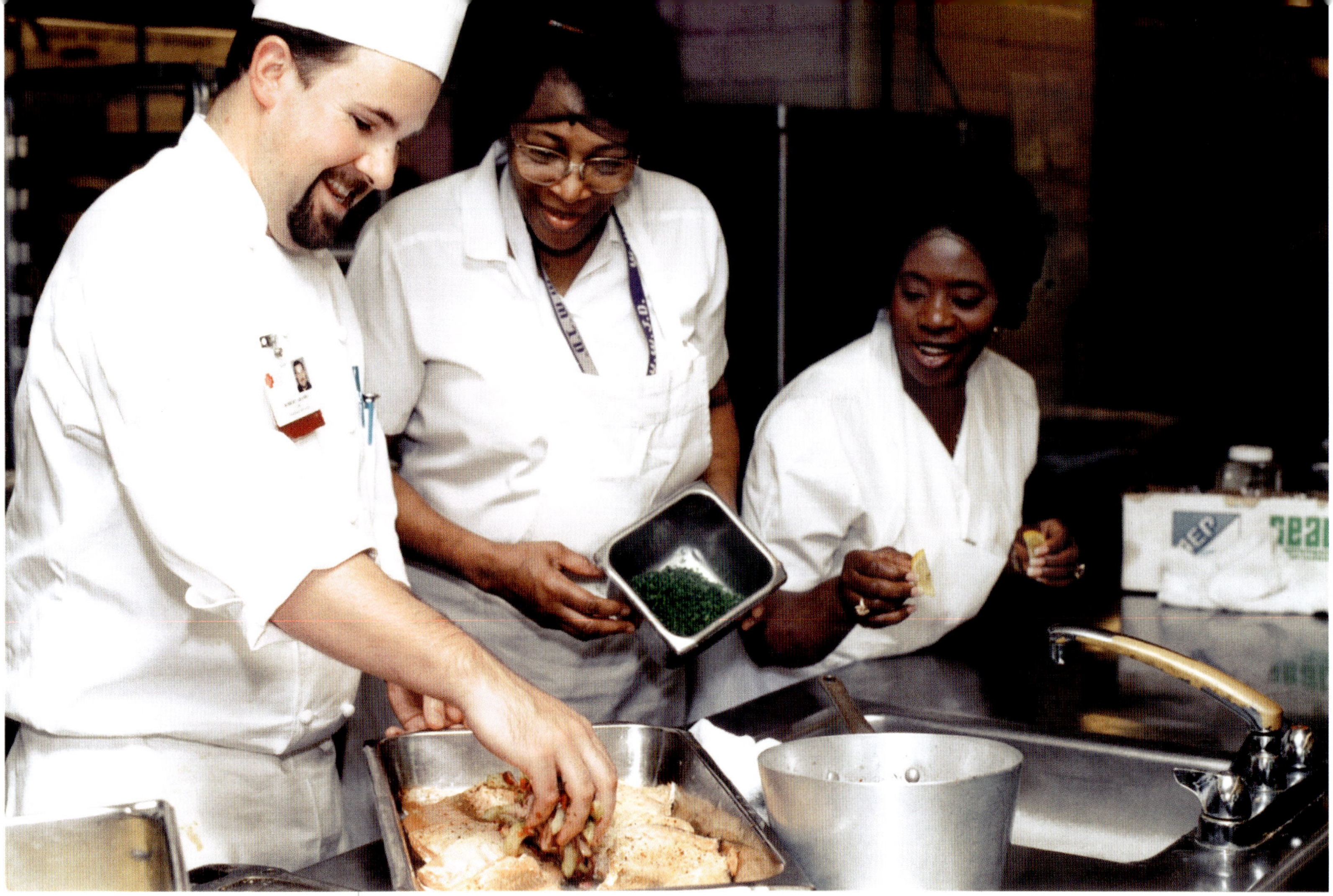

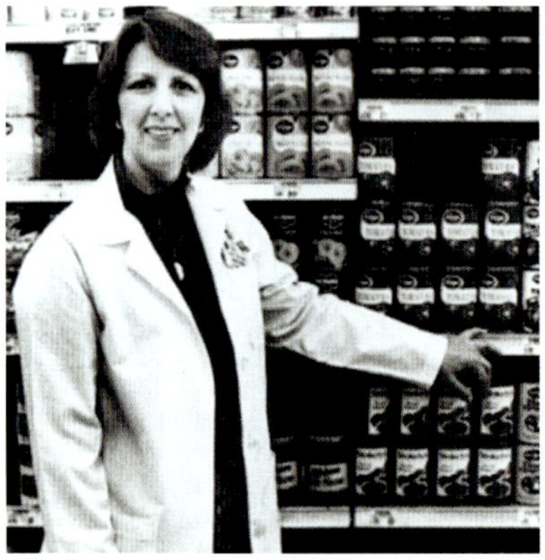

Top: Chef Robert Adamo prepares chicken with two of his coworkers. **Above:** Nancy Ward, RD, became the chief clinical dietician in 1978.

assist the patient in making selections.[21] He replaced the five-meal-a-day patient food plan with the "cook-chill" system. It was a labor-saving system in that food was prepared a day in advance, refrigerated in large containers, and heated with the microwave when ready to be served.[22]

He expanded the staff of dietitians to include five clinical and one teaching dietitian. When Gail Shackelford stepped down as chief clinical dietition in 1978, he named Nancy Ward, RD, as her successor.[23] Ward helped create the Nutrition Support Team in collaboration with the Pharmacy. The team initially included a pharmacist, a nurse, and a dietitian. The position of nurse later was dropped, and the number of dietitians and pharmacists was increased. The team worked with patients whose nutritional needs were unique and based on the severity and complexity of trauma and disease.[24]

Dennis Ryan died in an accident in 1985 when a tree fell on him as he was assisting a friend who owned a tree service.[25] Tony Ford succeeded Ryan as director of Food Services, and Ford remained director from 1986–1993. Before coming to DeKalb General, Tony Ford served for six years as head of food services at West Paces Ferry Hospital in Atlanta. He recruited Bob Heim as his assistant director.[26]

Ford initiated measures to make the hospital's cafeteria and patient food "more interesting, tastier and healthier." He discontinued the use of microwaves and kitchens on the patient floors and placed patients' plates on carts equipped with heating wires that warmed the food.[27] Dietary began baking its own breads, cookies, and pastries.[28] There were weekly "surprises" in the cafeteria that might include a

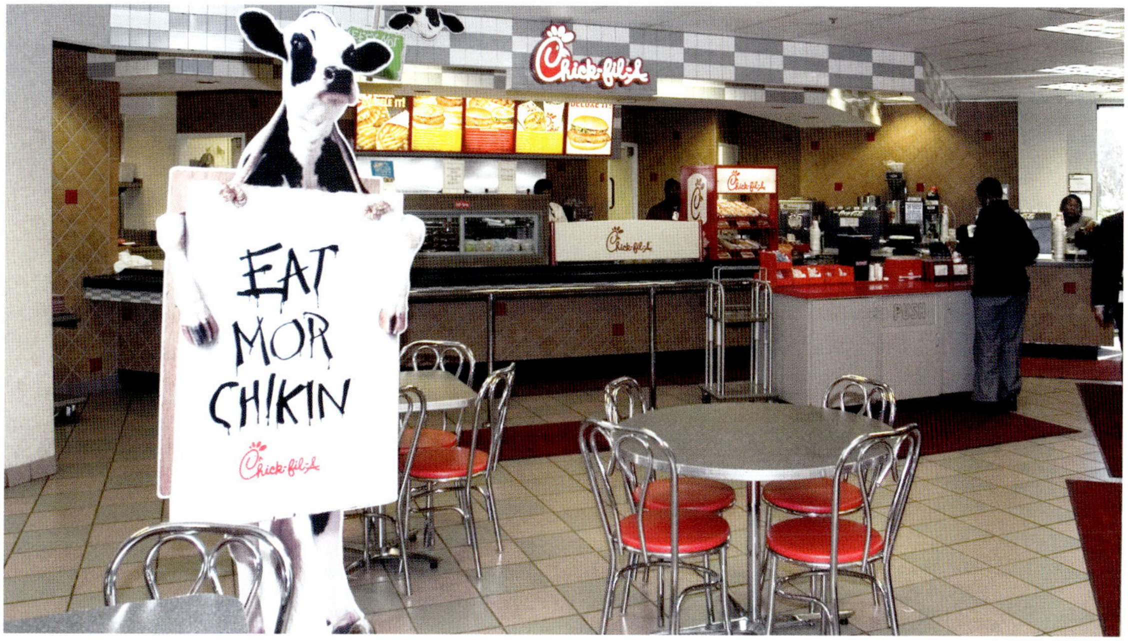

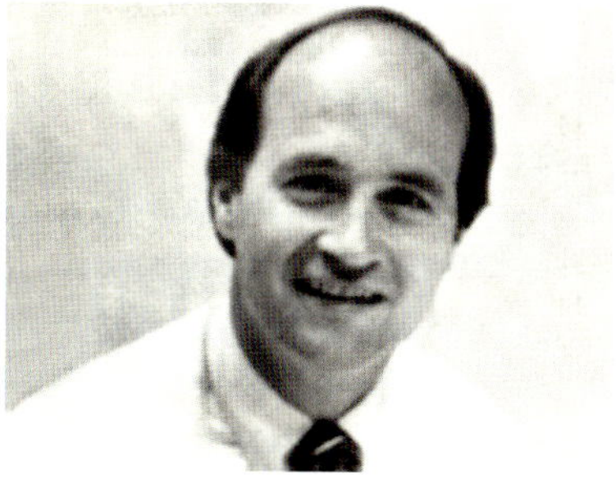

Left: The Chick-Fil-A snack bar is a popular eatery in the professional office building. **Above:** Tony Ford succeeded Dennis Ryan as director of Food Services in 1986. He was responsible for making the food more interesting, tastier, and healthier. He also introduced weekly surprises and created monthly themes for the cafeteria.

take-out pizza service, hot dogs, a salad bar, or a taco bar. He created monthly themes for the cafeteria such as the "Orient Express" featuring Chinese cuisine, "Octoberfest" with hearty German dishes, Halloween brew, Mexican dishes, Cajun cooking, and other surprises. He also oversaw the renovation and enlargement of the cafeteria to increase its seating capacity from 175 to 275, expanded the food stations, and converted the serving lines to self-serve.[29] During Ford's tenure, the name of the department was changed from Dietary to Nutrition Services.[30]

The first Professional Office Building was completed during Tony Ford's tenure, and he established a snack bar in the space now occupied by Chick-Fil-A. Both the snack bar and Chick-Fil-A were managed by Nutrition Services.[31] Ford also put into operation a computer system that Dennis Ryan had purchased but not activated. It was one of the first in Atlanta to be used by Nutrition Services. The computer printed menus that conformed more specifically to patients' diet orders, and it provided dietitians with better information that assisted them in their work. Later, through the hospital Intranet, Nutrition Services was able to place the diet manual on the computer, making it available to all the staff.[32]

Marty Tulley succeeded Tony Ford as director of Nutrition Services. In 1998 Tulley oversaw another renovation and expansion of the cafeteria, and in 2002 undertook a major renovation of the kitchen when asbestos was found in the ceiling.[33] During the ninety days of kitchen renovation, all cooking was done in two trailers parked outside the dining area.[34] One of Tulley's most notable achievements was to hire Robert Adamo as chef. Adamo came to DeKalb Medical from the Hyatt Regency in Atlanta where he was executive chef, bringing with him culinary skills that enhanced the patient and cafeteria food.[35]

Barbara Mayfield followed Marty Tulley as director of Nutrition Services in 2004. During her tenure, Nutrition Services assumed the additional oversight for food services at the DeKalb Medical's hospitals at Downtown Decatur and at Hillandale.[36] When Mayfield resigned in 2007, DeKalb Medical negotiated a contract with Sodexho Incorporated, formerly of the Marriott Corporation, to assume management of Nutrition Services on all three campuses, including patient meals, all three cafeterias, the Azalea Bistro in the Women's Center and Surgery Center, and the Chick-Fil-A service in the North Decatur Professional Office Building.[37]

Occupational Health and Infection Control

Occupational Health and Infection Control currently are each responsible for many demanding duties. Occupational Health performs preemployment and annual examinations for approximately four thousand employees in DeKalb Medical's three hospitals. It ensures compliance with the many regulations prescribed by the Occupational Safety and Health Administration (OSHA), the Centers for Disease Control and Prevention (CDC), the Joint Commission on the Accreditation of Healthcare Organizations (JCAHO), the Centers for Medicare and Medicaid Services (CMS), Medicare, Medicaid and other agencies. It manages employee exposures to blood and body fluids and tuberculosis (TB); provides TB testing and annual influenza vaccine to employees, volunteers, and medical staff; manages Workers' Compensation; and deals with many other responsibilities.

Infection Control monitors surgical site infections, bloodstream infections, central-line infections, ventilator-associated pneumonias and other infections; plans and oversees the prevention of infections in the hospital; documents and reports infections that do occur; and works with and educates physicians, nurses, and all the hospital staff (including those such as Environmental Services, Dietary, Laundry, and Maintenance) in understanding, appreciating, and implementing the role of each in preventing and containing infections.

Yet when Sally Williams, RN, was named director of the combined Occupational Health and Infection Control Department in 1973, she was told, "The other employees will hate you for your cream-puff, do-nothing job."[1]

There was, indeed, a time when the responsibilities of the two services were minimal and easily managed. Margaret Ford, RN, who later became DeKalb General's second director of Nursing, was director of Employee Training and Health Services in 1961. She had time to make house calls. The employee newsletter warned the staff, "She may visit any employee on sick leave to see if that employee is actually sick."[2] It was not until 1970 that the workload began to increase when the Georgia Department of Public Health mandated that all hospital employees undergo a medical examination, including a chest X-ray, upon employment and annually thereafter.[3] Flu shots were offered as a free fringe benefit for the first time in 1971.[4] In 1972 available records make the first reference to an Infection Control service. In that year Pat Vinton, RN, was referred to as "Health Nurse and Surveillance Officer."[5] Infection Control as a distinct, recognized hospital service had its birth a year later, in 1973, when Sally Williams was named director of Occupational Health and Infection Control.

The two services were included in one department from 1972 until 1975 when the JCAHO recommended that they be separated.[6] In 1995 the hospital recombined the two services into one department,[7] where they remained until 2007 when they were separated again due to the increasing responsibilities assigned to each.[8]

Occupational Health

Occupational Health has had a series of leaders. When Margaret Ford resigned in 1962, Olive Ann Koporec, RN, became the "Supervisor of Employee Health Services."[9] She was succeeded by Charlotte

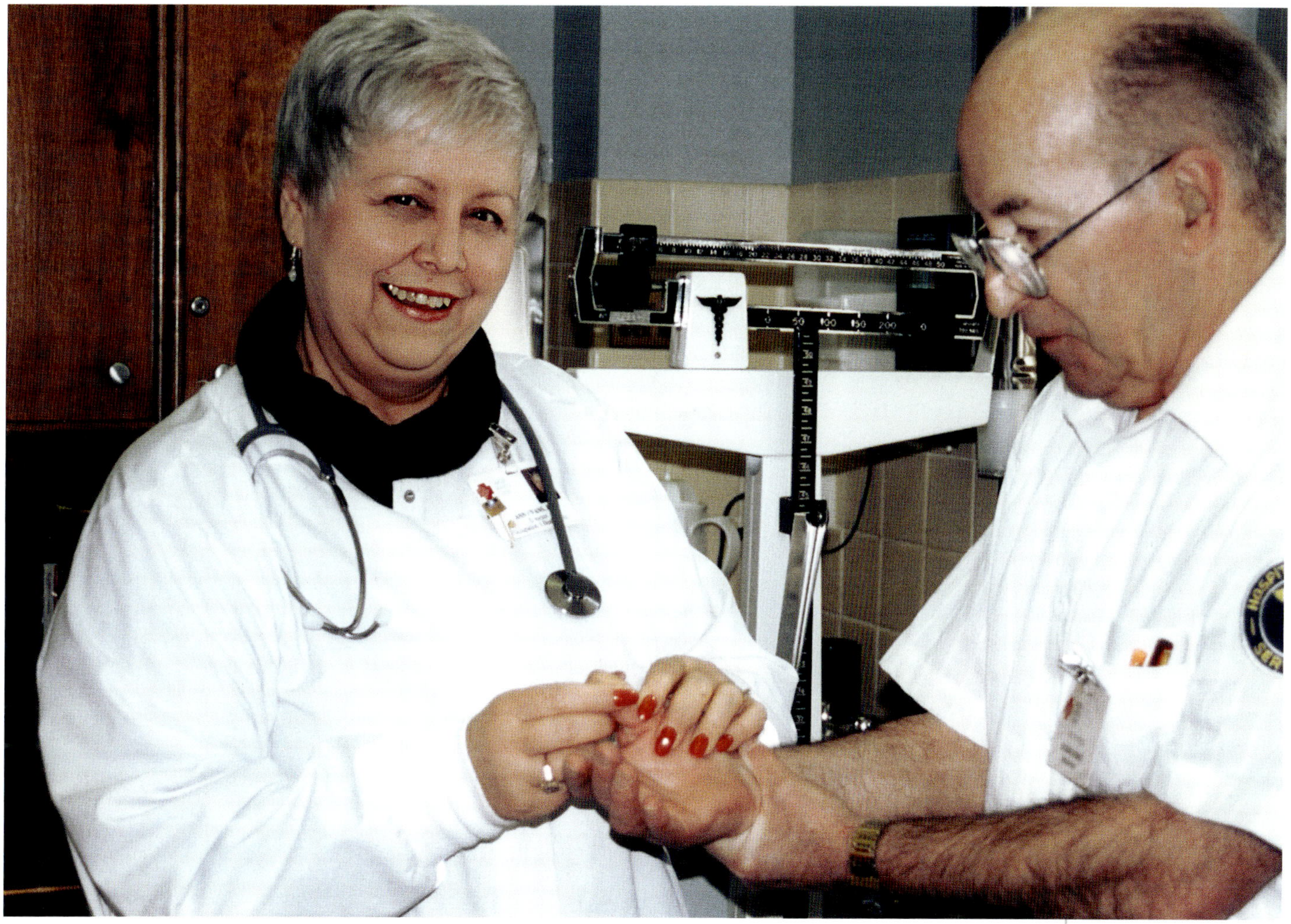

Davis (later Courtois), RN, in 1971,[10] Judy McCumber, RN, in January1972,[11] and Pat Vinton, RN, in November 1972.[12]

When Pat Vinton was assigned to another position in 1973, she recommended Sally Williams as her replacement.[13] Williams served as director of the department, and Ann Evans, RN, (described in the employee newsletter as "the one with the pleasant smile"[14]) was "Infection Control and Health Nurse."[15] When the services were separated in 1976, Evans became coordinator of Occupational Health and remained in that position until 1995 when the services were once again combined into one department, and she took a part-time position. Connie Wilbanks, RN, became manager of Occupational Health in 1995,[16] Cathy Boyles, RN, in 1997,[17] Kathy Pickard, RN, in 2002,[18] and Gay Newton, RN, in 2003.[19] Yasmine Bandali, RN, is the current manager.[20]

The responsibilities of Occupational Health have increased over time. Margaret Ford, in addition to calling on sick-leave employees at home to see if they really were sick, encouraged all employees to take the free oral Sabin type 2 polio vaccine even if they had received the full series of Salk polio shots.[21] Her successor, Olive Ann Koporec, reminded employees how illnesses and accidents are to be handled:

"Smiling" Ann Evans, RN, director of Occupational Health attending to Eugene Furey, foreman of Preventive Maintenance in Building Services.

While an employee is at work, accidents are handled by the house doctor or a specialist if the house doctor deems it necessary, and the hospital will pay for it. Illnesses are seen by the house doctor at request of the [nursing] supervisor to determine if the employee should continue working that day, and the hospital pays. If the employee needs to be sent to a physician for treatment, the employee pays."[22]

Ann Evans instituted a modified work program that allowed injured employees to return to work sooner than previously was the case. The program allowed them to perform modified or lighter duties until they were able to resume their normal duties.[23]

When Cathy Boyles was manager, in addition to handling the usual employment physicals, she began administering the annual flu shots, dealing with on-the-job illnesses and injuries, and helping with stressful situations. Managing employee exposure to blood and body fluids became a frequent safety issue. Testing for the proper fitting of masks used in tuberculosis isolation became a time-consuming responsibility. She also began offering more employee training in better lifting techniques, proper posture, appropriate seating positions, and other aspects of ergonomics.[24]

The responsibility for Workers' Compensation and regulatory requirements from the CDC, OSHA, and other agencies became demanding and burdensome. OSHA required that employee records be kept for thirty years from the time of employment. Ann Evans, Cathy Boyles, Kathy Pickard, and Gay Newton each had responsibility for Occupational Health and Workers' Compensation. Eventually, Workers' Compensation responsibilities called for a dedicated person. Elizabeth Carroll, RN, Jean Smith, RN, and Dawn Manning were, in succession, assigned that role. Once Occupational Health and Infection Control were separated in 2007, Dawn Manning became manager of Workers' Compensation.[25]

Infection Control

Infection Control had a meager beginning at DeKalb General. In 1973 Sally Williams gladly applied for the job that Pat Vinton was vacating. She thought she was applying only for the position of health nurse, and she liked the idea of being of service to the employees. It was not until a week after being named to the position that Martha "Cookie" Nodal (Kalember), RN, assistant director of Nursing, told her that she also was to be in charge of Infection Control. Surprised, Williams admitted she did not know what Infection Control was supposed to do. Nodal suggested that she attend a scheduled meeting of Atlanta-area hospital infection control nurses to learn more about the job. Williams went, but she was embarrassed when the Emory representative asked her the "nosocomial rate" at DeKalb General. Williams had no idea that the nosocomial rate referred to the rate of hospital-acquired infections. She was relieved that the Emory nurse was called away before she had to give her an answer.[26]

Williams soon discovered that Infection Control at DeKalb at that time amounted to recording mostly "meaningless data." Attending physicians were required to check a box on the front sheet of their patient's charts to indicate whether or not a patient had an infection, and to check a second box to indicate if a patient acquired an infection while in the hospital. The Infection Control nurse was expected to accept as accurate the "yes" or "no" checked by physicians even when a particular physician checked "no infection" for the patient he admitted with a diagnosis of urinary tract infection.[27]

The early approach to infections focused mainly on proper diagnosis and treatment rather than prevention and control. One urologist irrigated his patients' catheters three times daily with tap water.

Neither did he consider it important to keep irrigation systems closed. When Williams advocated practices aimed at prevention and control, one physician referred to her as the "witch doctor practicing voodoo."[28]

The importance of an effective Infection Control program, however, soon became apparent. The JCAHO introduced infection control requirements with which hospitals had to comply to remain accredited. The medical staff's Infection Control Committee, chaired by such respected physicians as Knox Kinlaw, MD, Donald Printz, MD, and Norman Jacobs, MD,[29] supported the concerns and recommendations of Infection Control. Printz, Jacobs, and Robin Dretler, MD, in addition to being held in high regard, were trained and experienced in infectious diseases. They helped educate the medical staff on the importance of prevention and control as well as accurate documentation, diagnosis and proper treatment. The prevention and control of infections gradually was seen not only as a nursing issue, but one that involved the physicians, nurses, and every service that directly or indirectly affected patient care. Eventually Infection Control, with physician support, extended beyond information, education, and recommendation to that of actual intervention in critical situations.

Sally Williams, who once did not know what Infection Control was supposed to do or the meaning of "nosocomial infection rate," emerged as a recognized leader in the field. She was in the first group in the nation to become certified infection control nurses; she became a leader in local, state, and national infection control organizations; and she was named "Infection Control Nurse of the Year" by the state organization.[30]

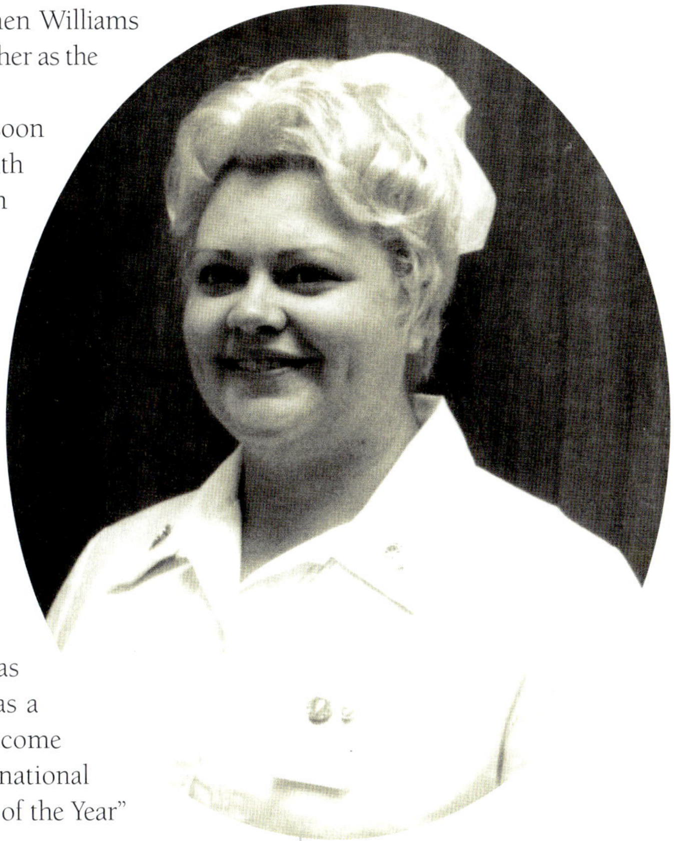

Sally Williams, RN, was DeKalb General Hospital's first Infection Control Nurse in 1973. She went on to become a recognized leader in the field of Infection Control.

When Williams resigned in 1994, she encouraged her friend at Emory Hospital, Helen Ebaugh, RN, to apply for the position.[31] Ebaugh served as director for thirteen years, including the period beginning in 1995 when Infection Control and Occupational Health were recombined into a single department. She worked with Norman Jacobs who was chairman of the Infection Control Committee, medical director of Infection Control, and epidemiologist. This latter position gave him the informal authority not only to recommend but to intervene with the hospital or physicians when risky circumstances arose.[32]

During Ebaugh's tenure, the prevention of hospital-acquired infections took on an increased financial significance in addition to the primary goal of keeping the hospital safe for patients, their families, doctors, and employees.[33] New federal regulations dictated that as of October 2008, Medicare and Medicaid will no longer pay for certain infections that develop after a patient is admitted to the hospital. The list of those conditions includes central-line bloodstream infections, urinary tract infections, and infections following orthopedic surgery, the insertion of pacemakers and other heart surgery procedures. The regulations deem those infections to be avoidable and refer to them as "never events."[34] Hospitals will have to bear the cost of managing them. Other types of hospital-acquired infections are to be added to the "never-events" list in 2009.

In addition to the financial impact of receiving no reimbursement for managing hospital-acquired infections, the courts increasingly are awarding multimillion-dollar judgments to plaintiffs who acquire infections in the hospital. They contend that there is "proof that nearly all hospital infections are avoidable when doctors and staff clean their hands and rigorously practice proper hygiene and other preventive measures."[35] They cite Beth Israel Hospital in New York City, Johns Hopkins Medical Center in Baltimore, and Sutter Medical Center in Sacramento as having reached the goal of zero central line bloodstream infections.

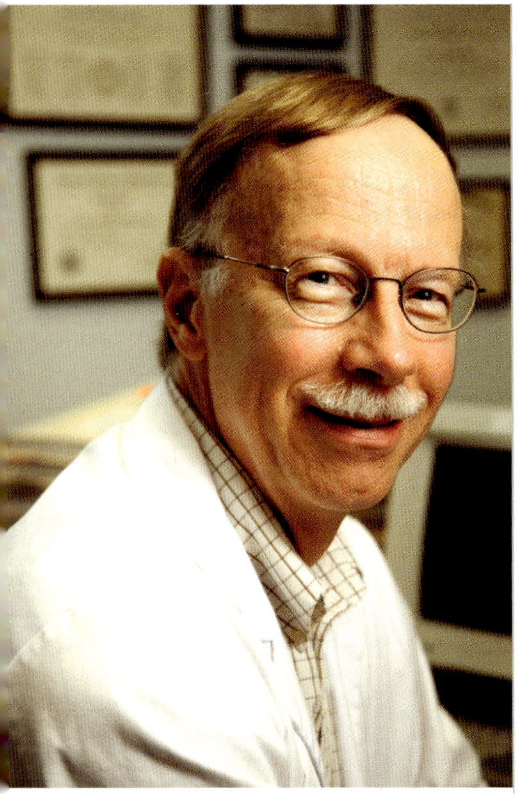

Norman Jacobs, MD, served as chairman of the Infection Control Committee, medical director of Infection Control, and epidemiologist.

In addition to the financial issue, the seriousness and extent of infections has taken on a new dimension. There was a time when *Staphylococcus aureus* (Staph) infections were not thought of as major threats. In 1962 a nurse entered the following note in the employee newsletter:

> *"Staph" is short for* Staphylococcus aureus, *a germ that is responsible for many infections. In hospitals we come in contact with many different types of patients and pick up germs on our skin, in our noses and on our clothing. These germs do not harm us if we are in good health. If we have a positive culture, we may be carrying the germ to a patient who may be susceptible to them and get an infection from us. The Infection Committee of our hospital recommends using Bacitracin ointment in the nose 3 times a day and frequent washing of the face and nose with Phisohex... Staph will clear up in ten days to two weeks.... Most people outside the hospital do not know enough about Staph to understand it. We as employees can cause unfavorable public relations to the hospital if we share with the outside [community] problems such as this.*[36]

Currently 85 percent of Staph infections in the hospital are methicillin-resistant-Staph-aureus (MRSA) infections,[37] and there is an increasing number of multi-drug-resistant-organisms (MDRO).[38] Worrisome is the fact that Staph infections are becoming resistant to vancomycin, an antibiotic once relied upon to treat effectively most MRSA infections. In addition, virulent strains of MRSA are becoming widespread in the community so that individuals admitted to the hospital may be carriers of infections.[39] This alarming finding has led DeKalb Medical to make plans to test every patient being admitted to the Intensive Care Unit (ICU), and possibly other areas, for MRSA infections.[40]

Marti Jaynes, RN, succeeded Helen Ebaugh in 2007 as senior Infection Control specialist. Now, appropriately, her title has been changed to "Infection Preventionist."[41] Prevention has become an imperative. And basic hand washing remains a key prerequisite. Jaynes created a poster contest entitled "Wash Lively, DeKalb Medical," utilizing the name of Wash Lively, one of the seven original hospital trustees. The winning poster was printed, laminated, and located throughout the hospitals.[42]

The implementation of the electronic medical record has been an enormously helpful aid to Infection Control's ability to access patient records and to monitor hospital infections as they occur. The challenge at DeKalb Medical, as at most hospitals, remains that of convincing all members of the healthcare team to endorse and follow required procedures. As an example of success, Beth Israel Medical Center went over one thousand days without a central-line bloodstream infection because it had a checklist that all doctors and nurses followed, including rigorous hygiene, clean hands, sterile drapes, and cleansing the insertion site.[43] It is a goal to which DeKalb Medical is committed and toward which it is progressing.

Challenges remain, but Norman Jacobs observed that DeKalb's Infection Control program "has enabled the hospital to have a major ICU, cancer service, Neonatal Intensive Care Unit (NICU), orthopedic, vascular and other programs with good outcomes and good infection rates."[44] It is an accomplishment that reflects the commitment, the tenacity, and the creativity of the organization's leadership to address this crucial issue.

Pastoral Services

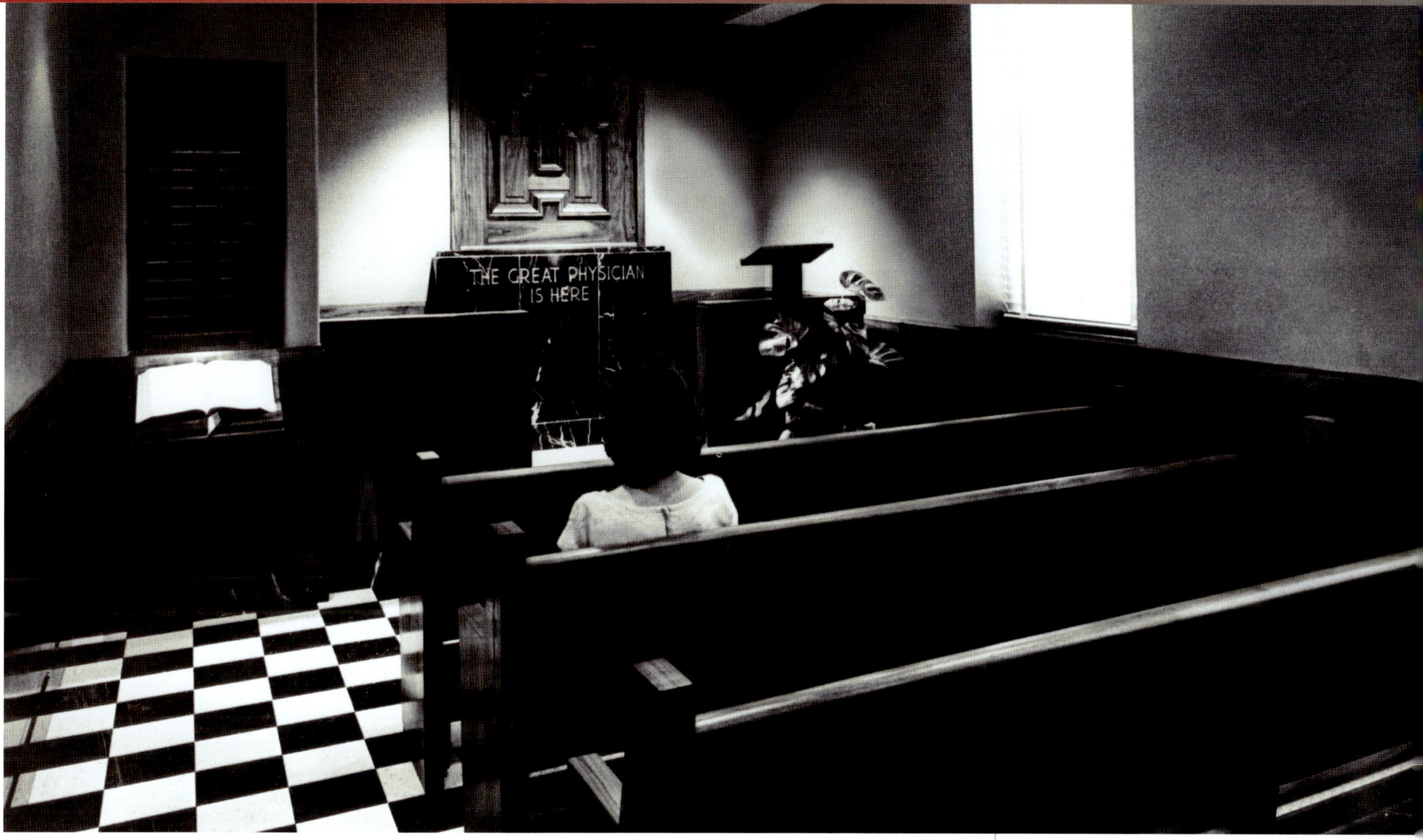

DeKalb General Hospital's 1961 chapel, acknowledging "The Great Physician is here."

It was inevitable that someday DeKalb Medical would have its own chaplains. Those involved in planning the new hospital and those responsible for its operation openly confirmed the importance of the spiritual life of the institution.

When, in 1958, trustee J. Ross McCain wrote to William Thrasher, a candidate for the position of hospital administrator, he asked Thrasher to send his ideas on "how may we provide for a strong Christian influence at the hospital."[1] The trustees included a chapel in the original hospital plans, and the marble wall behind the chapel's pulpit was inscribed with the words, "The Great Physician is here." At the groundbreaking ceremony in 1959, McCain said, "We believe that God is still the Great Physician, and we would not wish to operate any hospital which does not recognize His presence and guidance."[2] The two songs sung at the dedication ceremony in April 1961 were "God Bless America" and "Bless This House, O Lord, We Pray."[3] The plaque displayed at the dedication ceremony was inscribed with the words, "To the Glory of God and the Improved Health of Mankind."[4] Two of the questions on the original employee application form asked: "Do you have regular Sunday School attendance?" and "Do you have regular church attendance?" The hospital's admission form asked for the patient's religious preference and asked if the patient wanted a visit from a minister. In a 1970 interview with the local press, Administrator William Thrasher said, "Since the hospital has been in existence, we have tried to operate it on Christian principles."[5]

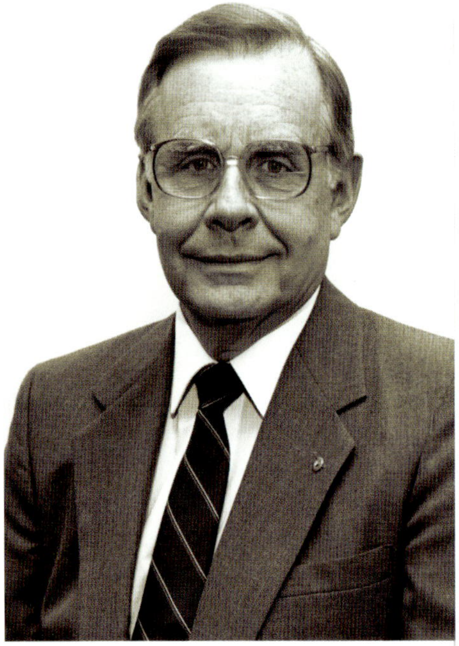

Above: Wayne E. Spangler, MDiv, was hired as the first chaplain at DeKalb General in 1978. He stayed on as chaplain until his retirement in 1992. **Right inset:** Betty Castellani, DMin, was hired as associate chaplain in 1987. When Spangler retired, she became director of Pastoral Services.

The trustees considered the possibility of having a chaplain prior to the hospital's opening. In the summer of 1960, Chaplain Charles Gerkin of the Grady Chaplaincy Division of the Greater Atlanta Council of Churches, offered to establish a chaplaincy program at DeKalb General. The trustees replied that they appreciated the offer but would have to wait until the hospital was financially able to hire a chaplain.[6]

Community ministers provided the hospital's pastoral services for the first seventeen years. They visited their own hospitalized parishioners, called on other patients requesting a visit by a minister, and conducted religious services at the hospital. In 1963 the Authority asked Administrator Thrasher and trustee McCain to investigate the possibility of having a hospital chaplain.[7] They recommended that the Authority include the position of a chaplain in the 1963–1964 budget.[8] The Authority approved their recommendation but did not include money for a chaplain in the next several budgets. The trustees were still trying to get DeKalb General "in the black" financially.

In 1972 local ministers urged Thrasher to hire a chaplain,[9] and the Medical Staff Executive Committee made a similar recommendation.[10] The Authority, however, did not act on either of those requests. Rather, four years later Authority minutes stated that "nothing [for a chaplain] was included in the 1976–1977 budget since we were unable to identify a need based on patient requests."[11]

In 1977, at a quarterly meeting of the medical staff, physicians voted by a wide margin to ask the Authority to hire a chaplain.[12] The Authority's Professional Service Committee supported the request; and the Authority directed administration to define the qualifications for a hospital chaplain, develop a job description, include the position in the 1977–1978 budget, and begin the process of looking for a qualified person.[13]

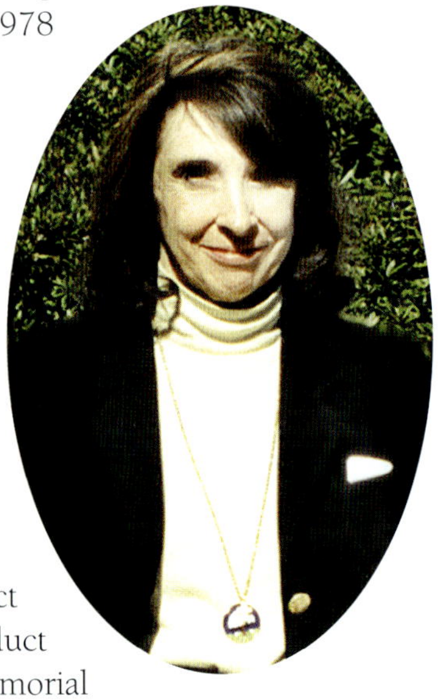

In the fall of 1978, DeKalb General Hospital selected Wayne E. Spangler, MDiv, as its first chaplain.[14] Betty Castellani, DMin, was hired in the spring of 1987 as associate chaplain,[15] and she became director of Pastoral Services when Spangler retired in 1992. McClellon Cox, MDiv, joined the staff as associate chaplain in the fall of 1996.[16] Currently, in addition to Castellani and Cox, the full-time Pastoral Services staff includes Joyce Young, MDiv, and McGiffert Townley, MDiv.[17]

The chaplains carry a heavy load. They cover DeKalb Medical's three hospitals and are on call twenty-four hours a day, seven days a week for any emergency requiring the services of a chaplain. They make regular rounds in the Emergency Department, critical care units, and other areas of the hospital. They offer counseling and personal support, conduct prayer services, and respond to patient requests for a chaplain. They conduct ecumenical services as well as weddings, funerals, communion services, memorial services, and baptisms. They conduct support and bereavement groups, and they represent DeKalb Medical at various community events.

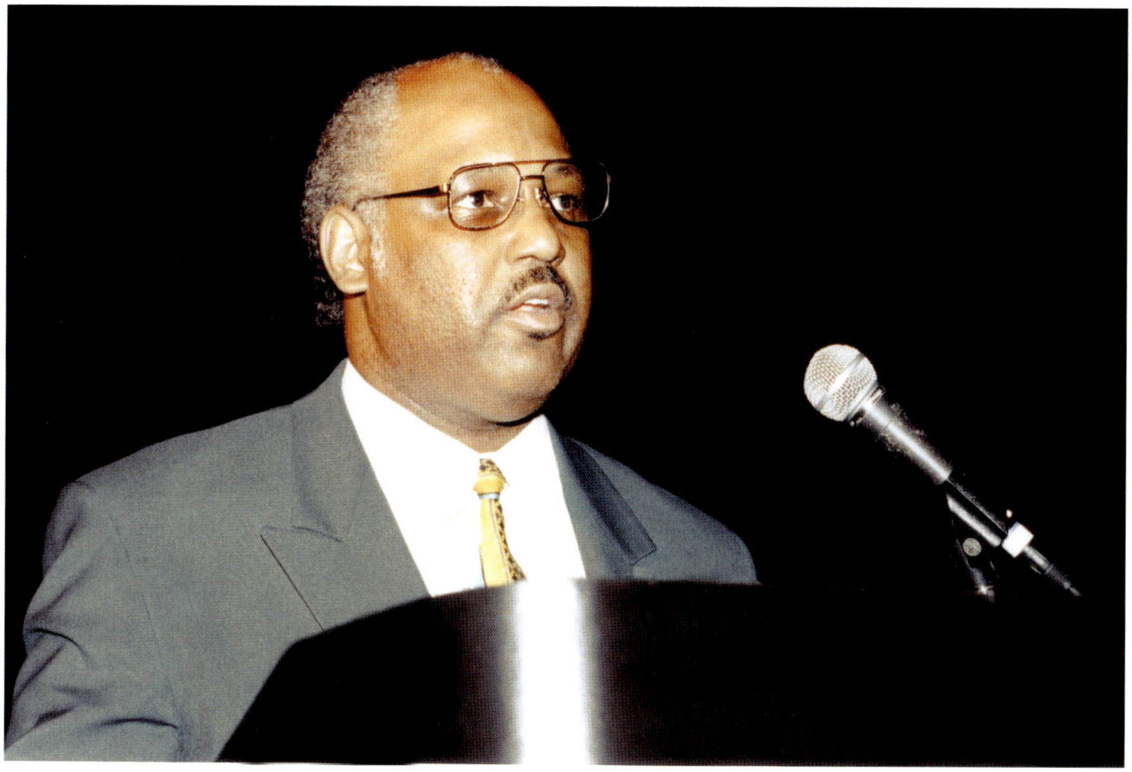

McClellon Cox, MDiv, was hired as associate chaplain in 1996.

The original hospital chapel on the North Decatur campus was located near the entrance to the administrative offices. It was relocated to a site closer to the front entrance during the hospital's 1993 renovation and expansion. In 2001 it was completely restored and named in honor of Pete and Jerri Pike in recognition of their major gift for its restoration. The Pikes said they wanted to repay DeKalb Medical Center for its excellent service to their family and the community over the previous thirty years.[18] The chapel is used by patients, their families, and staff for meditation, prayer, baptisms, communion services, memorial services, and weddings.

When DeKalb Medical at Hillandale opened in 2005, the chaplains conducted a service to bless the hands of the staff and physicians.[19] Pete and Jerri Pike made another major donation to construct and furnish the chapel in that facility.

Pastoral Services recognizes, respects, and supports the religious, national, and cultural diversity that characterizes DeKalb Medical's community, patients, staff, and physicians. The newly completed chapels are designed to be used by all faiths. Chaplains offer their services to the diverse staff, patients, and their families; and they reach out in a spirit of cooperation with the religious leaders of all congregations. At the heart of their service is the core value envisioned by the early leaders of the hospital that the spiritual life of the patients, staff, physicians, and institution will always go hand in hand at DeKalb Medical with the healing touch that is directed at the mind and body.

Pharmaceutical Services

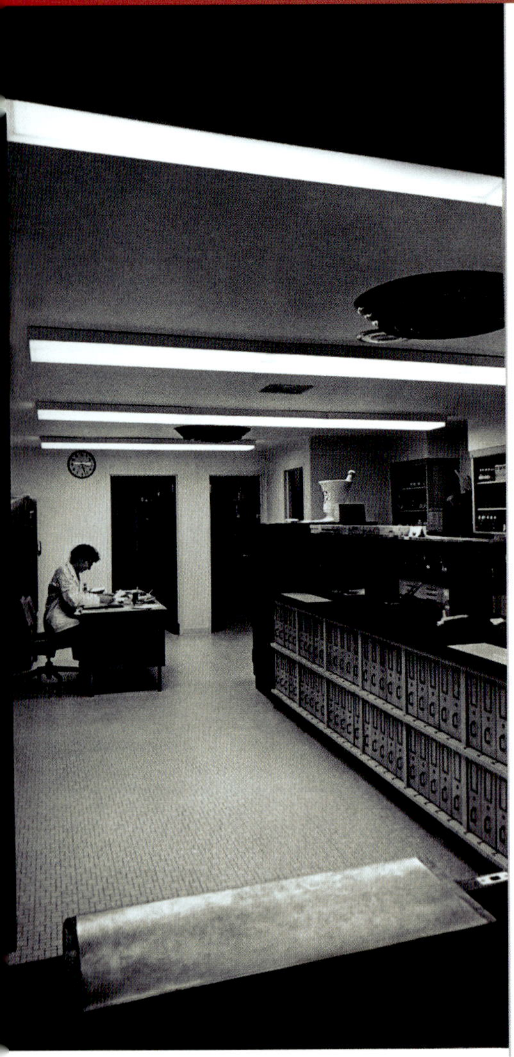

When the Pharmacy Department opened in 1961, it had 550 square feet and a two-person staff.

The 1961 DeKalb General Pharmacy Department occupied 550 square feet, was open from 7 AM until 11 PM, and the staff consisted of a director and an assistant director. Medication orders were sent from the nursing stations on cards, and all records were kept manually.[1] In 1962, when the hospital's purchasing agent resigned, as a cost-saving measure the DeKalb County Hospital Authority transferred many of the purchasing agent's responsibilities to the pharmacist and changed his title to director of Pharmacy and Supply Services.[2]

The year 1965 brought good news and bad news to the pharmacy. The good news was that John R. Gerlach, later to become DeKalb Medical's chief executive officer, came to work at DeKalb General as a part-time pharmacist while completing his master's degree in hospital administration at Georgia State University. The bad news was that Administrator Thrasher had to fire the director of Pharmacy and Supply Services. The director confessed to having conspired with a hospital supplier over a two-year period to embezzle money from the hospital.[3]

Patricia Twiggs became the second director of Pharmacy in 1965 but remained in the position for only a few months.[4] She was followed by Nancy Rowe.[5] James Briscoe, RPh, became director in 1967, and the responsibility for purchasing was returned to a director of the Purchasing Department.[6]

Briscoe was director of the Pharmacy Department for six years, during which time he spearheaded several major innovations. He and Stanley Aldridge, MD, chairman of the medical staff Pharmacy and Therapeutics Committee, streamlined the administration of medications. They reviewed the existing process by which medications were ordered, processed, and delivered to the patient and, to their dismay, discovered the procedure involved fifteen separate steps that required unnecessary labor and that created an increased risk for error. They developed a new, simplified drug distribution program that benefited the hospital, staff, and patients.[7]

In 1971 Briscoe expanded pharmacy hours to include the eleven pm to seven am hours. Lee Underwood, RPh, who joined the staff in 1970, was the first pharmacist for the night shift.[8] Briscoe also established a five-week clinical rotation program for senior pharmacy students from the Mercer University School of Pharmacy.[9] And he initiated a new program for preparing intravenous (IV) medications under completely sterile conditions.[10]

James Briscoe was elected president of the State Hospital Pharmacy Association in 1970,[11] and in 1972 he was named Georgia Hospital Pharmacist of the Year.[12] *Hospital Pharmacy Notes*, a national hospital pharmacy publication, ran a feature story on the innovations that he brought to the DeKalb General pharmacy.[13]

In 1971, during Briscoe's tenure, the IV (intravenous) Team was created. Administrator William Thrasher reported to the Authority that the medical staff and Briscoe advocated the creation of a team of nurses to start and maintain IV fluids for patients.[14] Robert Gibbs, MD, chief of staff, added that such a service would provide better patient care and would relieve the floor nurses for other important patient care responsibilities.[15]

Thrasher presented a plan for a hospitalwide IV service that required fourteen nurses. Wash W. Lively, chairman of the Finance Committee, said such a program was not financially feasible.[16] The

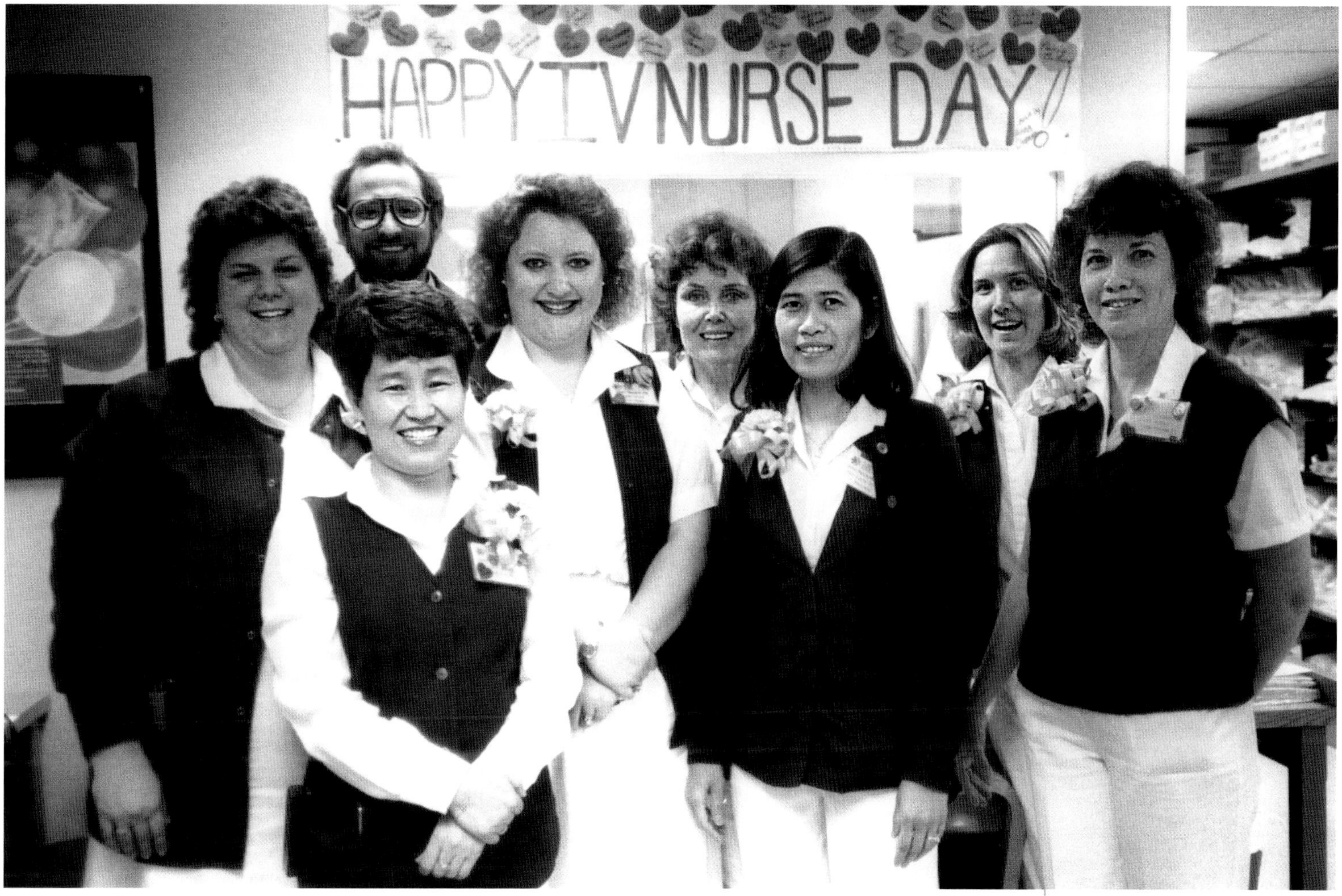

IV Team; back row: Joe Chapman, unidentified colleague, Judy Lewis Sheppard; middle row: Lynn Boyd Dixon, Ellen Hargett, Chitra Petchrawises, Judy Guthrie; and front row: Sook Cheoun.

trustees, instead, approved a pilot plan for four nurses who would be assigned to the pharmacy staff and who would provide IV services on the fourth floor on a trial basis.

The hospital charged a $1 fee for each IV fluid started.[17] After two months, Thrasher reported that the program was going well with great patient, physician and nursing satisfaction, and that it was paying for itself. The trustees expanded the program to include the second floor, using the same four nurses.[18] In August 1972 the Authority approved the medical staff's recommendation that more nurses be added to serve the third floor,[19] and by October 1972 the program was producing such positive reviews and financial results that it was made hospitalwide with a full staff of fourteen nurses.[20] The IV Team had six different coordinators.[21]

By 1985 DeKalb General employed more than fifty IV nurses, one of the largest teams in the southeast. They performed an average of 75,000 procedures each month, administering IV fluids, IV medications, blood and blood products, and chemotherapy.[22] In addition to starting and maintaining IVs, the team trained nurses and emergency medical technicians in the proper way to start IVs, and they responded to all Blue Alerts for cardiac or respiratory arrests. Seeing the success of the program at DeKalb General, ten other Atlanta hospitals had established IV teams by 1989.[23]

In 1993 administration announced a plan to return the responsibility for IV services to the floor nurses as a cost-reduction measure. The announcement met with such distress and resistance on the part of physicians, the floor nurses, and the IV Team that the proposal temporarily was shelved.[24]

In 1995 members of the IV Team were transferred from the Pharmacy staff to Nursing Services, and the duties of the team were significantly modified. Team members continued starting IVs, but staff nurses were trained to administer the IV fluids, medications, chemotherapy, and blood and blood products. More than six hundred staff nurses were trained and tested in their ability to provide IV therapy to their patients. Former IV Team coordinator, Ellen Hargett, wrote a comprehensive manual called the IMAG (Intravenous Medication Administration Guide) which provided in detail all the information needed for IV therapy. A copy of the manual was placed on every nursing unit and was made accessible online the following year by Chris Davis, RN. It exists today and is maintained by the Nursing and Pharmacy Committee. The process, known as "IV Transition," took place over two years. It was one of the most outstanding training programs ever undertaken by Nursing Services. For the nursing staff, it developed new skills, refined existing ones, and enhanced continuity of care and a sense of pride in the nurses' ability to care for the complete needs of their patients.[25]

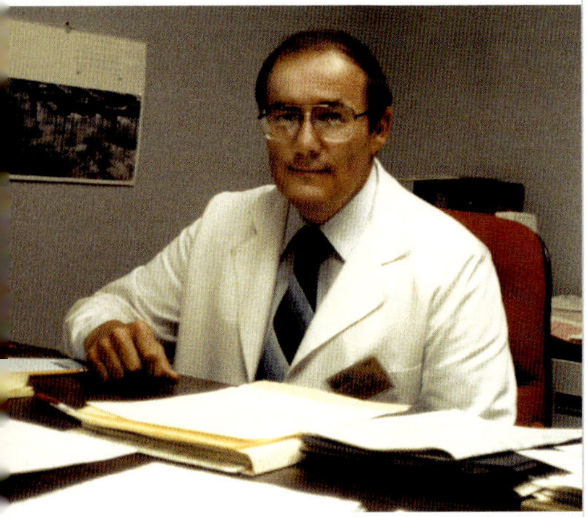

Walter J. (Jack) Linn, RPh, director of Pharmaceutical Services from 1973–1988.

In 2006 the IV Team transition went one step further, and the role of starting IVs also was transferred to staff nurses. The IV team retained only a skeletal crew to start IVs when floor nurses encountered difficulties.[26] In July 2006 Leigh Ann Miller, RN, and Rayna Ashburn, RN, two former IV Team members formed a PICC Team to place IV lines that previously could be placed only by physicians in Interventional Radiology. The team has been successful and remains active today.

Walter J. (Jack) Linn, RPh, succeeded James Briscoe as director of Pharmacy in 1973.[27] Jack Linn came to DeKalb General as a Mercer pharmacy student in 1966, remained on the staff after he was graduated in 1968, and was appointed assistant director of Pharmacy in 1970. As director, he was instrumental in establishing the innovative "unit dose drug distribution program" in 1974[28] and a pharmacy home health program in 1984.[29]

Lee Underwood, RPh, became director of the Pharmacy in 1988. He recalled that when he joined the staff in 1970 there was a director, an assistant director, four other pharmacists, a department secretary, four part-time pharmacy students, and two technicians. When he retired in 2005 the pharmacy had sixty-three full-time employees, nearly half of which were pharmacists and most of the others technicians.[30]

In 1989 the Pharmacy Department changed its name to Pharmaceutical Services to reflect its expanded scope of services. Initially only administering drugs, it now offered nutritional support; pharmacokinetics information regarding the absorption, distribution, metabolism and excretion of drugs; oncology support; drug information and interaction alerts; and anticoagulation management. Those services were divided into five basic areas: clinical pharmacy services, nutritional support services, drug dispensing, intravenous admixture, and the IV Team.[31]

Clinical pharmacy services used, among other sources of information, the Micromedex computerized drug information software. It provided information on drugs, potential adverse drug reactions, drug interactions, and drug identification. Clinical pharmacists circulated throughout the hospital to provide one of Pharmaceutical Services' most important services by offering important drug information to physicians, nurses, and patients.[32]

Nutritional support was responsible for preparing the prescribed ingredients for patients receiving nutrition by way of IV administration or feeding tubes in the stomach. Today the dietitians who are members of the Nutrition Support Team are a part of the pharmacy staff.[33]

The drug dispensing area prepares, dispenses and maintains records on all patient drugs, including the preparation of IV fluids, IV medications, and chemotherapy.[34]

In addition to witnessing expanded services, Lee Underwood saw drug costs and charges increase. When he became director in 1988, drugs cost the hospital $3.19 million annually for which the hospital charged (and were mostly paid) $9.56 million. In 2005, the year of his retirement, annual drug costs amounted to $15.5 million and charges totaled $108 million. In 2005, however, when revenue depended on per diem and other fixed payments from Medicare, Medicaid, managed care and other third-party payers, charges correlated very poorly with payments for inpatient services. Pharmaceutical Services today realizes a small net operating margin for its outpatient services, but inpatient services seeks at best to break even by performing service in the most efficient way possible.[35]

Pharmacy inaugurated more teaching programs in the 1990s. In addition to James Briscoe's program whereby senior Mercer pharmacy students rotated through DeKalb pharmacy services, Lee Underwood added senior students from the University of Georgia School of Pharmacy. He also enrolled in a one-year postgraduate residency program those who had completed a doctor of pharmacy degree in the Mercer University School of Pharmacy.[36] DeKalb Medical Center's postgraduate residency program was the only one in the state other than one at the University of Georgia.[37] Currently the pharmacy accepts senior pharmacy students from Mercer and from the University of Georgia who spend five-week clinical rotations at the North Decatur campus. Approximate seventy students per year rotate through the program, most of whom come from Mercer School of Pharmacy.[38]

In addition to rotating senior students, pharmacy now has two independent, accredited residency programs that Mercer helped establish in 1992. One is a one-year General Pharmacy Practice residency program in which graduate students rotate through the various clinical services. The other is an Advanced Oncology Residency in which graduate students concentrate on all aspects of oncology and hematology.[39]

During Lee Underwood's administration, the pharmacy added two major technological advances. The first was the Pyxis system to house and dispense drugs on the nursing units utilizing specialized storage cabinets. In the early 1990s, however, DeKalb's Pyxis system was limited. At that time Pharmacy leased just enough cabinets to house only a few of the medications used on the nursing units. There was only one cabinet on each unit that held primarily narcotics to control pain and drugs to control nausea and vomiting. The system also lacked a security component to control and monitor drugs removed from the cabinets.[40] Pyxis at that time, therefore, had limited capacity and value.

In 1999 DeKalb Medical Center added another technological advancement when it installed McKesson's robot system to dispense drugs. Named "D'Spenser" by the pharmacy staff, the robot was linked to the pharmacy computer from which it read orders, slid along a track, gathered drugs from bar-coded bags hanging from pegs attached to the walls, and deposited the drugs into a patient's bar-coded box at the end of the track. Drugs then were taken from the bar-coded box to the appropriate nursing unit.[41]

The pharmacy found, however, that using both the limited Pyxis system and the robot dispensing system led to problems of inefficiency, delays in getting drugs to the nursing stations, difficulties for the nurses to locate ordered and delivered drugs, repetition when nurses reordered "lost" drugs (most of which already were somewhere on the unit), and strained nursing-pharmacy relations.[42] In addition, the robot system was expensive to lease and labor-intensive to operate, requiring five technicians seven days

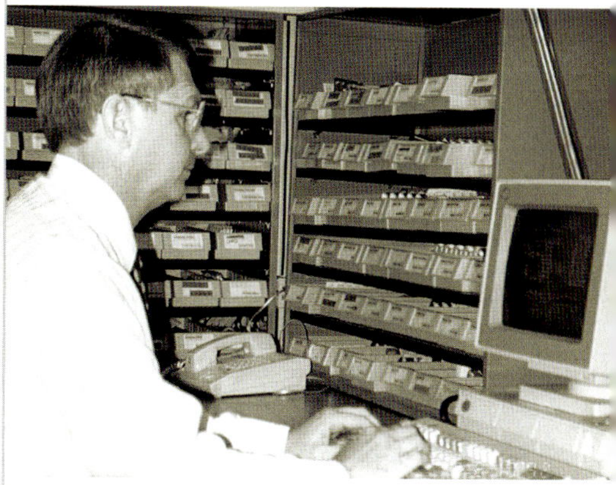

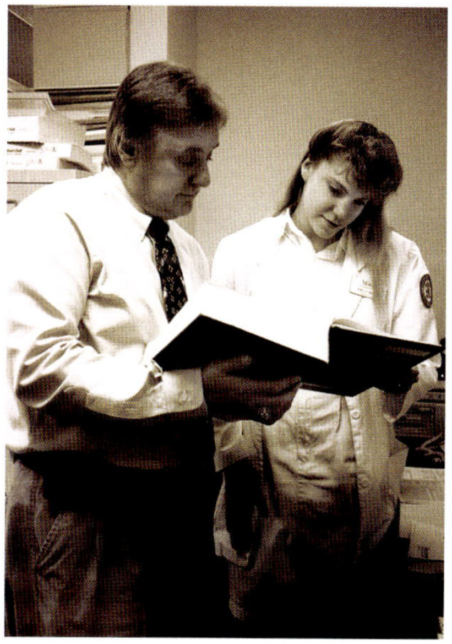

Top: Lee Underwood, RPh, was director of Pharmaceutical Services from 1988–2005. **Above:** Clinical pharmacist Martin Job, DPh, with Mercer University pharmacy student Emily Smith.

a week to run it.[43]

The hospital engaged a Georgia Volunteer Hospital Association (VHA) consulting pharmacist in May 2004 to conduct an assessment of pharmacy operations and to make recommendations for improving the efficiency of staffing and medication distribution. The consultant recommended having only one medication distribution system.[44]

The pharmacy chose to discontinue McKesson's robot system when its lease expired in 2006 and to use the savings to add more Pyxis cabinets. With that change, as much as 95 percent of the medications used within a given unit were on that unit in its Pyxis cabinets and readily available once an order was received, reviewed, and approved by the pharmacist. In addition, the expanded Pyxis system had more control and safety measures to reduce the risk of administering the wrong medication or the wrong dosage. Pharmacy trained more technicians in the use of the Pyxis machine and made technicians available on every shift to handle Pyxis-related problems.[45]

In 2003 the pharmacy installed McKesson's Meds Manager Computer System to interface Pharmaceutical Services with the hospital's new Sunrise Clinical Manager (SCM) system that would include the Computerized Physician Order Entry (CPOE) system.[46] While the McKesson system was a sophisticated and comprehensive system, it also presented challenges once the CPOE system was activated. It could interface with the CPOE system but was not integrated with it. The result of having two systems that were not integrated once again led to inefficiencies and delays. The need for integration led to the decision to replace the McKesson system. It will be replaced in 2009 with the Eclipsys Pharmacy System, which will be fully integrated with the SCM and CPOE systems.[47]

When Lee Underwood retired as director of Pharmaceutical Services in 2005, Scott McAuley, RPh, became director.[48] McAuley joined the pharmacy staff in August 2000 as the associate director. Pharmacy managers at the Hillandale campus and the Downtown Decatur campuses now report to him.[49]

In addition to expanding the Pyxis system, replacing the robot system, and making plans to replace the McKesson pharmacy system with the Eclipsys Pharmacy System, Pharmaceutical Services has established other initiatives. It has focused on enhancing its customer service orientation to give nurses and physicians what they need to do their jobs and to create a more collegial relationship. When Nursing Services rated its support systems, pharmacy rose from an earlier 30-percent approval rating to a score in the 80 percent range.[50]

Prior to the addition of the Eclipsys Pharmacy system in 2009, plans call for the installation of the electronic medical administration record (eMAR) system. Currently, nurses keep medication records on paper, which is time consuming and poses a risk for the record being lost, incomplete, or misread. The eMAR system will integrate with CPOE and computerize the processes of ordering, approving, distributing, and administering drugs in a safer and more-efficient manner.[51]

A third advancement that may be achieved in the next three years involves bedside barcode scanning of medications being administered to patients. By scanning the barcode on the medication and the barcode on the patient's identification bracelet, the administering nurse confirms that the drug to be administered is the right drug, in the right dose, and being administered at the right time.[52] A record of the administered medications is automatically recorded and compared with the order for its use to confirm accuracy and appropriateness.

Quality Care for Every Patient

It has been said glibly that "quality" is achieved when the right people do the right thing, the right way, for the right reason, at the right time, the first time. The challenge of that simplified definition is how to know if they are the right people, if it is the right thing, if it is the right way, if it is the right reason, and if it is the right time. Added to that quandary is whether those to whom a service is provided perceive it to be the right thing, provided by the right people, the right way, for the right reason, at the right time. Achieving quality, and having it perceived as such by the recipient is a challenging, complex quest.

In certain sectors, that task may be easier than in others. A machine shop may be able to determine if all the bolts and nuts it manufactures meet their prescribed specifications; and if the products are shipped to the right customers, in the right amount, at the agreed upon price, and arrive intact when promised; and if it receives five-star satisfaction ratings from all its customers. That machine shop may lay legitimate claim to having achieved quality and service excellence in the production and distribution of its products.

Health care is a different story. There are no precise or consistent criteria for defining the right thing, the right people, the right reason, or the right time for many health services. And the expectations of those receiving those services may range from objective reality to total fantasy. Yet every healthcare institution, including DeKalb Medical, is expected to—and strives to—provide quality care with service excellence. The measurements by which quality and service are attained in health care, however, will of necessity always be to some degree arbitrary, limited, and imprecise.

DeKalb Medical has consistently contended that providing quality health care was its reason for being. At the 1961 DeKalb General Hospital dedication ceremony, Administrator William Thrasher pledged "to give the best care at the least cost to the patient."[1] The 1971–1972 hospital objectives said, "The primary concern of DeKalb General is for the welfare, comfort, and safety of the patient."[2] DeKalb Medical Center's 1991 mission statement declared that it would "contribute to the well-being and quality of life of our community by providing, in partnership with our physician practices, high-value health and wellness services for those whom we serve."[3] Its 2001–2002 performance improvement plan declared, "Our ultimate vision of success . . . is to provide the best possible care with the best possible service and least possible cost for our patients."[4] The 2003 revised mission statement said, "The mission of DeKalb Regional Healthcare System is to improve lives through the delivery of excellent health and wellness services in partnership with its physicians."[5]

Each of those statements reflects a commitment to quality care, perceived as such by its recipients, as DeKalb Medical's reason for being and an acknowledgment that quality care is essential to good patient outcomes. Yet, in its early years, neither DeKalb General nor most other hospitals had systems in place to measure or determine if it was indeed providing quality care or excellent service.

DeKalb General Hospital in its early days received from patients and their families many tributes to the quality of service offered. A patient told Administrator Thrasher that an employee saw that he did not have the morning paper and went to get one for him. When another patient asked if the hospital could launder his pajamas since he had no one at home to do it, a nurse took his pajamas to her home

A patient told Administrator Thrasher that an employee saw that he did not have the morning paper and went to get one for him. When another patient asked if the hospital could launder his pajamas since he had no one at home to do it, a nurse took his pajamas to her home and washed them herself.

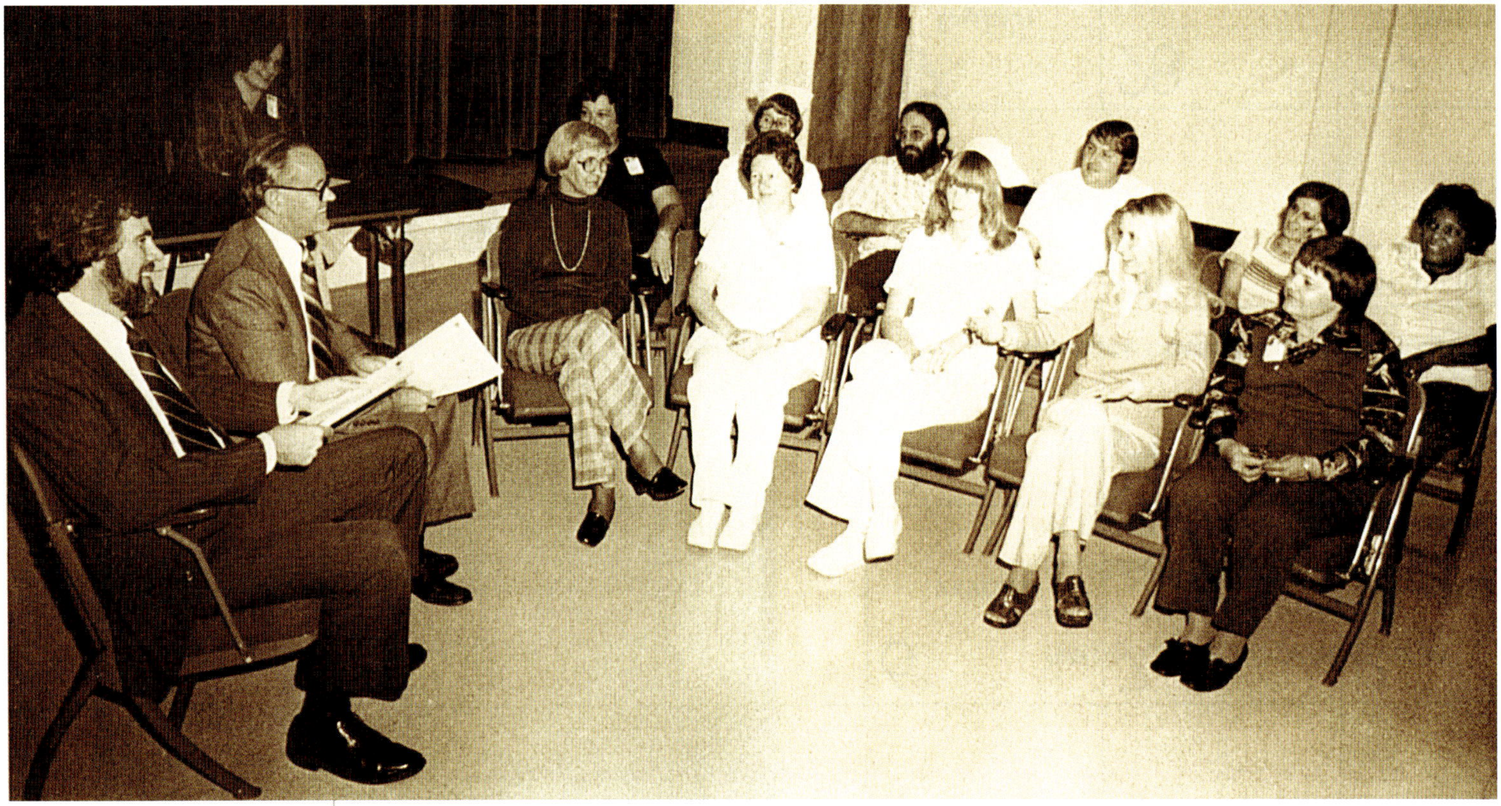

Bill Sublett, director of Administrative Services (left) and Perry Stephens, director of Personnel (right) meet with the Employee Council composed of representatives from many of the hospital departments.

and washed them herself.[6] A husband wrote that when his wife spent ten days in DeKalb General, from the moment of her entry to her discharge, the spoken word was, "May we help you?" but the spirit of the question was "We will help you."[7] Two surveys were conducted in 1970 to determine patient satisfaction—one for nursing and one for food—and the administrator reported to the trustees that "both appeared very favorable."[8]

Of course not everyone was satisfied. One patient called Medical Records to say that he did not get enough gravy on his roast beef. The representative answering the phone told him he must have the wrong number because he was speaking with the Medical Records Department. He replied, "Yes, I know. I just wanted it on my record that I did not get enough gravy on my roast beef."[9]

There were personal opinions, concerns, and complaints. In August 1961 Chief of Staff L. C. Buchanan, MD, told the trustees that physicians were concerned about the quality of patient care and the cost of care to patients.[10] There were reports of sentinel events such as operating on the wrong patient or a patient death as a result of the wrong medication. There was a contest and prize of $600 offered for the best staff idea to "bring improvement and savings to DeKalb General Hospital."[11] The trustees established an Employee Council in 1969 through which representatives from most departments met monthly to share suggestions and voice concerns about the hospital's services and operation. In the 1970s the nursing staff instituted nursing audits, and the medical staff created physician audits to compare the level of care provided against a few selected criteria.[12]

In the meantime, a quality revolution was taking place in another part of the world. Edward Deming, a statistician, and Joseph Juran, a management consultant, went to Japan as part of the allied occupational forces after World War II to teach the Japanese industrial world the application of statistical quality concepts and tools for improving processes. Deming taught a fourteen-point plan, a philosophy of management, and a method for insuring quality performance. Juran developed the quality trilogy: quality planning, quality control, and quality improvement. Deming and Juran are credited with the invention of the Total Quality Management (TQM) concept.

Despite their revolutionary achievements in Japan's industrial world, those men were relatively unknown in this country for thirty years until they were discovered by the media in 1980. The concept of quality management then exploded in the United States, and a veritable new industry emerged with consultants and "experts on every corner." Two of the better-known American quality gurus were Philip B. Crosby and Tom Peters. Crosby is best known for his concepts of "Quality Is Free" and "Zero Defects" that focused on financial indicators to document the excessive cost of poor quality. Peters identified leadership as central to the quality improvement process, substituted the term leadership for management, and depicted the leader's role to be one of managing by walking around (MBWA) to listen, teach, and facilitate.[13]

American industries across the board—manufacturing, retail, education, service, and healthcare—quickly adapted quality improvement processes. Hospitals like DeKalb General finally had tools available to them and a mechanism to examine if they were indeed providing the quality and service to which they were committed.

Soon, however, participating in the quality improvement process was not just something hospitals wanted to do; it was something they were required to do. They were externally as well as internally motivated. They had to participate in the quality improvement process or risk penalties. The Joint Commission on Accreditation of Healthcare Organizations (JCAHO) made hospital accreditation contingent upon demonstrating quality-improvement activities. Medicare and Medicaid made participation a requirement for reimbursement eligibility. The Department of Health and Human Services (HHS) and the Centers for Medicare and Medicaid Services (CMS) announced the Hospital Quality Initiative (HQI). CMS encouraged hospitals to report the results of a standardized set of core quality measures. Those reports demonstrated how well a hospital compared with others, and the reports were available to the public on an Internet website. While hospitals were not required to report their results, those who chose not to could expect a reduction in their Medicare and Medicaid reimbursements.[14] Managed-care organizations, insurers and employers increasingly based their contracts with hospitals and physicians on their ability to document quality of care, patient safety, and service excellence.

In 1980 JCAHO published a new requirement that all hospitals must have in place a quality assurance program by January 1981. DeKalb General complied by establishing a Quality Assurance Committee to design and implement a quality assurance plan.[15] The initial requirements were fairly simple and rudimentary, such as patient length of stay, mortality rates, readmissions for the same diagnosis, and complications. By 1991 the JCAHO required hospitals to address at least ten performance improvement measures to be in compliance.[16]

As described in chapter 10, in 1997 CEO John Gerlach and Chief of Staff Michael Hartman, MD, advised the board of directors that the JCAHO and third-party payers contracting with the hospital now were looking for something more than what DeKalb Medical Center was doing. The JCAHO wanted an integrated approach to quality improvement that reached across department lines and that quantified evidence of quality performance. While the hospital was engaged in acceptable departmental quality improvement activities, the JCAHO considered those activities to be fragmented and isolated. Insurers also said they lacked quantifiable, measurable documentation.[17] The board approved the formation of a multidisciplinary Quality Council to "establish a state-of-the-art, organization-wide quality measurement system, a mechanism for setting aggressive targets for ever-higher levels of quality and customer satisfaction and a process for involving all employees and medical staff in the continuous improvement of all that we do."[18] The name of the council later was changed to Performance Improvement Council,[19] and Steve Mayfield was named director.[20] He was succeeded by Debbie King, RN,[21] then Ellen Hargett.[22]

The Performance Improvement Council elevated DeKalb Medical's quality initiatives to a new level. It satisfied the accreditation requirements of JCAHO, provided third-party payers with quantified documentation of quality performance and produced data on "core measures" (the management of heart attacks, pneumonia, and congestive heart failure) that could be shared with the public via the Internet as a part of the CMS hospital reporting initiative. It focused on enhancing the quality of care, patient safety, operational effectiveness and efficiency, and physician partnership. The council established priorities to improve care and assigned teams to address those priorities. It provided data to and received input from the DeKalb Physician-Hospital Organization(DPHO). It worked with members of the medical staff and DPHO to create order sets for managing a variety of specific diseases/conditions based on the latest scientific evidence for best practices. Those order sets would be needed when the Computerized Physician Order Entry (CPOE) system "went live" in 2005. It developed departmental and management scorecards that reflected customer satisfaction, safety, clinical performance, and operational performance.[23]

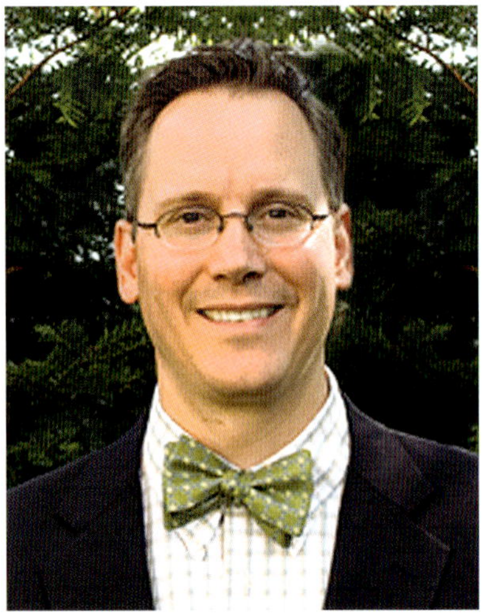

Steven Meurer, PhD, was named executive director of the DeKalb County Institute in 2004.

DeKalb Medical Center formed a Service Excellence Committee,[24] also known as Team EXCEL (Extraordinary Customer Excellence and Leadership) "to create an organizational culture that better supports the patient healing process and empowers employees to have a customer-oriented focus in their work."[25] Acknowledging that every day in the organization there are fifty thousand "moments of truth" when a patient, family member, employee, or physician draws a conclusion about service or the lack thereof,[26] the team's goal was to improve the level of patient, physician, and employee satisfaction.

There emerged, however, an even greater need and opportunity to demonstrate precisely the quality of care provided. In 2003 PROMINA relinquished back to its member organizations the responsibility for negotiating contracts with managed-care organizations and other third-party payers. The DPHO, a major player in securing contracts, negotiated pay-for-performance agreements and created a need to integrate hospital goals and objectives with those of the DPHO. DeKalb Medical was one of five hospital systems in Georgia to sign on with Blue Cross/Blue Shield's pilot Q-HIP (Quality-in-sights: Hospital Incentive Program) initiative to reward hospital systems that met or exceeded quality indicators in fifty measures of patient safety, results, and satisfaction.[27]

As described in chapter 10, in 2004 CEO Eric Norwood and his team envisioned the concept of clinical integration as the way to bring all the parties together, and they proposed the establishment of the DeKalb Quality Institute as the research and development vehicle to make clinical integration possible and to provide documentation for pay-for-performance contracts.[28] The institute would address the quality of care, service excellence, patient safety, and operational performance of all three of DeKalb Medical's hospitals, physicians, and the DPHO. Its stated mission was "to differentiate DeKalb Medical and its medical staff and the DeKalb Physician-Hospital Organization from their competitors in terms of enhanced quality, service and patient safety."

Steven Meurer, PhD, was named executive director.[29] He created the structure of the institute, mobilized its components, and established it as an essential tool in DeKalb Medical's quest for clinical integration, quality care, service excellence, and continuous improvement. Recognizing that quality in healthcare is always a moving target, the institute served as a vital research initiative, seeking to identify best practices in health care.

According to Steve Meurer's successor, Cathleen Wheatley, RN, MS, the institute under Meurer's leadership created a new organizational culture that made DeKalb Medical excited about quality, that launched it ahead of the current quality concept, and that made it known in the community for its focus on quality.[30] It took quality beyond being just another tiresome performance improvement project. The institute brought the DPHO and the DRHS hospitals together to research and develop new standards of clinical practice that spanned inpatient, outpatient, and ambulatory practice environments. It integrated information technology into the quality initiative. It collected and analyzed data from throughout the organization that related to operations, patient care, patient satisfaction, and safety. It utilized 1,200 indicators and eighty-five scorecards. It compared DeKalb's performance with that of peer institutions, its own past performance, and established targets (benchmarks). It shared its findings with the DPHO, the medical staff, the organization's departments, committees, managers, senior executives, and governing bodies. It identified opportunities for improvement and demonstrated to third-party payers in a quantified manner the quality of care provided.[31] It improved core quality measures from the fiftieth percentile range to the ninetieth percentile range in a short period of time.[32] It enabled the organization to report its data for public scrutiny.

Cathleen Wheatley succeeded Steven Meurer in 2007 and was named senior vice president for Quality, Care Management, Information Technology, and Infection Control.[33] She joined the DeKalb nursing staff in 2003, was made director of Medical-Surgical Services, became director of Patient Care at DeKalb Medical at Hillandale, interim administrator at Hillandale following the resignation of Julia Jones, and served unofficially as vice president for Patient Care and chief nursing officer at DeKalb Medical at North Decatur following the resignation of Brent Robinson, RN, in 2007.

Building on the foundation laid by Steven Meuer, she has focused on integrating quality, informatics, care management, and infection control into one cohesive initiative. The institute is moving from seeing and communicating data to understanding it, applying it, and finding solutions to problems it reveals. It is demonstrating to the DeKalb Medical organization the interrelatedness of best practices to clinical quality, appropriate length of stay, appropriate financial reimbursement, improved patient satisfaction, decreased readmissions, and enhanced patient safety.[34]

The DeKalb Medical Board established a Quality Committee that is chaired by a physician board member and composed of representatives from the board, administrative executives, and medical staff. The Quality Committee will "own" the board's quality issues as the Finance Committee owns its financial matters, bringing to the board quality issues that warrant its knowledge and consideration.[35]

While recognizing that the measurement of quality and service excellence in health care will always be somewhat limited, arbitrary, and imprecise, the DeKalb Quality Institute has catapulted DeKalb Medical in a quantum leap from the early days of individual complaints and compliments, sentinel events, random surveys, and audits to a level of meaningful information, a mechanism for continual improvement, new energy, commitment, instrumentation, integration, and vision. It was because of this new capability that the institute was able to share a documented level of performance with the public that allowed DeKalb Medical to receive in 2007 the five-star rating referenced in chapter 10 for its treatment of stroke, heart attack, hip replacement, hip fracture repair, peripheral vascular bypass, pneumonia, and sepsis and to be ranked in the top 5 percent of nearly five thousand U. S. hospitals in providing those services.[36]

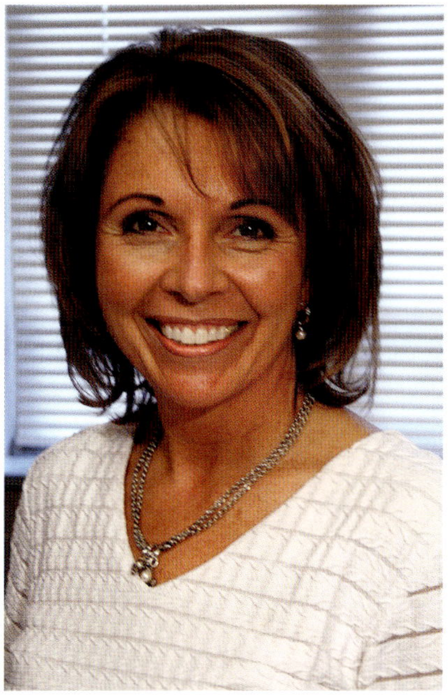

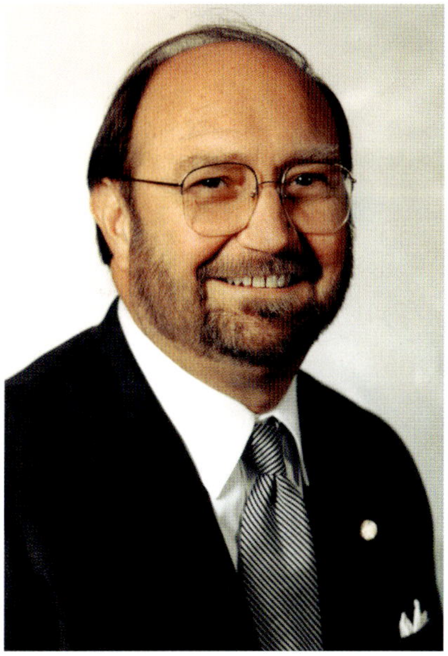

Top: In 2007, Cathleen Wheatley, MS, RN, was named senior vice president of Quality, Care Management, Information Technology and Infection Control. **Above:** Roy Vandiver, MD, neurosurgeon, former chief of staff, is a long-time member of the DeKalb Medical Board of Directors, first recipient of the DeKalb Medical Foundation Charles B. Eberhart Award, and chairman of DeKalb Medical Board's Quality Committee.

Radiology (Imaging) Services

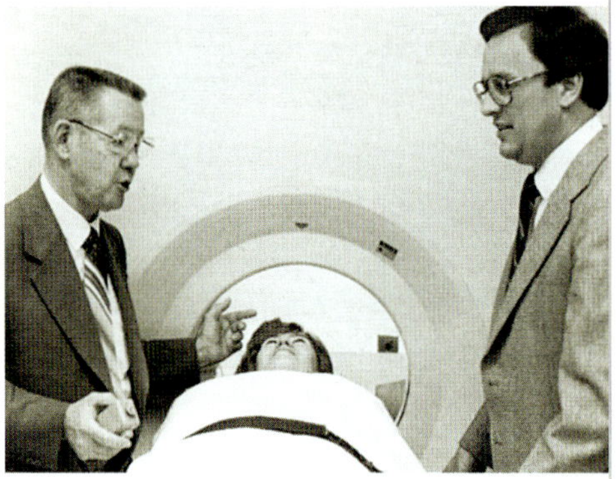

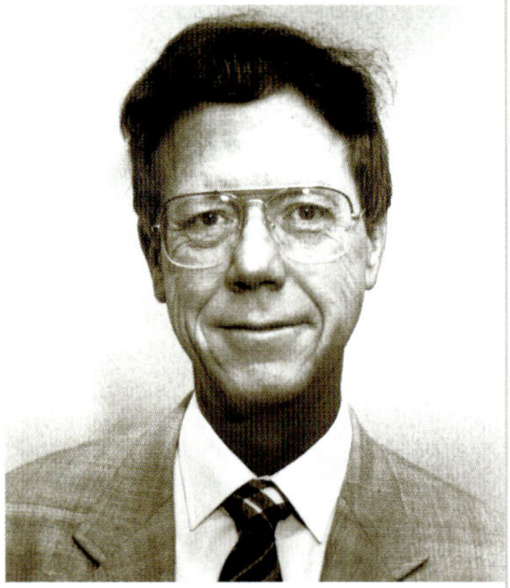

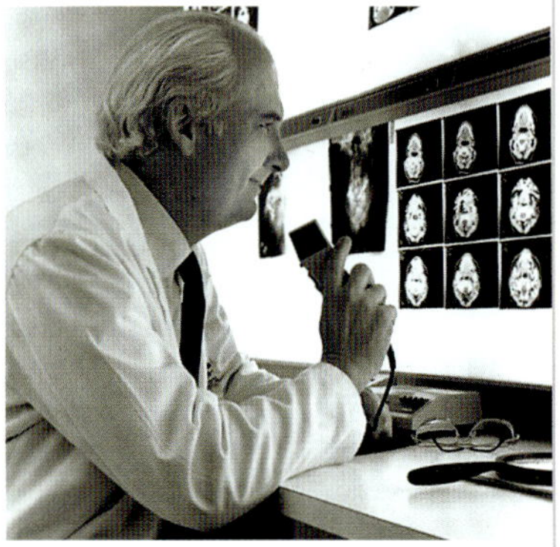

Top: Frank Morgan, MD, (left) was the first radiologist at DeKalb—here he discusses the CT scanner with John GerLach, then director of Patient Services. **Center:** Donald Minor, MD, became the second radiologist in July of 1961. **Above:** Robert Stephenson, MD, joined the staff in 1976.

When the DeKalb County Hospital Authority met in November 1958, Administrator William Thrasher "suggested that in the very near future consideration should be given to contracting with a radiologist. . . . A discussion followed, and it was the opinion of those present [that] such action should be delayed until construction [of the hospital] was actually started."[1] The following May, however, the trustees agreed that the time had come to ask the Authority chairman and the administrator, with the advice of the DeKalb Medical Society's Advisory Committee, to contract with a radiologist.[2]

Several physicians applied for the position, and the advisory committee investigated each candidate.[3] In August 1959 Authority Chairman J. Rufus Evans reported to the trustees that the committee recommended Frank E. Morgan Jr., MD, a radiologist with an office in downtown Decatur, and that a contract was being negotiated with him.[4]

Morgan's contract stipulated that he would be the hospital's radiologist, medical director of the Radiology Department, and chief of the medical staff's Department of Radiology. He would be an independent contractor, would receive 30 percent of the professional fees charged as his compensation, and would be responsible for paying the salary of any other radiologists added to the staff. The hospital would provide the facility, equipment, and technical staff who would be hired only with the radiologist's approval. The contract would be reviewed every six months, and it could be terminated by either party with ninety days' notice.[5]

Morgan was the sole radiologist when the hospital opened in May 1961. Donald Minor, MD, joined him in July. James Milsaps, MD, came on board in 1965, but moved to Piedmont Hospital in 1967. Jay Coffsky, MD, replaced Milsaps in 1967 as the third radiologist. Tom Daley, MD, joined the staff in 1970, Robert Davies, MD, in 1971, Michael Luckett, MD, in 1972, Clifford (Mack) Kerley, MD, in 1973, Gary Lasky, MD, in 1974, Robert Stephenson, MD, in 1976, and William Whitaker, MD, in 1977.

Evelyn Bates, RT, helped Morgan plan the department, and she recommended the equipment to be purchased and the technical staff to be hired. When the hospital opened, she was the first director of Technical Radiology. She remained in that position, however, for only a month because she married and moved to California. Before leaving she recommended Jo Ann Kilpatrick, RT,[6] as her replacement. She referred to Kilpatrick as a friend in whom she had great confidence.

Jo Ann Kilpatrick (later Morgan) served as the second director of Technical Radiology from 1961 to 1973.[7] Della Johnson, RT, became her successor in 1973. Johnson joined the radiology staff in 1964, became chief technologist in 1968 and technical director in 1973. She had been a member of the Radiology staff for forty-three years and director of the department for thirty-four years when she retired in 2007.[8] On the occasion of her retirement, she said, "If you want to make it to forty-three years, you must love your institution, love the people you work with, and always put your patients first."[9] Michele P. Grose, RT, succeeded Della Johnson, and is the current director of Imaging Services (the current name for the department).

When the hospital opened in 1961, there were two diagnostic X-ray rooms, one radiation therapy room, an X-ray unit for use in the orthopedic and cystoscopy operating room, and one mobile

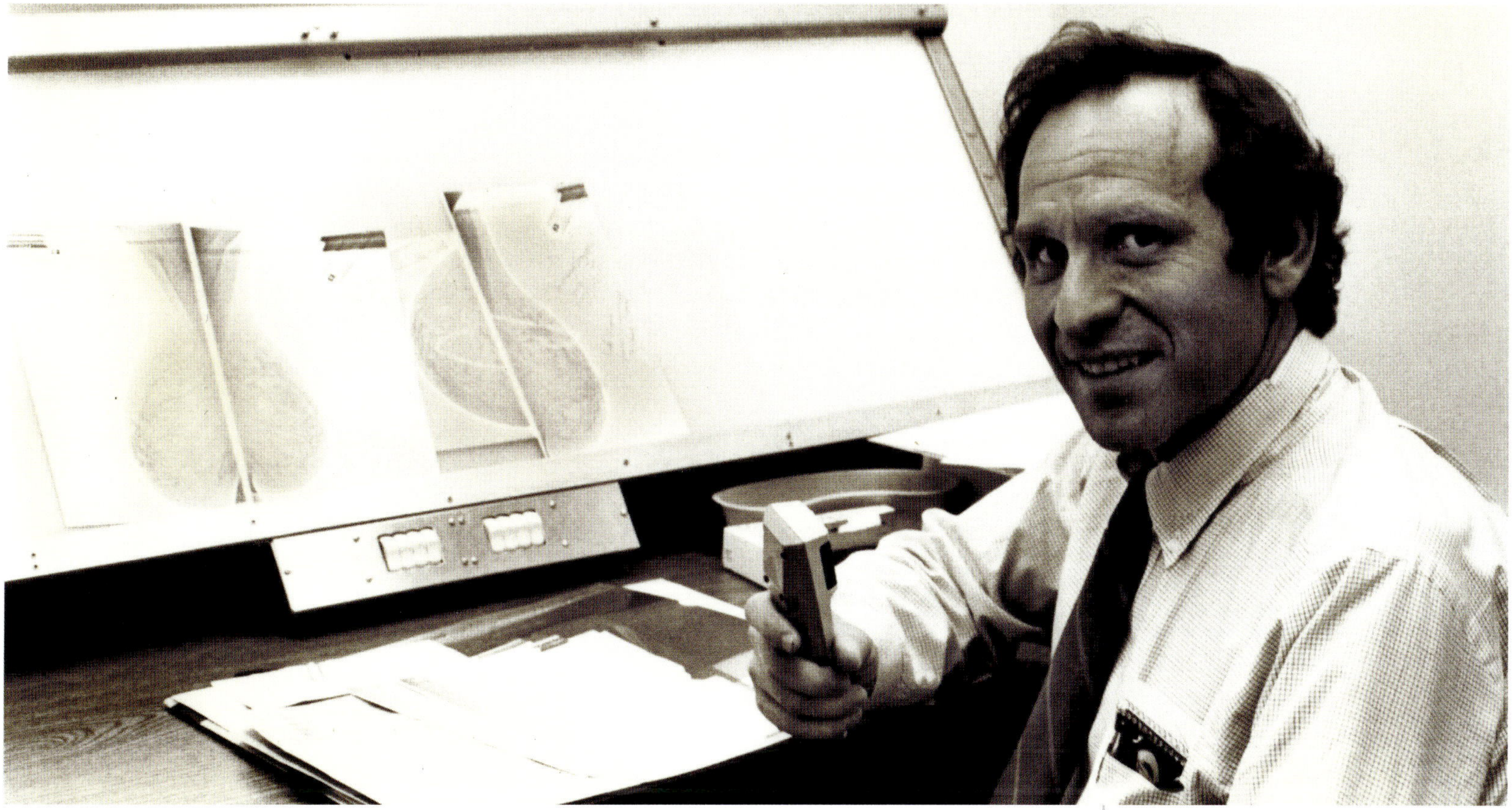

X-ray unit. The hospital bought the latest automatic developer that reduced film processing time from the usual one hour required for wet readings to only six minutes. The total cost of equipping the entire Radiology Department at that time, including filing cabinets and miscellaneous supplies, was $116,728.34.[10] In 1981, twenty years later, it cost $310,275 to replace the obsolete equipment in just one of those rooms.[11]

Radiology averaged fourteen patients a day the first month that the hospital was open. Following the major expansion that was completed in 1971, the department had nine X-ray rooms, X-ray equipment for three operating rooms, and an average of 214 patients per day.[12]

The Radiology Department quickly recognized the need for "growing its own" technical staff. In 1965 it established the two-year DeKalb General Hospital School of X-ray Technology and named Jo Ann Kilpatrick Morgan as the director.[13] She served as the director of both the school and the technical department until her retirement in 1973. The school began with four students, but within three years enrolled twelve students in each of the two-year classes.[14] It has maintained an enrollment of twenty-four as of 2007.

The school not only provided the department with some of its most loyal and outstanding technicians and leaders, but has been recognized as a program of excellence. In 1967, just two years after the school opened, six of the ten awards presented at the state convention of radiology schools went to DeKalb's radiology students.[15] When the school was surveyed in 1968 by the American College of Radiology, it was accredited "with an excellent rating, superior in all respects."[16]

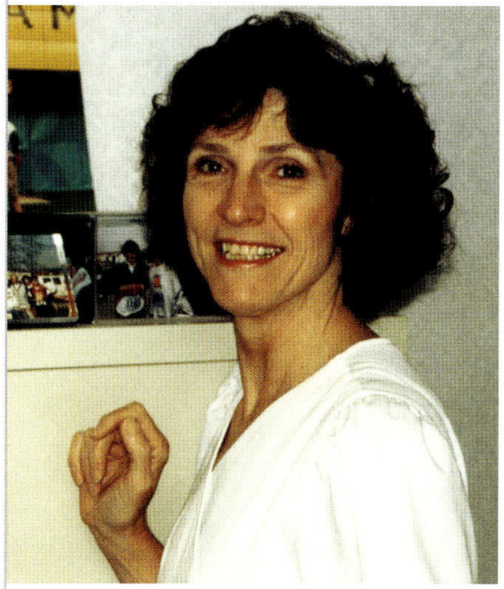

Top: Jay Coffskey, MD, dictates a radiology report. He has been on the DeKalb Medical staff since 1967. **Above:** Della Johnson, RT, was director of Radiology (Imaging) Services from 1973–2007.

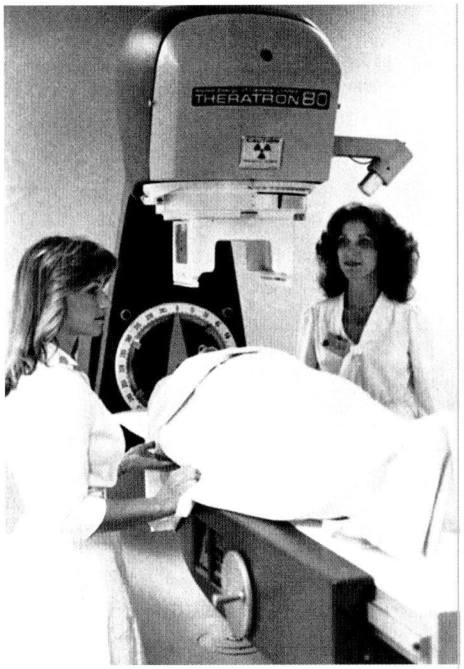

Della Johnson, RT, technical director (right) and Deborah Boyd, RT, working with the upgraded cobalt unit acquired when the state denied a DeKalb General Hospital application for a linear accelerator.

When Jo Ann Morgan retired as director of the school in 1973, Carolyn Yensen, RT, succeeded her, followed by Patricia Martin, RT, and then Lashaun Taylor, RT, the current manager of the School of Radiology.[17]

Radiation Therapy was initially a part of the Radiology Department, and the radiologists provided treatment with a cobalt unit. Radiologists were trained in radiation therapy as part of their residency program. In 1973 the medical staff recommended that Radiation Therapy be made either a subdepartment of the Radiology Department or an independent department.[18] The Hospital Authority approved the concept of its being a subdepartment of the Radiology Department[19] and discussed recruiting a radiation oncologist. No action, however, was taken on either of those matters for a year. At the October 1974 meeting of the trustees, Chief of Staff LaMar McGinnis expressed disappointment at the delay. The Authority then appointed a committee to study what should be done about radiation therapy at DeKalb General.[20]

As discussed in the segment on Cancer Services, the committee explored the possibility of having a shared radiation therapy service with Georgia Baptist Hospital, Crawford W. Long Hospital, and Emory Hospital, but the medical staff advised against that plan.[21] In 1977 the medical staff recommended replacing the cobalt unit with a linear accelerator and recruiting a radiation oncologist.[22] The hospital agreed with the recommendation. It filed a certificate of need (CON) application with the state to purchase a linear accelerator. Two radiation oncologists, Frank Critz, MD, and John McLaren, MD, joined the medical staff. The state, however, denied the hospital's application for a linear accelerator.[23] The Authority, therefore, upgraded its cobalt unit, made Radiation Therapy a department independent of the Radiology Department and named Frank Critz as its medical director of Radiation Therapy.[24]

Frank Morgan reported to the medical staff in 1967 that he had obtained ultrasound equipment on a trial basis to see how well it worked and how useful it might be.[25] Ultrasound technology provided the ability to see internal body structures with the use of reflected sound waves. A month later, he reported to the physicians that he considered the equipment unsatisfactory and had returned it.[26] It was not until eight years later that Radiology purchased and kept its first ultrasound equipment which, by then, had been vastly improved and refined.[27]

The Radiology Department steadily increased the number of individuals it served, the types of services it provided, and the technology it acquired to provide those services. It obtained its first mammography equipment in 1970,[28] and in 1975 purchased new and improved mammography equipment.[29] In 1984 the department opened a separate Diagnostic Breast Center on the ground floor of the 800 wing of the hospital. The breast center's technology included xeromammography, that provided better details than traditional mammography, transluminal light scanning, and ultrasound technology.[30] In 1996 the Diagnostic Breast Center moved into new and expanded space in the second Professional Building. In 2002 it added state-of-the-art digital mammography to its armamentarium at a cost of $1.8 million that was provided by the DeKalb Medical Center Foundation. In that same year the Diagnostic Breast Center performed 37,000 procedures.[31] It established an MRI Breast Program that offers another dimension to its available breast studies in that the MRI has identified an additional 5 percent of abnormalities that otherwise might have been missed.[32]

In 2000 the Diagnostic Breast Center partnered with the Osteoporosis Center to offer bone-density studies, another service especially for women but also for men.[33] The Osteoporosis Center conducts bone-density studies by either the DEXA bone scanner or the simpler, faster, and less-expensive ultrasound scan of the heel.[34]

Many revolutionary developments have taken place in the field of radiology technology. In 1974 the British company EMI Central Research Laboratories developed a computerized tomography machine, known today as the CT scanner, but at that time referred to as the EMI scanner. EMI Laboratories, incidentally, was funded by the Beatles musicians with the enormous profits generated from the sale of their music.[35]

The Radiology Department considered buying an EMI scanner that would allow radiologists to see inside the patient's body with detail and clarity never before possible.[36] The scanner generated a three-dimensional image by taking a large series of two-dimensional X-ray images of an organ.[37] The disadvantage of the EMI scanner was that it could examine only the head. Regardless, the radiologists were enthusiastic about the potential benefits of this advanced technology, and Morgan asked the Authority to buy one. In May 1974 the Authority approved $400,000 for an EMI scanner but asked Morgan and his associates first to investigate what else might be under development that would not have the limitation of examining only the head.[38]

DeKalb General's neurosurgeons and neurologists offered to buy an EMI scanner and place it in the hospital. The trustees considered their offer and consulted with the radiologists who were concerned about a potential conflict of interest and about their liability if nonradiologists interpreted studies in their department. The Authority expressed appreciation for the offer but decided the hospital should buy its own equipment.[39]

In the meantime, Ohio Nuclear Company announced a Delta Scanner-50 CT scanner capable of examining the whole body. The neurosurgeons and neurologists discarded their plans for an EMI scanner and purchased the Delta machine for their office. In 1975 DeKalb General paid $550,000 for the hospital's own Delta Scanner-50.[40] Despite the advanced nature of this new technology, the Delta Scanner-50 was obsolete five years later, and the hospital purchased a new CT scanner for $1.2 million.[41]

In 1970 Radiology added nuclear medicine to its services. Nuclear medicine permits the study of the body's organs by administering radioisotope agents that are selectively taken up by specific organs from which radiation is emitted, detected and displayed.[42] Within two years nuclear medicine was performing more than four hundred procedures a month.[43]

In 1984 the Radiology Department petitioned the trustees to purchase one of the new and exciting Magnetic Resonance Imaging (MRI) machines, considered by many to be the most important diagnostic imaging discovery in medicine since the discovery of X-ray by Roentgen in 1890.[44] The first commercial MRI scanner was manufactured in Europe by Picker, Ltd., and installed in the University of Manchester Medical School in 1983. The MRI scanner creates a powerful magnetic field that aligns the nuclei of the hydrogen atoms found in the body's water. Those nuclei act as microscopic compass needles that line up in order when exposed to the MRI's magnetic field, and they release energy in the form of weak microwaves that are detected, amplified, and measured by the scanner. The scanner constantly alters its magnetic fields, thus producing different perspectives and a three-dimensional view of the structure being examined.[45]

The hospital initially considered contracting with a company to provide a mobile unit,[46] but decided to purchase its own. The construction of the Diagnostic Imaging Center for DeKalb Medical Center's outpatient radiology services already was in the planning stages. It would house an MRI scanner as well as an outpatient CT scanner, traditional X-rays, ultrasound, nuclear medicine, and vascular lab. The state approved the project, including the MRI scanner, and the Imaging Center was completed in 1988.[47]

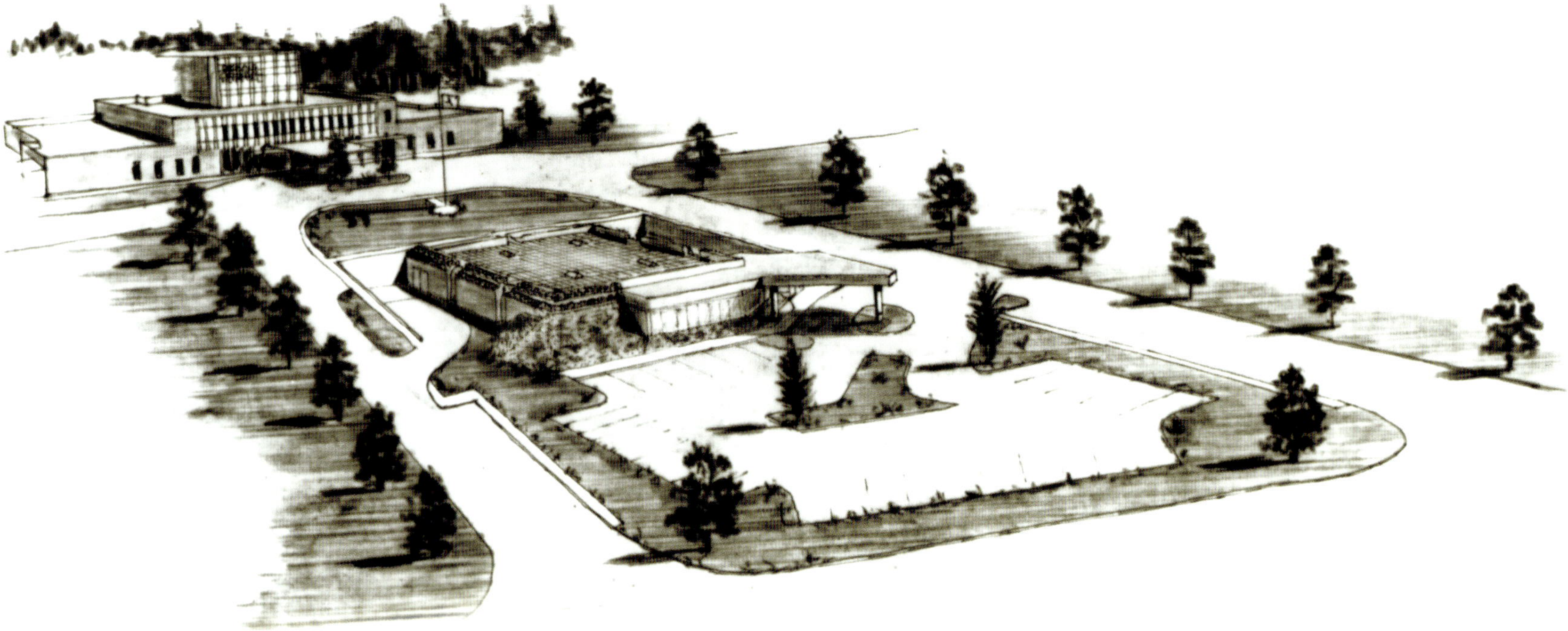

Above: Architectural rendering of the planned Diagnostic Imaging Center. **Below:** Groundbreaking for the Diagnostic Imaging Center. **Below right:** Diagnostic Imaging Center construction is well underway.

DeKalb Medical Center purchased a second, open MRI in 1999[48] to accommodate more comfortably larger patients and those with claustrophobia.[49] It acquired a third MRI in 2005 that it placed in the hospital near the Emergency Department, making it more readily accessible to emergency and hospitalized patients.[50]

In 2001, DeKalb Medical Center contracted with a vendor to provide a mobile Positron Emission Tomography (PET) scanner to be at the hospital once each week. The PET scanner added another dimension to the diagnosis of cancer, cardiac disease, various brain disorders, and other conditions.[51] While X-ray, ultrasound, CT scanning, and MRI scanning visualize structural anatomy, PET scanners identify metabolic activity. The PET scanner is particularly useful in diagnosing cancer. The procedure

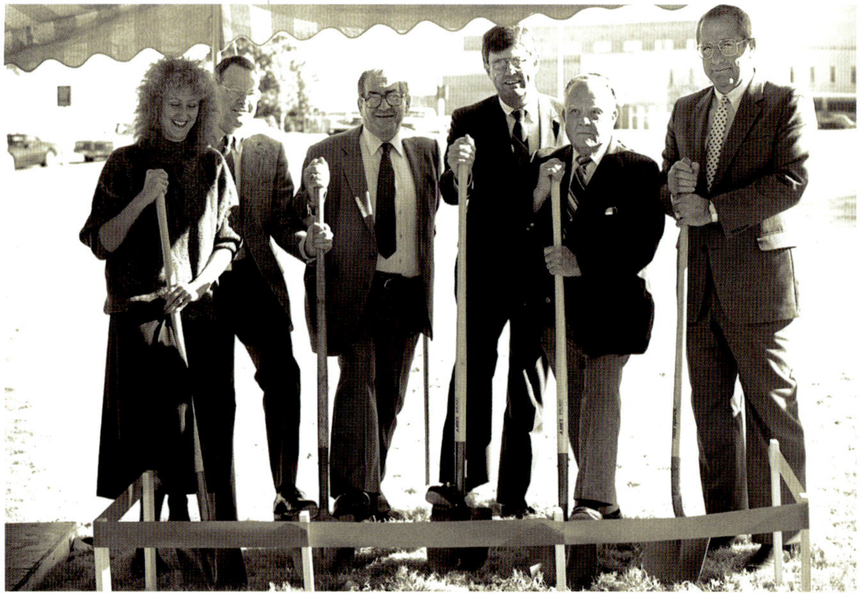

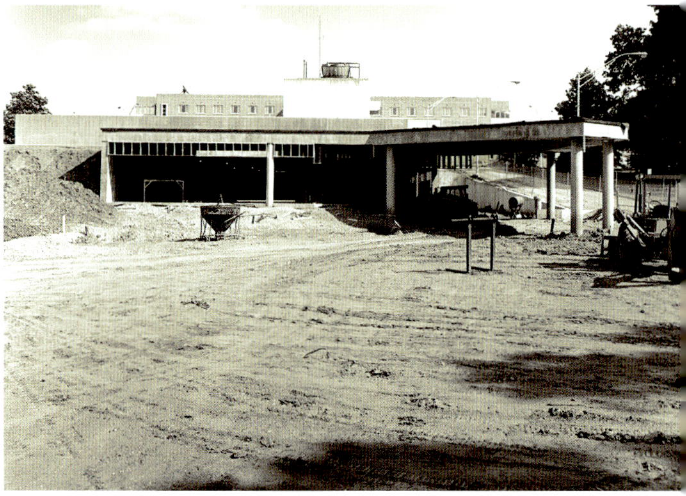

includes the intravenous administration of a form of glucose that accumulates in diseased cells. Since most cancers metabolize glucose at a higher rate than normal tissue, malignant cells may often be detected on the PET scan before they can be seen by the other imaging modalities.[52]

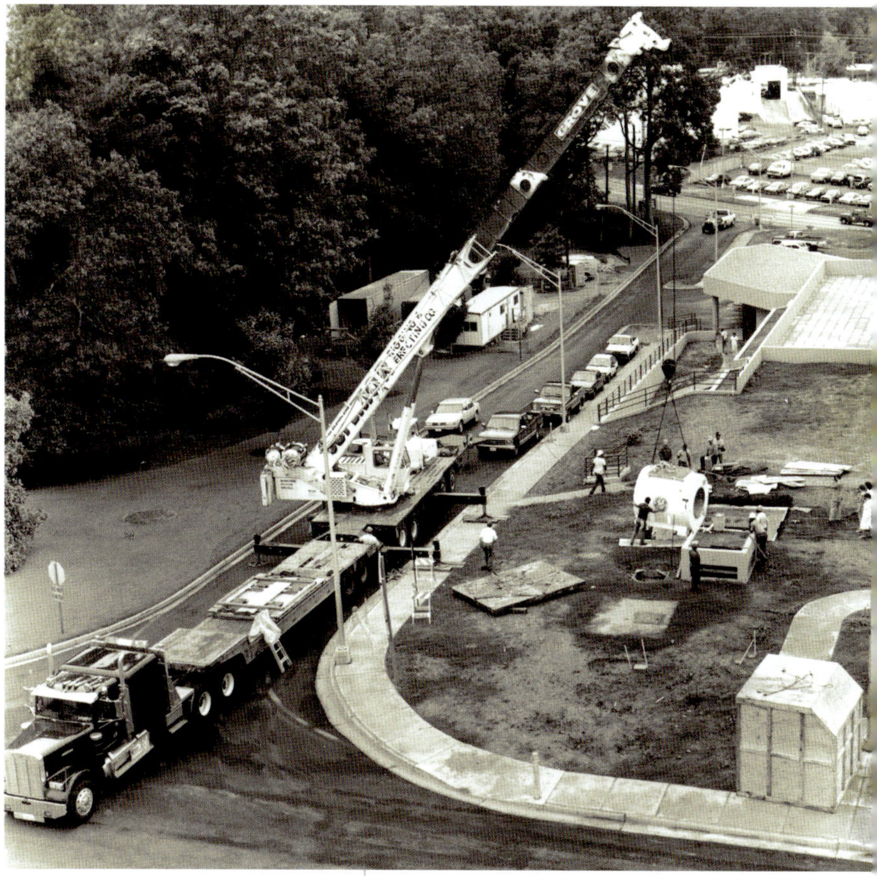

The hospital in 2004 acquired its own combined PET/CT scanner. The $2.5 million equipment was funded by the DeKalb Medical Foundation, $1.5 million of which was donated by sisters Bobbie Bailey and Audrey Morgan. The hospital spent an additional $1 million to renovate space for the unit.[53] The PET/CT combined unit "marries" anatomy and function, producing three-dimensional images of the affected body parts.[54] The scans reveal unusual metabolic activity and pinpoints where abnormalities are located, helping identify disease as well as its stage and progression.[55]

The Radiology Department also advanced the scope of its services when it initiated what is today referred to as "interventional radiology." The department began offering interventional radiology in 1973 when it set aside two rooms to be used for "special procedures." Michael Luckett, MD, and Tom Daley, MD, were in charge of these procedures.[56] They injected contrast materials into blood vessels or lymph channels and looked for abnormalities in the vessels leading to or from the brain, kidneys, lymph nodes, and other parts of the body. Early on, before the availability of the CT, MRI, and PET scanners, Luckett and Daley examined the brain with a technique called the pneumoencephalogram that replaced some of the spinal fluid in the brain with air, oxygen, or helium to show more clearly the structure of the brain on an X-ray picture.[57] In 1984 the hospital spent $1.1 million to enhance its special procedures technology with the addition of "digital subtraction angiography" that "subtracted" images which interfered with the view of specific structures under study.[58]

For most of interventional radiology's first twenty-five years, its procedures were used primarily for diagnostic purposes. In the 1990s special procedures moved to a new level when the technology was used to treat as well as diagnose disease processes. That is when "special procedures" became known as "interventional radiology." Interventional radiologists, guided by X-rays, ultrasound, CT scans, MRIs, fluoroscopy, and other instruments, insert catheters through vessels to perform studies and treat vascular and nonvascular disorders with balloons, stents, filters, or medications. They perform such procedures as "uterine artery embolization" to block the flow of blood to fibroid tumors in the uterus to shrink them without traditional surgery. They inject "clot-busting" medications into obstructed vessels to dissolve blood clots. They perform "balloon angioplasty" to unblock clogged arteries and place catheters in large veins to infuse drugs or nutrition over a period of time.[59]

Thus, from 1961 with its one radiologist, ten staff members, two X-ray rooms, one cobalt therapy room, and less than $117,000 in equipment, Radiology (Imaging) Services has grown in personnel, technology, expertise, and scope of services to be a major player in the DeKalb Medical health system. When Jay Coffsky joined the medical staff in 1967, the three radiologists with a support staff of a dozen viewed about one hundred X-rays each day. In 2007 twelve radiologists at work in DeKalb Medical's three

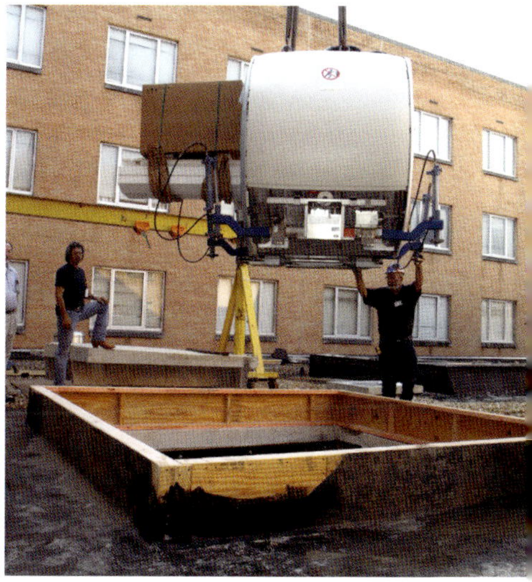

Above: A new MRI machine is lowered by crane into the Diagnostic Imaging Center.

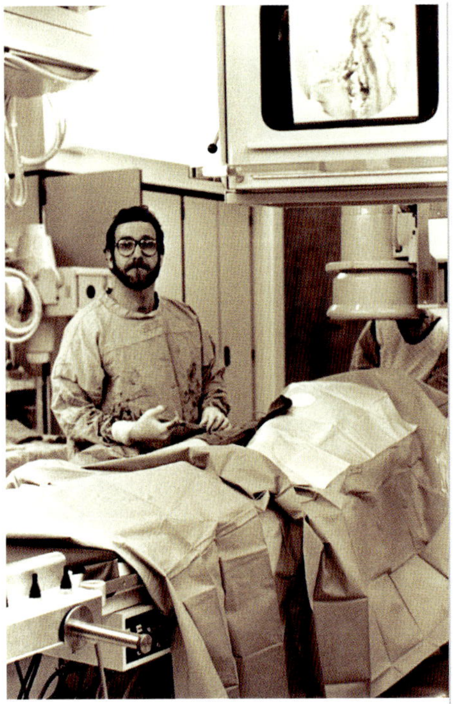

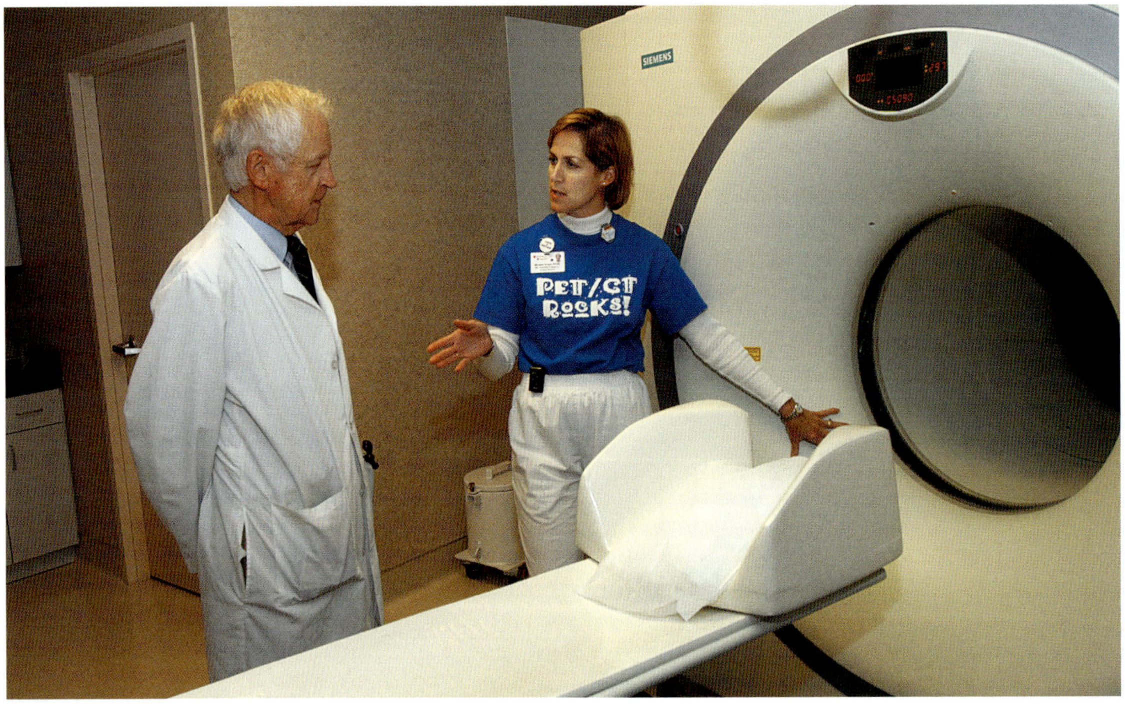

Above: Michael Luckett, MD, conducts a study in the special procedures room.
Above right: Michele Grose, RT, describes the PET/CT scanner to Benjamin Okel, MD.

hospitals, its Diagnostic Imaging Center, and its Diagnostic Breast Center, with a support staff of 250, use approximately sixty viewing rooms to examine more than nine hundred diagnostic studies daily. Their studies include X-rays, CT scans, mammograms, ultrasound studies, MRIs, and PET/CT scans.[60] Those diagnostic studies are in addition to the activities that may be underway in the special procedures/interventional radiology arenas or those that others may be performing in the localization of tumors in operating rooms.

In 1967 X-rays were developed on plain film and reports were delivered to referring physicians through the U. S. Postal Service.[61] Today those studies are performed digitally, and the images as well as the reports can be delivered instantly online to the ordering physician. In 2002 Radiology entered the digital age when it spent $2.6 million to install the Picture Archival Communication System (PACS) that allowed diagnostic exams conducted in the department to be viewed and interpreted by physicians via computer workstations in the Radiology Department and other clinical areas.[62] It took that capability a step further in 2004 when it linked its PACS system with the hospital's Sunrise Clinical Manager (SCM) central system and the physicians' portal system so that an authorized user can view via the computer reports and images from any remote site with Internet capability.[63]

DeKalb radiologists have not only served DeKalb Medical with their professional knowledge and expertise, but they have made enormous contributions as citizens of the medical community. They recently made a major donation to fund the renovation of the Diagnostic Imaging Center reception area, they have served as sponsors of the annual Nightingala and the annual Charles B. Eberhart Golf Classic fund-raising events, and they donate their services to read the radiographic studies performed by the mobile Wellness on Wheels for prisons and underserved communities and those that are provided by the Physicians' Care Clinic for the county's uninsured. They have been good citizens as well as valued professionals since the hospital first opened it doors in 1961.

Rehabilitation Services

In 1995 DeKalb Medical Rehabilitation Services chose a new name, Rehab Results Group. It proudly announced that its staff consisted of nearly 150 specialists including physical therapists, occupational therapists, recreational therapists, speech-language pathologists, audiologists, exercise physiologists, certified athletic trainers, nurses, social workers/case managers, and physicians. Those specialists, they said, could be found throughout the organization's facilities, providing an extensive range of services to all age groups from premature babies to the elderly who present with a wide variety of needs and disorders. And, they added, they are doing it very well with "a comprehensive program that is a benchmark for all other rehabilitation services in the state."[1]

That description of the organization's rehabilitation services was a "far cry" from those of the early days or the most recent days. The need for rehabilitation services at DeKalb General Hospital was not even discussed in the first six years. It was not until 1967, when a major hospital expansion was being planned, that the Medical Staff Executive Committee appointed a "Physiotherapy Committee," chaired by Baker Huff, MD, to investigate whether the hospital should establish a "physiotherapy service."[2] The committee consulted with the orthopedists and other physicians and reported back to the medical staff that it saw no need for a physiotherapy service at DeKalb General since orthopedist Edgar Howell, MD, offered that service in his Decatur office.[3]

The DeKalb County Hospital Authority accepted the physicians' recommendation and asked Administrator William Thrasher to work out a service agreement with Howell.[4] The two of them agreed on an arrangement whereby Howell's physical therapist, Margaret Worst, would see patients in the hospital one afternoon a week and on an emergency basis when requested by a physician.[5]

That arrangement lasted for four years until the physicians decided DeKalb General should have its own Physical Therapy (PT) Department. In 1971 the Authority approved the medical staff's recommendation and authorized the creation of a PT Department operated by a qualified physical therapist who would serve under the direction of the medical staff's Physical Therapy Committee.[6]

The PT Department opened in March 1972 under the direction of Dilys Jagger, PT. Jagger had trained at the Birmingham Hospital School of Physiotherapy in England, had served as a physical therapy instructor in Massachusetts, and had established a physical therapy department in New Mexico.[7]

The PT Department's hours were from 9 AM to 3 PM Monday through Friday for inpatient and outpatient services.[8] The hours and services were expanded as the need arose and additional staff members were hired. Patients came for therapy from Gwinnett County, Forsyth County, and Clark County.[9] By 1978 the department saw an average of one hundred patients a day, and the staff included eighteen employees.[10] It offered Saturday morning hours and evening services three days a week. In addition to traditional techniques, it used biofeedback for headaches, transcutaneous nerve stimulation for chronic pain, and galvanic electrical stimulation for edema. It also offered classes on injury prevention to the community and to hospital employees.[11]

Later in 1972 the hospital established an Occupational Therapy (OT) Department under the direction of Joanne Willis, OT.[12] Occupational therapy used a variety of modalities to help impaired individuals diminish their impairment and return to optimal physical and psychosocial status for independent living.[13] It trained individuals either to perform tasks of daily life and work, or to compensate and adapt to residual physical and mental limitations using appropriate aids.[14]

In 1974 DeKalb General hired Betsy Gerault, ST, speech pathologist, to establish a Speech Therapy (ST) Department[15] and work with patients who had voice impairment caused by such conditions as stroke, brain injury, removal of the vocal cords, cleft palate, and other disorders.

In 1981, as part of a hospital expansion project, the PT, OT, and ST departments were relocated from individual sites into a central center, and the functions of the three departments were merged into one Rehabilitation Services Department.[16]

Rehabilitation Services has had to make significant changes over time in response to the conditions imposed by the healthcare market. In the early years, the department established services that met a need, that had a sufficient patient volume, and that were fiscally viable. Many of those programs no longer exist or have been modified for a variety of reasons. Competition from other rehabilitation practices often reduced patient volume. Shrinking reimbursement from managed-care and other third-party payers made some services unsustainable. Regulatory restrictions for Medicare and Medicaid patients reduced or eliminated some services.

In 1974 the staffs of PT, OT, and ST joined together to provide a structured program for stroke patients. Within a short period of time, that program was seeing as many as twelve patients a day.[17] Rehabilitation Services continues to see stroke patients on an outpatient and acute inpatient basis, but the stroke program is no longer a separate service.[18]

In 1984 occupational therapist Robin Underwood, ROT, formed a multidisciplinary Adapt Team (Activating the Differently Abled for Productive Tasks) to assist adults with disabilities from cerebral palsy, spina bifida, epilepsy, muscular dystrophy, and numerous other causes to achieve lifestyle rehabilitation, to master their environment, and to gain control over their lives. The team included representatives from speech pathology, social services, occupational therapy, physical therapy, and mental health that functioned as an integrated service to rehabilitate the physical, emotional, and social capabilities of these patients.[19] While those patients still are seen in the current services, the ADAPT Team as such no longer exists.[20]

In 1985 DeKalb General established a WorksWell program to offer comprehensive health services to business and industry that focused on prevention of on-the-job injuries and the rehabilitation of injuries that did occur. In 1991 WorksWell opened a new, 10,000-square-foot facility at the Snapfinger Woods Industrial Park in South DeKalb County with Robin Underwood as manager.[21] It featured a simulated work environment, including a 1946 DeSoto automobile, and prepared employees to return to work sooner with confidence in their readiness to perform job-related duties.[22] By 1992 WorksWell had four thousand enrolled employees.[23] Today WorksWell has two reduced components. The physician component is located in the Stonecrest primary care facility in South DeKalb County. The rehabilitation component has been relocated from the 10,000-square-foot facility at Snapfinger Woods to the ground floor of the North Decatur hospital.[24]

In 1988 DeKalb Medical Center contracted with ArthritisCare Centers of America (ACCA) and established an inpatient ArthritisCare Center. In 1990 it expanded the service by creating an outpatient program on the second floor of the Decatur FamilyCare Center.[25] The center offered total arthritis care services to arthritis patients, including educational and family programs, counseling, pain management, physical and occupational therapy, and medical and surgical treatment. It provided

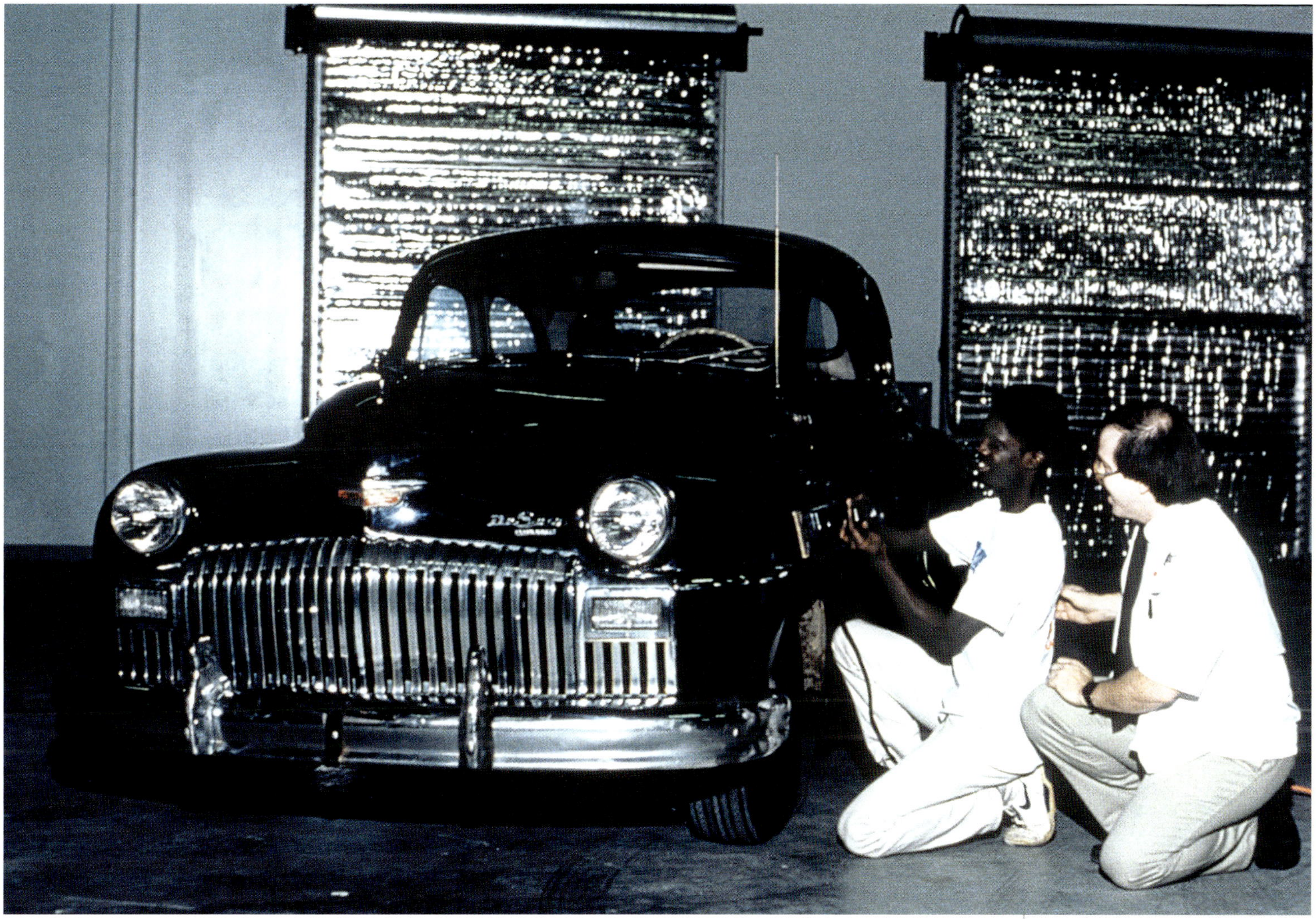

This 1946 DeSoto at the Works-Well Facility at Snapfinger Woods is part of the real-life work environments used to retrain injured workers. Physical therapist John Watkins instructs an auto body repair worker in the correct way to position his body while sanding a car.

self-help courses and classes on joint replacement surgery, fibromyalgia, osteoporosis, rheumatoid arthritis, osteoarthritis, and other arthritis-related subjects. Referring physicians prescribed PT and OT services for their patients.[26] Three rheumatologists, Gary Botstein, MD, Sanford Hartman, MD, and Hugh Spruell, MD, served as co-medical directors of the center.[27] In 2004 decreasing patient volume and reimbursement led to the closing of the ArthritisCare Center as a freestanding entity. Services to patients with arthritis now are offered in the Outpatient Rehabilitation Departments on the North Decatur and Hillandale campuses.[28]

In 1989 DeKalb Medical Center established an Inpatient Rehabilitation Unit on the east wing of the 3700 nursing unit.[29] It was one of the first in Atlanta. Mark Feeman, DO, a physiatrist (a physician who specializes in rehabilitation medicine) was named medical director of the eight-bed unit.[30] The unit provided an intensive inpatient program for patients of all ages suffering from a variety of disorders and conditions, including joint replacements, strokes, amputations, swallowing disorders, musculoskeletal injuries, and neuromuscular diseases such as brain tumors and injuries,

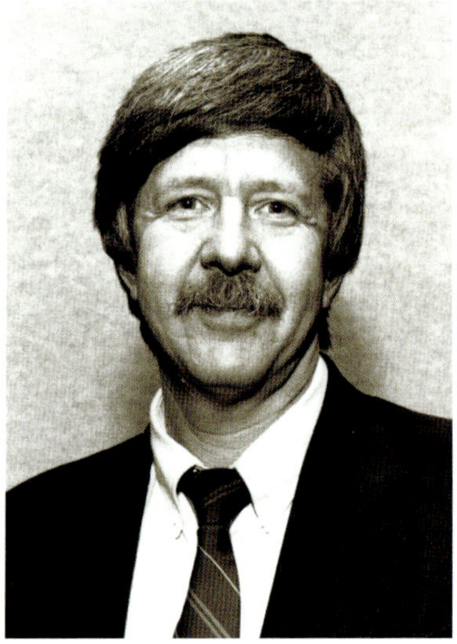

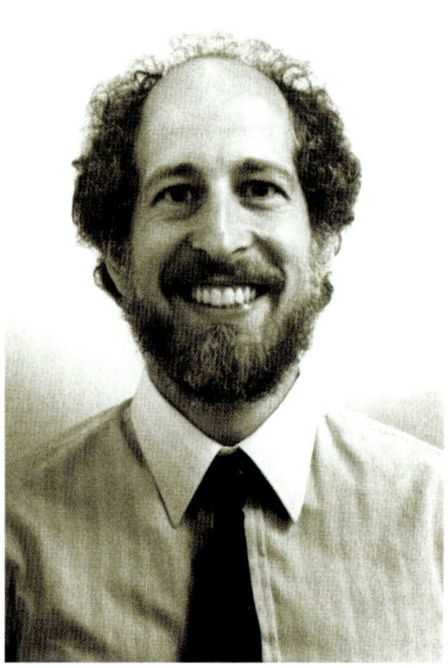

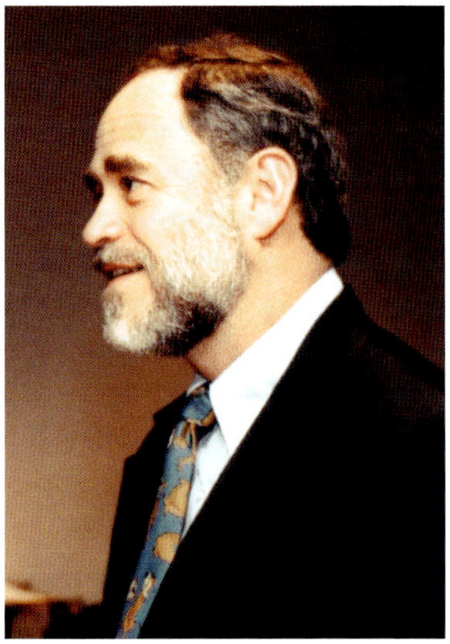

Right: In 1988 DeKalb Medical established an inpatient ArthritisCare Center that later added an outpatient program. Three rheumatologists were co-directors (left to right), Hugh Spruell, MD, Gary Botstein, MD, and Sanford Hartman, MD. **Below:** Mark Feeman, DO, was named medical director of the inpatient rehabilitation center established in 1989.

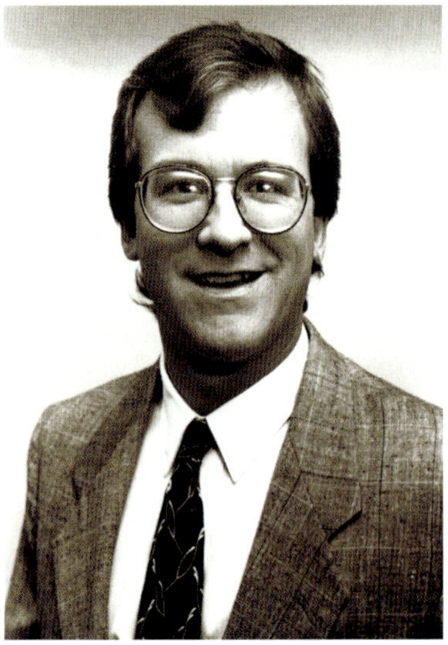

multiple sclerosis, and Guillain-Barre syndrome. In 1994 it was one of only four facilities in the nation to be awarded a three-year accreditation for its compliance with the demanding and stringent standards of the Commission on Accreditation of Rehabilitation Facilities (CARF).[31]

Because of a heavy demand, the inpatient unit was expanded from eight to twenty beds and later to twenty-five beds.[32] It subsequently was licensed for as many as thirty beds should the need arise.[33] Changes in the rules pertaining to reimbursement and services covered, however, limited the patients who qualified for admission. The federal Center for Medicare and Medicaid Services (CMS) enacted the "75 percent" rule that eliminated many of the patients who had been eligible for treatment in the unit. CMS published an approved list of diagnoses that qualified for care in an inpatient rehabilitation facility. In order to be recognized as an inpatient rehabilitation facility for Medicare and Medicaid purposes, a facility must document that at least 75 percent of its patients are on the approved list.[34] Many of DeKalb's previous inpatient rehabilitation patients had a single joint replacement, but that diagnosis was not on the approved list. Only those with bilateral joint replacement qualified. Thus the DeKalb Medical Inpatient Rehabilitation Unit could no longer provide its services to that large group of patients. Currently the hospital contracts with the Milestone Corporation for marketing and management services for the unit to enhance its success in today's competitive and challenging environment.[35]

In 1990 DeKalb Medical Center opened a new Pediatric Rehabilitation Center on Winn Way. The center consolidated all of DeKalb's pediatric rehabilitation services. It treated approximately 140 patients per month and served children from birth to age fifteen with a variety of conditions including developmental delays, learning disabilities, Down syndrome and other mental retardations, head injuries, neurological impairment, speech/language disorders, cerebral palsy, orthopedic problems, and other disorders.[36] Children's Healthcare of Atlanta and other facilities subsequently expanded their rehabilitation services to the extent that the need for a freestanding pediatric facility eventually ceased to exist.[37]

In 1993 DeKalb Medical Center's outpatient rehabilitation service established a program for multiple sclerosis (MS) patients. The program taught MS patients how to recognize their limitations while achieving their maximum level of independence. Russell Wallace, MD, was medical director of the MS program until his retirement,[38] after which the program was integrated into the Outpatient Departments.

DeKalb Medical Center purchased operation rights to Decatur Hospital in 1994. The hospital initially functioned as a general acute-care facility. In 1996 it was made primarily a long-term acute care facility, and rehabilitation services were provided for two years by a contract service. In 1998 the rehabilitation service was brought "in house" so that now PT, OT, and ST are provided by the Downtown Decatur Rehabilitation Department under the supervision of Lorry Lewis, ST.[39]

In 1999 the Rehab Results Group, the new name adopted by Rehabilitation Services in 1995, recognized that many patients did not need an intensive inpatient rehabilitation program but instead needed more than traditional outpatient services. It organized a Day Treatment Program for individuals who fit that category. The Day Treatment Program offered a full range of rehabilitation services to patients in four-to-eight-hour increments of therapy a day rather than the usual one-to-two-hour sessions available in the outpatient sessions.[40] Once again, a reduction in patient volume and reimbursement for those services did not justify continuing a stand-alone program. Those services now are provided as needed in the Outpatient Departments.[41]

Competition has been a significant factor in shaping Rehab Results Group's current services. Children's Healthcare of Atlanta expanded its services which diminished DeKalb's pediatric program and its sports medicine program for high school athletic events. Private rehabilitation facilities now surround the DeKalb Medical facilities. In 2001 the United States Department of Health and Human Services released its "Stark II Regulations" that allow physicians under certain conditions to refer patients to their own rehabilitation facilities or to those in which they have a financial interest. Whereas orthopedic referrals once constituted a major portion of Rehab Results Group's outpatient services, most of those patients now are seen in their orthopedists' own facilities or in those facilities in which orthopedists have a vested interest.

Kevin McMullen, PT, came from the Rockdale Health System in 2005 to be the director of DeKalb Medical Rehabilitation Services, and he has helped Rehab Results Group meet the challenges of the times. The group continues to provide comprehensive inpatient acute care and an inpatient rehabilitation unit at the North Decatur campus, as well as basic and specialized outpatient services at the North Decatur and Hillandale campuses and the Killian Hills Medical Center. The group has creatively refined and restructured its organization and services to meet existing needs and those that are financially viable. It found, for example, a significant need to assist patients with lymphedema (swollen limbs due to fluid accumulation) and those needing aquatic therapy. It found a great need to assist amputee patients and those with problems of balance and dizziness. The rehabilitation staff has enhanced its expertise in those service areas, and it continues to look for and meet remaining, unmet needs and opportunities.

While the challenges imposed by the current healthcare environment have led to a streamlining of its services and structure, the Rehab Results Group continues to offer a quality and variety of services that have made it one of the rehabilitation leaders in the Atlanta community. Its commitment to patient care, its competent staff and leadership, and its track record of creative management give every assurance that it will continue to be a benchmark for other rehabilitation services in the days to come.

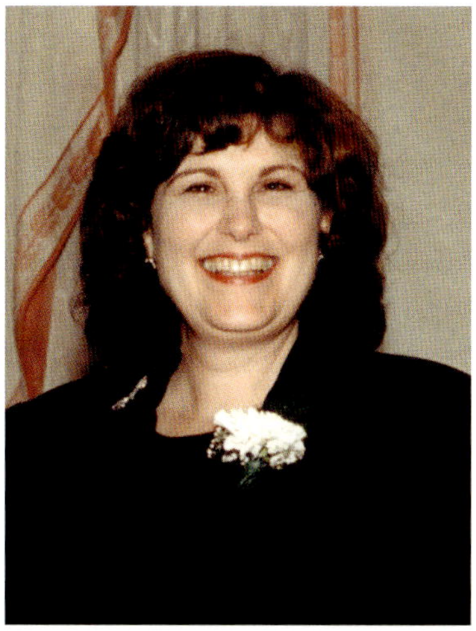

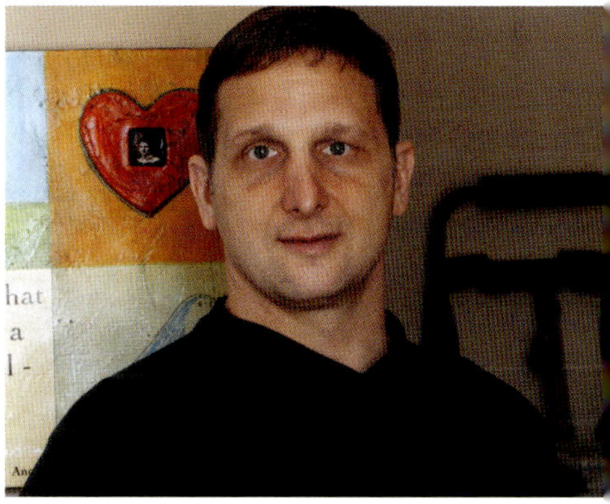

Top: Kathy LaPorte, RN, CCRN, MSN, was a member of the DeKalb Medical Staff from 1993 to 2003, serving as director of Rehabilitation Services and as administrator of the Skilled Nursing Facility. **Above:** Kevin McMullen, PT, was named director of DeKalb Medical Rehabilitation Services in 2005.

Respiratory Care Services

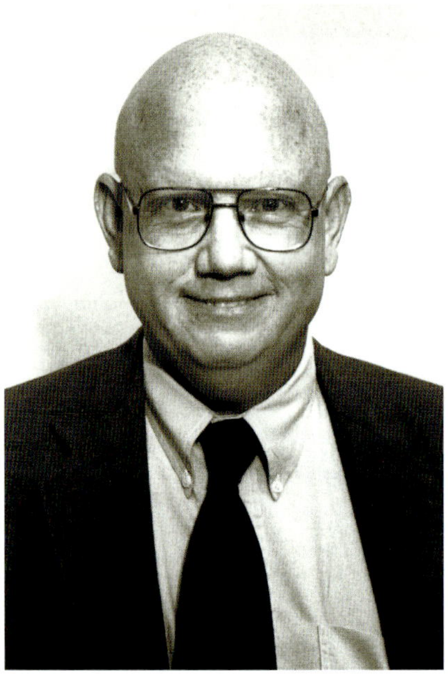

Above William Reichert, MD, pulmonologist, was named first medical director of Respiratory Care Services at DeKalb General in 1974. **Right:** Clare Hart, RPFT, who was hired in 1974 as pulmonary function technologist—a position she still holds today at DeKalb Medical—administers a pulmonary function test while Reichert reads the results.

When DeKalb General Hospital opened in 1961, there was no in-house respiratory service, no piped-in oxygen in the intensive care unit or other patient rooms, and no in-house respiratory staff. DeKalb General's respiratory services and staff positions were provided by contract with an outside company.

Stansell's O_2 Service had the first contract, and it was known at DeKalb General as Stansell's Inhalation Therapy Department.[1] Stansell's changed the name to the Respiratory Therapy Department in 1973 on the recommendation of the American Association for Respiratory Therapy.[2]

The company boasted of "providing continuous twenty-four-hour service with a technician on duty at all times."[3] It supplied portable oxygen tanks for the intensive care unit and patient rooms as well as some portable gases for the operating rooms. It offered educational programs and invited "any interested" employee or physician to attend its Inhalation Therapy Technical Conference held every other Monday morning.[4]

In 1972 the medical staff recommended that DeKalb General purchase equipment to perform pulmonary function tests for patients with known or suspected pulmonary problems. It said the hospital could purchase the equipment for as little as $1,620, and that the service could be located in the EKG Department. Stansell's, however, made a counter offer to provide the equipment and perform

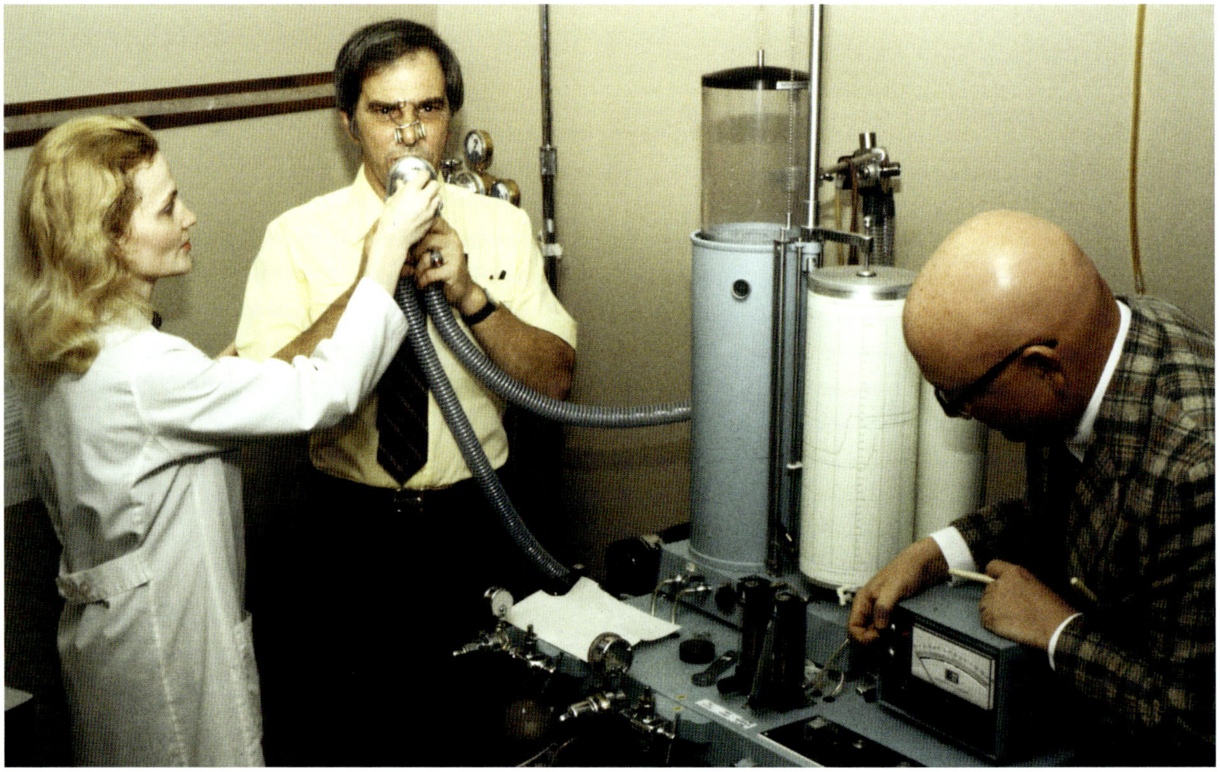

pulmonary function tests for $10 each, and the DeKalb County Hospital Authority accepted Stansell's offer.[5] Two years later, in 1974, the medical staff again petitioned the hospital to have its own pulmonary function laboratory and its own medical director of respiratory services. Administration agreed and converted part of a storage area on the ground floor into a pulmonary function laboratory.[6] William Reichert, MD, became the medical director of the Pulmonary Function Laboratory and Respiratory Services, and Clare Hart, RPFT, became the pulmonary function technologist, a position she continues to hold in 2007.[7] In 1976 the DeKalb General Auxiliary donated $20,000 toward the construction of a full-capacity Pulmonary Function Laboratory that was located on the first floor in Room 1775.

In 1982 DeKalb General changed respiratory service vendors and awarded the contract to the PMS Company based in Orlando, Florida.[8] PMS also provided respiratory services to Scottish Rite Hospital and other Atlanta medical facilities. In 1990 DeKalb Medical Center changed once more and awarded its respiratory service contract to the CPR Company with headquarters in Tennessee. In 1995 DeKalb Medical Center terminated the contract with CPR Company, brought the service in-house,[9] and changed the name of the department to the Respiratory Care Department.

Jack Wooten, RRT, became the first in-house director in 1995.[10] He was followed by John Walsh, RRT,[11] then by William (Bill) Townsend, RRT, in 2002.[12] Bill Townsend remains the director at the time of this writing in 2007. During Townsend's tenure, Stephen Parkman, RRT, became adult care supervisor and Lawrence Wade, RRT, neonatal care supervisor.[13]

Townsend recalled that working at DeKalb was like being a part of a big family. He also said that respiratory therapy students who rotate through the service from Gwinnett Technical College and Georgia State University say it still is the friendliest service in town.[14]

In 1990 DeKalb Medical Center contracted with Sleep Services of America to assess and manage such conditions as obstructive sleep apnea, sleep deprivation, and other sleep disorders. At the time, the service was independent of the Respiratory Care Department. James Wellman, MD, who was then the only physician in Atlanta certified in sleep disorders, owned sleep Services of America. His laboratory at DeKalb consisted of two beds on the ground floor of the hospital. Mark Pollock, MD, was a member of Wellman's group and was working toward certification in sleep disorders.[15]

In 1992 the laboratory was relocated to the first Professional Office Building, was expanded to four beds,[16] and the contract was awarded to Southeastern Lung Care (SELC) owned by Thomas DeMarini, MD. Pollock had, by then, attained certification, had joined SELC, and was designated as the medical director of the laboratory at DeKalb.[17]

The contract with SELC was terminated in 2001 and awarded to Pollock who had left the SELC group.[18] DeMarini, in turn, established an independent sleep laboratory on Winn Way. In 2004 the contract was once again awarded to DeMarini's SELC, renamed Sleep Disorders Center, and located in the second Professional Office Building. Rana R. Hasan, MD, a member of SELC, became the medical director and Valerie Reid, CST, the manager.[19] Pollock, in turn, established his independent sleep laboratory on Winn Way and another at DeKalb Medical at Hillandale. The hospital's sleep laboratory, therefore, has spawned three independent sleep laboratories in the area as the contracts have been renegotiated from time to time.

As of 2007 the Respiratory Care Department at North Decatur has responsibility for oversight of respiratory therapy, the sleep laboratory, the pulmonary function laboratory, obtaining arterial blood gases and providing a representative to respond to Blue Alerts for cardiopulmonary arrests. It also has an advisory relationship with its sister hospital departments at Hillandale and at Downtown Decatur.

Social Services and Care Management

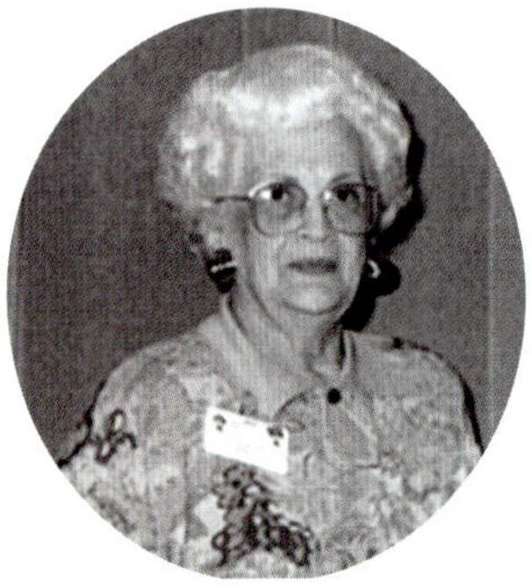

Esther Russell, MSW, was the first director of the Social Services Department at DeKalb General Hospital.

At the June 1971 meeting of the Medical Staff Executive Committee, Clyde Rountree, MD, chief of the Psychiatry Department, announced that "a part-time psychiatric social worker had been engaged and was now working on the [mental health] unit."[1] That individual was Esther Russell, MSW, DeKalb General Hospital's first social worker. Six months later, John Gerlach, director of Patient Services, sent a memorandum to Administrator William Thrasher, stating that

> *The requirements of the Joint Commission of Accreditation of Hospitals have recently been revised to include as one of its principles that "Social Services must be available to patients accepted for care, as well as to the family, in order to promote optimal social functioning of the patient."...A formally organized social service department under the direction of a qualified social worker should be established at large general hospitals....*
>
> *Since June of 1971, a social worker has been working three days a week in the Mental Health Unit, providing services to the psychiatric patients.... I propose at this time to establish a Social Services Department.... Esther Russell, MSW, shortly will be named director of the Social Services Department, and although she will only be working three days a week, she will be responsible for [all] the activities of this department.*[2]

Esther Russell continued her work in the Mental Health Unit while establishing, developing, and supervising the hospital's Social Services Department. Mary Lou Bothwell Fountain worked with Russell in the new department for the next two years.[3] Fountain was well known in DeKalb General for, a decade earlier, she had been the first director of Admissions who had helped Thrasher get the hospital ready for opening in 1961.[4]

Physicians, nurses, patients, and their families immediately welcomed and utilized Social Services. The department's staff served on many hospital and medical staff committees. They counseled with patients and their families who had concerns about financial problems, illness and death, changes in lifestyle imposed by illness or injuries, and other traumatic issues. Social workers also helped patients and their families identify and access available community resources for their posthospital care.[5]

Russell established a Patient Representative program in the Emergency Department as one of her earliest initiatives in 1973. She hired a staff of representatives to be on duty in the Emergency Department twenty-four hours a day, seven days a week, to serve as patient advocates. Patient representatives later also worked with the patients and their families in the critical care units. They functioned as liaisons between the medical staff, administration, patients and their families, often a difficult role to fill.[6] They counseled patients and their families when under stress, provided status reports to family members waiting on news about patients, assisted with the admission process, kept families and patients informed when waiting for tests and procedures, assisted in transfers to other facilities, and helped families deal with the impact of trauma and death.[7] They often were the ones designated to notify family members of a patient's accident or emergency.[8]

Russell also established a support group for stroke survivors. In 1975, at the urging of stroke survivors Caryl Reilly and Pat Palmer, she organized the DeKalb Stroke Club. It may be Georgia's oldest patient-run stroke support group. They gather monthly to deal with the physical and emotional challenges imposed by their illness;[9] they learn how to minimize the risk of recurrences; and they encourage one another to adhere to prescribed exercises, to optimize self-care, to utilize community resources, and to relate to others. The club has donated equipment and supplies to the hospital to help rehabilitate stroke patients.[10] And they demonstrate courage and a zest of life. Palmer, one of the club's cofounders, described the challenges of renewing poststroke relationships in a poignant essay entitled, "On Being Green." Reilly, the other cofounder, at the age of seventy-four participated in a half marathon in Hawaii, walking more than thirteen miles in six hours, nineteen minutes, and eleven seconds.[11]

In 1980 Russell recommended that the hospital establish an Employee Assistance Program. The hospital agreed and placed the program under the auspices of Social Services to offer confidential, short-term personal counseling and referral services at no cost to employees. The program later became an employee benefit provided through Mental Health Services, and it was expanded to include family members or partners living in the employee's household.[12]

Esther Russell was a creative leader and an energetic and tireless worker, and she was also a director who ran a "tight ship." She insisted on knowing everything that was going on with her staff. Paula Simon (Eissner), LMSW, joined the Social Services staff in 1979 and recalls that at the end of each day, the staff members were required to sit in

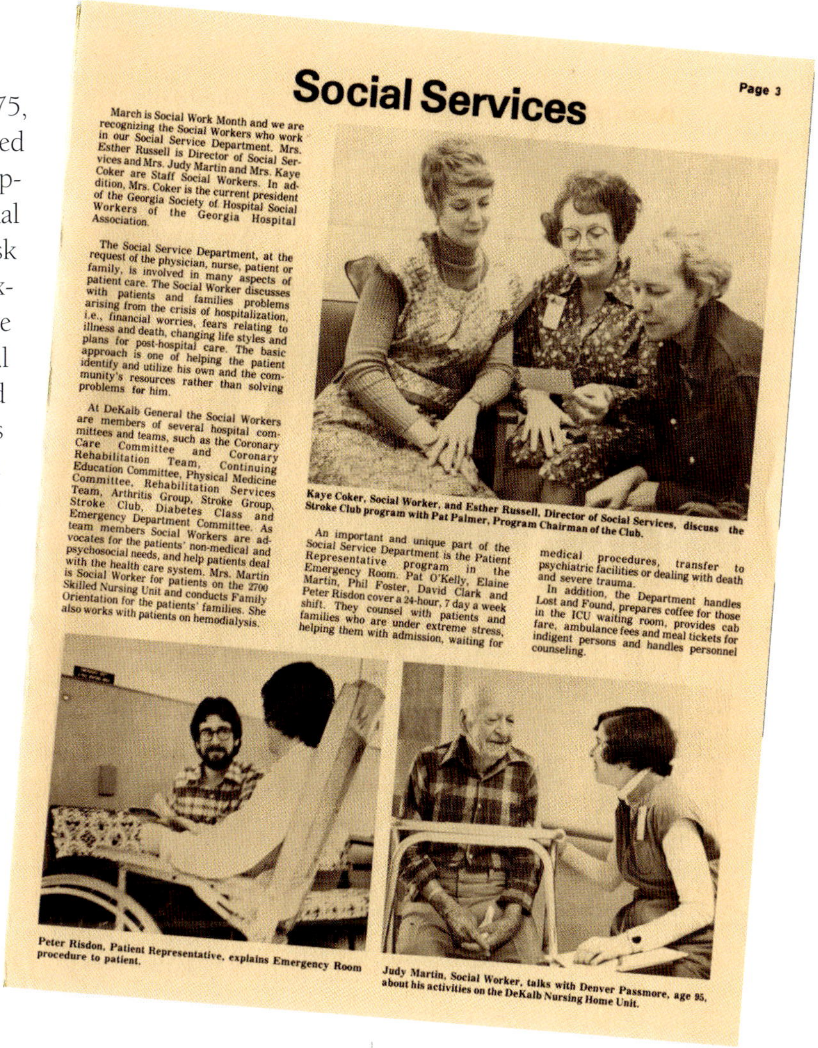

Social Services

Page 3

March is Social Work Month and we are recognizing the Social Workers who work in our Social Service Department. Mrs. Esther Russell is Director of Social Services and Mrs. Judy Martin and Mrs. Kaye Coker are Staff Social Workers. In addition, Mrs. Coker is the current president of the Georgia Society of Hospital Social Workers of the Georgia Hospital Association.

The Social Service Department, at the request of the physician, nurse, patient or family, is involved in many aspects of patient care. The Social Worker discusses with patients and families problems arising from the crisis of hospitalization, i.e., financial worries, fears relating to illness and death, changing life styles and plans for post-hospital care. The basic approach is one of helping the patient identify and utilize his own and the community's resources rather than solving problems for him.

At DeKalb General the Social Workers are members of several hospital committees and teams, such as the Coronary Care Committee and Coronary Rehabilitation Team, Continuing Education Committee, Physical Medicine Committee, Rehabilitation Services Team, Arthritis Group, Stroke Group, Stroke Club, Diabetes Class and Emergency Department Committee. As team members Social Workers are advocates for the patients' non-medical and psychosocial needs, and help patients deal with the health care system. Mrs. Martin is Social Worker for patients on the 2700 Skilled Nursing Unit and conducts Family Orientation for the patients' families. She also works with patients on hemodialysis.

Kaye Coker, Social Worker, and Esther Russell, Director of Social Services, discuss the Stroke Club program with Pat Palmer, Program Chairman of the Club.

An important and unique part of the Social Service Department is the Patient Representative program in the Emergency Room. Pat O'Kelly, Elaine Martin, Phil Foster, David Clark and Peter Risdon cover a 24-hour, 7 day a week shift. They counsel with patients and families who are under extreme stress, helping them with admission, waiting for medical procedures, transfer to psychiatric facilities or dealing with death and severe trauma.

In addition, the Department handles Lost and Found, prepares coffee for those in the ICU waiting room, provides cab fare, ambulance fees and meal tickets for indigent persons and handles personnel counseling.

Peter Risdon, Patient Representative, explains Emergency Room procedure to patient.

Judy Martin, Social Worker, talks with Denver Passmore, age 95, about his activities on the DeKalb Nursing Home Unit.

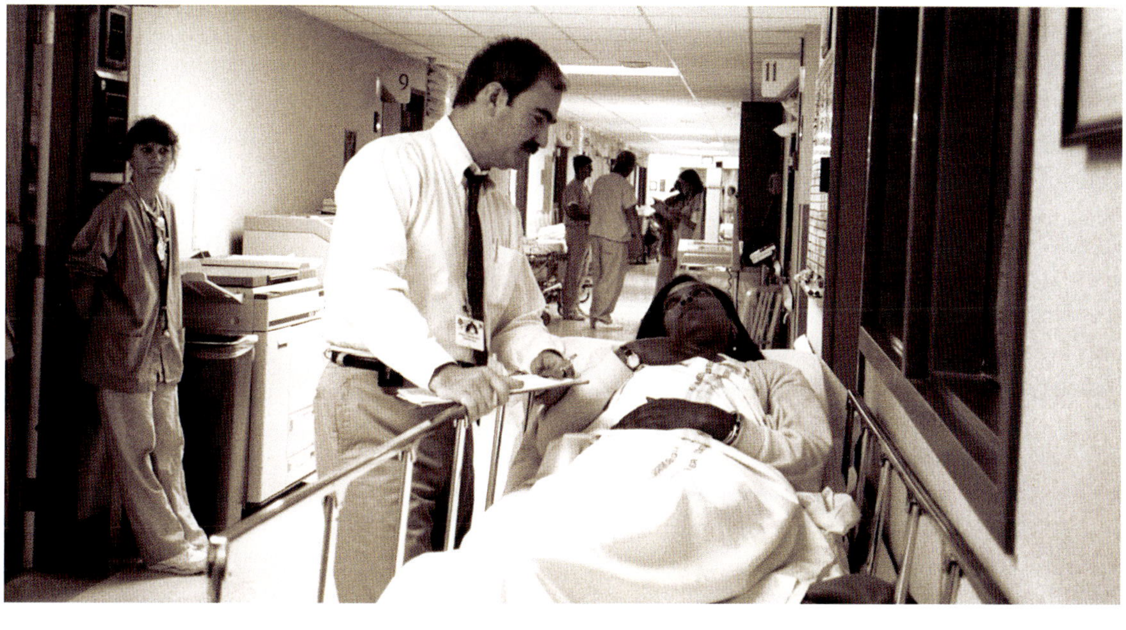

Above In the March 1977 issue of the *InDecatur*, the Social Services Department was highlighted for all its wonderful work. Featured were Esther Russell, director of Social Services,, Kaye Coker, social worker, Pat Palmer, program chairman of the Stroke Club, Peter Risdon, patient representative, and Judy Martin, social worker. **Left:** John Hall, patient representative talks with a patient.

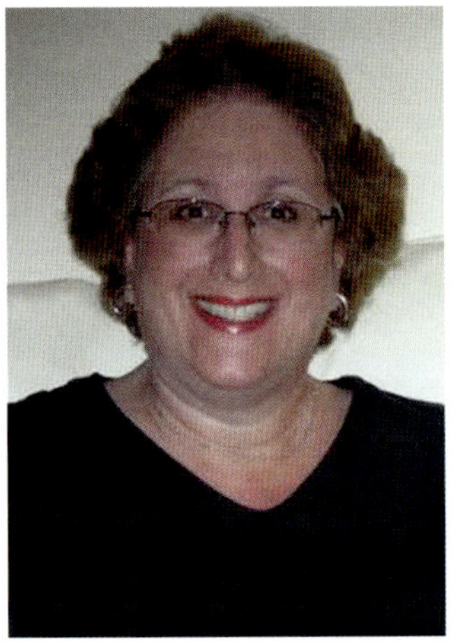

Paula Eissner became the new Social Services director when Esther Russell retired in 1991.

Russell's office and write a report, giving the details of all they had done that day.[13]

When Russell retired in 1991, Paula Eissner succeeded her as director. However, the department subsequently underwent major changes. Discharge planning, one of Social Services's responsibilities, was transferred to Utilization Review nurses with a significant reduction in the size of the Social Services staff. In 1996 the Patient Representatives program was transferred to the Emergency Department where staff functioned less as social workers and more as assistants to the Emergency Department staff.

In 1997 the hospital merged Social Services, Utilization Review, Discharge Planning and Case Management, once separate functions or departments, into one department, Medical Management.[14] Medical Management was later renamed Case Management[15] and eventually Care Management.[16]

Glen Richmond was the first director of the combined department,[17] followed by John Dorenbush,[18] Mimi Wallace Jones,[19] Beth Manza Carrillo,[20] and, in 2006, Paul Olander who already was serving as director of Behavioral Health (the new name of Mental Health Services).[21]

Care Management now integrates functions previously provided by separate staffs. It determines if patients are assigned to the appropriate level of care, obtains authorization for hospital care from third-party payers, provides continued-stay reviews for third-party payers, assesses patients' needs to qualify for being discharged, coordinates discharge planning referrals and transportation services, provides patients and their families with the information they need to access appropriate community resources, serves as liaison between the healthcare team and patients and their families, provides support and counseling as well as crisis intervention for patients and their families, identifies patients in need of financial assistance and refers them to appropriate resources, and provides assistance with advance directives and end-of-life issues.[22]

Olander modified and integrated existing staffing assignments[23] and added certain specialized assignments. Among these specialized assignments is a case manager of Disease Specific Care who focuses on the ten diagnostic-related groups (DRGs) where there is the greatest variance between DeKalb Medical practices and Medicare standards, such as patient length of stay.[24] Another case manager serves as a Denial Coordinator, and another has the responsibility of giving all Medicare patients two notices, as required by Medicare, that they have the right to appeal plans for their discharge.[25]

Moving patients through the hospital system in an appropriate, effective, safe, and efficient manner has always been a priority but a difficult goal to achieve. Olander was placed in charge of a reorganized "Throughput Team" that is working to reduce the time lag between the time when a decision is made to discharge a patient, the time the patient leaves, and the time that Environmental Services says "the room is ready for the next patient." A planned "electronic bed board" will assist this process by showing the team the location of all patients who are in a bed, the category of each patient, the anticipated discharge date of each patient; and all such data will be in one place rather than, as in the past, recorded with pen and paper "all over the place."[26]

Consultants recommended that DeKalb Medical's director of Care Management should be a registered nurse, which Paul Olander is not. He was a trained geologist and an attorney in his earlier life, and he has a master's degree in social work, but he is not a registered nurse. Administration followed the consultants' advice and undertook a national search for a qualified registered nurse to replace him as director of Care Management. After a six-month search, administration concluded it already had the best person for the job and appropriately reoffered it to Paul Olander who accepted.[27] He subsequently was named Leader of the Year for DeKalb Medical.[28]

Surgical Services

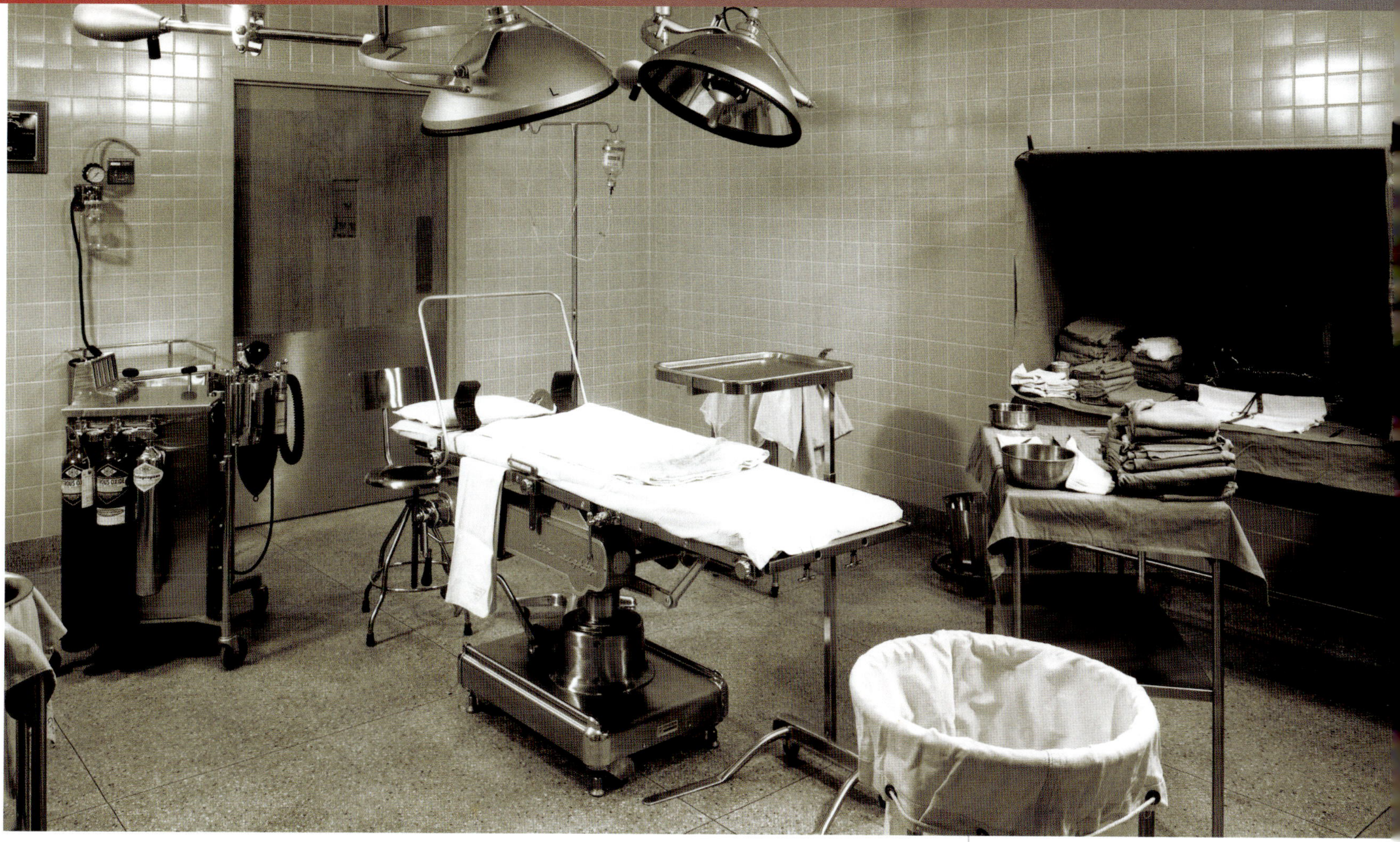

One of the operating rooms at DeKalb General Hospital when it first opened in 1961.

There were representatives of five surgical specialties on the medical staff when DeKalb General Hospital opened in 1961. James Anthony, MD, Manuel Artime, MD, Earnest Atkins, MD, H. Duane Blair, MD, L. C. Buchanan, MD, Herbert Girardeau, MD, Richard Smoot, MD, and Angier Wills, MD, were the eight general surgeons. Betty Ann Brooks, MD, Richard Castle, MD, Byron Dunn, MD, Catherine Foster, MD, John Fristoe, MD, and Lawrence Matthews, MD, were the six obstetricians and gynecologists. Albert Fregosi, MD, and Edwin McDowell, MD, were the urologists; Ed Johnson, MD, the lone orthopedist; and Hobson Rice, MD, the ophthalmologist.

The surgical support staff was fully represented. George Sessions, MD, and Anibal Adan, MD, were the anesthesiologists; Webster Sherrer, MD, was filling in as pathologist for Frank Matthews, MD, who was waiting to be released from the armed forces; and Frank Morgan, MD, soon to be joined by Donald Minor, MD, was the radiologist.

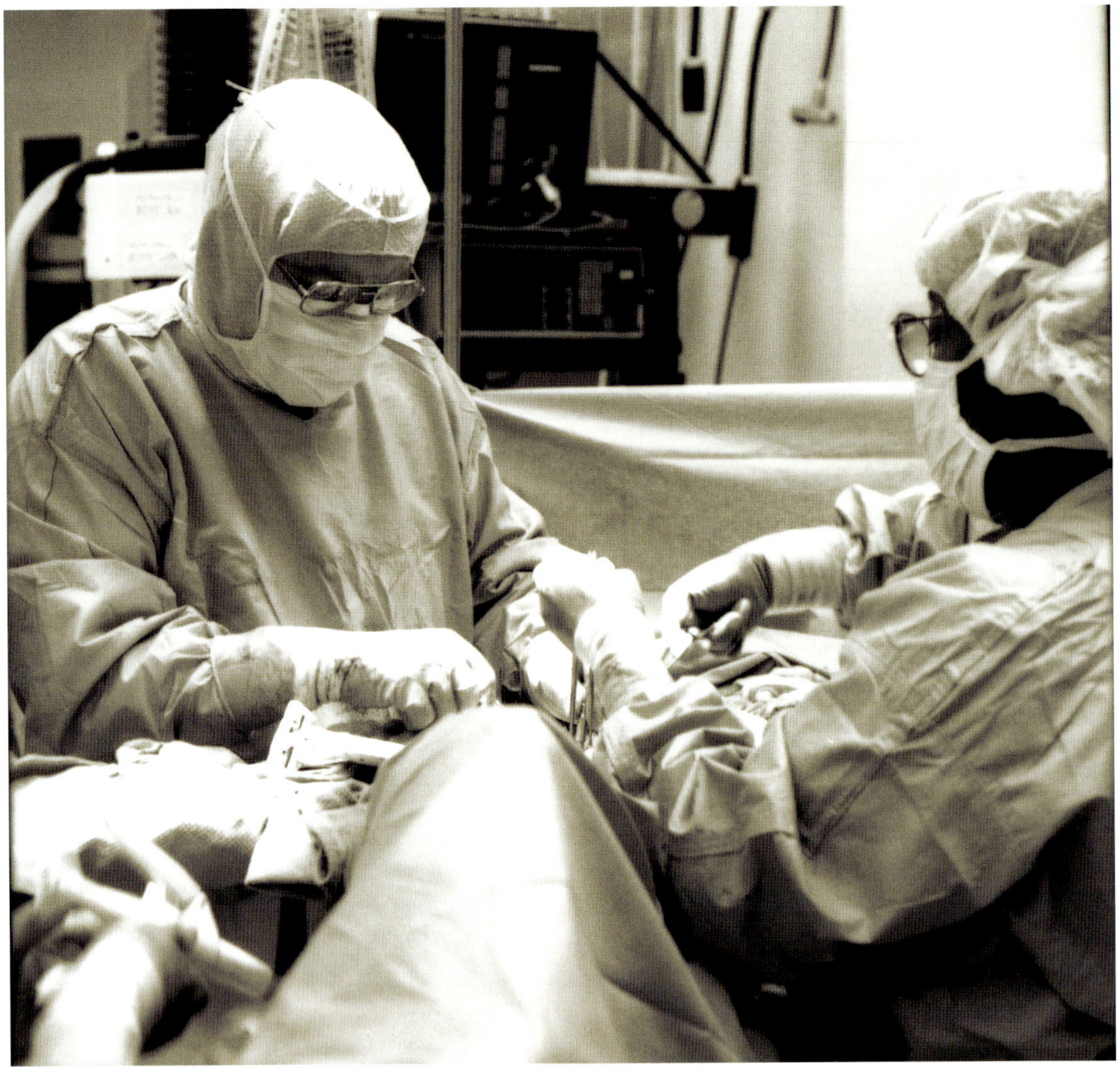

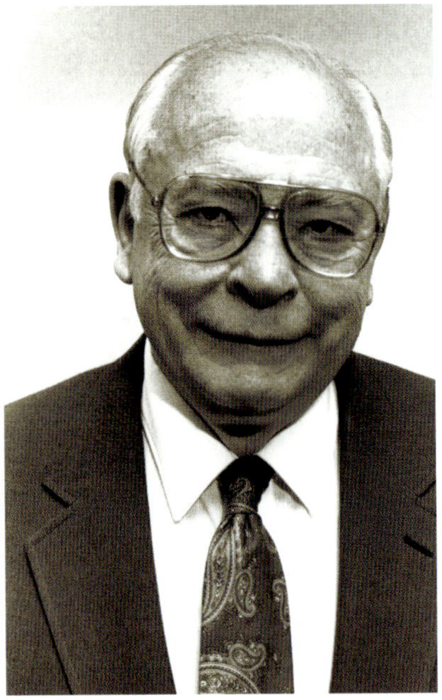

Above: Earnest Atkins, MD, general surgeon, twice invited L. C. Buchanan, MD, to join him for a meal in appreciation for Buchanan's having monitored Atkins's surgery, but each time Buchanan wound up having to pay. **Above right:** An operation in progress at DeKalb General Hospital.

Other surgeons rapidly joined the medical staff, including neurosurgeons, plastic surgeons, oral and maxillofacial surgeons, thoracic surgeons, otolaryngologists (ENT), vascular surgeons, pediatric surgeons, gynecological oncologists, colon and rectal surgeons, and (the last specialty to be accepted) podiatrists.

L. C. Buchanan performed DeKalb General's first surgery, a thyroid procedure, on Martha Ivey the day after the hospital opened, and Anibal Adan administered the anesthesia. Each surgeon on the staff was monitored by a peer on every procedure performed for the first two years. Earnest Atkins recalled that Buchanan often monitored him and served as his assigned assistant. To show his appreciation, Atkins invited Buchanan to be his guest for breakfast at a local restaurant. When checking out, Atkins realized he had left his wallet at home. Buchanan insisted on paying. To make amends, Atkins later asked Buchanan to join him for lunch at the club where he was a member and where he could sign for the meal. When they arrived, they found that the club did not serve lunch on Monday, so they went to a restaurant only to discover that Atkins once again did not have his wallet, and Buchanan had to pay.

Terribly embarrassed, Atkins invited Dr. and Mrs. Buchanan to be his guests for dinner. Atkins said Buchanan graciously declined the invitation.[1]

There were five general operating rooms, one cystoscopy room, and six surgical nurses.[2] Dale Harrell, RN, was the hospital's first operating room supervisor.[3] She was succeeded by Edna Howell, RN, Arlene Burton, RN,[4] and Margaret Panter, RN,[5] who remained in that position until her retirement in 1990 after which Susan Bales Harris, RN, was named director of Surgical Services. Harris holds that position today.[6]

The 1971 hospital expansion project doubled the number of general operating rooms to ten. In May 1982 DeKalb General completed a $7.3 million expansion that created the Ambulatory Surgery Center[7] for which Kay Meads, RN, was named manager.[8] In 1993 DeKalb Medical Center opened a three-story surgical and maternity pavilion with more than 107,000 square feet of new and renovated space at a cost of $15.6 million.[9] The project replaced the inpatient and outpatient surgery areas, the operating rooms, and the recovery and preadmission areas, as well as the maternity and nursery areas.[10] It provided fourteen new operating rooms and a room in the maternity area where caesarean sections could be performed. In 2005 construction got underway for a new five-story, 163,000-square-foot, $55-million Women's Center and Surgery Center that had a grand opening in January 2007. The surgical area provides computer-guided navigation for outpatient neurosurgery, orthopedics, and ENT procedures, and it has thirty private, surgical preparation and recovery rooms.[11]

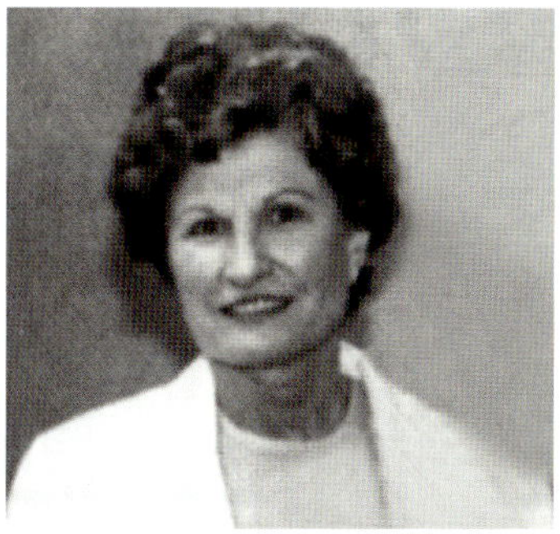

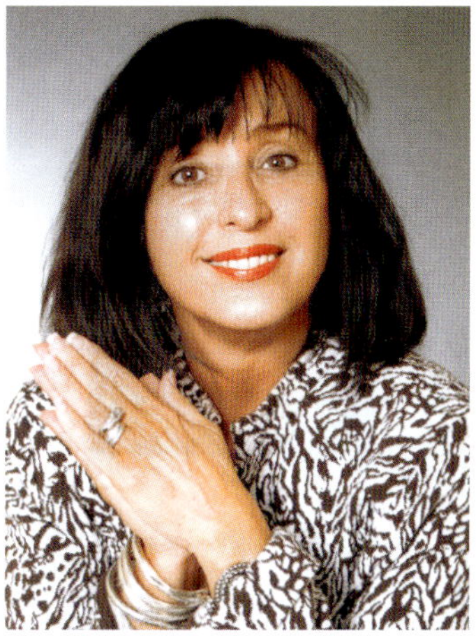

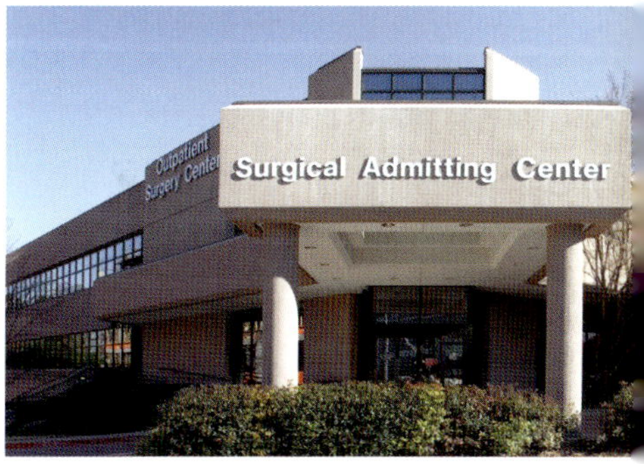

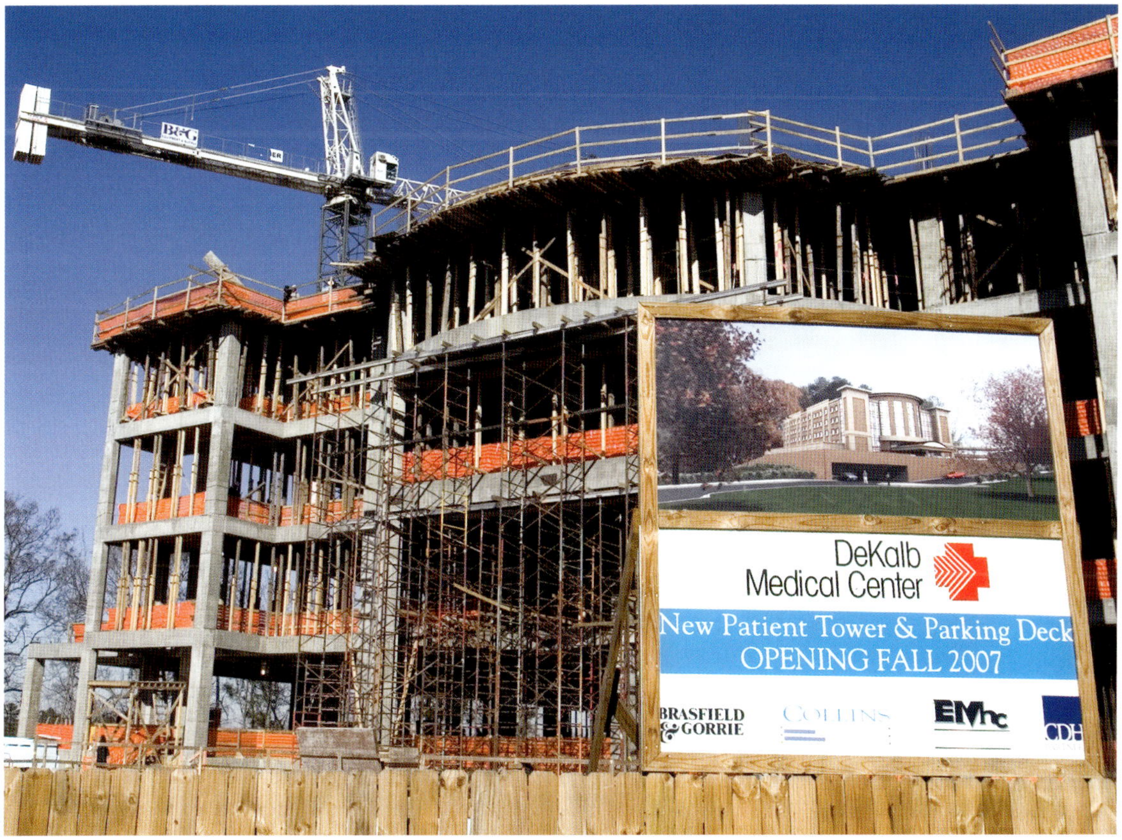

Top: Margaret Panter, RN, became OR supervisor in 1969 and remained in that position until she retired in 1990. **Center:** Susan Bales Harris, RN, succeeded Panter as director of Surgical Services and remains in that position today. **Above:** DeKalb Medical Center's new Surgery and Maternity Center opened in 1993. **Left:** The new Women's Center and Surgery Center under construction. It was completed in 2007.

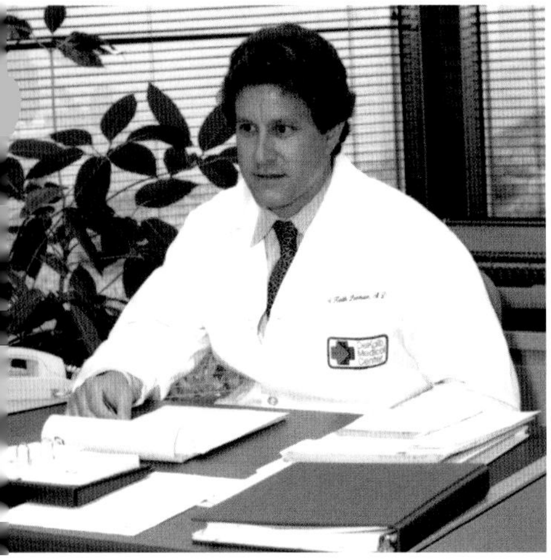

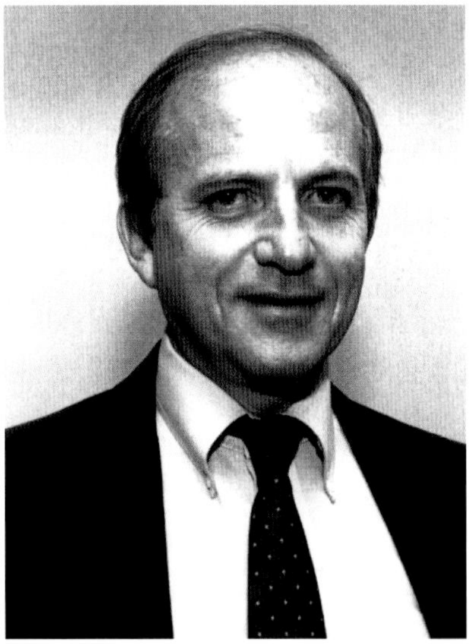

Top: Keith Levinson, MD, DeKalb Medical urologist. **Above:** Sidney Appel, MD, general surgeon who performed the first laparoscopic gall bladder surgery at DeKalb Medical Center and who initiated bariatric surgery.

DeKalb surgeons acquired new technology, new techniques, and new expertise with which they provided their services. For example, in managing renal stones, urologists progressed from the traditional open surgery to pulverizing stones with ultrasound devices,[12] and then pulverizing them with laser beams.[13] In 1988 the hospital purchased a Candella laser for $200,000,[14] and in 1990 a KTP laser for $90,000 that all surgeons could use for a variety of surgical procedures.[15] To treat prostate cancer, urologists went from the traditional total radical prostatectomy and external beam radiation to the nerve-sparing surgical technique that minimized incontinence and sexual impotence, the use of radioactive iodine seed implants in and around tumors, and cryotherapy with frozen needle implants.[16] At one point in time, the urologists, in collaboration with radiation oncologist Frank Critz, MD, had the largest number of patients treated with radioactive seed implants of any hospital in the nation.

Neurosurgeons reach brain tumors deep within the brain guided by stereotactic images. They manage movement disorders such as Parkinson's disease by placing stimulating electrodes in target sites in the brain. They treat painful, collapsed, or injured vertebrae by inserting and inflating balloons to restore the shape of the vertebrae, and then inserting a special cement to secure the repair.[17]

In 1982 plastic surgeons began removing excessive body fat with liposuction. Ophthalmologists introduced refractive cataract surgery that replaced the affected lens with an artificial lens, which also corrected other visual problems such as astigmatism, nearsightedness, or farsightedness. They offered LASIK (laser-assisted *in situ* keratomileusis) surgery that surgically changed the shape of the cornea to correct nearsightedness or astigmatism and that helped individuals become less dependent on glasses or contact lens.[18]

General surgeons, initially led by Sidney Appel, MD, performed bariatric surgery on morbidly obese patients for whom all other measures at losing weight had failed. The surgery involved banding or stapling portions of the stomach, or a gastric bypass procedure to restrict the size of the stomach and alter the small intestine's ability to absorb calories. The American Society for Bariatric Surgery designated DeKalb Medical Center's Surgical Weight Loss Center, now under the medical direction of Scott Steinberg, MD, as a Bariatric Surgery Center of Excellence.[19]

One of the most significant advances now used by nearly all surgical specialists was the inauguration of laparoscopic surgery. This technique revolutionized the entire field of surgery—and it was one in which DeKalb Medical Center became a regional leader.

This surgical technique had a long history before it made its way to DeKalb Medical Center or to any other American hospital. In 1901 Georg Kelling of Dresden, Germany, inserted a cystoscope into a dog's abdominal cavity and insufflated the cavity with room air. He coined the term "celioscopy."[20] Nine years later Hans Christian Jacobaeus, a Swedish physician, performed the same procedure on a man and coined the term "laparoscopy." These early procedures were purely diagnostic since appropriate operative instruments were not available at that time.[21] Harry Hopkins, after World War II, invented the rod lens system and fiberoptics that laid the foundation for current laparoscopy; and Courtney Clarke, a physician in Trinidad in the 1960s, designed operative instruments to be used in laparoscopic surgery.[22] The culminating piece of technology came in 1986 when a computer-chip television camera was developed and attached to the end of the laparoscope. That invention ushered in the era of video-laparoscopy, which moved the technology from being a "blind" procedure to one in which the surgeon visualized his procedure on a screen. That achievement proved to be the critical factor that led to the widespread acceptance of laparoscopy in the surgical armamentarium.[23]

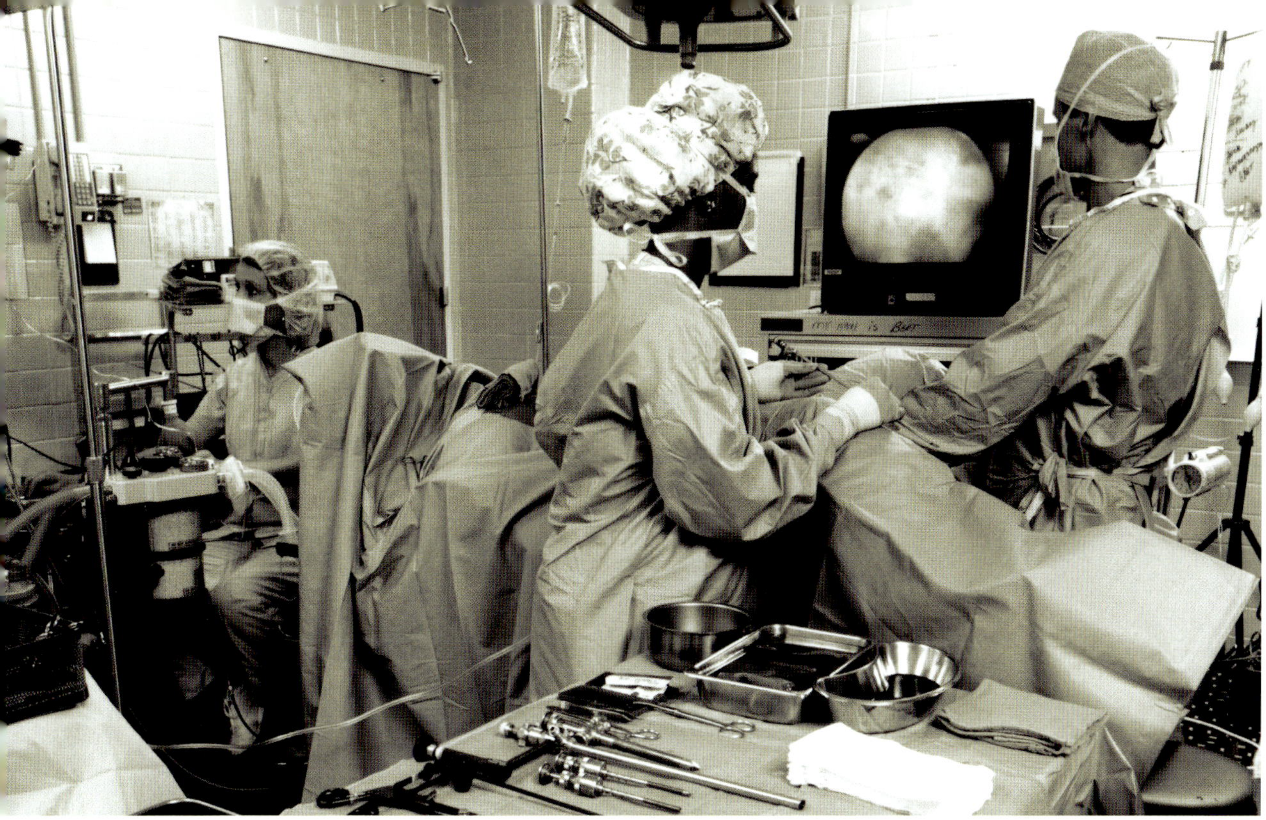

Orthopedists used arthroscopy for joint procedures and gynecologists used laparoscopy for gynecologic surgery such as tubal ligations before general surgeons developed confidence in the new technology. Liver biopsies were the first laparoscopic procedures attempted by general surgeons.[24] Mauret and Francois Dubois in France each performed the first cholecystectomies for the removal of diseased gallbladders in patients in 1987,[25] and McKernam and Saye performed the first laparoscopic cholecystectomy in the United States in 1988.[26] When Jacque Perissat of Bordeaux, France, used the recently developed videoscopic technology and performed a video-laparoscopic cholecystectomy in June1989, he provided the stimulus for the rest of the world to perform the procedure in that manner.[27]

In the early 1990s, gynecologists at DeKalb Medical Center, led by David Bryan, MD, and Jay Kulkin, MD, ushered in this new technology for DeKalb's surgical services.[28] They not only demonstrated and encouraged the other surgical specialists to become trained in laparoscopic surgery, but they helped establish the only accredited hands-on training laboratory in Atlanta to provide surgeons with on-site instruction and experience. They even guided hospital CEO John H. Gerlach in performing a laparoscopic cholecystectomy in the laboratory. Gerlach may be the only non-physician hospital CEO in the country who has successfully removed a gallbladder via the laparoscope, even if the procedure was performed on a pig.

What once was a strange and new surgical technique is now a standard of care for all the surgical specialists in nearly all their procedures. Three or four small openings are made in the abdomen to permit the insertion of laparoscopes and other instruments to visualize structures and perform surgery.

Sidney Appel, assisted by David Bryan, performed the first laparoscopic cholecystectomy at DeKalb Medical Center.[29] Gallbladder surgery currently is an outpatient procedure. In addition, patients undergoing hysterectomies, which formerly required days in the hospital postoperatively and as many as six weeks recovery, now are released from the hospital within twenty-four hours and resume normal activity within two weeks.[30]

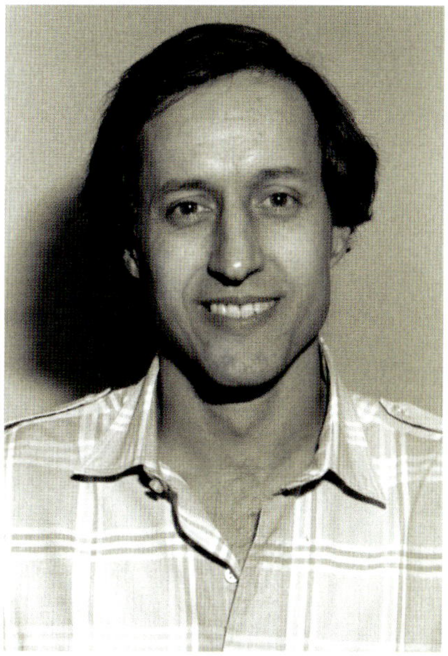

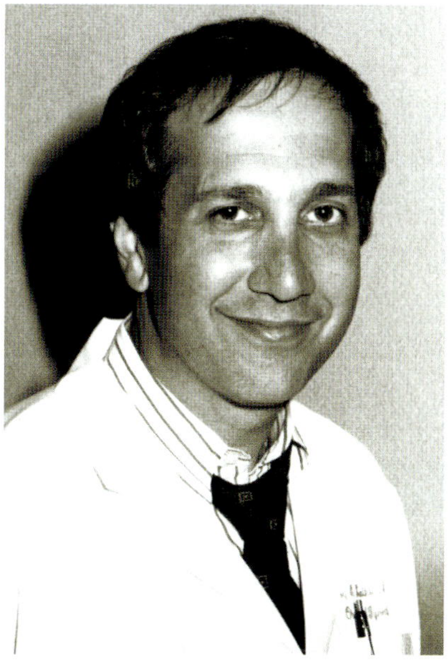

Top left: A surgeon performing video laparoscopic surgery in 1991. **Above:** David Bryan, MD, (above top) and Jay Kulkin, MD, (above lower), pioneered laparoscopic surgery at DeKalb Medical Center and provided hands-on laboratory training for other surgeons..

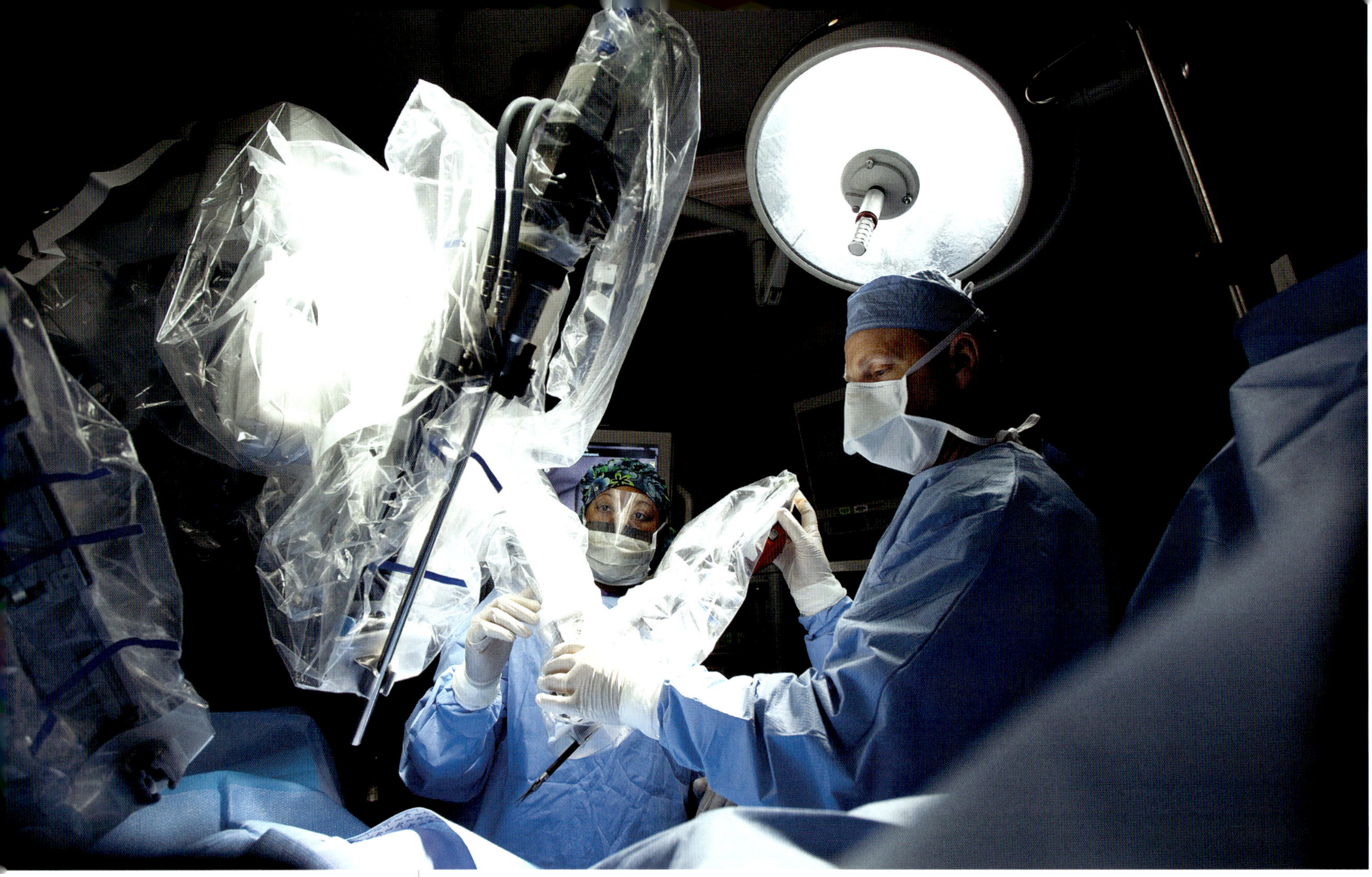

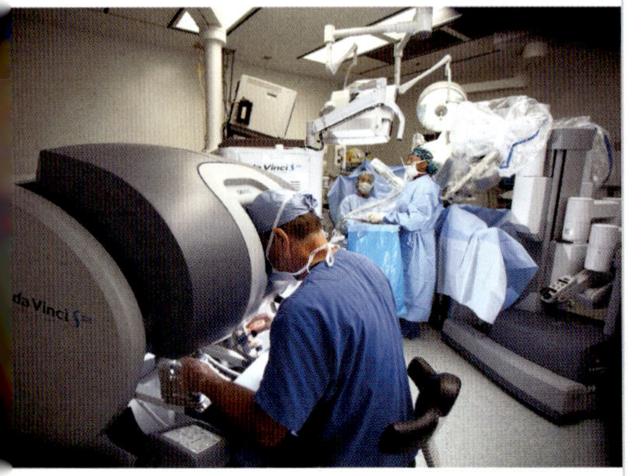

Charles Dixon, RN, demonstrates the use of the da Vinci robot in performing medical procures.

The story of new surgical initiatives and new technology, however, goes on. Orthopedists, led by Maurice Jove, MD, are looking at new methods for performing hip joint replacement with the Birmingham Hip Resurfacing procedure.[31] Robotic surgery has entered the surgical scene, and DeKalb Medical has acquired the da Vinci remote control technology with a major donation made by Bobbie Bailey.[32] Like laparoscopic surgery, robotic surgery also uses small access openings, but the procedure is performed with direct visualization whereas laparoscopic surgery works with mirror images. The same robotic equipment can be used for cardiovascular, general, gynecological, and urological surgery.[33]

In addition to staying abreast of new technology, DeKalb Medical continues to look for new ways to enhance its services and its physician relationships. All surgery will be relocated from the Downtown Decatur campus to the North Decatur campus so that Downtown Decatur can become primarily a rehabilitation and long-term acute-care facility.[34] DeKalb Medical formed a joint venture with its general surgeons and dedicated four of the operating rooms to their exclusive use.[35] It will renovate the former labor and delivery areas of the old maternity pavilion to create three operating rooms dedicated exclusively to the orthopedists; and it will renovate the patient rooms on the 2200 nursing unit to be used by orthopedic patients. The goal is to create a "world-class Orthopedic Center of Excellence."[36]

DeKalb Medical demonstrated from the day it first opened its doors that it was committed to providing the best surgical services available, and it continues to demonstrate that commitment.

The Wellness Center

On October 28, 1985, DeKalb General Hospital held a grand opening for its Women's Wellness Center, the first wellness center for women in the southeastern United States.[1] It occupied 2500 square feet in a portion of the area previously used by Mental Health Services, and it promoted a "holistic" approach to women's health. As a "holistic" center, it focused on a woman's lifestyle and her emotional, spiritual, intellectual, and physical needs.[2] Manager Holly Wolfe, RN, and her team had surveyed the community, other healthcare facilities, and the literature, and they found the field to be "wide open" for this kind of facility.

The center was "a step beyond traditional spas, fitness facilities, and other hospital-based wellness centers in that it offered services to women who wanted to implement lifestyle changes with a positive impact on their health."[3] It was open to women of all ages and all walks of life.[4] Its programs were tailored to the individual's specific needs based on an interest assessment, a fitness assessment, and a complete health-risk appraisal.[5] Its mission supported DeKalb General's commitment to provide the best possible care for the sick and to keep people healthy and out of the hospital.[6]

The Women's Wellness Center provided an important community service, but it also introduced the hospital to many citizens in the community. Surveys showed that women make almost 70 percent of the decisions concerning their family's health care.[7] If DeKalb County women were happy with the Wellness Center, they might bring the rest of their family to DeKalb General when other health-related services were needed.

The center offered exercise programs; lifestyle programs such as smoking cessation, weight control, and stress management; childbirth classes that included prenatal sessions and information about caesarean section births, natural childbirth and obstetrical anesthesia; courses on parenting; and classes dealing with issues such as hormonal therapy, menopause, premenstrual syndrome, and surgical hysterectomy.[8] The staff included registered nurses, physical therapists, social workers, exercise specialists, and dieticians.[9]

Not surprisingly, within six months men began asking, "What about us?" Having heard women brag about the center, men requested comparable services. In 1987 the center became coeducational, and the name was changed to The Wellness Center.[10]

In 1988 the center developed an Employee Wellness Program as a hospital benefit. Hospital employees, volunteers, medical staff, and the office staff of DeKalb's physicians could participate in all of the center's programs at substantial discounts.[11]

The Wellness Center was enormously popular, and soon was "bursting at the seams."[12] In April 1996 it was relocated to a new facility in the second Professional Office Building. It now occupies 18,000 square feet, contains an indoor track, an indoor pool maintained at a comfortable water temperature, two spacious aerobic rooms with impact-resistant flooring, treadmills, stair-climbers, stationery bikes, other cardiovascular equipment, classrooms, a demonstration kitchen, Cybex weight equipment, a free-weight room with a complete weight circuit, a massage therapy room, a sports medicine area for training and rehabilitation, locker rooms and showers, free towel service, a consumer health library, and free parking.[13] The facility is open seven days a week.

In the new facility The Wellness Center expanded its program to fifty-four classes and services,

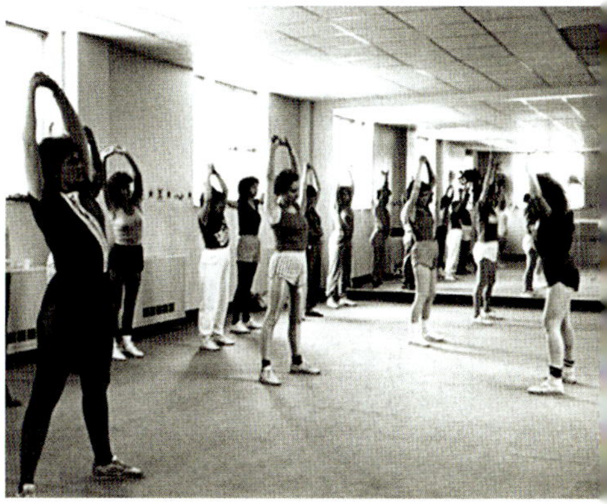

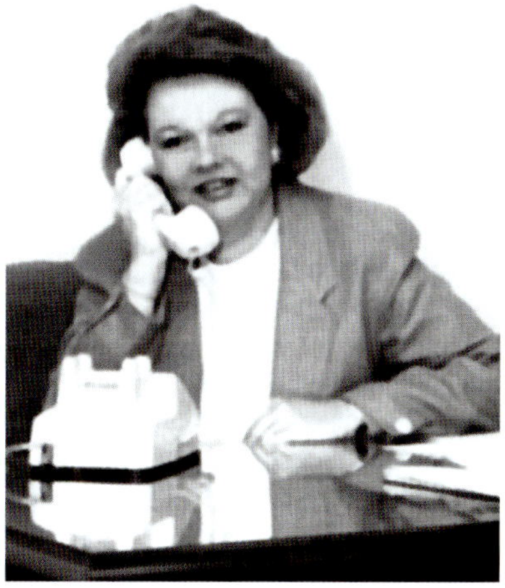

Top: An exercise class at the Wellness Center. **Above:** Holly Wolfe, RN, worked with a team to develop the Wellness Center and was its first director.

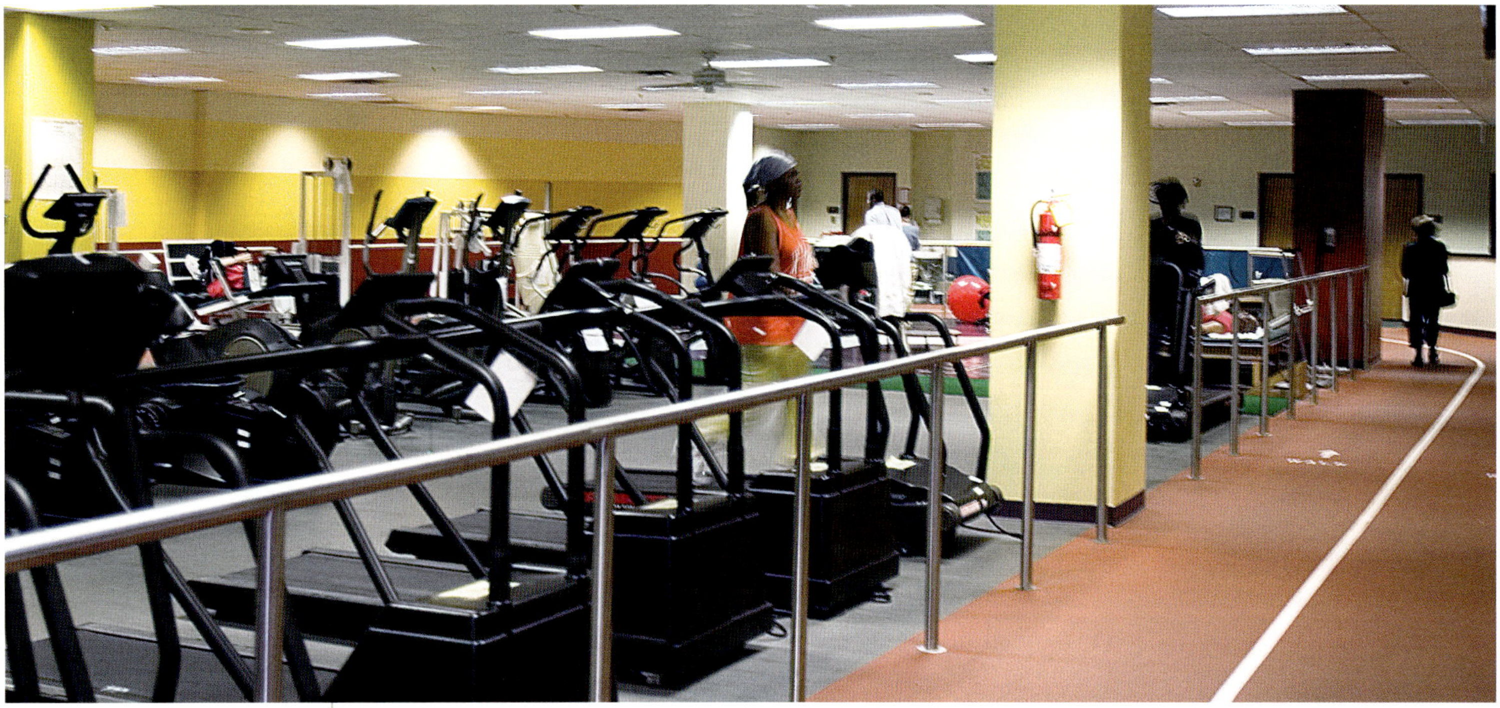

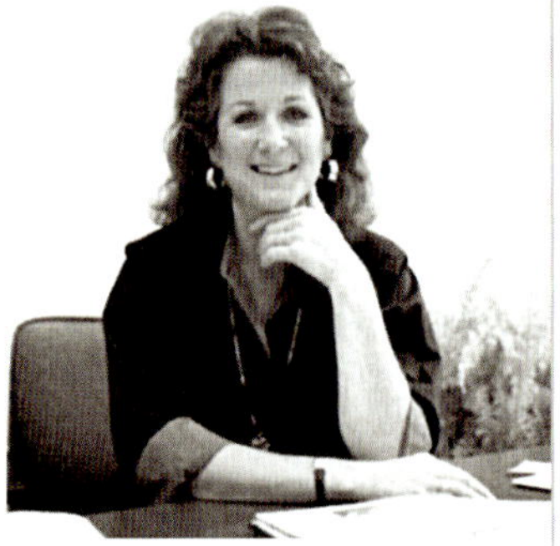

Top: The Wellness Center is considered one of the top fitness centers in Atlanta according to *The Atlanta Business Chronicle*. **Above:** Gail Winfrey Winston, RN, MSN, was the second director of the Wellness Center, and the well-known early radio voice of DeKalb General Hospital in the 1980s.

including tai ji for patients with arthritic joints and problems of balance, reflexology, healing touch, meditation, yoga, massage therapy, belly dancing lessons and a sports medicine program.[14] *The Atlanta Business Chronicle* recognized The Wellness Center as one of the top fitness centers in Atlanta.[15]

It instituted an annual Fitness Challenge for all employees to encourage a healthier lifestyle.[16] Participants underwent an initial assessment of weight, body fat, and cardiovascular endurance. The challenge included three, three-month rounds. Employees could join one or all three rounds, and they could participate as teams or as individuals. The team with the most improvement received $1,000 as first prize and $500 as second prize, and the individual with the most improvement at the end of a round won $200. More than six hundred employees have participated.[17]

Holly Wolfe retired as director of The Wellness Center in the fall of 2003, and Gail Winfrey Winston, RN, MSN, became her successor as director of Health Promotion. Winston had been a member of the hospital staff since 1973 and The Wellness Center staff since it opened in 1985.[18] For several years Gail Winfrey Winston was the voice of DeKalb Medical Center's most memorable and effective radio ads. As director of Health Promotion, she is responsible for Health Promotion, The Wellness Center, Cardiac Rehabilitation, the Senior Spectrum program for senior citizens, and DeKalb Medical's sponsorship of a School Nurse Program in two of the five City of Decatur Schools.

From its 2,500-square-foot facility on the ground floor of the hospital with its program for women, to its present, state-of-the-art 18,000-square-foot facility with fifty-four classes and services for men and women of all ages, needs and interests, The Wellness Center has fulfilled and exceeded the dream that Holly Wolfe, Gail Winston, and their team envisioned in 1985. The center is one of DeKalb Medical's most visible and significant symbols and instruments of its commitment to the community's health and wellness.

Women's and Infants' Services

DeKalb General Hospital had been open for only six hours when its first baby arrived. John Fristoe, MD, delivered six-pound, eleven-ounce Stacey Elizabeth Stull to the proud parents, Mr. and Mrs. T. E. Stull. The community celebrated this historic event, and the Decatur Business and Professional Association showered Stacy and her parents with gifts, including a box of "It's A Girl" cigars from Stacy's Pharmacy (not the baby's pharmacy).[1] Stacey Stull returned for the hospital's fifteenth anniversary celebration and again in 1993, at the age of twenty-two, for the opening of the hospital's new maternity center.

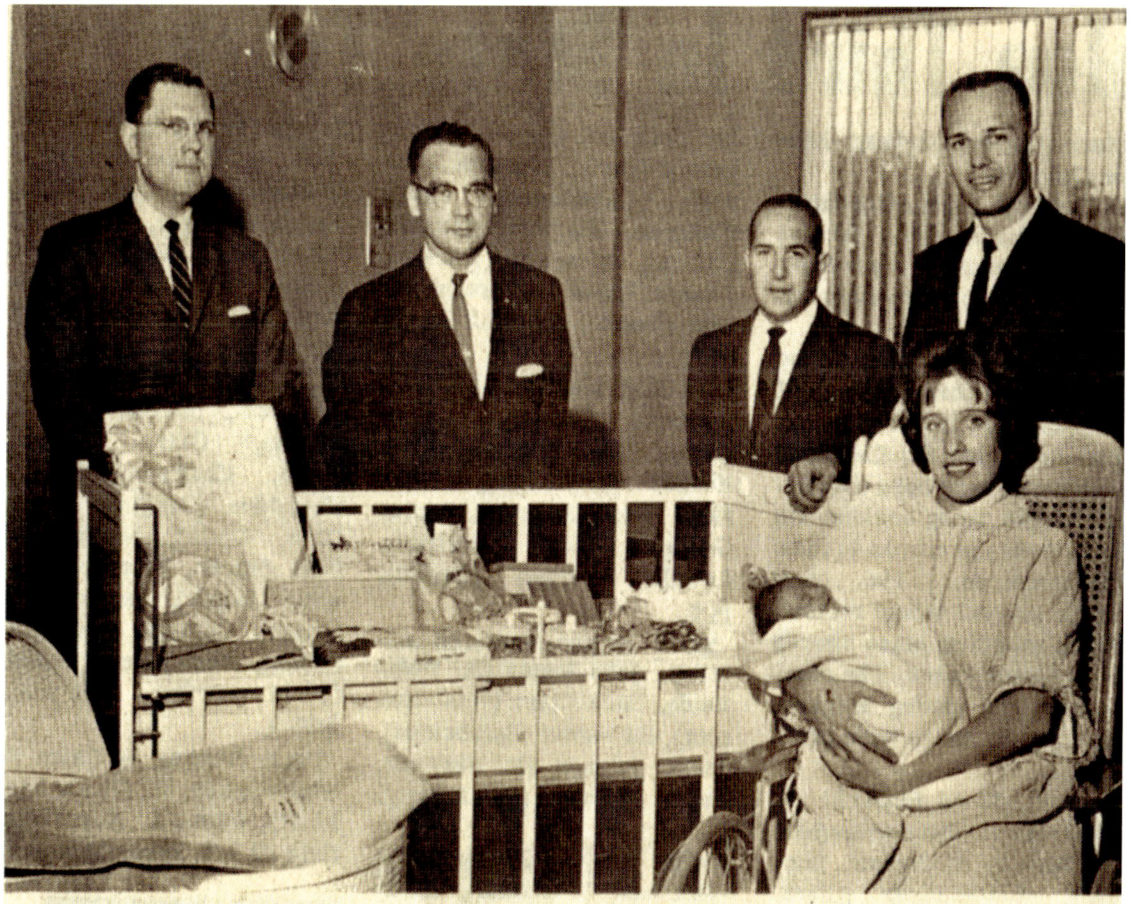

GOING HOME -- Stacey Elizabeth Stull, first baby born at DeKalb General Hospital, is shown as she leaves the hospital with her gifts from the Decatur Business & Professional and Park & Shop Association. Left to right are David Morris, Ray Esary, and Joe Maas of the Association, and Mr. & Mrs. Stull. A total of 25 babies were born at the hospita durings its first week of operation.

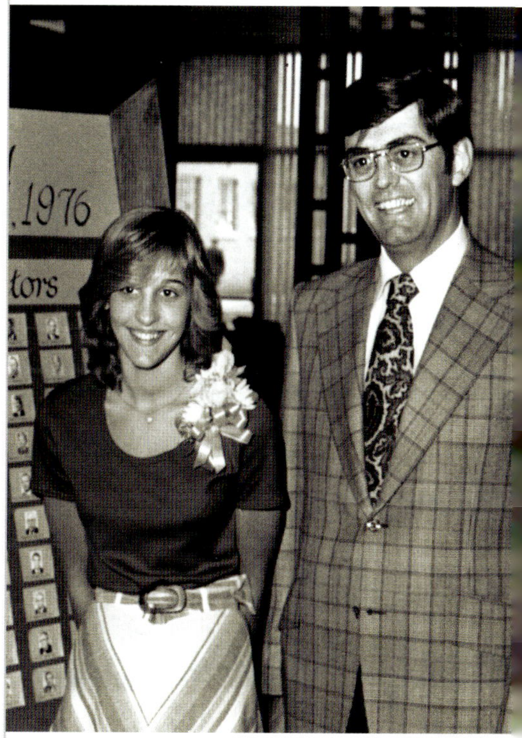

Left: A news clipping celebrates the first baby born at DeKalb General Hospital, Stacey Elizabeth Stull. **Above:** Administrator Charles Eberhart greets Stacey Stull as she returns to the hospital for its fifteenth anniversary. She also returned when she was twenty-two to celebrate the hospital's new maternity center.

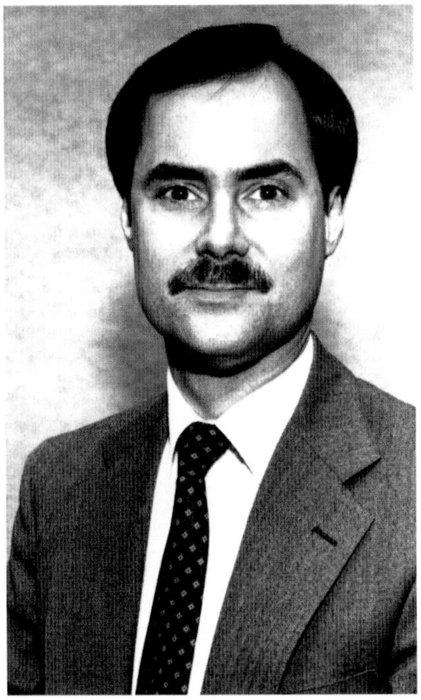

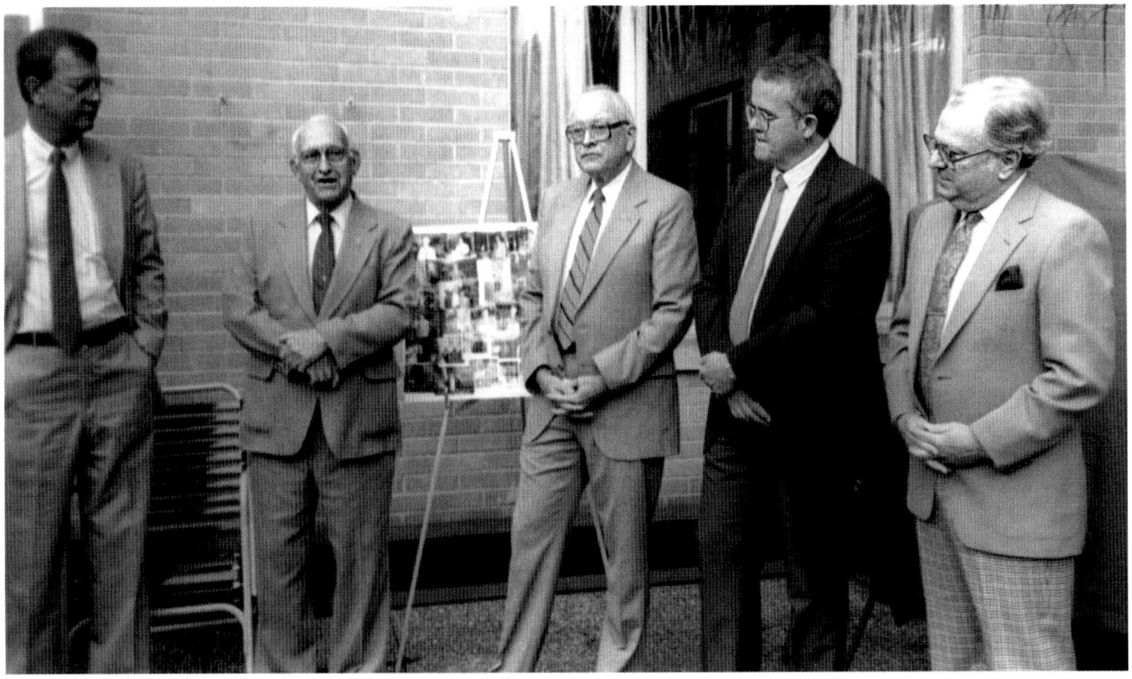

Above right: Former chiefs of the Obstetrics and Gynecology Department: Elliott Moon, MD, L. P. Matthews, MD, Ralph Tillman, MD, Wallace Hardy, MD, and John R. Castle, MD. **Above:** William Hutchinson, MD, who delivered DeKalb General Hospital's first quadruplets.

In 1961 Lawrence Matthews, MD, was chief of Obstetrics and Gynecology, Mary Chambers, RN, was the head nurse on Labor and Delivery, and Carmen McKoon, RN, was the head nurse in the nursery. Mary Chambers joined the staff a month before the hospital opened to order supplies, write policies and procedures and get Labor and Delivery ready for action.[2]

The six original obstetricians on the medical staff delivered twenty-five babies during the hospital's first week.[3] By 2001, forty years later, DeKalb Medical's seventy obstetricians and thirteen specialists were delivering more than 6,300 babies a year, second in number only to Atlanta's Northside Hospital.[4]

DeKalb Medical's maternity services had its share of celebrity and unusual births, including former President and Mrs. Jimmy Carter's grandbaby who was delivered to their daughter, Amy.[5] DeKalb General's first twins were born in August 1961 to parents who did not know they were going to have twins.[6] In 1975 an expectant mother and her husband came to the hospital thinking they would take home a baby brother to their five-year-old daughter. Her obstetrician, John McLane, MD, suspected twins, but the mother delivered triplet girls. The five-year-old sibling at home said that would be no problem since they could keep one and give the others to two of their neighbors who didn't have any children. The parents elected to keep all three.[7] In 1985 William Hutchinson, MD, delivered quadruplets to a mother who had taken the fertility drug, clomiphene. Two boys and two girls arrived ten weeks early but did well in DeKalb's neonatal intensive care unit.[8]

In 1999, in 2000, and again in 2003 DeKalb Medical delivered babies from abdominal pregnancies in which the fertilized egg implanted somewhere in the abdominal cavity. It is a rare condition, according to the Centers for Disease Control and Prevention, occurring in one out of every ten thousand live births with a mortality rate of 50 percent for the pregnant mother.[9] Two of DeKalb's abdominal-birth babies and all three of the mothers survived and did well.

Two of DeKalb's most challenging births involved infants delivered to mothers on life support. In

January 2003 a twenty-nine-year-old expectant mother who had been stabbed in the head and abdomen was brought to DeKalb Medical Center in a coma. She required continued life support for the ensuing eleven weeks. In her thirty-third week of pregnancy, while still in a coma, she delivered a healthy, four-pound-six-ounce baby boy by caesarean section. The mother's parents, who had nine other grandchildren, took the baby to their home in New Jersey when he was ready for release from the hospital, and he did well.[10] The baby's mother eventually came off life support but died at a later time.

In November 2003 a teenage freshman college student in her twelfth week of pregnancy sustained a head injury, convulsed, and went into a coma. At DeKalb Medical Center she was placed on life support that was maintained in the hope of saving the baby. Four months after admission, the comatose expectant mother spontaneously gave birth to a fourteen-week-premature baby boy. He had a significant congenital heart valve deformity that needed surgery, eye problems that needed surgery, kidney failure, and a life-threatening bacterial infection. His prognosis was grim, but he was resuscitated and placed on a respirator in the neonatal intensive care unit. For two days after giving birth to the baby, the mother was evaluated several times by physicians, determined to be brain-dead, and, in accordance with Georgia law, was taken off life support. All cardiac and respiratory functions ceased within thirty minutes.[11]

To everyone's amazement, the baby lived. His bacterial infection responded to antibiotics, his kidneys returned to normal function, he breathed on his own, and doctors were able to surgically repair his damaged heart valve and to operate on his eyes. A little over two months after his birth, he went home with his grandmother and appeared to be healthy and doing well.[12]

Unfortunately, the baby's grandmother disputed the doctors' findings that the baby's mother was brain-dead; and she sued the hospital and the physicians on behalf of the baby for having removed life support from the mother without the family's consent.[13] Georgia law stipulates that when two physicians evaluate a patient on two occasions and declare the patient to be brain-dead, the patient is dead. Under the law, the final decision to discontinue treatment remains with physicians and not the family. The grandmother's suit remains pending before the Georgia Supreme Court.[14]

Over the years, DeKalb Medical enhanced its women's and infants' facilities and its services. The original obstetrical facility had labor and delivery rooms for normal, vaginal deliveries on the second floor, while caesarean sections were performed in one of the surgical operating rooms on the first floor. Fathers remained in the waiting room and were excluded from either of these procedures. In 1983 the hospital opened a dedicated obstetrical operating room in the delivery area for mothers requiring caesarean section, allowing expectant mothers to retain the same nurses throughout the delivery process[15] and allowing fathers to be a part of the birthing process.[16]

In 1974 DeKalb General became the only hospital in the South to have all of its newborn infants tested for hearing impairment. Stanley Tenenbaum, MD, chief of Pediatrics, developed the program in coordination with the Cotillion Club of Decatur and the DeKalb County Board of Education.[17]

In 1978, when Egleston Childrens Hospital said it could no longer assure DeKalb that it could receive and provide care for all its sick newborns, DeKalb General Hospital became only the second community hospital in Atlanta to obtain the full-time services of a neonatologist.[18] Michael Armand, MD, a pediatrician with advanced training in the care of high-risk newborns, of premature newborns, of newborns in distress, and other newborns with special medical needs, established DeKalb General's Neonatal Intensive Care Unit (NICU).[19] The unit was equipped with ventilators, respiratory support systems, and monitoring devices to check respiration, heart rate, temperature, and blood pressure. Abdul Ahmed, MD, joined Armand in 1989 as DeKalb's second neonatologist.[20] More than 12 percent

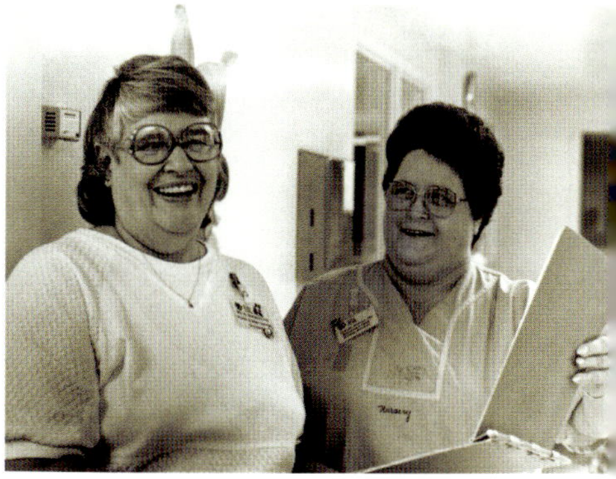

Mary Chambers, RN, head nurse in Labor and Delivery (left) reviews a chart with Carmen McKoon, RN, head nurse in the nursery.

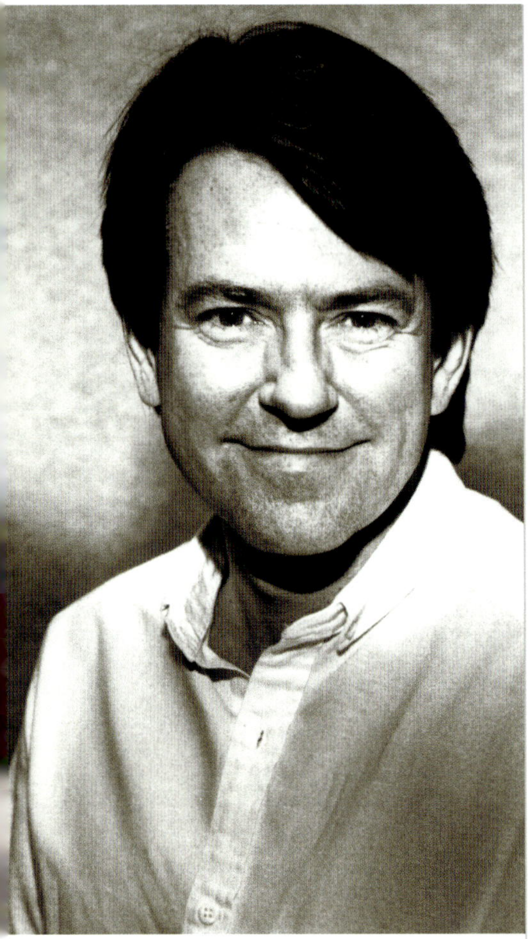

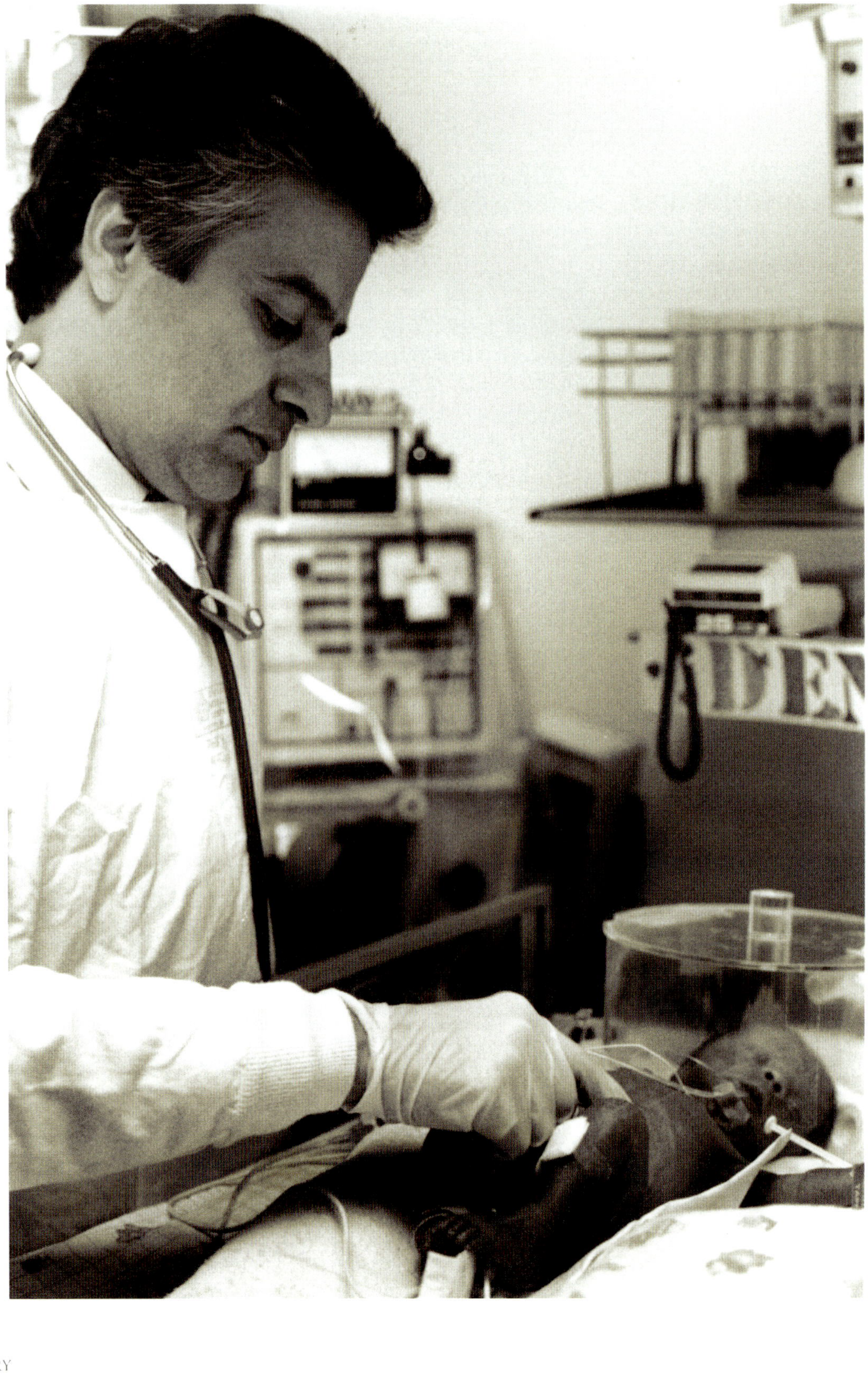

Above: Michael Armand, MD, pediatrician and neonatologist established DeKalb General Hospital's Neonatal ICU to care for premature infants and others with special medical needs. **Right:** Abdul Ahmed, MD, joined Dr. Armand in 1989 as the hospital's second neonatologist.

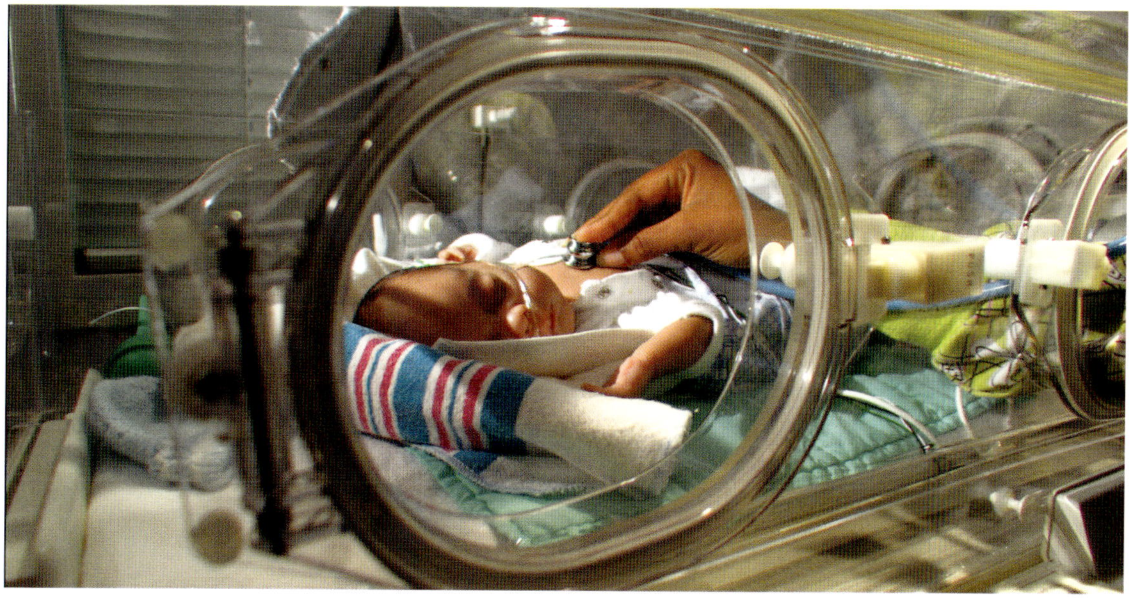

Left: A premature infant in the Neonatal Intensive Care Unit. **Below:** Women's and Infants' Services, in collaboration with The Wellness Center, offers classes in postpartum fitness for mothers with young babies. **Bottom:** Margie Hunter, RN, was named director of Women's and Infants' Services in 2003.

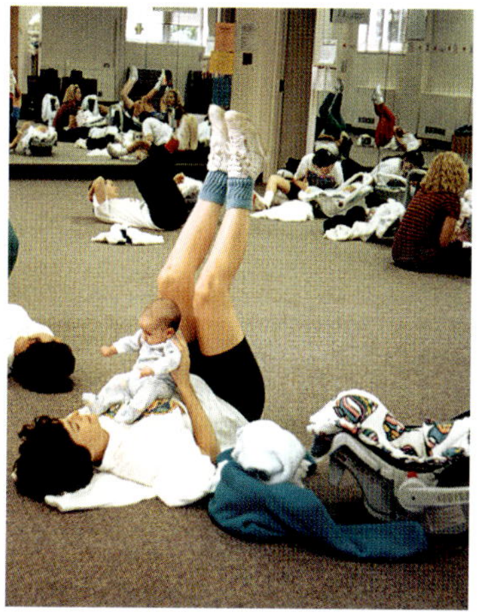

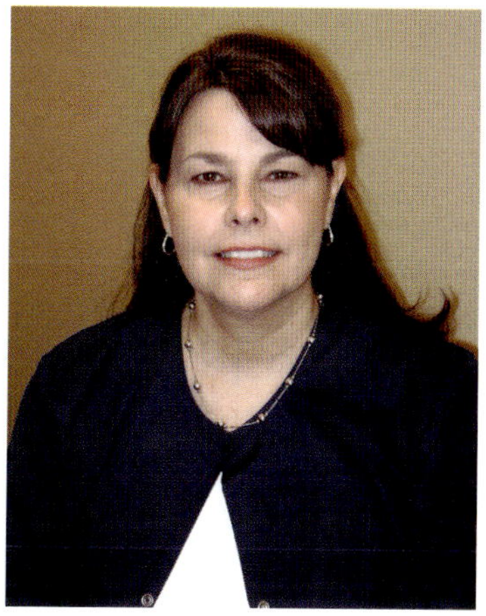

of DeKalb's deliveries go to the NICU,[21] and the unit has been a key factor in DeKalb Medical's ability to provide state-of-the-art maternity care to mothers and their babies. A member of Armand's group is in the hospital twenty-four hours a day, seven days a week, a level of service found in no other hospital in Atlanta.[22] The NICU is undergoing a complete renovation that will be completed in 2008.[23]

In 1979 DeKalb General ventured into a new concept of family-centered maternity care with the creation of a "birthing room" where fathers and mothers could remain together during labor, delivery, and recovery for uncomplicated pregnancies and deliveries. The birthing room concept also afforded the mother the choice of having a natural childbirth without the aid of anesthesia.[24] The Labor-Delivery-Recovery (LDR) room was so popular that all future expansions incorporated and expanded the concept.

In 1987 DeKalb General Hospital's maternity services "went to the movies." A made-for-TV movie, "Kids Like These," starring Richard Crenna and Tyne Daly, was filmed at DeKalb General. The movie was based on the true story of a family's coping with a child born with Down syndrome. Mary Chambers, Dixie Wilson, Susan Bales (Harris), Jim Courtney, and Henry Elder were among the familiar DeKalb General faces seen in the movie. The experience created a great deal of excitement and fun for the employees, and, as Mary Chambers said, "was one of the OB highlights of that era."[25]

Women's and Infants' Services has collaborated with The Wellness Center to provide extensive obstetrical education and counseling services. It has offered preconception counseling, childbirth preparation, baby talk and baby sign language, newborn baby care, how to raise a smart and emotionally healthy baby, mom and baby fitness, breast feeding, and many other classes.[26] Doris Vorce, RN, was the first certified lactation consultant in the state of Georgia and the first to practice in the obstetrical department of a hospital. She joined DeKalb General's staff in 1969, and under her guidance, encouragement, and instruction, 70 percent of all women who delivered at DeKalb breast-fed their babies.[27] She retired in 1999 after thirty years of service at DeKalb Medical. Jamie Ray, RN, IBCLC, is the current manager of the Lactation Department and Obstetrical Community Education.[28]

In 2003 Margie Hunter, RN, was named director of Women's and Infants' Services.[29] Hunter reorganized Women's and Infants' Services shortly after her appointment, was in charge of establishing the service on the Hillandale campus, and organized the service in the new Women's Center that was completed in 2007. In addition, she convened a task force that developed a coordinated approach to bereavement care to acknowledge, assist, and support with respectful, and compassionate services parents expecting or experiencing the loss of a newborn. Sharon Gregory, RN, was named Perinatal Bereavement coordinator.[30]

In 1990, the medical staff and governing body approved the addition of certified nurse midwives who were employed by and who would work under the supervision of obstetrician members of the medical staff.[31] Numerous mothers with low-risk pregnancies enjoyed the prenatal care, the personal support, and the delivery experience provided by nurse midwives.

In the fall of 1991, DeKalb Medical Center negotiated a contract with Paul C. Browne, MD, an Emory Clinic perinatologist, to provide on a part-time basis diagnostic tests and maternal-fetal services to DeKalb's high-risk obstetrical patients.[32] In February 1993 Browne became the full-time medical director of the Perinatal Center at DeKalb Medical Center[33] to provide obstetrical care to high-risk expectant mothers with such conditions as diabetes, high blood pressure, and mothers carrying babies with high-risk conditions; and to offer advanced diagnostic tests to reveal otherwise unsuspected conditions of the mother-to-be and her unborn child.[34]

In 1992 the state approved a certificate of need application for a $15.3 million project to renovate and replace the existing surgical and the obstetrical areas.[35] The three-story, 107,000-square-foot addition was completed in 1993. The second floor housed the maternity unit and included twelve additional Labor-Delivery-Recovery-Postpartum (LDRP) rooms, three operating-delivery rooms, an expanded neonatal intensive care unit, and space for the Perinatal Center. In 1999 the hospital added six new LDRP rooms and two new operating-delivery rooms. In 2003–2004 the facility underwent another $1.6 million renovation with the addition of 4,500 square feet of new space.[36]

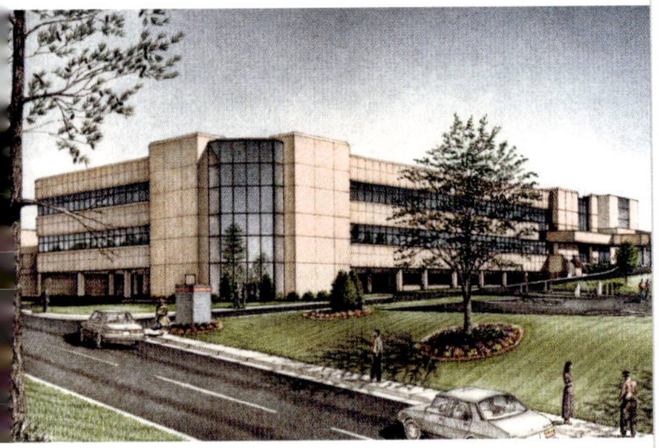

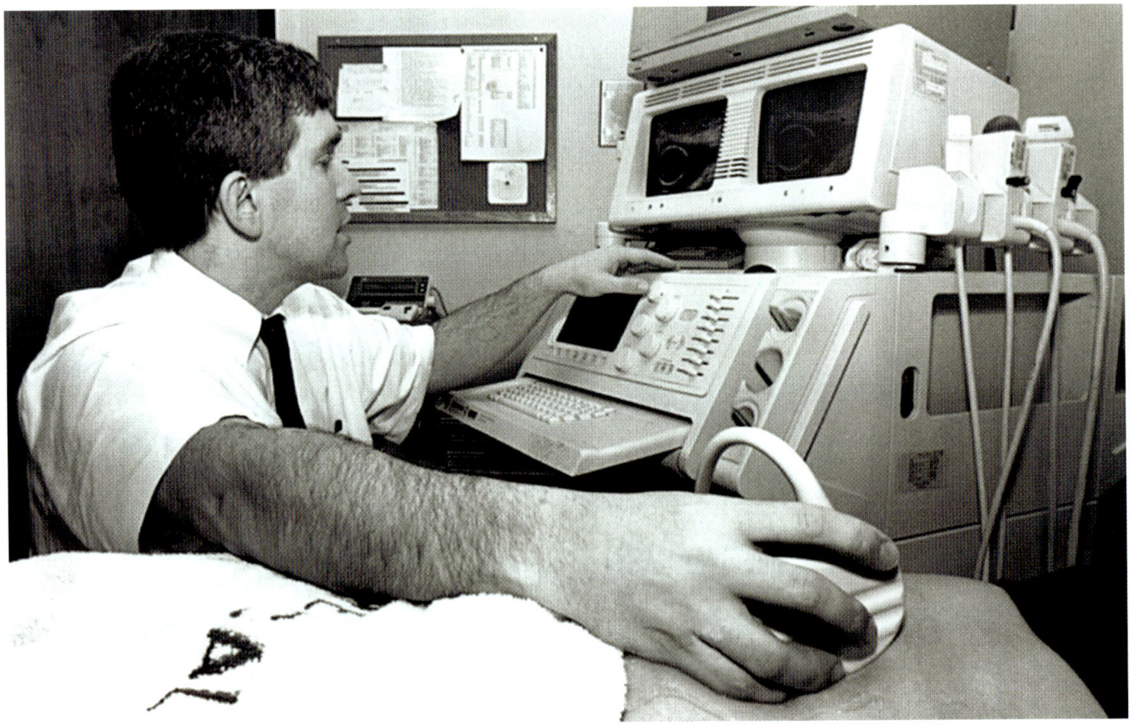

Above: Artist rendering for the new 107,000 square-foot Surgery and Maternity Center completed in 1993. **Right:** Paul C. Browne, MD, perinatologist, performing an ultrasound examination on a high risk maternity patient.

DeKalb Medical at Hillandale opened in 2005 and included a maternity unit with five antepartum rooms for expectant mothers who require hospitalization before delivery, six obstetrical assessment rooms, eight Labor-Deliver-Recovery rooms, a ten-bed special care nursery and twenty-five mother-baby postpartum rooms. As of 2007 Hillandale is delivering approximately 1,400 babies a year.[37]

Despite the new and renovated facilities, the Department of Obstetrics and Gynecology asked the hospital to build an entirely new women's center.[38] The DeKalb County Hospital Authority and the board of directors approved the sale of revenue anticipation certificates to fund the project, and in 2004 the state approved the certificate of need application to construct a $55 million, five-story, 163,000-square-foot Women's Center (later named Women's Center and Surgery Center) with a three-level parking garage underneath to accommodate 425 parking spaces.[39] The Women's Center included eighteen new labor-delivery-recovery (LDR) suites, private family waiting areas adjacent to the LDR suites, ten obstetrical assessment rooms, three caesarean delivery suites, and a thirty-six-bassinet well-baby nursery. There are sixty-two postpartum mother-baby rooms with amenities such as high-speed Internet access, refrigerators, private bathrooms, and window seat couches spacious enough for guests to sleep over. The NICU and the Growing Preemie nursery stayed in the main hospital. The new Women's Center and Surgery Center had a grand opening in January 2007.[40]

DeKalb Medical's Women's and Infants' Services has a trained, experienced, and dedicated staff of physicians, nurses, and support personnel, including specialty services, that has made its maternity care among the best available anywhere. The rapid population growth in South DeKalb County and the explosive influx of young couples and families in the greater Decatur community, coupled with the new facilities and enhanced service capabilities, present DeKalb Medical's North Decatur campus, its Hillandale campus, and its physicians with a unique opportunity to become one of the region's preeminent Women's and Infants' Services.

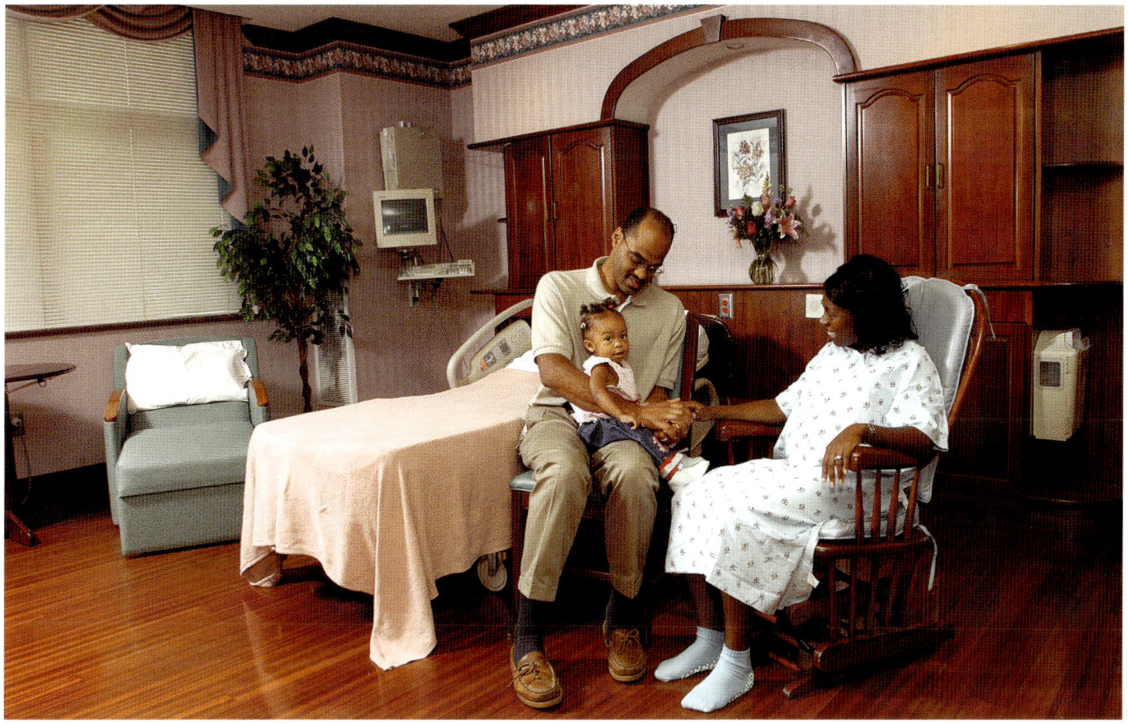

Julia H. Jones and her husband, Bernard and family enjoy one of the new Labor-Delivery-Recovery rooms completed in 1993.

DeKalb County Hospital Authority

2007 Members

Gregory Levett, Sr. —Chairperson
Georgia Barker—Vice Chairperson
John R. Gerlach—Secretary-Treasurer

Duane Blair, MD	Oliver Lee
Mereda Johnson	Albert Scott, MD
William Hardcastle, MD	Coleman Seward

MEMBER	TERM		REPLACED BY
J. Rufus Evans, MD	1957–1969	Chr 1957-1969	William E. Lewis
J. Ross McCain	1957–1965		Floyd Sanders, MD
Julius A. McCurdy	1957–1964		A. Waldo Sowell
Wash W. Lively	1957–1987		H. Duane Blair, MD
M. E. Smith	1957–1969		Rufus Camp
Hugh Rowland	1957–1964		William P. Tatum
R. L. Mathis, Jr.	1957–1974		Pat Mathis
A. Waldo Sowell	1964–1976	Chr 1969–1976	Ralph Birdsong
William P. Tatum	1964–1992	Chr 1976–1992	(Not replaced, number reduced by 3)
Floyd Sanders, MD	1965–1997	Chr 1995–1996	Albert Scott, MD
Rufus Camp	1969–1975		Charles Ginden
William E, Lewis	1969–1973		L. C. Buchanan, MD
Pat Mathis	1974–1995	Chr 1992–1995	Alex Y. Wu
H. Duane Blair, MD	1987–		
L C Buchanan, MD	1973–1991		Roy Vandiver, MD
Charles Ginden	1975–1992		(Not replaced, number reduced by 3)
Ralph Birdsong	1976–1990		Warren Jobe
James Goodman (2 added)	1985–1988		Oliver Lee
Judy McMahan (2 added)	1985–1996		Richard W. Jones
Gregory Levett, Sr. (3 added)	1994–	Chr 2005–	
Alex Y. Wu	1996–2002		Coleman Seward
Albert Scott, MD	1998–		
Oliver Lee	1989–	Chr 1996–2005	
Warren Jobe	1991–1992		(Not replaced, number reduced by 3)
Roy Vandiver, MD	1991–2006		William Hardcastle, MD
Georgia Barker (3 added)	1994–		
Richard Jones	1998–2002		John R. Gerlach
Coleman Seward	2002–		
Cornelius Flowers, MD (3 added)	1994–2007		Mereda Johnson
John R. Gerlach	2002–		
Mereda Johnson	2007–		

Appendix B

DeKalb Medical Center, Inc., Board of Directors

2007 Members
Oliver Lee—Chairperson
Terry Duis—Vice Chairperson
Roy Vandiver, MD—Secretary
David Jollay—Treasurer
Eric Norwood—President and CEO
Charles Clifton, MD—Chief of Staff, DeKalb Medical at North Decatur
Michael Quinones, MD—Chief of Staff, DeKalb Medical at Hillandale

MEMBER	TERM		REPLACED BY
William P. Tatum	1992–1993	Chr 1992–1993	Audrey Morgan
Pat L. Mathis	1992–1998	Chr 1993–1998	Biff Wilson
Charles Ginden	1992–2000		Terry Duis
Charles B. Eberhart	1992–1995		Bonnie Phipps
John R. Gerlach	1992–2003		Eric Norwood
Judy McMahan	1992–2005	Chr 2000–2004	Terry Duis
Floyd Sanders, MD	1992–1997		Gulshan Harjee, MD
Warren Jobe	1992–1999		James Young
Oliver Lee	1992–	Chr 2007–	
H. Duane Blair, MD	1992–2007	Chr '98–'00, '04–'07	David Jollay
Roy Vandiver, MD	1992–		
Audrey Morgan	1993–2003		Daniel Thompson
Bonnie Phipps	1995–2001		Don Smith
Gulshan Harjee, MD	1997–2004		(Not replaced, transferred to DRHS)
Biff Wilson	1999–2003		David Jollay
James Young	1999–2001		Gregory Levett, Sr.
Terry Duis	2000–2004		(Not replaced, transferred to DRHS)
Eric Norwood	2003–		
Gregory Levett, Sr.	2001–2004		(Not replaced, transferred to DRHS)
Don Smith	2002–2004		(Not replaced, transferred to DRHS)
Daniel Thompson	2003–2004		(Not replaced, transferred to DRHS)
David Jollay	2003–2004		(Not replaced, transferred to DRHS)
Terry Duis	2006–		

EX OFFICIO MEMBERS AS CHIEF OF STAFF, DEKALB MEDICAL AT NORTH DECATUR

R. H. "Tim" Almeroth, MD	1992–1992
Julian Fred Fuerst, MD	1992–1994
Catherine Huggins, MD	1994–1996
Michael Hartman, MD	1996–1998
Sanford Hartman, MD	1998–2000
Jay Coffsky, MD	2000–2002
William Hardcastle, MD	2002–2004
Albert Scott, MD	2004–2006
Thomas DeMarini, MD	2006–2006
Charles "Chip" Clifton, MD	2006–2008

EX OFFICIO MEMBERS AS CHIEF OF STAFF, DEKALB MEDICAL AT HILLANDALE

Cornelius Flowers, MD	2005–2006
Michael Quinones, MD	2006–2008

Appendix C

DeKalb Regional Health System, Inc., Board of Directors

2007 Members

Oliver Lee—Chairperson
Terry Duis—Vice Chairperson
Roy Vandiver, MD—Secretary
David Jollay —Treasurer
Eric Norwood, President and CEO
Charles "Chip" Clifton, MD, Chief of Staff, DeKalb Medical at North Decatur
Michael Quinones, MD, Chief of Staff, DeKalb Medical at Hillandale

Robert Wilson
Peter Gordon, MD
Gulshan Harjee, MD
Gregory Levett, Sr.
Don Smith
Daniel Thompson

MEMBER	TERM		REPLACED BY
William P. Tatum	1992–1993		Audrey Morgan
Charles Ginden	1992–2000	Chr 1992–2000	James Young
Warren Jobe	1992–1999		Biff Wilson
H. Duane Blair, MD	1992–2007	Chr 2000–2007	Michael Quinones, MD
Judy McMahan	1992–2005		Robert Wilson
Oliver Lee	1992–	Chr 2007–	
Roy Vandiver, MD	1992–		
Charles B. Eberhart	1992–1995		John R. Gerlach
Audrey Morgan	1993–2004		Peter Gordon, MD
John R. Gerlach	1995–2003		Eric Norwood
Biff Wilson	1999–2003		Don Smith
James Young	2000–2001		Terry Duis
Robert Wilson	2005–		
Michael Quinones, MD	2007–		
Terry Duis	2002–		
Eric Norwood	2003–		
Don Smith	2003–		
Peter Gordon, MD	2004–		
Gulshan Harjee, MD (From DMC)	2004–		
Gregory Levett Sr. (From DMC)	2004–		
Daniel Thompson (From DMC)	2004–		
David Jollay (From DMC)	2004–		

CHIEFS OF STAFF
DEKALB MEDICAL AT NORTH DECATUR

R. H. "Tim" Almeroth, MD	1992–1992
Julian Fred Fuerst, MD	1992–1994
Catherine Huggins, MD	1994–1996
Michael Hartman, MD	1996–1998
Sanford Hartman, MD	1998–2000
Jay Coffsky, MD	2000–2002
William Hardcastle, MD	2002–2004
Albert Scott, MD	2004–2006
Thomas DeMarini, MD	2006–2006
Charles "Chip" Clifton, MD	2006–2008

DEKALB MEDICAL AT HILLANDALE

Cornelius Flowers, MD	2005–2006
Michael Quinones, MD	2006–2008

Appendix D

Decatur Health Resources, Inc., Board of Directors

2007 Members
Oliver Lee—Chairperson
Terry Duis—Vice Chairperson
Roy Vandiver, MD—Secretary
David Jollay —Treasurer
Eric Norwood—President and CEO
Charles "Chip" Clifton, MD, Chief of Staff, DeKalb Medical at North Decatur
Jeffery Michaelson, MD, Chief of Staff, DeKalb Medical at Downtown Decatur

MEMBERS	TERM		REPLACEMENT
Charles Eberhart	1993–1995	Chr 1993–1995	Ninfa Saunders, RN
John R. Gerlach	1993–2003	Chr 1995–2003	Eric Norwood
Bonnie Phipps	1993–1997		Ken Robinson
Carol Nikola	1994–1996		Richard Schmidt
Judy Turner	1994–2004		Roy Vandiver, MD
Ninfa Saunders, RN	1995–2001		Bill Sublett
Richard Schmidt	1996–2002		Skip Wright
Ken Robinson	1997–1999		Susan Sciullo
Eric Norwood	2003–	Chr 2003–2004	
Susan Sciullo	1999–2004		Oliver Lee
Bill Sublett	2001–2004		John Shelton
Skip Wright	2002–2004		Judy McMahan
Oliver Lee	2004–	Chr 2007–	
John Shelton	2004–2004		H. Duane Blair, MD
Judy McMahan	2004–2005		Terry Duis
Roy Vandiver, MD	2004–		
H. Duane Blair, MD	2004–2007	Chr 2004–2007	David Jollay
Terry Duis	2005–		
David Jollay	2007–		

DEKALB MEDICAL AT DOWNTOWN DECATUR	
Stephen Leff, MD	2002–2004
David Snyder, MD	2004–2006
Jeffrey Michaelson, MD	2006–2008

Appendix E

Other Boards and Committees — 2007

DeKalb Medical Foundation Board of Trustees

Robert E. Wilson, Chairperson
Robin H. Dretler, MD, Medical Vice Chairperson
Diane P. Harden, CPA, Treasurer
C. Leigh Minter, Director
H. Duane Blair, MD
J. Randall Carroll
Julie Childs
Grover Evans, Jr.
J. David Ewing
J. Nelson Geter
Thomas E. Gould, JD
Shirley A. Grainger
Richard B. Herzog, Jr.
Beverly Hutchinson
Dee Keeton
John S. Kennedy, MD
Ann T. McCrory
Judy R. McMahan
Audrey B. Morgan
Eric Norwood
Angelia Russell
John A. Shelton, Jr.
Judy F. Sherman
Leonard Thibadeau
Judy B. Turner

DeKalb Medical at Hillandale Community Committee

Gregory B. Levett Sr., Chairperson
Duane Barclay, DO
Cornelius Flowers, MD
Clay Fowler
Willie Hinton
Julia H. Jones
Oliver Lee
Delphyne Lomax
Michael A. Quinones, MD
John A. Shelton, Jr.
Theresa Walker
Cathleen Wheatley, RN

DeKalb Medical at Downtown Decatur Community Committee

Peter Gordon, MD, Chairperson
Dennis Byerly
Jan Eastman, RN
Jeffrey Michaelson, MD
John A. Shelton Jr.
Judy Turner

DeKalb Medical at North Decatur Community Committee

Gulshan Harjee, MD, Chairperson
Sherri Bruenig
Charles Clifton, MD
Bill Crane
Phyllis Edwards
Judy R. McMahan
Lyn Menne
Eloise Ragsdale
John A. Shelton Jr.
Demetrice Williams
Judy Yates

DeKalb Medical At Hillandale Advisory Board

Cornelius Flowers, MD, Chairperson
Duane Barclay, DO
Duane Blair, MD
Chris Jarrett, MD
Gregory B. Levett, Sr.
Eric Norwood
Michael Quinones, MD
Albert Scott, MD
Gavin Warner, MD

DeKalb Medical Auxiliary Board of Managers

Shirley Grainger, President
Betty Osborn, President Elect
Joann Bakay, First Vice President
Sally Houghton, Second Vice President
Janot Sauerbrey, Third Vice President
Jean D'Englere, Fourth Vice President
Inez Autrey, Secretary
Dave Mathieson, Treasurer
Nancy Reed, Dogwood Shop Representative
Frechia Barrett, Parliamentarian

Appendix F

Executive Leadership

2007

Eric P. Norwood—President and Chief Executive Officer
John A. Shelton Jr. —Executive Vice President and Chief Operating Officer
Diane Harden—Senior Vice President and Chief Financial Officer
Cathleen Wheatley, RN—Senior Vice President for Quality, Care Management, Information and Infection Control
Lynne Anderson—Vice President of Patient Relations and Compliance
Duane Barclay, DO—Vice President of Physician Support Services
Tom Crawford—Vice President of Human Resources
Cheryl Iverson—Vice President of Business Development and Marketing
Clay Fowler—Vice President and Administrator of DeKalb Medical at Hillandale
Phileda Seda, RN—Assistant Administrator Patient Care Services at Hillandale

LEADERSHIP POSITION	LEADER	TERM
Administrator/CEO	William H. Thrasher	1958–1973
	Charles B. Eberhart	1973–1995
	John R. Gerlach	1995–2003
	Eric P. Norwood	2003–
Assistant to Administrator	Ted Barner	1960–1962
	John R. Gerlach	1968–1970
Chief Operating Officer	John R. Gerlach	1990–1995
	Ninfa Saunders, RN	1998–2001
	Eric P. Norwood	2002–2003
	John A. Shelton	2004–
Financial Officer	Charles Anderson	1960–1986
	Bonnie Phipps	1986–1996
	Kenneth Robinson	1997–1999
	Susan Sciullo	1999–2005
	Diane Harden	2005–
Administrative Services	Charles B. Eberhart	1970–1973
	Douglas Buchner	1973–1978
	Bill Sublett	1978–2003
Patient Care Services	John R. Gerlach	1970–1994
	Ninfa Saunders, RN	1994–2001
	Susan Parry, RN	2001–2004
	Brent Robinson, RN	2004–2007
Nursing	Opal Hopkins Fyffe, RN	1960–1965
	Margaret Ford, RN	1965–1969
	Naomi Harman, RN	1969–1992
	Ninfa Saunders, RN	1993–2001
	Susan Parry, RN	2001–2004
	Brent Robinson, RN	2004–2007

LEADERSHIP POSITION	LEADER	TERM
Hospital Relations/Risk Mgmt	William H. Thrasher	1974–1983
	Martha Nodal Kalember, RN	1983–1992
	Mary Kay Keisling	1993–2000
	Jerilyn Bing	2000–2001
	Lynne Anderson	2001–
Public Relations/Marketing	Monnie Mitchell	1965–1985
	Pam Willoughby	1985–1986
	Al Curran	1986–1992
	Blaine Wyatt	1992–1994
	Laurie Poeppleman	1994–2003
	Cheryl Iverson	2003–
Human Resources	Mary Lou Hurt	1961–1970
	Bill Sublett	1970–1978
	Perry Stephens	1978–1994
	Tom Crawford	1994–
Medical Affairs	John Harrel, MD	1974–1987
	Wytch Stubbs, MD	1988–1996
	R. Paul Crank, MD	1996–2001
	Nancy Rampell, MD	2002–2004
	Duane Barclay, DO	2004–
DeKalb Medical at Downtown Decatur		
	Carol Nikola	1994–1996
	Richard Schmidt	1996–2002
	Skip Wright	2002–2007
DeKalb Medical at Hillandale	Julia Hunter Jones	2005–2007
	Clay Fowler	2007–
Legal Counsel	George Dillard	1958–1970
	Ed Dorsey	1970–1978
	James Rawls	1978–

Appendix G

1961 DeKalb General Hospital Medical Staff and Officers

Department of Anesthesia

George P. Sessions, MD
Anibal Adan, MD

Department of General Practice

John H. Affleck, MD (Courtesy)
Charles A. Allard, MD
H. Homer Allen, MD
Robert B. Ansley, MD
Joe D. Beasley, MD
Eleanor E. J. Bundy, MD
Henry G. Carter, MD
Leon Carter, MD
C. E. Cunningham, MD
G. A. Duncan, MD (Courtesy)
Robert F. Eaves, MD
J. Rufus Evans, MD
Lawrence L. Freeman, MD
John P. Heard, MD
Houston W. Kitchin, MD
Howard B. Lee, MD
James H. Litton, MD
Malcolm M. Lockhart, MD
W. A. Mendenhall, MD
Floyd R. Sanders, MD
John M. Schreeder, MD
M. Freeman Simmons, MD
Thomas Q. Spitzer, MD
John F. Trotter, MD
T. O. Vinson, MD (Consulting)
Luther M. Vinton, MD

Department of Medicine

H. Harper Butterworth, MD
C. Warren Davidson, MD
Robert I. Gibbs, MD
Timothy Harden, MD
Robert W. Hubbell, MD
Thomas McGeachy (Courtesy)
Zebulon V. Morgan, MD
Chester W. Morse, MD
Benjamin B. Okel, MD
Rosemonde S. Peltz, MD
Fincher C. Powell, MD
W. Patrick Smith, MD
Jean S. Staton, MD
Virginia M. Tuggle, MD
Peter D. Walz, MD

Department of Obstetrics/Gynecology

Betty Ann Brooks, MD
John R. Castle, MD
Byron H. Dunn, MD
Catherine E. Foster, MD
John W. Fristoe, MD
Lawrence P. Matthews, MD

Department of Pathology

Webster A. Sherrer, MD (Consulting)
Frank Matthews, MD

Department of Pediatrics

William J. Brannan, MD
Carlos Duarte, MD (Courtesy)
J. Thomas Leslie, MD

Department of Radiology

Frank E. Morgan, MD

Department of Surgery

James E. Anthony, MD
Manuel E. Artime, MD
Earnest C. Atkins, MD
H. Duane Blair, MD
Leslie C. Buchanan, MD
Herbert G. Girardeau, MD
Richard H. Smoot, MD
S. Angier Wills, MD

Department of Surgery/Ophthalmology

M. Hobson Rice, MD

Department of Surgery/Orthopedics

Edward L. Johnson, MD

Department of Surgery/Urology

Albert H. Fregosi, MD
Edwin H. McDowell, MD
James W. Morgan, MD (Courtesy)

The Authority appointed the following medical staff officers and department chiefs to serve from March 22, 1961 through September 30, 1962:

Chief of Staff	Leslie C. Buchanan, MD
Vice-Chief of Staff	Homer H. Allen, MD
Secretary of Staff	Henry G. Carter, MD
Chief, Department of Anesthesiology	George P. Sessions, MD
Chief, Department of Pathology	W. Frank Matthews, MD
Chief, Department of Radiology	Frank E. Morgan, MD
Chief, Department of General Practice	M. Freeman Simmons, MD
Chief, Department of Medicine	Robert I. Gibbs, MD
Chief, Department of OB/Gyn	Lawrence P. Matthews, MD
Chief, Department of Pediatrics	J. Thomas Leslie, MD
Chief, Department of Surgery	Richard H. Smoot, MD

Appendix H

DeKalb Medical Chiefs of Staff

DeKalb Medical at North Decatur	
L. C. Buchanan, MD	1961–1962
Floyd Sanders, MD	1962–1964
Fincher Powell, MD	1964–1966
Earnest Atkins, MD	1966–1968
Fincher Powell, MD	1968–1970
Robert Gibbs, MD	1970–1972
LaMar McGinnis, MD	1972–1974
Duane Blair, MD	1974–1976
Clyde Rountree, MD	1976–1978
Ralph Tillman, MD	1978–1980
William Ward, MD	1980–1982
Edwin Galler, MD	1982–1984
Angier Wills, MD	1984–1986
Elliott Moon, MD	1986–1988
Roy Vandiver, MD	1988–1990
Robert "Tim" Almeroth, MD	1990–1992
Julian F. Fuerst, MD	1992–1994
Catherine Huggins, MD	1994–1996
Michael Hartman, MD	1996–1998
Sanford Hartman, MD	1998–2000
Jay Coffsky, MD	2000–2002
William Hardcastle, MD	2002–2004
Albert Scott, MD	2004–2006
Thomas DeMarini, MD	2006–2006
Charles "Chip" Clifton, MD	2006–2008

DeKalb Medical at Downtown Decatur	
Charles "Chip" Clifton, MD	1994–1996
Jackie Garringer, MD	1996–1998
Sheldon Lincenberg, MD	1998–2000
Stephen Leff, MD	2000–2004
David Snyder, MD	2004–2006
Jeffery Michaelson, MD	2006–2008

DeKalb Medical at Hillandale	
Cornelius Flowers, MD	2005–2006
Michael Quinones, MD	2006–2008

Appendix I

Presidents of the DeKalb Medical Society

Year	President
1950	Lawrence P. Matthews, MD
1951	Richard H. Smoot, MD
1952	William P. Smith, MD
1953	W. A. Mendenhall, MD
1954	Chester W. Morse, MD
1955	W. Freeman Simmons, MD
1956	Fincher C. Powell, MD
1957	John T. Leslie, MD
1958	John E. Beck, MD
1959	Robert B. Ansley, MD
1960	Floyd R. Sanders, MD
1961	Leslie C. Buchanan, MD
1962	John F. Trotter, MD
1963	Robert I. Gibbs, MD
1964	Howard B. Lee, MD
1965	James E. Anthony, MD
1966	Luther M. Vinton, MD
1967	M. Hobson Rice, MD
1968	H. Harper Butterworth, MD
1969	Catherine F. Foster, MD
1970	Timothy Harden Jr., MD
1971	Frank E. Morgan, MD
1972	Earnest C. Atkins, MD
1973	John P. Heard, MD
1974	Benjamin B. Okel, MD
1975	Lawrence L. Freeman, MD
1976	LaMar S. McGinnis, MD
1977	Stanley P. Aldridge, MD
1978	H. Duane Blair, MD

Year	President
1979	Charles W. McDowell, MD
1980	O. Wytch Stubbs, MD
1981	Ernest C. Fokes, MD
1982	Douglas Smith, MD
1983	William R. Hardcastle, MD
1984	William J. Rawls, MD
1985	Clyde B. Rountree, MD
1986	Roy W. Vandiver, MD
1987	Frank Matthews, MD
1988	William F. Keeton, MD
1989	William G. Whitaker, MD
1990	Walker L. Ray, MD
1991	Gary R. Botstein, MD
1992	Stanley W. Sherman, MD
1993	Joy A. Maxey, MD
1994	John S. Kennedy, MD
1995	Andrew P. Morley, MD
1996	Robert L. Davies, MD
1997	Elliott C. Moon, MD
1998	Stephen P. Leff, MD
1999	Kenneth A. Hoose Jr., MD
2000	Lewis F. Green, MD
2001	Peter A. Gordon, MD
2002	Nancy Rampell, MD
2003	Nancy Rampell, MD
2004	Michael G. Hartman, MD
2005	Charles F. Clifton Jr., MD
2006	Robin H. Dretler, MD
2007	Joseph Weissman, MD

Appendix J

Recipients of the Julius A. McCurdy Citizenship Award

This award was established in 1973 to recognize outstanding community service by a DeKalb County physician or outstanding citizen. The award is presented at the Society's Annual Meeting in honor of Julius A. McCurdy who was founder of Decatur Federal Savings and Loan Association.

1973	Philip E. Christopher, M.D.
1974	Leslie C. Buchanan, M.D.
1975	Theodore C. Mosley, M.D.
1976	O. Wytch Stubbs Jr., M.D.
1977	Ralph A. Tillman, M.D.
1978	Luther M. Vinton Jr., M.D.
1979	Russell W. Wallace Jr., M.D.
1980	Roy W. Vandiver, M.D.
1981	Alexander T. Parkinson, M.D.
1982	M. Virginia Tuggle, M.D.
1983	John P. Heard, M.D.
1984	Earnest C. Atkins, M.D.
1985	H. Duane Blair, M.D.
1986	Tom R. Raaen, M.D.
1987	Don W. Printz, M.D.
1988	Harry R. Foster, M.D.
1989	W. Mark Coppage, M.D.
1990	Benjamin B. Okel, M.D.
1991	S. Perry Brickman, D.D.S.
1992	G. Douglas Talbott, M.D.
1993	Gary R. Botstein, M.D.
1994	Charles Eberhart
1995	Martha H. Crenshaw, M.D.
1996	LaMar S. McGinnis, M.D.
1997	Floyd Sanders, M.D.
1998	Stephen P. Leff, M.D.
1999	J. W. "Hank" Holderfield
2000	Sheldon M. Lincenberg, M.D.
2001	R. Paul Crank, M.D.
2002	Paul W. Wiesner, M.D.
2003	Walker L. Ray, M.D.
2004	Jean S. Staton, M.D.
2005	Hugh Spruell, M.D.
2006	Roger Rowell, M.D.
2007	Betty Castellani, D. Min.

Appendix K

Recipients of the William H. Thrasher Good Samaritan Award

The award is named after William H. Thrasher, DeKalb Medical's first administrator. It is awarded each year to the employee who, by his or her words, acts and deeds best represents the characteristics displayed by the Good Samaritan in the biblical parable. DeKalb Medical employees nominate co-workers for the award. Members of the senior management team review the nominations and choose the recipient. The recipient receives a monetary gift and his or her name is placed on the Thrasher Award plaque displayed on the first floor of the hospital.

1984	Ruby Dobbs, Unit Clerk, Diagnostic and Treatment Center
1985	Prebble Mitchell, RN, Enterostomal Therapy
1986	Betty Frost, RN, 4700 Staff Nurse
1987	Clare Hart, R-CRP, Pulmonary Function Laboratory
1988	Dottie Gelderman, RN, 2700
	Ralph W. Aldridge Jr., Clinical Laboratory
1989	Joyce Garmon, Business Office
1990	Patty Pilger, RN, Labor & Delivery (Posthumous)
	Louise Hinesley, Emergency Department
1991	Robin Underwood, Rehabilitation Services
1992	John Hall, Patient Representative, Social Services
1993	Rose McKeever, LPN, Charles B. Eberhart Cancer Center
	Travis Wilhite, Imaging Services
1994	Barbara French, RN, 3200 Nursing Unit
1995	James Solomon, Environmental Services
1996	Cynthia Burgess, RN, 4200 Medical Oncology Unit
1997	Martha Williams, RN, Diagnostic and Treatment Center
1998	Teresa Jordan-Hamilton, Emergency Department
1999	Ramiro Tamez, Security Services
2000	Doris Adams, Financial Services
2001	Ray Darden, Environmental Services
2002	McClellon D, Cox, Pastoral Services
2004	Barbara Kleynen, RN, Critical Care Services
2006	Greg Hinesley, RN, Human Resources
2007	Donna Lawson Cannon, RN, Charles B. Eberhart Cancer Center

Appendix L

Recipients of the DeKalb Medical Foundation Charles B. Eberhart Award

This award, named in memory of Charles B. Eberhart, is given to the individual who has demonstrated outstanding commitment and service to the DeKalb Medical Foundation, DeKalb Regional Healthcare System and the community.

1995	Roy Vandiver, M.D.
1996	Judy McMahan
1997	Jim Underwood
1998	Judy Sherman
1999	Maureen Vandiver
2001	Gayle M. Lindsay and Teresa S. Avant
2002	Dee Keeton
2003	H. Duane Blair, M.D.
2007	Robert E. Wilson

Charles B. Eberhart Cancer Center Hero of the Year Award

The Charles B. Eberhart Cancer Center Hero Award, named in memory of Charles Eberhart, is awarded to the cancer survivor who is recognized for overcoming his or her struggle with illness, displaying courage in the face of adversity and making his or her community a better place.

1998	Helen Gene Eberhart
1999	Caraker Paschal
2000	Darrie B. Wohlman
2001	Susan and Jim Watson
2003	Milt Mogren
2005	Janet Shoemaker

DeKalb Medical Recipients of The Georgia Hospital Association Distinguished Service Award

Each year the Georgia Hospital Association presents its Distinguished Service Award to two Georgia hospital trustees or community leaders who have made significant contributions to improving health care in Georgia.

1972	J. Rufus Evans, MD
1995	Charles B. Eberhart (Posthumous)
2001	Judy McMahan
2006	H. Duane Blair, MD

Appendix M

Red Cross Volunteers

Year	Chairman	Hours Donated
1975–1976	Frances Stukes	
1976–1977	Mary Kate Jones	
1977–1978	Edith Dewitt	39,043
1978–1979	Jessie Walker	
1979–1980	Isabelle Carter	33,728
1980–1981	Rose Bruhn	
1981–1982	Joyce Kenna	
1982–1983	Sunny Fraser	
1983–1984	Barbara Moriarity	
1984–1985	Ann Hord	
1985–1986	Alice Swygert	
1986–1987	Marjorie Ware	27,363
1987–1988	Edith Henderson	
1988–1989	Edith Henderson	25,392
1990–1991	Nancy Reed	26,983
1991–1992	Nancy Reed	23,775
1992–1993	Ivy Lois Hubert	21,012
1993–1994	Ivy Lois Hubert	20,824
1994–1995	Bernice Smith	18,160

Appendix N

DeKalb Medical Auxiliary

YEAR	ADULT VOLUNTEERS	YOUTH VOLUNTEERS	PRESIDENT	ADULT HOURS	YOUTH HOURS	TOTAL HOURS	HOSPITAL & FOUNDATION DONATIONS	NURSING SCHOLARSHIP DONATIONS	CANCER & WISH LIST DONATIONS
1973-1974	127	8	Ree Stamps	12,000	1,000	13,000	$5,000		
1974-1975	125		Annie Ruth Anderson (Brown)			10,773	$12,000		
1975-1976	126	45	Betty Botdorf			14,011	$51,000		
1976-1977	123	27	Frances Statham			15,101	$40,000		
1977-1978	123	65	Jackie McCloud			13,595	$46,000		
1978-1979	165	110	Tina Newman	18,125	12,101	30,226	$54,000		
1979-1980			Tina Newman	16,847	13,677	30,524	$68,000		
1980-1981	144	115	Gail Lawrence	22,039	10,780	32,819	$82,000	$40,000	
1981-1982	188	108	Gail Lawrence	23,513	9,515	33,028	$90,000	$40,000	
1982-1983	185	118	Beth Glennon	26,733	12,840	39,213	$100,000	$40,000	
1983-1984	185	118	Beth Glennon	30,037	10,727	40,767	$120,000	$40,000	
1984-1985	171	125	Jean Newman	30,597	10,019	40,616	$100,000	$40,000	
1985-1986	187	130	Jean Newman	31,602	11,095	42,697	$100,000	$40,000	
1986-1987	174	120	Jo Rawls	31,850	11,118	42,958	$100,000	$40,000	
1987-1988	174	120	Jo Rawls	30,849	7,205	38,054	$102,000	$40,000	
1988-1989	168	100	Coral Stone	34,766	8,502	43,268	$140,000	$40,000	
1989-1990	155	90	Coral Stone	35,718	6,326	42,044	$145,000	$40,000	
1990-1991	191	100	Mary Meek	38,480	8,692	47,172	$145,000	$40,000	
1991-1992	163	100	Mary Meek	36,405	9,196	45,601	$150,000	$40,000	
1992-1993	169	85	Claire Petersen	36,322	8,743	45,065	$155,000	$40,000	
1993-1994	149	65	Claire Petersen	35,629	8,238	43,867	$150,000	$40,000	
1994-1995	130	85	Marilyn Yancey	31,859	8,124	39,983	$155,000	$40,000	
1995-1996	203	129	Frances Cowan			48,681	$155,000	$40,000	
1996-1997	211		Frances Cowan			46,569	$155,000	$40,000	
1997-1998	193		Janot Sauerbrey	41,240	4,465	45,705	$160,000	$40,000	
1998-1999	178	88	Janot Sauerbrey	40,093	4,783	44,876	$175,000	$40,000	
1999-2000	180		Ann Hord	40,583	3,406	43,989	$175,000	$40,000	
2000-2001	180	101	Ann Hord	37,069	4,233	41,302	$177,500	$40,000	
2001-2002	163		Inez Autry			38,649	$177,500	$15,000	
2002-2003	162		Marlene Barnes			41,332	$120,000		$23,500
2003-2004	159		Marlene Barnes			39,710	$150,000		$22,121
2004-2005	123	25	Frechia Barrett			38,401	$50,000		$30,960
2005-2006	116	22	Frechia Barrett			34,020	$50,000		$34,280
2006-2007	130		Shirley Grainger			38,401	$75,000		$32,701
						1,222,244	$3,730,000	$855,000	$120,062

DIRECTORS

1978	Kathy Hayes
1980	Brenda Coker
1984	Joyce Bowman (Sanders)
1999	Dan Williams
2006	Linda Dacey-Caban

Endnotes

Chapter One

1 Alabama Department of Archives and History, Montgomery, Alabama. Alabama History Timeline: From Prehistory to Modern Day, "1798: Mississippi Territory," Nathan H. Glick pen and ink drawings, LPR92, (http://www.archives.state.al.us/timeline/1800/gig3.gif); Golden Ink, About North Georgia, "American Indian Land Cessions In Georgia," (http://ngeorgia.com/history/indianla.html); *The New Georgia Encyclopedia: History and Archeology*, "Yazoo Land Fraud," (http://www.georgiaencyclopedia.org/nge/Article.jsp?id=h-663).

2 Larry Worthy, Ed., "North Georgia Creek History," About North Georgia (http://ngeorgia.com/history/creekhistory.html).

3 Brenda Pierce, "Atlanta Timeline," A GaGenWeb Project Site (http://www.rootsweb.com/~gafulton/atlantahistorystuff.html).

4 "DeKalb County," CVIOG, (http://www.cviog.uga.edu/Projects/gainfo/histcountymaps/dekalbhistmaps.htm).

5 "Archives of DeKalb County," *Roadside Georgia*, (http://roadsidegeorgia.com/county/dekalb.html.

6 "DeKalb History," *DeKalb County, Georgia*, (http://www.co.dekalb.ga.us/history.htm).

7 "Hightower Trail History," Boy Scouts of America, (http://www.hightowertrail.com/Highs.htm).

8 *Roadside Georgia*.

9 "The History of the City of Doraville," (http://www.doravillega.us/History/history.htm); Jim Perkins, "The Hightower Trail Revealed," first printed in the Dunwoody Crier, Nov. 3, 2004, and reprinted with editing in The Hightower Trail, (http://www.hightowertrail.com/HighTrail map.htm).

10 "DeKalb County, Georgia History," The Georgia Gen Web Project, (http://bellsouthpwp.net/m/s/msaffold/dekalb%20history.htm).

11 "Creek Indians," Buckhead, (http://www.buckhead.org/history/creek-indians.htm).

12 Jeanne Osborne Gibbs, "From Cowslip to Cobalt: A Century and a Half of Medicine in DeKalb County, Georgia." Research and Romance in Medicine, DeKalb County Medical Auxiliary, For the Medical Association of Georgia, February, 1971.

13 Calvin Weaver, MD, *The History of Medicine in DeKalb County*.

14 Jean Osborne Gibbs.

15 Calvin Weaver.

16 "DeKalb County Courthouses 1823-1967," The Georgia Gen Web Project, (http://personal.atl.bellsouth.net/m/s/msaffold/Cthouses.htm).

17 Vivian Price, "Time Line DeKalb," *Decatur/DeKalb News Era: A News/Sun Exclusive Historical Edition*, 1991.

18 *Roadside Georgia*, Vivian Price.

19 Vivian Price.

20 *Roadside Georgia*.

21 "Georgia Railroad" (http://www.railga.com/georgia.html).

22 "DeKalb County," Georgia Snapshots.

23 Boy Scouts of America.

24 Brenda Pierce.

25 Brenda Pierce, "History of Georgia's Capital Cities," Georgia Government, (http:www.georgia.gov/00/article/0,2086,4802_4987_15252433,00.html).

26 "DeKalb History," *DeKalb County, Georgia*.

27 "This Century In DeKalb County. DeKalb's 1900s: A County Comes Of Age," *The Atlanta Journal-Constitution*, (http://nl.newsbank.com).

28 "The Richard F. Sams Farm," DeKalb History Center, (http://www.dekalbhistory.org/02_history/02_ c08.html).

29 Vivian Price and Brenda Pierce, "The History of the City of Doraville;" *The Atlanta Journal-Constitution*, "This Century In DeKalb County. DeKalb's 1900s: A County Comes Of Age;" DeKalb History Center, "Before Fulton County, There Was DeKalb County; Before Atlanta, There Was Decatur: Celebrating 182 Years of History," (http://www.dekalbhistory.org/02_history/02.html).

30 Vivian Price, "DeKalb County Schools, 1903-1936)," DeKalb History Center, (http://www.dekalbhistory.org/02_history/02_c06.html).

31 Georgia Government.

32 Brenda Pierce and Gary S. Hauk, "Emory University: A Brief History," (http://emoryhistory.emory. edu/history/index.html).

33 "History of Oglethorpe University," Oglethorpe University, (http://www.oglethorpe.edu/about_us/ history/brief.asp).

34 "Agnes Scott College," New Georgia Encyclopedia, (http://www.georgiaencyclopedia.org/nge/Article.jsp?id=h-1451).

35 "Columbia Theological Seminary," The New Georgia Encyclopedia, (http://www.georgiaencyclopedia.org/nge/Article.jsp?id=h-1633).

36 "DeKalb County Historical Population Profile," *The Atlanta Journal-Constitution*; CVIOG, (http://www.cviog.uga.edu/Projects/gainfo/countypop/dekalbpop.htm).

37 *The Atlanta Journal-Constitution*.

38 "The History of the City of Doraville," The Atlanta Journal-Constitution; "Biography of Scott Candler," DeKalb County Public Library, (http://www.dekalb.public.lib.ga.us/branches/scandler.htm).

39 Biographical File: Candler, Scott ,DeKalb History Center; Fran Fossett, "Scott Candler, Sr. Turns 85, Still Watching DeKalb Closely," Decatur DeKalb News, June 28, 1972.

40 "Saint Joseph's History of Healing," Saint Joseph's Caring for Atlanta 125 Years, (http://stjosephs.chainreactionweb.com/index.php?src=gendocs&link=history&category=Main).

41 Brenda Pierce, "Hirsch Hall," The City of Atlanta Online, (http://www.atlantaga.gov/government/urbandesign_hirsch.aspx); "Grady Health System," The New Georgia Encyclopedia, (http://www.georgiaencyclopedia.org/nge/Article.jsp?id=h-1216)

42 "History," Georgia Baptist Health Care Ministry Foundation, (http://www.gbhcs.org/history.html; Monroe F. Swilley, Jr. Library, "History of the Georgia Baptist College of Nursing/Mercer University," (http://swilley.mercer.edu/speccoll/nursing_history.asp); "The Tabernacle Infirmary," Material History of American Religion Project, (http://www.materialreligion.org/documents/sept98doc.html)

43 M. J. Dewey, "The Early History of Emory University Hospital," J Med Assoc Ga 1952 Oct;41(10):462-5; Anna Tyszkiewicz, "Candler, Asa Griggs," Learning To Give, (http://www.learningtogive.org/papers/index.asp?bpid=79); "Emory University Hospital," Emory Healthcare, (http://www.emoryhealthcare.org/departments/EUH/about_us.html); "Emory University Hospital Kicks Off Centennial Year With Call For Memorabilia," Emory Healthcare, (http://www.emoryhealthcare.org/press_room/ehc_news/2005/Feb/Emory_University_Hospital_kick.html.

44 Diane Hopper Schmidt, *Piedmont Hospital: A Century of Better Care*. Published by Piedmont Hospital, 2004, pp. 12, 30, 34, 51, 58, 61.

45 Ren Davis, *Caring for Atlanta: A History of Emory Crawford Long Hospital*. Wings Publishers, 2003, pp. 10, 11, 36.

46 "Emory Crawford Long Hospital," Emory Healthcare, (http://www.emoryhealthcare.org/departments/ECL/about_us/about_us.html).

47 "Scottish Rite Hospital," (http://www.masonic info. com/srchildh.htm).

48 "Scottish Rite Hospital;" Brenda Pierce.

49 "Georgia Elks Aidmore History," Georgia Elks Association, http://www.georgiaelks.org/aidmore/aidmorehist.htm).
50 "Donor Gives $18 million to Grady's Children's Hospital," AJC.Com, (http://www.ajc.com/hp/content/metro/atlanta/0405/20grady.html).
51 "Centers for Disease Control and Prevention," The New Georgia Encyclopedia, (http://www.georgiaencyclopedia.org/nge/Article.jsp?id=h-1209).
52 "Emory University School of Medicine," The New Georgia Encyclopedia, (http://www.georgiaencyclopedia.org/nge/Article.jsp?path=/ScienceMedicine/Medicine/Institutions); "History: A Brief History of Emory University School of Medicine," Emory University School of Medicine, (http://med.emory.edu/information/history.cfm).
53 "The Emory Clinic: Celebrating 50 Years of Care," *Emory Report*, (http://www.emory.edu/EMORY_REPORT/erarchive/2003/February/er Feb.3/2_3_03clinic. cfm).

Chapter Two

1 Biographical File: J. Rufus Evans, MD, DeKalb History Center; "J. Rufus Evans: DeKalb's Doctor of the Year Still Makes House Calls," *The Decatur-DeKalb News*, May 2, 1973, p. 15A.
2 Erica Hatchett, "Julius A. McCurdy Jr., 89, DeKalb lawyer, co-founder of S&L" *The Atlanta Journal-Constitution*, May 10, 1993, p. B4 (http://nl.newbank.com/nl-search/we/Archives ....).
3 Still Makes House Calls.
4 Minutes, DeKalb County Hospital Authority, February, 1960.
5 Biographical File: Evans; "Retired Health Chief: He Envisioned DeKalb's Hospital," *The Decatur-DeKalb News*, September 4, 1968.
6 Biographical File: Evans.
7 Hatchett.
8 Levi Willard, "DeKalb General Hospital: A Dream From The Early 1950s Became Reality," *The DeKalb News/Sun*, July 22, 1981.
9 Willard.
10 Willard.
11 Georgia Law 1941, p. 241; O.C.G.A. 31-7-70 to 31-7-96.
12 Constitution of the DeKalb County Hospital Authority.
13 Minutes, DeKalb County Hospital Authority, September 25, 1957.
14 "Ground Broken for DeKalb's Hospital; Expansion Seen," The DeKalb New Era, May 21, 1959.
15 Minutes, DeKalb County Hospital Authority, January 1958.
16 The General InDecatur, December 22, 1961.
17 Minutes, DeKalb County Hospital Authority, March 7, 1958.
18 Minutes, DeKalb County Hospital Authority, May, 1958.
19 J. Ross McCain letter to W. E. Uzell, Hospital Services Division, State Health Department, January 7, 1958.
20 Minutes, DeKalb County Hospital Authority, September 1958.
21 Minutes, DeKalb County Hospital Authority, February 1958
22 J. Ross McCain letter to William H. Thrasher, February 13, 1958, with attached document, "DeKalb County Hospital Authority Advance Planning."
23 McCain letter to Thrasher.
24 "A Plan to Erect, Equip and Put Into Operation a 200-Bed General Hospital in DeKalb County, Georgia," by William H. Thrasher, Administrator, Athens General Hospital, Athens, Georgia, February, 1958.
25 "Hill-Burton Community Service Obligations," (http://www.hpolicy.duke.edu/cyberexchange/conversion/gchap75.html).
26 Minutes, DeKalb County Hospital Authority, August 1959.
27 Minutes, DeKalb County Hospital Authority, August 1961.
28 Minutes, DeKalb County Hospital Authority, August 1961.
29 Minutes, DeKalb County Hospital Authority, April 1959.
30 Minutes, DeKalb County Hospital Authority, February 1960.
31 Minutes, DeKalb County Hospital Authority, June 1958.
32 Minutes, DeKalb County Hospital Authority, February 1959.
33 Minutes, DeKalb County Hospital Authority, June 1959.
34 "DeKalb Hospital Unit Takes Bids on 200-Bed Project," The DeKalb New Era, April 16, 1959.
35 McCain, J. Ross, "Some Notes As to Groundbreaking, DeKalb General Hospital," May 15, 1959.
36 McCain, "Some Notes".
37 "Decatur Firm Gets DeKalb Hospital Job," The DeKalb New Era, April 23, 1959.
38 Minutes, DeKalb County Hospital Authority, January 1959.
39 Minutes, Medical Advisory Committee, July 27, 1959.
40 Minutes, Medical Advisory Committee, November 30, 1959.
41 Minutes, DeKalb County Hospital Authority, March 1961.
42 "New Hospital Names Director of Nursing," DeKalb General Hospital Press Release, September 15, 1960.
43 Opal Fuller Hopkins Application for Employment, DeKalb General Hospital, March 8, 1961.
44 Opal Hopkins Fyffe interview, March 3, 2006.
45 Minutes, DeKalb County Hospital Authority, February 1959; September 1959; October 1959; May 1960.
46 Fyffe interview.
47 Minutes, DeKalb County Hospital Authority, February 1960; March 1960.
48 Hopkins Application.
49 Minutes, DeKalb County Hospital Authority, February 1960.
50 Minutes, DeKalb County Hospital Authority, March 1960; April 1960.
51 Minutes, DeKalb County Hospital Authority, April 1960.
52 Minutes, DeKalb County Hospital Authority, April 1960.
53 "Assistant Administrator Accepts New Position," The General InDecatur, May 25, 1962.
54 Minutes, DeKalb County Hospital Authority, April 1962.
55 Minutes, DeKalb County Hospital Authority, June 1960.
56 Minutes, DeKalb County Hospital Authority, October 1960.
57 Minutes, DeKalb County Hospital Authority, February 1960.
58 Minutes, DeKalb County Hospital Authority, March 1961.
59 Minutes, DeKalb County Hospital Authority, December 1960.
60 Levi Willard; "Hospital Opens Monday; Medical, Administrative Staff Told," *The DeKalb New Era*, April 26, 1961.
61 MEK (name of author unknown), "DeKalb General History," February 10, 1976.
62 Shorty Lorentzson, "DeKalb General Hospital Staff Is 'Trained To Care'," *The DeKalb New Era*, April 26, 1961.
63 Fyffe interview.
64 Fyffe interview.
65 Minutes, DeKalb County Hospital Authority, January 1961.
66 Minutes, Medical Advisory Committee, January 22, 1960.
67 Lorentzson.

68 Willard, "Hospital Opens Monday."
69 Lorentzson.
70 Lorentzson.

Chapter Three

1 Mary Thomas, "D.G.H. History 1961-1976, 15th Anniversary," *The Atlanta Journal*, May 1, 1976.
2 "Gifts Welcome First Baby At Hospital," *The Atlanta Journal-Constitution*, May 3, 1961; "Stull Baby Is First For DeKalb Hospital," Newspaper article, source and date unknown.
3 Original schedule for May 2, 1961 as posted in the Anesthesia Department office.
4 Minutes, DeKalb County Hospital Authority, May 24, 1961.
5 Minutes, DeKalb County Hospital Authority, July 26, 1961.
6 Opal Fyffe letter to William H. Thrasher, July 12, 1965.
7 Request For Proposal sent to each candidate for position of Administrator: "DeKalb County Hospital Authority Advance Planning."
8 George Hutcheson, "DeKalb Hospital Growing," *Decatur-DeKalb News*, 1963.
9 Minutes, DeKalb County Hospital Authority, July 26, 1961.
10 Minutes, DeKalb County Hospital Authority, April 26, 1961.
11 Minutes, DeKalb County Hospital Authority, July 26, 1961.
12 Minutes, DeKalb County Hospital Authority, December 11, 1961.
13 Minutes, DeKalb County Hospital Authority, April 8, 1963.
14 Minutes, DeKalb County Hospital Authority, February 11, 1963.
15 Minutes, DeKalb County Hospital Authority, December 9, 1963.
16 Minutes, DeKalb County Hospital Authority, August 30, 1961.
17 Minutes, DeKalb County Hospital Authority, February 10, 1964.
18 Minutes, DeKalb County Hospital Authority, October 9, 1961.
19 Minutes, DeKalb County Hospital Authority, September 14, 1964.
20 Minutes, DeKalb County Hospital Authority, April 8, 1963.
21 Minutes, DeKalb County Hospital Authority, January 8, 1962.
22 Minutes, DeKalb County Hospital Authority, May 14, 1962.
23 Minutes, DeKalb County Hospital Authority, November 13, 1961.
24 Minutes, DeKalb County Hospital Authority, July 27, 1960.
25 Minutes, DeKalb County Hospital Authority, September 9, 1963; February 10, 1964.
26 Minutes, DeKalb County Hospital Authority, January 14, 1963.
27 Minutes, DeKalb County Hospital Authority, February 12, 1968.
28 Minutes, DeKalb County Hospital Authority, June 11, 1962.
29 Minutes, DeKalb County Hospital Authority, May 14, 1962.
30 Minutes, DeKalb County Hospital Authority, May 14, 1962.
31 Minutes, DeKalb County Hospital Authority, September 13, 1961.
32 Minutes, DeKalb County Hospital Authority, June 11, 1962.
33 Minutes, DeKalb County Hospital Authority, November 14, 1966.
34 Minutes, DeKalb County Hospital Authority, December 11, 1961.
35 Minutes, DeKalb County Hospital Authority, October 8, 1962.
36 Minutes, DeKalb County Hospital Authority, October 14, 1963; March 9, 1964; April 20, 1964.
37 Minutes, DeKalb County Hospital Authority, October 12, 1964.
38 Minutes, DeKalb County Hospital Authority, March 14, 1966.
39 "History—DeKalb General," Author and date unknown, p. 5.
40 "Public Law 89-97: Medicare and Medicaid 1965," *Healthcare Professions Delivery Systems*, http://www.nvcc.edu./home/bhays/dogwood/medicareact.htm, 8/13/05.
41 Minutes, DeKalb County Hospital Authority, July 11, 1964.
42 Minutes, DeKalb County Hospital Authority, October 8, 1962.
43 Announcement for first DGH Christmas Open House.
44 Minutes, DeKalb County Hospital Authority, February 12, 1968.
45 Minutes, DeKalb County Hospital Authority, February 10, 1964.
46 Minutes, DeKalb County Hospital Authority, March 8, 1965.
47 Minutes, DeKalb County Hospital Authority, September 13, 1965.
48 Minutes, DeKalb County Hospital Authority, December 13, 1965.
49 Minutes, DeKalb County Hospital Authority, August 15, 1966.
50 Minutes, DeKalb County Hospital Authority, October 12, 1964.
51 Minutes, Annual Meeting, DeKalb County Hospital Authority, October 1, 1969.
52 Minutes, Medical Staff Executive Committee, September 1969.
53 Minutes, Medical Staff Executive Committee, September 1969.
54 Minutes, DeKalb County Hospital Authority, August 11, 1965; August 16, 1965.
55 "Dr. Evans, Area Doctor, Retires After 50 Years," *The Neighbor*, April 14, 1975.
56 "Dr. J. Rufus Evans to Receive Distinguished Service Award," *The General InDecatur*, November 10, 1972.
57 "Dr. Evans, Area Doctor . . . ."
58 The General InDecatur, November 10, 1972.
59 Minutes, DeKalb County Hospital Authority, July 2, 1962; September 10, 1962.
60 Minutes, DeKalb County Hospital Authority, July 8, 1963.
61 Minutes, DeKalb County Hospital Authority, February 8, 1965.
62 Minutes, DeKalb County Hospital Authority, June14, 1965.
63 Atkins, Ernie, MD, Lecture: "The History of DeKalb Medical Center."
64 Opal Fyffe letter to William H. Thrasher, July 12, 1965.
65 Cathleen Conway Johnson, "The Troubles with Angels of Mercy: The Mass Resignation of Registered Nurses at DeKalb General Hospital, Decatur, Georgia, January 22, 1969." A thesis submitted to the Faculty of the Graduate School of Emory University in partial fulfillment of the requirements for the degree of Doctor of Philosophy, The Graduate Institute of Liberal Arts, 1994.
66 Johnson, p. 43.
67 J. Ross McCain, "Some Notes As To Groundbreaking, DeKalb General Hospital," May 15, 1959.
68 Minutes, DeKalb County Hospital Authority, February 10, 1964.
69 Mary Thomas, "D.G.H. History 1961-1976, 15th Anniversary," *The Atlanta Journal-Constitution*, May 1, 1976.
70 Minutes, DeKalb County Hospital Authority, February 12, 1968; February 7, 1966.
71 Minutes, DeKalb County Hospital Authority, May 24, 1961.
72 Minutes, DeKalb County Hospital Authority, May 24, 1961; June 10, 1964.

73 Minutes, DeKalb County Hospital Authority, November 12, 1962.
74 Minutes, DeKalb County Hospital Authority, November 12, 1962.
75 Minutes, DeKalb County Hospital Authority, January 20, 1964.
76 Minutes, DeKalb County Hospital Authority, July 8, 1963.
77 Minutes, DeKalb County Hospital Authority, May 11, 1964.
78 Minutes, DeKalb County Hospital Authority, December 9, 1963.
79 Minutes, DeKalb County Hospital Authority, August 12, 1963.
80 Minutes, DeKalb County Hospital Authority, September 9, 1963.
81 Minutes, DeKalb County Hospital Authority, May 11, 1964; June 10, 1964.
82 Minutes, DeKalb County Hospital Authority, January 20, 1965.
83 Minutes, DeKa!b County Hospital Authority, August 15, 1966.
84 Minutes, DeKalb County Hospital Authority, October 10, 1966; November 14, 1966; December 7, 1966.
85 Minutes, DeKalb County Hospital Authority, April 10, 1967.
86 Minutes, DeKalb County Hospital Authority, January 20, 1965.
87 Minutes, DeKalb County Hospital Authority, February 10, 1964
88 Minutes, Joint Meeting of the DeKalb County Hospital Authority, DeKalb County Board of Commissioners, and the Community Council of the Atlanta Area, Inc., December 1, 1965; Minutes, DeKalb County Hospital Authority, December 13, 1965.
89 Minutes, DeKalb County Hospital Authority, December 13, 1965; Minutes, Joint Meeting of the DeKalb County Hospital Authority, DeKalb County Board of Commissioners, and the Community Council of the Atlanta Area, Inc., December 21, 1965.
90 Minutes, Joint Meeting of the DeKalb Count Board of Commissioners and the DeKalb County Hospital Authority, December 21, 1965.
91 Minutes, Joint Meeting of the DeKalb County Hospital Authority, DeKalb County Board of Commissioners, and the Community Council of the Atlanta Area, Inc., December 21, 1965.
92 Minutes, DeKalb County Hospital Authority, January 10, 1966; February 7, 1966.
93 Minutes, DeKalb County Hospital Authority, April 10, 1967.
94 Minutes, DeKalb County Hospital Authority, June 12, 1967.
95 Minutes, DeKalb County Hospital Authority, November 13, 1967.
96 Minutes, Special Meeting, DeKalb County Hospital Authority, December 11, 1967.
97 Minutes, DeKalb County Hospital Authority, January 8, 1968.
98 Minutes, DeKalb County Hospital Authority, March 11, 1968.
99 Minutes, Special Meeting, DeKalb County Hospital Authority, May 21, 1968.
100 Minutes, DeKalb County Hospital Authority, June 6, 1968; *The General InDecatur*, November 10, 1972.
101 L. G. Davis, Robert E. McKee General Contractors, Inc., letter to Bothwell Associates, July 2, 1968.
102 Minutes, DeKalb County Hospital Authority, October 21, 1968; January 13, 1969.
103 Mary Thomas; Minutes, DeKalb County Hospital Authority, July 16, 1970; October 5, 1970; September 13, 1971.
104 Minutes, DeKalb County Hospital Authority, October 4, 1971.
105 Minutes, DeKalb County Hospital Authority, March 2, 1970.
106 Minutes, DeKalb County Hospital Authority, May 12, 1969.
107 Minutes, DeKalb County Hospital Authority, May 12, 1969; Mattie L. Meadows, Director of Dietary, memorandum to William H. Thrasher, February 6, 1969, "Temporary Feeding Arrangements While the Contractor Has Possession of the Present Kitchen and Dining Facilities".
108 "New Addition Nearly Ready," DeKalb New Era, July 9, 1970.
109 "DeKalb Hospital Expansion Jumps Ahead of Schedule," *The Atlanta Journal*, January 14, 1970.
110 "DeKalb Hospital Expansion Jumps Ahead;" Mary Thomas.

Chapter Four

1 Opal Hopkins Fyffe interview, March 3, 2006; Minutes, DeKalb County Hospital Authority, April 9, 1962.
2 Fyffe interview.
3 Minutes, DeKalb County Hospital Authority, August 30, 1961.
4 Minutes, Special Meeting, DeKalb County Hospital Authority, May 28, 1962.
5 Minutes, DeKalb County Hospital Authority, June 11, 1962.
6 Minutes, DeKalb County Hospital Authority, November 13, 1961.
7 Minutes, DeKalb County Hospital Authority, June 11, 1962.
8 Minutes, DeKalb County Hospital Authority, November 8, 1965.
9 Minutes, DeKalb Hospital Authority, June 14, 1965.
10 Minutes, DeKalb County Hospital Authority, December 11, 1967.
11 Minutes, DeKalb County Hospital Authority, December 11, 1967.
12 Minutes, DeKalb County Hospital Authority, August 12, 1963.
13 Minutes, DeKalb County Hospital Authority, July 13, 1964.
14 Minutes, DeKalb County Hospital Authority, May 9, 1963.
15 Minutes, DeKalb County Hospital Authority, June 10, 1963.
16 Minutes, DeKalb County Hospital Authority, May 11, 1964.
17 Fyffe interview.
18 Fyffe interview.
19 Minutes, DeKalb County Hospital Authority, March 8, 1965.
20 Fyffe interview.
21 "60 Seconds With Naomi Harman," *InDecatur*, March 1996.
22 Fyffe interview.
23 Opal Fyffe letter to William H. Thrasher, July 12, 1965.
24 Richard F. Newcomb, "Should Nurses Strike? A Test Case In Georgia," *RN Magazine*, June, 1969, p. 42.
25 Minutes, DeKalb County Hospital Authority, November 8, 1965.
26 Newcomb, p. 42.
27 Minutes, DeKalb County Hospital Authority, March 14, 1966, April 11, 1966.
28 Minutes, DeKalb County Hospital Authority, June 13, 1966.
29 Minutes, Medical Staff Executive Committee, May, 1967.
30 Minutes, DeKalb County Hospital Authority, May 8, 1967.
31 Minutes, DeKalb County Hospital Authority, September 18, 1967.
32 Minutes, Finance Committee, DeKalb County Hospital Authority, , December 8, 1967.
33 Minutes, DeKalb County Hospital Authority, December 11, 1967.
34 Minutes, DeKalb County Hospital Authority, September 18, 1967; December 11, 1967.

35 Johnson, Cathleen Conway, *The Troubles with Angels of Mercy: The Mass Resignation of Registered Nurses at DeKalb General Hospital Decatur, Georgia, January 22, 1969*, a thesis submitted to the faculty of the Graduate School of Emory University in partial fulfillment of the requirement for the degree of Doctor of Philosophy, The Graduate Institute of Liberal Arts, 1994, pp. 20f.
36 Johnson, p. 39.
37 Johnson, p. 41.
38 Johnson, p. 44f.
39 Fyffe interview.
40 Johnson, p. 48.
41 Johnson, p. 63.
42 Johnson, pp. 48, 74.
43 Johnson, p. 40.
44 Johnson, pp. 50, 83.
45 Johnson, p. 40.
46 Johnson, p. 83.
47 Minutes, Finance Committee, DeKalb General Hospital, November 11, 1968.
48 Johnson, pp. 79-82.
49 Johnson, pp. 83-86.
50 Minutes, DeKalb County Hospital Authority, December 9, 1968.
51 Minutes, DeKalb County Hospital Authority, December 9, 1968.
52 Minutes, DeKalb County Hospital Authority, December 9, 1968.
53 Minutes, DeKalb County Hospital Authority, December 9, 1968.
54 Minutes, Finance Committee, DeKalb County Hospital Authority, December 16, 1968.
55 Minutes, Finance Committee, DeKalb County Hospital Authority, December 16, 1968.
56 Johnson, p. 95.
57 Johnson, p. 108.
58 Johnson, pp. 91-100.
59 Johnson, p. 101.
60 Johnson, p. 142.
61 Johnson, p. 104.
62 Johnson, pp. 106, 112.
63 Newcomb, p. 43, Johnson, p. 111.
64 Minutes, DeKalb County Hospital Authority, January 13, 1969.
65 William H. Thrasher letter to Stanley Kravit, Director, Economic Security Project, January 14, 1969.
66 Johnson, p.114.
67 Minutes, DeKalb County Hospital Authority, January 13, 1969.
68 William H. Thrasher press statement, January 13, 1969.
69 *The Atlanta Journal*, Thursday, January 16, 1969, Johnson, p. 120.
70 Johnson, p. 116.
71 Fyffe interview.
72 Fyffe interview.
73 Fyffe interview.
74 Johnson, p. 116.
75 Fyffe interview.
76 Johnson, p. 122.
77 Johnson, pp. 123f.
78 Newcomb, p. 43.
79 Johnson, p. 124.
80 Johnson, p. 124; Newcomb, p. 43.
81 Newcomb, p. 43.
82 Johnson, p. 125.
83 Minutes, Special Meeting, Executive Committee of the Medical Staff, January 18, 1969.
84 Minutes, Special Meeting, Executive Committee of the Medical Staff, January 19, 1969.
85 Johnson, p. 134.
86 Minutes, Special Meeting, DeKalb County Hospital Authority, January 19, 1969.
87 Minutes, Special Meeting, DeKalb County Hospital Authority, January 19, 1969.
88 Johnson, p. 134.
89 Newcomb, p. 44f.
90 Johnson, p. 139.
91 Johnson pp. 140f.
92 Minutes, Special Meeting, Executive Committee of the Medical Staff, February 1, 1969.
93 Johnson, p. 108.
94 Newcomb, p. 47.
95 Johnson, p. 135.
96 Johnson, p. 135.
97 Minutes, Medical Staff Executive Committee, February 24, 1969.
98 Minutes, DeKalb County Hospital Authority, October 13, 1969.
99 Minutes, DeKalb County Hospital Authority, April 21, 1969.
100 Minutes, DeKalb County Hospital Authority, September 8, 1969.
101 Johnson, pp. 144f.
102 Minutes, DeKalb County Hospital Authority, April 14, 1969.
103 Minutes, DeKalb County Hospital Authority, February 10, 1969.
104 Minutes, DeKalb County Hospital Authority, April 21, 1969.
105 Minutes, DeKalb County Hospital Authority, March 10, 1969.
106 Minutes, Medical Staff Executive Committee, February 24, 1969.
107 Minutes, DeKalb County Hospital Authority, March 10, 1969; July 7, 1969.
108 Minutes, Finance Committee, DeKalb County Hospital Authority, March 6, 1969.
109 Newcomb, p. 40.
110 Johnson, p. 159.
111 Johnson, p. 159.
112 Johnson, p. 160.

Chapter Five

1 *DeKalb Medical Center Analysis of Corporate Restructuring*, March 23, 1992, p.1.
2 DeKalb Medical Center Analysis, p. 5.
3 James C. Rawls, Attorney, letter to Charles H. Anderson, April 13, 1987.
4 Charles B. Eberhart, CEO, memorandum to W. P. Tatum, chairman, DeKalb County Hospital Authority, September 17, 1990.
5 Eberhart memorandum.
6 W. P. Tatum, chairman, memorandum to members, DeKalb County Hospital Authority, October 1, 1990.
7 *DeKalb Medical Center Analysis*, p. 24.
8 Unified Government of Athens-Clarke County et al. v. Hospital Authority of Clarke County Et Al. 278 Ga. 17, S04A0449.
9 Gail Hagans, "Hospital Panel To Get New Candidate: Unterman Agrees To Send Second Slate," *The Atlanta Journal/The Atlanta Constitution*, December 12, 1991; Scott Rafshoon, "Wall Seeks To Nullify Hospital Meeting," *The Gwinnett Daily News*, December 11, 1991.
10 1976 HB 445, "Hospital Authorities; Conflicts of Interest."
11 O.C.G.A. § 31-7-74 (a).
12 James C. Rawls, Attorney, letter to Jonathan Weintraub, Esquire, Re: "Downsizing of DeKalb County Hospital Authority," November 22, 1993; Minutes, DeKalb County Hospital Authority, November 1994.
13 Minutes, DeKalb County Hospital Authority, January 1997; John R. Gerlach, assistant secretary, DeKalb County Hospital Authority, attachment to letter to DeKalb County Commissioner Elaine Boyer, October 6, 1997.
14 Minutes, DeKalb County Hospital Authority, October 2001.
15 Theresa Racine, "Hospital Authority Members Needed," *The Champion*, November 10, 1993
16 Charles Eberhart, CEO, letter to James C. Rawls, Attorney, November 1, 1994.
17 Exempt minutes, called meeting DeKalb County Hospital Authority, March 28, 1991.
18 James C. Rawls, Attorney, letter to Internal Revenue Service Assistant Commissioner, May 27, 1993, p. 3.

19 "Lease and Transfer Agreement by and between DeKalb County Hospital Authority and DeKalb Medical Center, Inc.," *DeKalb Medical Center Lease and Transfer of Property and Assets as of April 1, 1992, by and Between The DeKalb County Hospital Authority as Lessor and Transferor and DeKalb Medical Center, In., as Lessee and Transferee*, March 23, 1992, Section 9.1; Rawls letter to Assistant Commissioner, p. 12; Exempt minutes, DeKalb County Hospital Authority, May 1992; Minutes, DeKalb County Hospital Authority, March, 1992.
20 "Lease and Transfer Agreement," Section 2.3.
21 Minutes, DeKalb County Hospital Authority, November, 1993.
22 Rawls letter to Internal Revenue Service Assistant Commissioner, p. 3.
23 Minutes, DeKalb Regional Healthcare System, Inc. Board of Directors, April 1993.
24 "DRHS Board Approves Changes in Hospital System Governance," DeKalb Medical Center - Intranet, http://intranet2.drhs.org/dept/index.cfm?p=msp&pg_id=5071, April 20, 2007.
25 "DRHS Moves Forward With New Governance and Medical Staff Structures," *InDecatur*, January/February 2004.
26 "DRHS Board Approves Changes . . ."
27 "DRHS Moves Forward. . . ": "DRHS Board Approves."

Chapter Six

1 Minutes, DeKalb County Hospital Authority, August 1965.
2 Minutes, DeKalb Healthcare Regional System, Inc., Board of Directors, November 1994.
3 Minutes, DeKalb County Hospital Authority, July 7, 1986.
4 Minutes, DeKalb Medical Center, Inc., Board of Directors, June 5, 1995.
5 Minutes, DeKalb Medical Center, Inc., Board of Directors, September 6, 1994.
6 Minutes, DeKalb Medical Center, Inc., Board of Directors, May 2, 1994.
7 Minutes, DeKalb Medical Center, Inc., Board of Directors, July 5, 1994.
8 Minutes, DeKalb Healthcare Regional System, Inc., Board of Directors, January 3, 1995.
9 Minutes, DeKalb Healthcare Regional System, Inc., Board of Directors, April, 1995.
10 Minutes, Combined DeKalb Medical Center, Inc., Board of Directors and DeKalb Regional Healthcare, Inc., Board of Directors, May 25, 1995; Minutes, DeKalb Healthcare Regional System, Inc., Board of Directors, July 10, 1995; Minutes, DeKalb Healthcare Regional System, Inc., Board of Directors, October 2, 1995.
11 Minutes, DeKalb Healthcare Regional System, Inc., Board of Directors, November 6, 1995.
12 Minutes, DeKalb Healthcare Regional System, Inc., Board of Directors, January 8, 1996.
13 Robert J. Baudino memorandum to the Board of Directors, DeKalb Regional Healthcare Systems, Inc., and DeKalb Medical Center, Inc., January 2, 1996, "Affiliation/Merger Initiatives".
14 Robert J. Baudino memorandum to the Board of Directors, DeKalb Regional Healthcare Systems, Inc., November 30, 1994, "Evaluation of Hospital Network Options".
15 Minutes, DeKalb Healthcare Regional System, Inc., Board of Directors, January 3, 1995; Minutes, DeKalb Healthcare Regional System, Inc., Board of Directors, February 6, 1995.
16 Minutes, DeKalb Healthcare Regional System, Inc., Board of Directors, February 6, 1995.
17 DeKalb Healthcare Regional System, Inc., Board of Directors, May 1, 1995.
18 Minutes, DeKalb Healthcare Regional System, Inc., Board of Directors, October 2, 1995.
19 Minutes, DeKalb Healthcare Regional System, Inc., Board of Directors, January 8, 1996.
20 Robert J. Baudino memorandum, January 2, 1996.
21 Minutes, DeKalb Healthcare Regional System, Inc., Board of Directors, November 6, 1995.
22 Minutes, DeKalb Healthcare Regional System, Inc., Board of Directors, December 4, 1995.
23 Minutes, DeKalb Healthcare Regional System, Inc., Board of Directors, March 4, 1996.
24 Summary Minutes of the DeKalb Regional Health Board Ad Hoc Horizontal Integration Committee, March 28, 1996; John R. Gerlach memorandum to the Ad Hoc DRHS Board Committee on Horizontal Integration, March 26, 1996, "Committee Meeting."
25 John R. Gerlach memorandum to DeKalb Regional Healthcare System, Inc., Board of Directors, April 1, 1996, "Management's Recommendations for Affiliation."
26 Gerlach memorandum, April 1, 1996.
27 Gerlach memorandum, April 1, 1996.
28 "Change is Good—You Go First: Promina Goes Virtual," *Hospitals & Health Networks Pacesetters: Supplement to Hospitals & Health Network, Fall, 1998*, Pages 10-15.
29 Gerlach memorandum, April 1, 1996.
30 Gerlach memorandum, April 1, 1996.
31 Gerlach memorandum, March 26, 1996.
32 Gerlach memorandum, April 1, 1996.
33 Minutes, DeKalb Healthcare Regional System, Inc., Board of Directors, April1, 1996.
34 Minutes, Special Meeting of the DeKalb Healthcare Regional System, Inc., Board of Directors to Study the Affiliation With PROMINA, August 16, 1996.
35 Minutes, DeKalb Healthcare Regional System, Inc., Board of Directors, May 6, 1996.
36 Minutes, May 6, 1996.
37 Bernard L. Brown, Jr., CEO, PROMINA Health System and Charles Krivenko, MD, Coordinator of Physician Integration Study Group for PROMINA's Health System memorandum to John R. Gerlach, CEO, DeKalb Regional Healthcare System, and Paul R. Crank, Jr., MD, Coordinator of Physician Integration Study Group for DeKalb Regional Healthcare System, June 24, 1996, "Response to Outstanding Issues in Physician Integration Study Group".
38 Brown, June 24, 1996.
39 "DeKalb Doctors Worry Promina Alliance Would Hurt Private Practices," *The Atlanta Business Chronicle*, August 19, 1996.
40 "DeKalb Doctors Worry . . .": "Promina Northwest Recruits 165 More Doctors," *The Atlanta Business Chronicle*, October 14, 1996.
41 "DeKalb Doctors Worry . . ."
42 "The Physicians Study Group Executive Report: A Feasibility Study on an Affiliation with PROMINA," Submitted to DeKalb Regional Healthcare System, Inc., Board of Directors, August 5, 1996.
43 "The Physicians Study Group . . ."
44 Minutes, Special Meeting of the DeKalb Healthcare Regional System, Inc., Board of Directors to Study the Affiliation With PROMINA, August 16, 1996.
45 Minutes, DeKalb Healthcare Regional System, Inc., Board of Directors, October 7, 1996.
46 Minutes, DeKalb Healthcare Regional System, Inc., Board of Directors, December 2, 1996.
47 Minutes, DeKalb Healthcare Regional System, Inc., Board of Directors, February 12, 1997.
48 Minutes, DeKalb Healthcare Regional System, Inc., Board of Directors, March 3, 1997.
49 Minutes, DeKalb Healthcare Regional System, Inc., Board of Directors, July 7, 1997.
50 John R. Gerlach, CEO, "DMC Finalizes PROMINA Affiliation," Medical Staff Communique, April, 1997.
51 News Release: "PROMINA Board of Directors Adopts Fiscal Year 1998 Budget," June 12, 1997.
52 "Change is Good—You Go First."
53 "Change is Good—You Go First."

54 "Change is Good—You Go First."
55 Gerlach, "DMC Finalizes PROMINA Affiliation."
56 "Change is Good—You Go First."
57 "Promina's CEO Says Integrated Delivery Works," *The Atlanta Business Chronicle*, January 18, 1999.
58 John Gerlach, "Current Issues," *InDecatur*, June 1998.
59 John Gerlach, "Current Issues," *InDecatur*, April 1999.
60 "Change is Good—You Go First."
61 "Change is Good—You Go First."
62 "Change is Good—You Go First."
63 "Change is Good—You Go First."
64 "Promina's CEO Says Integrated Delivery Works."
65 Bernard Brown, "Lasting Lessons," *Hospitals & Health Networks Pacesetters: Supplement to Hospitals & Health Network, Fall, 1998*, Pages 2-3.
66 "Change is Good—You Go First."
67 "Southern Regional Calls for Resignations," *The Atlanta Business Chronicle*, April 12, 2000.
68 "Bonnie Phipps Named PROMINA Chief Executive," *PROMINA System Update*, April 2001.
69 Minutes, DeKalb Regional Healthcare System, Inc., Board of Directors, August 5, 2002.
70 "Hospital CEOs Say Goodbye," *The Atlanta Business Chronicle*, December 24, 2001.
71 John R. Gerlach letter to DeKalb Medical Center Physicians, September 1, 1999.
72 "Hospital System Evolving," *The Atlanta Business Chronicle*, May 17-23, 2002.
73 James C. Rawls letter to John R. Gerlach, September 1, 1999.
74 "Hospital Systems' $9M Dispute Now A Lawsuit," *The Atlanta Business Chronicle*, September 17, 2001.
75 Minutes, DeKalb Regional Healthcare System, Inc., Board of Directors, December 3, 2001.
76 "Hospital System Evolving."
77 Minutes, DeKalb Regional Healthcare System, Inc., Board of Directors, November 4, 2002.
78 Minutes, Executive Session, DeKalb Regional Healthcare System, Inc., Board of Directors, October 7, 2002.
79 Minutes, DeKalb Regional Healthcare System, Inc., Board of Directors, September 2, 2003; "Piedmont Hospital's Ties to Promina Severed," *The Atlanta Business Chronicle*, August 27, 2003.
80 "Piedmont Withdraws from PROMINA; DRHS Pledges to Remain Active Member," *InDecatur*, December, 2002.
81 "'Quasi' Insurers Draw Attention From Regulator," *The Atlanta Business Chronicle*, February 11, 1002
82 Minutes, Finance Committee, DeKalb Regional Healthcare System, Inc., May 30, 2002.
83 Julie Bryant, "Promina Health System Exiting Managed Care," *The Atlanta Business Chronicle*, July 26, 2002.
84 "Amidst Changes, Hospital System's Future Uncertain," *The Atlanta Business Chronicle*, August 19, 2002.
85 Minutes, DeKalb Regional Healthcare System, Inc., Board of Directors, May 6, 2002.
86 Susan Shelton, DeKalb PHO, memorandum to Bonnie Phipps et al, March 20, 2002, "Reconciliation of Risk Contract Balances;" Minutes, DeKalb Regional Healthcare System, Inc., Board of Directors, June 18, 2002.
87 Minutes, DeKalb Regional Healthcare System, Inc., Board of Directors, March 4, 2002.
88 Minutes, Finance Committee, DeKalb Regional Healthcare System, Inc., October 1, 2002.
89 Minutes, Executive Session, DeKalb Regional Healthcare System, Inc., Board of Directors, October 7, 2002.
90 Minutes, Finance Committee, DeKalb Regional Healthcare System, Inc., November 26, 2002.
91 Julie Bryant, July 26, 2002.
92 Minutes, DeKalb Regional Healthcare System, Inc., Board of Directors, October 1, 2002; Minutes, DeKalb Regional Healthcare System, Inc., Board of Directors, December 2, 2002; DeKalb Regional Healthcare System, Inc., Board of Directors, April 7, 2003.
93 "Promina Aims to Standardize Patient Care," *The Atlanta Business Chronicle*, November 26, 2001.
94 "The State of the System," PROMINA Doctors and Hospitals, Spring, 2002.
95 Julie Bryant, "Doctors to Be Paid for Quality," *The Atlanta Business Chronicle*, May 23, 2002.
96 "Promina Restructures, Drops Managed Care Contracting," *The Atlanta Business Chronicle*, October 31, 2003.
97 Eric Norwood, President and CEO, memorandum to DRHS Physicians, Governing Board and Employee Partners, October 31, 2003, "Restructuring the PROMINA Health System."
98 Minutes, DeKalb Regional Healthcare System, Inc., Board of Directors, December 2, 2002.
99 Minutes, DeKalb Regional Healthcare System, Inc., Board of Directors, June 7, 2004.
100 Minutes, DeKalb Regional Healthcare System, Inc., Board of Directors, January 9, 2003; Minutes, DeKalb Regional Healthcare System, Inc., Board of Directors, March 3, 2003.
101 Minutes, DeKalb Regional Healthcare System, Inc., Board of Directors, February 2, 2004.
102 Eric Norwood interview, August 21, 2008.

Chapter Seven

1 Minutes, DeKalb County Hospital Authority, February 1, 1988.
2 *InDecatur*, April 1990.
3 Charles B. Eberhart, CEO, memorandum to DeKalb Medical Center, Inc., Board of Directors, July 29, 1993, "Professional Services Committee's Recommendation Regarding Acquisition of Primary Care Practices."
4 Frank Houser, MD, Medical Director, External Operations, The Emory University System of Health Care, letter to an unidentified DeKalb Medical Center family physician, August 18, 1993.
5 Minutes, DeKalb Medical Center, Inc., Board of Directors, August 2, 1993.
6 Primary Care Division Budget, DeKalb Medical Center, Inc. Board of Directors Packet, March 7, 1994.
7 Minutes, DeKalb Medical Center, Inc., Board of Directors, September 9, 1993.
8 CEO Strategic Update to the DRHS Board of Directors, October, 2006.
9 "DRHS Primary Care Physicians" in DeKalb Regional Healthcare System, Inc. Board of Directors Packet for July 1, 1996; "Emory, Promina Expanding to Meet Demand," *Atlanta Business Chronicle*, October 20, 1997.
10 "International Medical Center Opens Its Doors to Multicultural Community," *InDecatur*, December, 1997.
11 "DMC Opens Senior Health Center," *InDecatur*, September, 1999.
12 Author's personal notes of that meeting.
13 Andy Morley, MD, "Executive Summary for a Primary Care Initiative: the Establishment of Network Medical Services Inc., a Medical Service Organization, a Component of the Network Development Plan Affiliated with DeKalb Medical Center and Related Practices," 1994.
14 Network Medical Services, March 17, 2000.
15 Minutes, Finance Committee, DeKalb Regional Healthcare System, Inc., July 30, 2002.
16 Personal communication, the author and Frank Houser, M.D., Vice President for Physician Affairs, Nashville, Tennessee, 2002.
17 Andy Miller, "DeKalb Medical Center Cuts Docs' Pay," *The Atlanta Journal-Constitution*, January 29, 2003.
18 Minutes, Finance Committee, DeKalb Regional Healthcare System, Inc., January 10, 2001.

19 Minutes, Buildings and Grounds Committee, DeKalb Regional Health System, Inc., January 26, 2006.
20 Minutes, Finance Committee, DeKalb Regional Healthcare System, Inc., March 27, 2002.
21 Minutes, Finance Committee, DeKalb Regional Healthcare System, Inc., July 30, 2002.
22 Andy Miller; Minutes, Finance Committee, DeKalb Regional Healthcare System, Inc., March 27, 2002.
23 Minutes, DeKalb County Hospital Authority, October 3, 1983.
24 Minutes, DeKalb Medical Center, Inc., Board of Directors, March 1, 1993.
25 Minutes, DeKalb Medical Center, Inc., Board of Directors, February 1, 1993.
26 Minutes, DeKalb Medical Center, Inc., Board of Directors, April 5, 1993.
27 Wytch Stubbs, MD, from Director of Medical Affairs memorandum to Charles B. Eberhart, CEO, May 19, 1993, "PHO Vote."
28 Minutes, DeKalb Medical Center, Inc., Board of Directors, November 1, 1993.
29 Minutes, DeKalb Medical Center, Inc., Board of Directors, December 6, 1993.
30 Judy Mitchell, "Current Issues: DeKalb Physician Hospital Organization," *InDecatur*, September, 1995.
31 Minutes, DeKalb Medical Center, Inc., Board of Directors, July 1, 1995.
32 "DeKalb PHO Announces CEO, Board of Directors," *InDecatur*, January, 1995.
33 Minutes, DeKalb Medical Center, Inc., Board of Directors, November 2, 1994.
34 Minutes, DeKalb Medical Center, Inc., Board of Directors, April 4, 1994.
35 "DeKalb PHO Announces CEO, Board of Directors," InDecatur, January, 1995.
36 Judy Mitchell.
37 Minutes, DeKalb Medical Center, Inc., Board of Directors, November 2, 1994.
38 Minutes, DeKalb Medical Center, Inc., Board of Directors, November 6, 1995.
39 Minutes, DeKalb Medical Center, Inc., Board of Directors, August 7, 1995.
40 Minutes, DeKalb Regional Healthcare System, Inc., Board of Directors, February 5, 1996.
41 Minutes, DeKalb Regional Healthcare System, Inc., Board of Directors, June 3, 1996.
42 Minutes, DeKalb Regional Healthcare System, Inc., Board of Directors, April 1, 1996.
43 "The DeKalb Physician Hospital Organization: A Brief History."
44 Minutes, DeKalb Physician Hospital Organization Board of Directors, March 12, 1996.
45 Minutes, DeKalb Medical Center, Inc., Board of Directors, December 2, 1996.
46 Copy, check from DeKalb Physician Hospital Organization made out to DeKalb Medical Center in the amount of $596,543.83, dated December 11, 1996.
47 Susan Helton, Executive Director, DPHO, memorandum to John R. Gerlach, CEO, DeKalb Medical Center, February 1, 1999, "Assessment of Medical Management Agreement With DeKalb Medical Center."
48 Minutes, DeKalb Medical Center, Inc., Board of Directors, January 1, 2001.
49 Minutes, DeKalb Medical Center, Inc., Board of Directors, May 7, 2001.
50 Minutes, DeKalb Medical Center Finance Committee, February 25, 2003.
51 Minutes, DeKalb Medical Center, Inc., Board of Directors, May 7, 2001.
52 Minutes, DeKalb Regional Healthcare System, Inc., Board of Directors, January 14, 2005.
53 "Clinical Integration Participation Agreement Between DeKalb Medical Center, Inc., Decatur Health Resources, Inc. And DeKalb Physician Hospital Organization, Inc."
54 "Clinical Integration and the DeKalb Quality Institute," Performance Improvement Council Document, August 31, 2004.
55 Minutes, DeKalb Regional Healthcare System, Inc., Board of Directors, June 13, 2005.

Chapter Eight

1 Constitution of the DeKalb County Hospital Authority, September, 1957.
2 Kelly D. Hamborg and Robert J. Baudino, Jr., memorandum to the Board of Directors of DeKalb Regional Healthcare System, Inc., and DeKalb Medical Center, Inc., June 30, 1998, "Decatur Hospital."
3 Minutes, Professional Service Committee, September 13, 1971.
4 Robert J. Baudino, Attorney, memorandum to Members of the Board of Directors of DeKalb Medical Center, February 1, 1993, "Decatur Hospital/OrNda Healthcorp."
5 Baudino memorandum.
6 Baudino memorandum.
7 Baudino memorandum.
8 Baudino memorandum.
9 Baudino memorandum.
10 Baudino memorandum.
11 Charles Eberhart, CEO, letter to Charles N. Martin, Jr, President, and Douglas B. Lewis, Senior Vice President, OrNda Healthcorp, July 20, 1993.
12 Minutes, DeKalb Medical Center, In. Board of Directors, Executive Session, August 2, 1993.
13 Charles Eberhart, CEO, letter to Charles N. Martin, Jr., President, and Douglas B. Lewis, Senior Vice President, OrNda Healthcorp, November 3, 1993.
14 "Decatur Hospital Within the DeKalb Regional Healthcare System, Inc.," InDecatur, November 1994.
15 Minutes, DeKalb Regional Healthcare Systems, Inc., Board of Directors Called Meeting, December 17, 1993.
16 Charles B. Eberhart, CEO, memorandum to DeKalb Medical Center, Inc., Board Members, December 30, 1993, "Decatur Hospital."
17 Robert J. Baudino, Attorney, letter to Charles Eberhart, CEO, DeKalb Medical Center, April 4, 1994.
18 Robert J. Baudino, Attorney, letter to Douglas B. Lewis, Vice President, OrNda Healthcorp, April 13, 1994.
19 Minutes, DeKalb Regional Healthcare Systems, Inc., Board of Directors Called Meeting, June 6, 1994.
20 "DeKalb Medical Center Finalizes Decatur Hospital Purchase," *InDecatur*, May 31, 1994
21 Minutes, DeKalb Regional Healthcare Systems, Inc., Board of Directors Called Meeting, June 6, 1994.
22 Minutes, DeKalb Regional Healthcare Systems, Inc., Board of Directors Called Meeting, June 6, 1994; Minutes, DeKalb Regional Healthcare Systems, Inc., Board of Directors, July 1, 1996.
23 Minutes, DeKalb County Hospital Authority, October 28, 1996; Minutes, DeKalb Regional Healthcare Systems, Inc., Board of Directors, September 3, 1996.
24 Minutes, DeKalb Regional Healthcare Systems, Inc., Board of Directors, June 3, 2002.
25 Carol Nikola, CEO Decatur Hospital, memorandum to John R. Gerlach, COO DeKalb Medical Center and Bonnie Phipps, CFO DeKalb Medical Center, April 19, 1995.
26 Minutes, DeKalb Regional Healthcare Systems, Inc., Board of Directors, November 6, 1995.
27 "Decatur Hospital Offers New Services," *InDecatur*, July 1996.
28 Minutes, DeKalb Regional Healthcare Systems, Inc., Board of Directors, November 6, 2000.
29 Minutes, DeKalb Regional Healthcare Systems, Inc., Board of Directors, March 4, 2002.
30 Minutes, DeKalb Regional Healthcare Systems, Inc., Board of Directors, March 4, 2002;

"Wound Care Center Moves to 2665 Professional Building," *InDecatur*, August 2002; "Wound Care Center Introduces New Treatment," *InDecatur*, July 2003.
31 Minutes, DeKalb Regional Healthcare Systems, Inc., Board of Directors, August 3, 1998; "Decatur Hospital Offers New Services," *InDecatur*, July 1996.
32 "Decatur Hospital Offers New Services," *InDecatur*, July 1996.
33 Richard Schmidt, "Current Issues," *InDecatur,* September 1997.
34 Minutes, DeKalb Regional Healthcare Systems, Inc., Board of Directors, November 3, 1997.
35 Minutes, Decatur Health Resources, Inc., Board of Directors, June 17, 1997; Minutes, Decatur Health Resources, Inc., Board of Directors, October 21, 1997.
36 Minutes, DeKalb Regional Healthcare Systems, Inc., Board of Directors, September 8, 1998.
37 "Decatur Hospital Offers New Services," *InDecatur*, July 1996; Richard Schmidt.
38 "Decatur Hospital Expands LTAC Unit," *InDecatur*, May 1999.
39 Richard Schmidt.
40 Minutes, DeKalb Regional Healthcare Systems, Inc., Board of Directors, January 6, 1997.
41 Minutes, DeKalb Regional Healthcare Systems, Inc., Board of Directors, October 6, 1997.
42 Minutes, DeKalb Regional Healthcare Systems, Inc., Board of Directors, September 2, 1997.
43 Minutes, DeKalb Regional Healthcare Systems, Inc., Board of Directors, May 4, 1998.
44 Minutes, DeKalb Regional Healthcare Systems, Inc., Board of Directors, September 8, 1998; Minutes, DeKalb Regional Healthcare Systems, Inc., Board of Directors, December 7, 1998.
45 "Decatur Hospital Expands LTAC Unit," *InDecatur*, May 1999.
46 Richard Schmidt.
47 Minutes, DeKalb Regional Healthcare Systems, Inc., Board of Directors, September 8, 1998; Minutes, DeKalb Regional Healthcare Systems, Inc., Board of Directors, May 3, 1999.
48 Minutes, DeKalb Regional Healthcare Systems, Inc., Board of Directors, January 3, 2000; "Decatur Hospital Special Care Unit to Open This Month," *InDecatur*, July 2003.
49 "Decatur Hospital Special Care Unit to Open This Month," *InDecatur*, July 2003.
50 Minutes, DeKalb Regional Healthcare Systems, Inc., Board of Directors, September 2, 2002.
51 Minutes, DeKalb Regional Healthcare Systems, Inc., Board of Directors, January 9, 2003.
52 *Decatur Focus*, May 2006.
53 Minutes, Community Committee, DeKalb Medical Center at Decatur, November 15, 2006.
54 Hamborg and Baudino memorandum.
55 Minutes, DeKalb Regional Healthcare Systems, Inc., Board of Directors, September 2, 1997.
56 Minutes, DeKalb Regional Healthcare Systems, Inc., Board of Directors, July 6, 1998.
57 Minutes, DeKalb Regional Healthcare Systems, Inc., Board of Directors, August 3, 1998.
58 "The New DeKalb Medical—Focusing Beyond Your Expectations," *Communiqué: A Newsletter for the Medical Staff of DeKalb Medical*, August 2007.
59 "The New DeKalb Medical."
60 "Long Range Plan For The Development of Hospital and Hospital Related Facilities in DeKalb County, Georgia," developed and adopted by DeKalb County Hospital Authority, July 10, 1967.
61 Minutes, DeKalb County Hospital Authority, January 196.
62 Minutes, DeKalb County Hospital Authority, June 1969.
63 Minutes, DeKalb County Hospital Authority, May 1970; Minutes, DeKalb County Hospital Authority, July 1970.
64 Minutes, DeKalb County Hospital Authority, May 1970.
65 Minutes, DeKalb County Hospital Authority, March 1971.
66 Minutes, Special Meeting, DeKalb County Hospital Authority, August 31, 1970.
67 Minutes, Special Meeting, DeKalb County Hospital Authority, August 24, 1970.
68 Minutes, DeKalb County Hospital Authority, August 1971.
69 "A Resolution Offered by the South DeKalb Hospital Committee to the DeKalb Medical Society Executive Committee, April 28, 1970."
70 Minutes, DeKalb County Hospital Authority, June 1971.
71 Minutes, DeKalb County Hospital Authority, February 1972.
72 Minutes, DeKalb County Hospital Authority, August 1972.
73 Minutes, DeKalb County Hospital Authority, October 1973.
74 William Thrasher memorandum to Charles Eberhart, October 28, 1974.
75 A. Waldo Sowell letter to A. C. Guhl, September 18, 1974.
76 A Resolution, the DeKalb County Commission, October 8, 1974.
77 A Resolution, October 8, 1974.
78 "South DeKalb Hospital Plans Are Shown," *The Atlanta Journal,* October 16, 1974.
79 Minutes, DeKalb County Hospital Authority, February 1976.
80 Minutes, DeKalb County Hospital Authority, April,1976; Minutes, DeKalb County Hospital Authority, May 1976; Minutes, DeKalb County Hospital Authority, July 1976.
81 Minutes, DeKalb County Hospital Authority, September 1976.
82 Minutes, DeKalb County Hospital Authority, September 1973.
83 Minutes, DeKalb County Hospital Authority, June 1977.
84 "South DeKalb Development Just a Matter of Time, Now," *DeKalb Extra*, September 27, 1979.
85 Minutes, DeKalb County Hospital Authority, December 1978.
86 Minutes, DeKalb County Hospital Authority Executive Committee, November 20, 1980.
87 Minutes, DeKalb County Hospital Authority, April 1981.
88 Minutes, DeKalb County Hospital Authority, July 1984; Minutes, DeKalb County Hospital Authority, August 1984; "SE Hospital Decision Extension Granted," DeKalb News/Sun, December 12, 1984.
89 "Plan for New DeKalb Hospital Rejected;" "Proposed Community Hospital Receives Strong Local Support," *The DeKalb News/Sun*, November 21, 1984.
90 Minutes, DeKalb County Hospital Authority, February 1985.
91 "Plan for New DeKalb Hospital Rejected."
92 "Agency says southeast DeKalb hospital not needed," DeKalb Extra, October 25, 1984.
93 Minutes, DeKalb County Hospital Authority, October 1984.
94 Minutes, DeKalb County Hospital Authority, November 1984.
95 Minutes, DeKalb County Hospital Authority, September 1985.
96 Minutes, DeKalb County Hospital Authority, October 1985.
97 "Med Center 'On,' Hospital In Question," *The Lithonia Observer*, June 12, 1986.
98 John Heard, MD, "Et Tu, DeKalb General," *DeKalb Medical Society Newsletter*, November 1986.
99 "A Resolution Urging DeKalb General Hospital to operate an emergency care facility in southeast DeKalb County," H. R. No. 358, March 4, 1985.
100 "Rep. Workman's Resolution Tells DeKalb General 'Thanks, But No Thanks' In Regard To Ur-

gent Care Facility," *The Lithonia Observer*, March 10, 1985.
101 Minutes, DeKalb County Hospital Authority, February 1986; "DeKalb General Plans Hospital in Lithonia," *DeKalb News/Sun*, March 12, 1986.
102 *DeKalb News/Sun*, March 12, 1986.
103 Minutes, DeKalb County Hospital Authority, October 1985.
104 Charles S. Smith, Jr., Chairman, Rockdale County Board of Commissioners letter to Charles B. Eberhart, Administrator, DeKalb General Hospital.
105 James H. Millner, Director of Reviews, North Central Georgia Health Systems Agency, Inc., letter to Marquita McNeal, Project Analyst, Georgia State Health Planning Agency, March 20, 1986.
106 Millner letter.
107 "South DeKalb Hospital Ruling Expected By June," *The DeKalb News/Sun*, March 19, 1986.
108 Minutes, DeKalb County Hospital Authority, June 1986; Minutes, DeKalb County Hospital Authority, September 1986; Charles B. Eberhart, DeKalb General Hospital Administrator, letter to Manuel Maloof, CEO of DeKalb County, October 3, 1986.
109 Robert E. Lanier, DeKalb County Commissioner letter to Mrs. Annette Maxey, Director, State Health Planning Agency, August 15, 1986.
110 Minutes, DeKalb County Hospital Authority, September 1986; Eberhart letter to Maloof, October 3, 1986.
111 "He Urges New Hospital in South DeKalb," *The DeKalb News/Sun*, December 11, 1991.
112 Minutes, DeKalb County Hospital Authority, January 1992.
113 Minutes, DeKalb County Hospital Authority, February 1992.
114 Minutes, DeKalb County Hospital Authority, November 1993.
115 Pat Mathis, Authority Chairman, letter to Liane Levetan, CEO DeKalb County, September 20, 1993.
116 "Plans For South DeKalb Hospital Announced," *The Champion*, January 22, 1992.
117 "South DeKalb Residents Want a Full Fledged Hospital," *The Champion*, November 3, 1993.
118 "Lithonia Outpatient Medical Center 'Is a Start' for South DeKalb Area," *The Atlanta Journal Constitution*, November 4, 1993.
119 "Med Center Eyes S. DeKalb Facility," *The Decatur-DeKalbNews/Era*, November 4, 1993.
120 Exempt Minutes, DeKalb County Hospital Authority, April 6, 1992.
121 Charles Eberhart personal notes for DeKalb County Hospital Authority, April 6, 1992.
122 Minutes, DeKalb Medical Center, Inc., Board of Directors, November 1993; Jennings, Ryan & Kolb, Inc., letter to Charles B. Eberhart, President/CEO, DeKalb Medical Center, November 15, 1993.
123 Minutes, DeKalb County Hospital Authority, July 2001.
124 Minutes, DeKalb County Hospital Authority, June 1993.
125 "Med Center Eyes S. DeKalb Facility," *The Decatur-DeKalbNews/Era*, November 4, 1993.
126 Julia M. Hunter, South DeKalb Project Manager, memorandum to Charles Eberhart, CEO, March 29, 1993.
127 Minutes, DeKalb Medical Center, Inc., Board of Directors, July 6, 1993.
128 Minutes, DeKalb County Hospital Authority, July 1994.
129 Jennings, Ryan, Federa & Company, "Report on the Financial Feasibility of Constructing a Medical Office Building/Outpatient Diagnostic Center on Hillandale Road," prepared for DeKalb Medical Center, October 2, 1992.
130 Mathis letter; Charles B. Eberhart, CEO, letter to Pat L. Mathis, Chairman, DeKalb County Hospital Authority, December 30, 1992.
131 Minutes, DeKalb County Hospital Authority, July 1996.
132 Minutes, DeKalb County Hospital Authority, April 1997.
133 Minutes, DeKalb Regional Healthcare System, Inc., Board of Directors, July 1998.
134 Minutes, DeKalb Regional Healthcare System, Inc., Board of Directors, September 1998; Minutes, DeKalb Regional Healthcare System, Inc., Board of Directors, September 1998.
135 Minutes, DeKalb County Hospital Authority, October 1998.
136 "DeKalb Medical Center Files CON Request for Outpatient Hospital," DMC news release, April 5, 1999.
137 "Hillandale Outpatient Surgery Center, Minor Emergency Center Celebrate Grand Opening This Month," *InDecatur*, July 2001.
138 Minutes, DeKalb County Hospital Authority, April 2000; Minutes, DeKalb County Hospital Authority, October 2000; "DeKalb Medical Center Files CON Request for Outpatient Hospital," InDecatur, April 1999.
139 Minutes, DeKalb County Hospital Authority, January 2000.
140 "State Approves Hillandale Expansion Project," *InDecatur*, February 2000.
141 Minutes, DeKalb County Hospital Authority, October, 1999; Minutes, DeKalb County Hospital Authority, November 1999.
142 Minutes, DeKalb County Hospital Authority, January 2001.
143 Minutes, DeKalb County Hospital Authority, January 1999.
144 Minutes, DeKalb County Hospital Authority, June 2003; Minutes, DeKalb County Hospital Authority, October 2003.
145 Minutes, DeKalb County Hospital Authority, July 2001.
146 Minutes, DeKalb Medical Center, Inc., Board of Directors, July 2001.
147 DMC Planning Department, "South DeKalb Hospital Plan," October 23, 2001.
148 Minutes, DeKalb Medical Center, Inc., Board of Directors, January 2002.
149 Jennings Ryan & Kolb, "Report to the Board: Feasibility of Hillandale-Phase III," August 6, 2001.
150 Minutes, DeKalb County Hospital Authority, October, 2001.
151 Minutes, DeKalb County Hospital Authority, January, 2002.
152 "Pillow Fight: State Decision Expected Soon in Battle to Build Hospital in South DeKalb," *The Atlanta Journal-Constitution*, January 6, 2002.
153 "Pillow Fight."
154 "State Approves DeKalb Medical Center's Application to Build New South DeKalb Hospital," *InDecatur Extra*, February 14, 2002.
155 "DMC Hillandale, March 2002," DRHS Board Report, February 27, 2002.
156 "DMC Hillandale, April 2002," DRHS Board Report, March 28, 2002.
157 "DeKalb Medical Center Establishes Planning Board for South DeKalb Hospital," *InDecatur Extra*, February 14, 2002.
158 John R. Gerlach, CEO, letter to DRHS Care Partners, August 9, 2002.
159 "Agency Reaffirms License for South DeKalb Hospital," *The Atlanta Journal-Constitution*, November 23, 2002.
160 Mark W. Maguire, "South DeKalb Hospital Halted In Its Tracks," *Rockdale Neighbor*, April 23, 2002.
161 Mark W. Maguire, "DeKalb Medical Center to Build Hospital," *DeKalb Neighbor*, April 23, 2002.
162 Maguire, "DeKalb Medical Center to Build Hospital."
163 Gerlach, CEO, letter to DRHS Care Partners.
164 Minutes, DeKalb County Hospital Authority, August 2003.

165 Jennings Ryan & Kolb, "Report to the Board: Feasibility of Hillandale-Phase III," August 6, 2001; Minutes, DeKalb Medical Center, Inc., Board of Directors, July 2001.
166 Chandler Brown, "Tenet Drops Out, DeKalb Medical Center To Build In South," *The Atlanta Journal-Constitution*, January 30, 2003.
167 Exempt Minutes, DeKalb County Hospital Authority, January 23, 2003.
168 John R. Gerlach, CEO, letter to Charles Evans, President, HCA Southeast Division, February 18, 2003.
169 Minutes, DeKalb County Hospital Authority, April 2003; Minutes, DeKalb Medical Center, Inc., Board of Directors, June 2003.
170 "The Making of a Hospital," DeKalb Medical Center at Hillandale, http://www.dekalbmedicalcentr.org/ hillandale/history.asp.
171 Minutes, DeKalb Medical Center, Inc., Board of Directors, March 1993.
172 Minutes, DeKalb County Hospital Authority, April 2004.
173 "Construction Begins On New South DeKalb Hospital," *InDecatur*, October 2003.
174 "The Making of a Hospital;" "DeKalb Medical Center at Hillandale Celebrates First Anniversary, July 18," *datelineDeKalb*, July-August, 2006.
175 Minutes, DeKalb County Hospital Authority, July 2005.
176 "DMC at Hillandale's Long Journey Leads to New Heights in Patient Care," *InDecatur Special Edition*, July 2005.
177 Mae Gentry, "Toast a New Hospital's Health: Southside's State-of-the-Art Facility Hosts an Open House," *The Atlanta Journal-Constitution*, July 14, 2005.
178 Minutes, DeKalb Regional Healthcare System, Inc., Board of Directors, September 2005.
179 Minutes, Medical Staff Executive Committee at Hillandale, May 1, 2007; Minutes, Medical Staff Executive Committee, November 6, 2007; "New Hillandale Administrator Dedicated to Serving Community," DeKalb Medical news release, October 22, 2007.
180 "I Have 40 Acres of Red Clay; I Want You to Build a Hospital," by Brett Fayssoux, *The Champion*, November 10-16, 2005.
181 Minutes, DeKalb County Hospital Authority, July 2005.
182 "DeKalb Medical Center at Hillandale Now Open," *Communique: a Newsletter for the Medical Staff of DeKalb Medical Center*, August, 2005.
183 "DMC at Hillandale's Long Journey Leads to New Heights in Patient Care," *InDecatur Special Edition*, July 2005.
184 Brooke Stark, "Hospital Meeting Higher Demands," *Rockdale Citizen*, October 25, 2005.
185 Chandler Brown, "New Hospital Cures Doubters," *The Atlanta Journal-Constitution*, July 27, 2006; "DeKalb Medical Center at Hillandale Celebrates First Anniversary, July 18," *datelineDeKalb*, July-August, 2006.
186 Minutes, DeKalb County Hospital Authority, July 2001.
187 "Bad Debts Hinder Operations at Hillandale Hospital," *Crossroads*, December 29, 2005.
188 "Bad Debts."
189 "DeKalb Medical Center at Hillandale, One Year Anniversary Review," August, 2006.
190 Minutes, Hillandale Advisory Board, DeKalb Medical at Hillandale, November 14, 2007.
191 "DeKalb Medical Center Named to Prestigious National 'Most Wired' List," *Communique: A Newsletter for the Medical Staff of DeKalb Medical Center*, September/October 2005.
192 Minutes, DeKalb Regional Healthcare System, Inc., Board of Directors, November 2, 2007.
193 CEO Strategic Updates for the DeKalb Regional Healthcare, Inc., Board of Directors, October, 2006.
194 Minutes, Medical Staff Executive Committee at Hillandale, July 3, 2007.

Chapter Nine

1 "Hospital Plans," *The Decatur-DeKalb News*, February 15, 1959.
2 Minutes, DeKalb County Hospital Authority, February 2, 1961; "Auxiliary History," DeKalb Medical Center—Intranet, http://xintranet.drha.org/dept/index.cfm?p=dept_page&pg_id=902.
3 "Gray Ladies Service for DeKalb General Hospital," DeKalb General Hospital Press Release, March 6, 1961.
4 "Red Cross Volunteers: In Appreciation of Years in Service, 1961-1995, A Touch of Class."
5 "DeKalb Medical Center Volunteers Celebrate One Million Hours of Service," DeKalb Medical Center News Release, November 30, 2001.
6 "A History of the DeKalb Medical Center Red Cross Unit."
7 "Gray Ladies Service for DeKalb General Hospital."
8 *The General InDecatur*, July 6, 1962.
9 "A History of the DeKalb Medical Center Red Cross Unit;" "Red Cross Volunteers Celebrate 30 Years With DMC," *InDecatur*, September 1991.
10 "Youth Contribute," *InDecatur*, July 2, 1976.
11 "DMC Wins for Most Pints Collected," *InDecatur*, September 2004.
12 "Red Cross Volunteers: In Appreciation of Years in Service, 1961-1995, A Touch of Class."
13 *The General InDecatur*, November 10, 1961.
14 "No. 1 In Blood Donations," *DeKalb Medical Pushing Forward*, Spring 2008, p. 5.
15 "Volunteer Section," DeKalb Medical - Intranet, December 4, 2007, http://intranet2.drhs.drhs.org/dept/index.cfm?p=dept_page&pg_id=900.
16 "Auxiliary History," DeKalb Medical Center—Intranet, http://xintranet.drha.org/dept/index.cfm? p=dept_page&pg_id=902; "Handbook for Red Cross Volunteers," Revised edition, 1994.
17 Claudia Tinkle, Volunteer Program Coordinator, "DeKalb Medical Center Volunteer Programs;" "DeKalb Medical Center Red Cross Unit 1994-1995 Annual Report."
18 Joyce Bowman, director of Volunteer Services, memorandum to Jack Gerlach, CEO/Administrator, "Red Cross Volunteers," July 19, 1995.
19 Minutes, DeKalb Medical Center, Inc., Board of Directors, June 5, 1995; "Auxiliary History;" "Red Cross Volunteers: In Appreciation of Years in Service, 1961-1995, A Touch of Class."
20 "Junior League DeKalb County—Chronology," http://www.jldekalb.org/dekalb/npo.jsp?pg=about1&tab=1934 to 1979.
21 Minutes, DeKalb County Hospital Authority, August 24, 1960.
22 Floyd Sanders, MD, personal communication; "Junior League DeKalb County—Chronology;" Paula Austin, Manager of The Dogwood Shop, "In My Own Words," *InDecatur*, April 1991.
23 *The General InDecatur*, November 10, 1961.
24 Minutes, DeKalb County Hospital Authority, December 7, 1970.
25 "Junior League DeKalb County—Chronology."
26 Minutes, DeKalb County Hospital Authority, December 7, 1970.
27 "Junior League DeKalb County—Chronology."
28 Minutes, DeKalb County Hospital Authority, December 7, 1970.
29 "Junior League DeKalb County—Chronology."
30 Minutes, DeKalb County Hospital Authority, November 1, 1971.
31 Claudia Tinkle.
32 Council on Auxiliaries of the Georgia Hospital Association Scrapbook Questionnaire, September 1, 1974.
33 Minutes, DeKalb County Hospital Authority, February 5, 1990.
34 "Welcome to the 'Auxiliary of DeKalb General

Hospital,'" *The General In Decatur*, September 14, 1973.
35 Council on Auxiliaries.
36 "Who Are The Ladies In The New Pink Uniforms?" *The General InDecatur*, June, 1975.
37 Council on Auxiliaries.
38 "Auxiliary Wish List, A Gift to DeKalb Medical."
39 "DeKalb Medical Auxiliary Annual Report, October 1, 2006 – September 30, 2007."
40 DeKalb General Auxiliary Scrapbook, 1980–1981.
41 DeKalb General Auxiliary Scrapbook, 1973–1974.
42 DeKalb General Auxiliary Scrapbook, 1974–1975.
43 Minutes, DeKalb County Hospital Authority, July 6, 1976; DeKalb General Auxiliary Scrapbook, 1975-1976.
44 Minutes, DeKalb County Hospital Authority, December 6, 1976; DeKalb General Auxiliary Scrapbook, 1976-1977.
45 DeKalb General Auxiliary Scrapbook, 1977–1978.
46 DeKalb General Auxiliary Scrapbook, 1978–1979.
47 DeKalb General Auxiliary Scrapbook, 1984–1985.
48 DeKalb General Auxiliary Scrapbook, 1983–1984.
49 DeKalb General Auxiliary Scrapbook, 1999–2000.
50 Minutes, DeKalb County Hospital Authority, December 1, 1980.
51 DeKalb General Auxiliary Scrapbook, 1995-1996.
52 "Auxiliary Wish List, A Gift to DeKalb Medical."
53 Paula Austin, Manager of The Dogwood Shop, "In My Own Words," *InDecatur*, April 1991.
54 "DeKalb Medical Auxiliary Annual Report, October 1, 2006 – September 30, 2007;" "DeKalb Medical Auxiliary: Welcome to a Review of the Many and Varied Activities of the Auxiliary."
55 "Auxilians Honored for Service," *InDecatur*, December 1997.
56 "DeKalb Medical Auxiliary Annual Report, October 1, 2006 – September 30, 2007."
57 "DeKalb Medical Auxiliary Annual Report, October 1, 2006 – September 30, 2007."
58 "DeKalb Medical Auxiliary Annual Report, October 1, 2006 – September 30, 2007;" "Independent Volunteers," Volunteers in Action Annual Report, July 1, 2001 – June 30, 2002.
59 Council on Auxiliaries of the Georgia Hospital Association Scrapbook Questionnaire, September 1, 1974.
60 "DeKalb Medical Center Volunteers Celebrate One Million Hours of Service," DeKalb Medical Center News Release, November 30, 2001; Minutes, DeKalb Medical Center, Inc., Board of Directors, December 3, 2001.
61 DeKalb Medical Center Auxiliary Annual Report, October 1, 2001 – September 30, 2002.
62 "DeKalb Medical Auxiliary: Welcome to a Review of the Many and Varied Activities of the Auxiliary."
63 "Red Cross Volunteer Retires After 27 Years of Service," *InDecatur*, March 1989.
64 "Independent Volunteers," Volunteers in Action Annual Report, July 1, 2001 – June 30, 2002.
65 "Independent Volunteers."
66 "Mission of Love," DeKalb Medical News Release, January 24, 2008.
67 Minutes, DeKalb Medical Center, Inc., Board of Directors, December 3, 2001; "DRHS Care Corps Holds Membership Drive," *InDecatur*, November 2001.
68 "DMC Mission, Vision, and Values," *DeKalb Medical Center Employee Handbook*, p. 2.
69 Minutes, DeKalb County Hospital Authority, October 28, 1959.
70 Minutes, DeKalb County Hospital Authority, November 25, 1959; Press Release, November 7–11, 1960.
71 Minutes, DeKalb County Hospital Authority, September 23, 1959.
72 Minutes, DeKalb County Hospital Authority, June 9, 1960.
73 Minutes, DeKalb County Hospital Authority, August 24, 1960.
74 Minutes, DeKalb County Hospital Authority, September 28, 1960.
75 Minutes, DeKalb County Hospital Authority, February 22, 1961.
76 Minutes, DeKalb County Hospital Authority, December 11, 1961; Minutes, DeKalb County Hospital Authority, January 5, 1970.
77 Minutes, DeKalb County Hospital Authority, December 6, 1960.
78 Minutes, DeKalb County Hospital Authority, August 24, 1960.
79 Minutes, DeKalb County Hospital Authority, August 24, 1960.
80 Press Release, October 10, 1960.
81 Minutes, DeKalb County Hospital Authority, October 19, 1960.
82 Minutes, DeKalb County Hospital Authority, May 14, 1962.
83 Minutes, DeKalb County Hospital Authority, February 22, 1961.
84 Minutes, DeKalb County Hospital Authority, September 16, 1958.
85 Minutes, DeKalb County Hospital Authority, October 15, 1858.
86 "The Good Samaritan Fund," *The General InDecatur*, November 10, 1961.
87 *The General InDecatur*, November 12, 1971; *InDecatur*, January 1990.
88 Minutes, DeKalb County Hospital Authority, July 2, 1990; "Premier Nightingala Raises Funds for Nursing Education," *InDecatur*, June 1989.
89 "Coppage Scholarship Established," *InDecatur*, November 1993.
90 "Local Nursing Students are Awarded $16,000 in Scholarship Funds from DeKalb Medical Foundation," *DeKalb Medical Pushing Forward*, Spring 2008, p. 19.
91 "Two Scholarship Opportunities," *datelineDeKalb E-Digest*, March 10, 2008; "DMC Foundation Receives Special $1.5 Million Gift," *InDecatur*, June–July 2005.
92 "Two Scholarship Opportunities."
93 "Tatum Donation Endows Oncology Nursing at DMC," *InDecatur*, November–December 2003.
94 "The History of the DeKalb Medical Center Foundation," http://www.dekalbmedicalcenter.org/foundation.
95 Minutes, DeKalb County Hospital Authority, March 7, 1988.
96 Charles B. Eberhart, Administrator, letter to James C. Rawls, Attorney, Powell Goldstein Frazer & Murphy, March 23, 1989.
97 Minutes, DeKalb County Hospital Authority, August 6, 1990.
98 Articles of Incorporation, DeKalb Medical Center Foundation, 1990.
99 Minutes, DeKalb County Hospital Authority, October 1, 1990.
100 "The History of the DeKalb Medical Center Foundation."
101 "W.H.A.T. Gets A Makeover," *W.H.A.T.'s Happening*, Spring, 2005.
102 "W.H.A.T. Employee Giving Campaign Raises More Than $770,000 for DMC Foundation," *InDecatur,* November, 2005, p. 1.
103 "W.H.A.T. Awards 2005 Community Health Grants," *W.H.A.T.'s Happening*, September, 2005, p.2.
104 "Fun Fact," *W.H.A.T.'s Happening*, Winter, 2004.
105 "The History of the DeKalb Medical Center Foundation."
106 "Other Foundation News," *W.H.A.T.'s Happening*, Winter 2006/2007, p.2.
107 "The History of the DeKalb Medical Center Foundation;" "Foundation Reaches Five-Year Milestone," *InDecatur*, July 1996; John Gerlach,

"Current Issues," *InDecatur*, July 1996.
108 "The History of the DeKalb Medical Center Foundation."
109 "DMC Foundation Project Earns Healthcare Award," *InDecatur*, June-July 2000.
110 "Contributions Lead to Successful Completion of Community Parnership/2000," *InDecatur*, April 2002.
111 "New Pete and Jerri Pike Chapel Opens at DMC After Renovation," *InDecatur*, April 2001.
112 "Dr. H. Duane and Emy Evans Blair: Building a Legacy," DeKalb Medical – Intranet, http://intranet.drhs.org/dept/index.cfm?p=msp&pg¬_id =6863.
113 "Gift Benefits Cancer Center, Honors Castellani," *InDecatur*, October.
114 "DMC Foundation Receives Special $1.5 Million Gift," *InDecatur*, June–July 2005.
115 "DMC Foundation Receives Special $1.5 Million Gift," *InDecatur*, June–July 2005.
116 "DeKalb Medical Foundation Thanks Dr. Bobbie Bailey—Record Gift of $3.3 Million," DeKalb Medical – Intranet, http://intranet.drhs.drhs.org.
117 John Gerlach, CEO, "Current Issues," *InDecatur*, July 2002.
118 "Touching the Community: DeKalb Medical Center Foundation Reaches Landmark 10th Anniversary," *Health Lines 1961–2001: 40th Anniversary,* Summer/Fall 2001, p. 14.
119 Program for Judy R. McMahan's Retirement, DeKalb Regional Health System Board, December 11, 2005.

Chapter Ten

1 Opal Hopkins Fyffe interview, March 3, 2006.
2 Minutes, DeKalb County Hospital Authority, February 10, 1964.
3 Duane Blair, MD, interview, December 9, 2008.
4 John R. Gerlach interview, December 11, 2008.
5 Shorty Lorentzen, "DeKalb General Hospital is 'Trained to Care'," by *The DeKalb New Era*, April 26, 1961.
6 "DGH Honors Memory of W. H. Thrasher," *The InDecatur*, December 22, 1983.
7 Charles Eberhart, "My Prayer for DMC;" Charles B. Eberhart letter to M. Scott Peck, M.D., October 13, 1994.
8 "Wood Carving Hobby of Hospital Exec," *The DeKalb News/Sun*, July 14, 1982.
9 "60 Seconds With Charles B. Eberhart," *InDecatur*, January, 1989.
10 Charles B. Eberhart resume.
11 Charles Eberhart personal communications with the author.
12 "60 Seconds With Charles B. Eberhart."
13 "1996 GHA Distinguished Service Award: Charles Eberhart: 'An Outstanding Leader, a Caring Person and a Very Special Friend,'" *Georgia Hospitals Today*, January, 1996.
14 "1996 GHA Distinguished Service Award."
15 "Eberhart Receives McCurdy Citizenship Award," *InDecatur*, March 1993.
16 "Cancer Center to be Named for Eberhart," *The Decatur–DeKalb News/Era*, May 4, 1995.
17 "1996 GHA Distinguished Service Award."
18 "Saying Goodbye to a Leader and a Friend," *In Decatur*, July 1995.
19 "Wood Carving Hobby of Hospital Exec," *The DeKalb News/Sun*, July 14, 1982.
20 Bill L. Sublett interview, March 6, 2008.
21 Mark S. Davis, M. D., "Thank You, Mr. Eberhart."
22 Julia Hunter Jones interview, June 5, 2007.
23 Charles B. Eberhart, Chief Executive Officer, memorandum to DeKalb Medical Center, Inc. Executive Committee and DeKalb Regional Healthcare System, Inc. Executive Committee, August 15, 1994.
24 Charles B. Eberhart, Chief Executive Officer, memorandum to DeKalb Medical Center, Inc., Executive Committee and DeKalb Regional Healthcare System, Inc., Executive Committee.
25 John R. Gerlach interview.
26 John Gerlach, CEO, "Current Issues" (his last newsletter column on the occasion of his retirement), *InDecatur*, July, 2003.
27 Gerlach, "Current Issues," 2003.
28 "CEO John R. Gerlach Announces Retirement Plans," *InDecatur Extra*, June 3, 2003.
29 Gerlach, "Current Issues, 2003."
30 "John R. Gerlach, President and CEO: 35 Years of Achievement," *InDecatur*, July, 2003.
31 Gerlach: 35 Years of Achievement.
32 "DRHS Makes Staffing Changes as Part of Labor Management Plan," *InDecatur*, January 15, 2003.
33 John R. Gerlach, "Current Issues," *InDecatur*, July 2002
34 "DRHS Makes Staffing Changes as Part of Labor Management Plan," *InDecatur*, January 15, 2003; "DRHS Completes Labor Management Changes," InDecatur, March 20003.
35 "Work Group Formed to Redesign Revenue Cycle," *InDecatur*, April 2000.
36 John R. Gerlach, President and CEO and Michael Hartman, MD, memorandum to the DMC Board of Directors, "Proposal for the Establishment of a Multi-disciplinary Quality Council at DMC," May 28, 1977; Minute, DeKalb Medical Center, Inc., Board of Directors, September 2, 1997.
37 John R. Gerlach, "Current Issues," *InDecatur*, November 2001.
38 Betty Castellani, "The John R. Gerlach Legacy," John Gerlach Retirement Reception, July, 2003.
39 Eric Norwood interview, August 21, 2008.
40 Norwood interview.
41 Norwood interview.
42 Minutes, DeKalb Regional Healthcare System, Inc. Board of Directors, December 12, 2005.
43 Minutes, Finance Committee, DeKalb Regional Healthcare System, Inc., August 29, 2006.
44 Minutes, DeKalb Regional Healthcare System, Inc. Board of Directors, July 9, 2007.
45 Jacqueline Palank, "Hospitals face Big Challenge Making Profit," *The Wall Street Journal*, April 30, 2008, p. B7B.
46 Andy Miller, "South Fulton Hospital Files for Chapter 11," *The Atlanta Journal Constitution*, May 1, 2000.
47 Urvaksh Karkaria, "Rockdale Medical Center Close to $90M Sale," *The Atlanta Business Chronicle*, November 23, 2007; Urvaksh Karkaria, "Troubled Rockdale Medical Back at Square One," *Atlanta Business Chronicle*, May 20, 2008.
48 Andy Miller and Craig Schneider, "Grady Expects Record Deficit This Year," *The Atlanta Journal Constitution*, October 12, 2007.
49 Minutes, Medical Staff Executive Committee, March 28, 2006.
50 "New Contract Broadens Healthcare Access in DeKalb County," DeKalb Medical news release, May 30, 2007; "DeKalb Medical and Kaiser Expand Access to Health Care," *datelineDeKalb*, June/July, 2007.
51 Eric Norwood, "The New DeKalb Medical: Pushing Beyond Your Expectations," *dateline DeKalb*, June/July 2007.
52 Norwood, "The New DeKalb Medical."
53 Eric Norwood, "Let's Talk About 'Excellence'," *InDecatur*, October 2003.
54 Eric Norwood, "Our Vision," *InDecatur*, January–February 2004.
55 Eric Norwood, "Our Values: Diversity, Respect, Healing and Service," *InDecatur*, March 2004.

Anesthesia Services

1 George Sessions, MD, interview, June 3, 2008.
2 Minutes, DeKalb County Hospital Authority, February 24, 1960.

3 Minutes, DeKalb County Hospital Authority, March 1961.
4 Sessions interview.
5 Sessions interview.
6 *InDecatur,* October 29, 1981.
7 William Keeton, MD, interview, June 4, 2008.
8 Keeton interview.
9 Keeton interview.
10 Keeton interview.
11 Charles "Chip" Clifton, MD, Interview, June 23, 2008.
12 Clifton interview.
13 Clifton interview.
14 Clifton interview.

Building Services and Material Management

1 *The General InDecatur*, June 8, 1962.
2 *The General InDecatur*, May 14, 1971.
3 *The General InDecatur*, May 1, 1970.
4 Dean Brown interview, October 28, 2008.
5 Brown interview; "Sebree Named Director of Materials Management," *InDecatur*, July 2004.
6 Richard "Rick" Carter personal communication, November 25, 2008.
7 "Did You Know," DeKalb Medical – Intranet.
8 Brown interview.
9 *The General InDecatur*, May 5, 1970.
10 *The General InDecatur*, January 9, 1970.
11 James Solomon personal communication, November 19, 2008.
12 Minutes, DeKalb County Hospital Authority, May 1969.
13 Minutes, DeKalb County Hospital Authority, June 1970.
14 *InDecatur*, February–March 1991.
15 Dan Callahan personal communication, November 19, 2008.
16 "Alexander Retired After 21 Years," The *InDecatur*, March 18, 1982.
17 "Maintenance Reorganization," *The General InDecatur*, August 4, 1972.
18 "Dedication Ceremony," *The General InDecatur*, September 3, 1971.
19 Clayton Bailey, "Inside Building Services," *InDecatur*, June 1991.
20 "Technical Maintenance Department Keeps Hospital Equipment Humming," *InDecatur*, January 1990.
21 Bill Sublett interview, March 6, 2008; Dan Callahan, Carl Lallerstedt, Mike Paul and Jackie Anderson interview, July 1, 2008.
22 Callahan et al interview, July 1, 2008.
23 Solomon communication; "Housekeeping Training Program Started," *The General InDecatur*, April 11, 1975.
24 *The General InDecatur*, June 8, 1962.
25 *The General InDecatur*, November 8, 1961.
26 "Housekeeping Training . . ."
27 "James Solomon Has Been Promoted Into the Position of Assistant Housekeeper," *The General InDecatur*, June 8, 1973.
28 Minutes, DeKalb County Hospital Authority, December 1969.
29 "James Solomon Has Been Promoted . . ."
30 *InDecatur*, September 1997.
31 "DMC Selects Sodexho to Manage Environmental Services," *InDecatur*, November–December 2003.
32 *The General InDecatur*, February 2, 1962.
33 *The General InDecatur*, May 12, 1972.
34 "Can You Imagine?" *InDecatur*, August 1985.
35 Grover Evans interview, November 20, 2008.
36 Mrs. Getswell, "As I See It," *InDecatur*, January 10, 1980.
37 "Grover Evans Earns Top State Honors," *InDecatur*, May 2003.
38 Minutes, DeKalb County Hospital Authority, June 1962; Minutes, DeKalb County Hospital Authority, November 2, 1970.
39 Evans interview.
40 Dorothy Nix, "Keeping It Clean Is Big Job for Him," *The Atlanta Journal-Constitution*, June 11, 1969.
41 Minutes, DeKalb County Hospital Authority, March 1969.
42 "Grover Evans Earns Top State Honors."
43 *The General InDecatur*, April 6, 1978.

Cancer Services

1 Betty Castellani interview, August 26, 2008.
2 "Cancer Center Recognized for Excellence," datelineDeKalb E-Digest, May 12, 2008; "Cancer Center Receives Outstanding Achievement Award," DeKalb Medical news release, May 8, 2008, http://www.dekalbmedical.com/News-Media/.../Default.aspx?aid=426.
3 Minutes, DeKalb Regional Healthcare System, Inc. Board of Directors, December 5, 2005; "Cancer Center Honored with Outstanding Achievement Award," *DeKalb Medical Center – Intranet*, http://www.dekalbmedicalcenter.org/shownews.asp?id=865.
4 "DMC Cancer Center Successfully Completes Accreditation Survey," DeKalb Medical Center – Intranet, http://intranet2.drhs.org/dept/index.cfm?p= msp&pg_id=5071.
5 Minutes, Medical Staff Executive Committee, February 5, 1969.
6 Minutes, Quarterly Medical Staff Meeting, October 24, 1970.
7 Minutes, DeKalb County Hospital Authority, July 6, 1973.
8 Minutes, DeKalb County Hospital Authority, March 3, 1975; Minutes, DeKalb County Hospital Authority, March 1, 1976.
9 *The General InDecatur*, November 24, 1961.
10 *The General InDecatur*, June 22, 1962.
11 Minutes, Medical Staff Executive Committee, September 9, 1968.
12 Minutes, DeKalb County Hospital Authority, October 21, 1968.
13 Minutes, DeKalb County Hospital Authority, December 9, 1968.
14 Minutes, DeKalb County Hospital Authority, December 6, 1971.
15 Minutes, DeKalb County Hospital Authority, January 3, 1972.
16 Minutes, DeKalb County Hospital Authority, September 5, 1977.
17 Minutes, DeKalb County Hospital Authority, March 4, 1985.
18 Minutes, DeKalb Medical Center, Inc. Board of Directors, October 4, 1993; Minutes, DeKalb County Hospital Authority, June 4, 1990; "DRHS Strengthens Smoking Policy," *InDecatur*, November–December, 2003.
19 Minutes, DeKalb Regional Healthcare System, Inc. Board of Directors, November 3, 2003.
20 Minutes, DeKalb County Hospital Authority, May 5, 1973; Minutes, DeKalb County Hospital Authority, September 4, 1973; Minutes, DeKalb County Hospital Authority, October 5, 1973.
21 Minutes, DeKalb County Hospital Authority, October 5, 1974.
22 Minutes, DeKalb County Hospital Authority, March 1, 1976.
23 Minutes, DeKalb County Hospital Authority, May 3, 1976.
24 Minutes, DeKalb County Hospital Authority, February 7, 1977.
25 Minutes, DeKalb County Hospital Authority, July 5, 1977.
26 Minutes, DeKalb County Hospital Authority, September 2, 1980.
27 Minutes, DeKalb County Hospital Authority, January 7, 1980.
28 Minutes, DeKalb County Hospital Authority, April 4, 1988.
29 *DeKalb General Hospital Cancer Program, 1984,*

p. 6.
30 Minutes, DeKalb County Hospital Authority, June 1, 1981; DeKalb General Hospital Cancer Program, 1984, p. 7; "Training Expands Department," *InDecatur*, March 19, 1981.
31 "Enterostomal Therapy Program At DeKalb General Hospital," *The General InDecatur*, February 14, 1975.
32 *DeKalb General Hospital Cancer Program, 1984*, p. 6.
33 Minutes, DeKalb County Hospital Authority, April 5, 1982.
34 Minutes, DeKalb County Hospital Authority, November 7, 1983; Minutes, DeKalb County Hospital Authority, December 5, 1983; Minutes, DeKalb County Hospital Authority, January 3, 1984; Minutes, DeKalb County Hospital Authority, October 1, 1984.
35 *DeKalb General Hospital Cancer Program, 1984*, p. 2.
36 Minutes, DeKalb County Hospital Authority, October 2, 1989.
37 Minutes, DeKalb County Hospital Authority, June 3, 1991.
38 Minutes, DeKalb County Hospital Authority, November 11, 1991.
39 "Kann Outpatient Treatment Center," The Wheels of Progress: 2004 Annual Report, DMC Cancer Center, p. 3; "Clinical Laboratory and Pathology: Stem Cell Transplants," DeKalb Medical Center – Intranet, http://intranet.drhs.org/dept/index.cfm?p=dept_page&pg_id=440.
40 Minutes, DeKalb County Hospital Authority, April 24, 2001.
41 "DMC's Stem Cell Transplant Program Receives National Accreditation," *InDecatur*, August 2003.
42 "Intensity Modulated Chemotherapy: Superior Radiation Therapy at DMC," Cancer Hope Line, Summer, 2002, p. 1; "Radiation Therapy," DeKalb Medical Center—Programs and Services, http://www.dekalbmedicalcenter.org/programs.asp?ps=76; "DeKalb Medical Center Offers Patients Access to the Most Advanced Cancer Treatments," DeKalb Medical news release, May 21, 2004, http://www.dekalbmedical.com/News Media/ViewAllStories/tabid/74/Default.
43 Castellani interview.
44 "Cancer Center Recognized for Excellence," *datelineDeKalb E-Digest*, May 12, 2008; "New Hope for Breast Cancer Patients," DeKalb Medical news release, March 19, 2007, http://www.dekalbmedical.com/NewsMedia/ . . . /Default.aspx?aid=336.
45 "Diagnostic Breast Center," *The Wheels of Progress: 2004 Annual Report: Charles B. Eberhart Cancer Center*, p. 9.
46 "Genetic Screening," DeKalb Medical Center – Programs and Services, http://www.dekalbmedicalcenter.org/programs.asp?ps=31; "Cancer Center Offers Genetic Testing," *InDecatur*, April 1999; "DMC Now Offers Testing for Hereditary Colon Cancer," *InDecatur*, February 2001.
47 *The General InDecatur*, November 24, 1961.
48 "Intraperitoneal Heated Chemotherapy," DeKalb Medical Center—Programs and Services, http://www.dekalbmedicalcenter.org/programs.asp?ps=44.
49 Castellani interview; "Cancer Center Continues to Lead in Advanced Treatment Support," *DeKalb Medical Center – Intranet*, http://www.dekalbmedicalcenter.org/shownews.asp?id=898; "Clinical Trials," The Wheels of Progress: 2004 Annual Report, DMC Cancer Center, p. 13.
50 Castellani interview.
51 "Kann Outpatient Treatment Center," *The Wheels of Progress: 2004 Annual Report, DMC Cancer Center*, p. 3; "Kann Treatment Center," *DeKalb Medical Center – Intranet*, http://xintranet.drhs.drhs.org/dept/index.cfm?p=dept_page&pg_id=6265.
52 "Cancer Center Honored with Outstanding Achievement Award," *DeKalb Medical Center – Intranet*, http://www.dekalbmedicalcenter.org/show news.asp?id=865.
53 "Cancer Center Continues to Lead in Advanced Treatment and Support," DeKalb Medical news release, June 27, 2006, http://www.dekalbmedical.com/NewsMedia/ViewAllNewsStories/tabid/74. . . .
54 Betty Castellani, Director of the Cancer Center, "Inside the Cancer Center," *InDecatur*, April 1991.
55 "Dedication to a Hero," *1994 Annual Report, Charles B. Eberhart Cancer Center, DMC*, p. 2.
56 "Cancer Survivors Offer Words of Hope," *InDecatur*, April 1990.
57 "DMC Offers Cancer Support Group for Children," *InDecatur*, October, 1993; "The Treehouse Gang," DeKalb Medical news release, August 23, 2007, http://www.dekalbmedical.com/ NewsMedia/. . ./Default.aspx?aid=351.
58 Betty Castellani, Director of the Cancer Center, "Inside the Cancer Center," *InDecatur*, April 1991.
59 "Radiation Oncology Program Still Growing," InDecatur, January, 1999; "Cancer Center Offers Genetic Testing," *InDecatur*, April 1999.
60 "DRHS Care Partners Honored With Community Healthcare Awards," *InDecatur*, July 2001.
61 "Two Employees Receive Good Samaritan Awards," *InDecatur*, August 1993.
62 "Donna Lawson Cannon, Champion of the Week," *The Champion*, Thursday, July 26–August 1, 2007, p. 6A.

Cardiovascular Services

1 Cardiology Agreement signed by Dr. Robert Hubble and Dr. Benjamin Okel, cardiologists, and Dr. J. Rufus Evans on behalf of DeKalb General Hospital, June 14, 1965; Minutes, DeKalb County Hospital Authority, June 14, 1965.
2 Minutes, DeKalb County Hospital Authority, February 12, 1968.
3 Minutes, DeKalb County Hospital Authority, May 12, 1969; Minutes, DeKalb County Hospital Authority, July 7, 1969.
4 Minutes, DeKalb County Hospital Authority, July 1, 1966.
5 Minutes, DeKalb County Hospital Authority, September 8, 1969; Minutes, Medical Staff Executive Committee, August 1970.
6 Minutes, DeKalb County Hospital Authority, March 4, 1974.
7 Minutes, DeKalb County Hospital Authority, March 5, 1973.
8 "Coronary Rehabilitation Program Completes First Year At DeKalb General," *The General In Decatur*, September 13, 1974.
9 "Cardiac Rehab Program Expands," *InDecatur*, January 1989; "Heart Wellness Center: Cardiac Rehabilitation," http://www.dekalbmedical.org/ProgramsServices/MoreServices/HeartWellnessCenter/tabid/279/Default.aspx,6/2/08; "CRP Team Helps Hearts Survive," *InDecatur*, April 26, 1984; "Heart to Heart," *InDecatur*, February 1986.
10 Minutes, DeKalb County Hospital Authority, October 1, 1984.
11 Minutes, DeKalb County Hospital Authority, November 2, 1987.
12 "DeKalb General Plans Cardiac Cath Unit," *InDecatur*, January 1989.
13 "DeKalb General Plans Cardiac Cath Unit."
14 Minutes, DeKalb County Hospital Authority, April 4, 1989.
15 "Staffing Highlights," *InDecatur*, October 1989.
16 "Cardiac Cath Technology Comes to DeKalb Medical Center," *InDecatur*, December 1989.
17 Patrick Green interview, August 28, 2008.

18 "DMC Unveils New Cardiac Catheterization Technology," *InDecatur*, February 2003.
19 "DMC Unveils New Cardiac Catheterization Technology."
20 Minutes, DeKalb Medical Center, Inc. Board of Directors, January 8, 1996.
21 "CHF Team Earns Top CARE Award," *InDecatur*, January 2001.
22 "CHF Team Earns Top CARE Award;" "DMC Opens Coumadin Clinic," *InDecatur*, August 2002.
23 "DMC Opens Coumadin Clinic," *InDecatur*, August 2002.
24 "DMC Opens Coumadin Clinic."
25 "DMC Wins Patient Safety Award for Coumadin Clinic," *InDecatur*, November 2002.
26 Charles B. Eberhart letter to Liane Levetan, Chief Executive Officer, DeKalb County (undated).
27 James C. Rawls letter to Charles B. Eberhart, CEO, November 23, 1993.
28 Minutes, DeKalb Regional Healthcare System, Inc. Board of Directors, February 14, 2005.
29 Thomas Aversano, MD, et al, "Thrombolytic Therapy vs Primary Percutaneous Coronary Intervention for Myocardial Infarction in Patients Presenting to Hospitals Without On-site Cardiac Surgery: A Randomized Controlled Trial," *JAMA*, Vol. 287 (15), 1945-1951, April 17, 2002.
30 Minutes, DeKalb Regional Healthcare System, Inc. Board of Directors, February 14, 2005.
31 DeKalb Regional Healthcare System, Inc. Board of Directors, April 11, 2005; DeKalb Regional Healthcare System, Inc. Board of Directors, June 13, 2005; DeKalb Regional Healthcare System, Inc. Board of Directors, July 11, 2005.
32 DeKalb Regional Healthcare System, Inc. Board of Directors, October 10, 2005.
33 CEO Strategic Update to the DRHS Board of Directors, October 2007.
34 "DeKalb Medical Invests $3.7 Million for Endovascular Lab," DeKalb Medical news release, July 16, 2008, http://www.dekalbmedical.org/NewsMedia/...Default.aspx?aid=435.
35 Green interview.

Child Care Center

1 Minutes, DeKalb County Hospital Authority, August 12, 1963.
2 Minutes, DeKalb County Hospital Authority, May 11, 1964.
3 Minutes, DeKalb County Hospital Authority, July 13, 1964; Minutes, DeKalb County Hospital Authority, September 9, 1963.
4 Minutes, Special Meeting, DeKalb County Hospital Authority, January 19, 1969.
5 Minutes, DeKalb County Hospital Authority, February 10, 1969.
6 Minutes, DeKalb County Hospital Authority, April 14, 1969.
7 John R. Gerlach, Assistant to the Administrator, memorandum to William H. Thrasher, Administrator, "Recommendation of Construction of DeKalb General Hospital Child Care Facilities," from April 21, 1969.
8 Minutes, DeKalb County Hospital Authority, May 22, 1969.
9 Minutes, DeKalb County Hospital Authority, July 6, 1970; Minutes, DeKalb County Hospital Building Committee, October 17, 1969; "Getting to Know Your Child Care Center," *The General InDecatur*, February 4, 1972.
10 "Day Care Center Opens," *The General InDecatur*, January 9, 1970; "Child Care Center Survey," *The General InDecatur*, April 14, 1972.
11 "Getting to Know Your Child Care Center."
12 "Child Care Center—Kindergarten," *The General InDecatur*, September 3, 1971.
13 "Getting to Know Your Child Care Center."
14 "New Day Care Schedule," *InDecatur*, October 10, 1975.
15 Minutes, DeKalb County Hospital Authority, October 6, 1975; Minutes, DeKalb County Hospital Authority, December 1, 1975.
16 Minutes, DeKalb Medical Center, Inc. Board of Directors, August 3, 1992.
17 Minutes, DeKalb Medical Center, Inc. Board of Directors, November 2, 1992.
18 Minutes, DeKalb Medical Center, Inc. Board of Directors, February 1, 1993.
19 Minutes, DeKalb Medical Center, Inc. Board of Directors, February 1, 1993; Minutes, DeKalb Medical Center, Inc. Board of Directors, August 2, 1993.
20 Minutes, DeKalb Medical Center, Inc. Board of Directors, December 5, 1994.
21 Minutes, DeKalb Medical Center, Inc. Board of Directors, August 3, 1998.

Communications: The DeKalb Medical Employee Newsletter

1 Unnamed employee newsletter, November 10, 1961.
2 "The Newspaper Is Names!," *The General In Decatur*, November 24, 1961; "The *InDecatur*'s Beginning," *InDecatur*, April 5, 1979.
3 "A Salute to the Second Floor Nurses," *The General InDecatur*, November 9, 1962.
4 *The General InDecatur*, June 8, 1961.
5 *The General InDecatur*, July 20, 1962.
6 *The General InDecatur*, July 20, 1962.
7 *The General InDecatur*, May 14, 1971.
8 *The General InDecatur*, November12, 1971; "Monnie Mitchell Retires," *InDecatur*, August, 1985
9 *InDecatur*, March, 1993.
10 *The General InDecatur*, February 2, 1962.
11 *The General InDecatur*, February 2, 1962.
12 "New Look at DeKalb General Hospital," *InDecatur*, August 1, 1975.
13 DeKalb General Hospital DeKalb Medical Center *Indecatur*, June 1984.
14 "DeKalb General Hospital," *Indecatur*, January 1986–July 1988; "*InDecatur* Sports A New Look," *InDecatur*, December 1988.
15 *InDecatur*, February 3, 1983.
16 "New *InDecatur* Newsletter Debuts," *InDecatur*, January 1999.

The Credit Union

1 Minutes, DeKalb County Hospital Authority, January 14, 1963.
2 Minutes, DeKalb County Hospital Authority, May 8, 1967.
3 Minutes, DeKalb County Hospital Authority, June 13, 1969.
4 Minutes, DeKalb County Hospital Authority, February 2, 1970.
5 "Credit Union," *The General InDecatur*, January 23, 1970.
6 "Credit Union," *The General InDecatur*, March 20, 1970.
7 Minutes, DeKalb County Hospital Authority, February 1, 1971.
8 Minutes, DeKalb County Hospital Authority, October 4, 1972.
9 "News From the Credit Union," *The General InDecatur*, June 11, 1971.
10 "C. O. I. N.," *The General InDecatur*, February 4, 1972.
11 "Great News from the Credit Union," *The General InDecatur*, October 13, 1972.
12 *InDecatur*, October 14, 1982.
13 Minutes, DeKalb Medical Center, Inc. Board of Directors, May 2, 1994.
14 "Credit Union," Wikipedia. The Free Encyclopedia, http://en.wilipedia.org/wiki/Credit_union, March 27, 2007.

15 "1994 Annual Report," DeKalb Medical Employees' Federal Credit Union; "DMC Credit Union Receives Highest Rating," *InDecatur*, November 1993.
16 "1994 Annual Report."
17 "1994 Annual Report;" Minutes, DeKalb Medical Center, Inc. Board of Directors, May 2, 1994.
18 "DeKalb Medical Employees' Federal Credit Union Expands to Better Serve Members," *InDecatur*, June 1994.
19 "About Us," MembersFirst Federal Credit Union, http://www.membersfirstga.com/asp/aboutus.asp, March 27, 2007.
20 "About Us."
21 "About Us;" "2006 Annual Report," MembersFirst Credit Union.

Demographic Changes with Rich Opportunities

1 John Gerlach, CEO, "DRHS Values Guide Our Mission," *InDecatur*, September 2000.
2 Eric Norwood, "Our Values: Diversity, Respect, Healing and Service," *InDecatur*, March 2004.
3 Minutes, DeKalb County Hospital Authority, November 2, 1970; Minutes, DeKalb County Hospital Authority, July 7, 1975.
4 Minutes, DeKalb Medical Center, Inc. Board of Directors, May 1, 1995.
5 John Gerlach, CEO, "Current Issues," *InDecatur*, August 1995.
6 "DMC Forms Diversity Committee," *InDecatur*, December 1995.
7 Minutes, DeKalb Regional Healthcare, Inc. Board of Directors, January 14, 2005.
8 "DMC Physicians Appoint New Leaders," and "DMC at Hillandale Names First Medical Staff Officers," *InDecatur*, December 2004–January 2005.
9 *InDecatur*, November 7, 1975.
10 *InDecatur*, July 1984.
11 "County Fact Sheet: DeKalb County, Georgia," Federation for American Immigration Reform, http://www.fairus.org/site/PageServer?pagename=research_research2b4f_sup.
12 "County Fact Sheet: DeKalb County, Georgia."
13 "County Fact Sheet: DeKalb County, Georgia."
14 "County Fact Sheet: DeKalb County, Georgia."
15 Mary Lou Pickel, "A Revolution in Diversity: Demographics in County Shifted Dramatically From 2000 to 2007," *The Atlanta Journal-Constitution*, August 7, 2008.
16 Pickel.
17 "Population 2005: DeKalb County, Georgia," epodunk, http://www.epodunk.com/cgibin/popInfo.php?locIndex=7908.
18 "DeKalb County Quick Facts from the U. S. Census Bureau," U.S. Census Bureau: State and County Quick Facts, http://quickfacts.census.gov/qfd/states/13/13/13089.html, December 10, 2007.
19 "DeKalb County, Georgia (GA)—Household income, demographics, local cities, towns and villages," http://www.muninetguide.com/states/Georgia/DeKalb.php, December 10, 2007.
20 "DeKalb County, Georgia – Wikipedia, the free encyclopedia," http://en.wikipedia.org/wiki/DeKalb_ County,_Georgia, December 10, 2007.

Diabetes Services

1 Minutes, DeKalb County Hospital Authority, June 3, 1985.
2 Minutes, DeKalb County Hospital Authority, August 5, 1985; Minutes, DeKalb County Hospital Authority, November 3, 1986.
3 "DeKalb General Announces Diabetes Medical Center Opening," *Indecatur*, January 1986.
4 "Diabetes Medical Center Celebrates 5-Year Anniversary," *InDecatur*, January 1991.
5 "Diabetes Medical Center Celebrates Birthday," *InDecatur*, February 1987.
6 "Diabetes Medical Center Celebrates 5-Year Anniversary."
7 "Diabetes Medical Center Celebrates Birthday."
8 Minutes, DeKalb Medical Center, Inc., Board of Directors, June 1, 1992.
9 "DeKalb Medical Center's Diabetes Education Program Lauded for Multicultural Efforts," DeKalb Medical Center—News and Media, http://www.dekalbmedicalcenter.org/shownews.asp?id=801.
10 "Foundation Projects: Building a Healthier Tomorrow," http://www.dekalbmedical.org/Foundation Giving/Projects/…/183/Default.aspx .
11 "DeKalb Medical Center at Hillandale Offers Type II Diabetes Classes," DeKalb Medical news release, September 24, 2003, http://www.dekalbmedical.org/NewsMedia/…/Default.aspx?ai. . . .
12 "Diabetes," DeKalb Medical - Intranet, http://www.dekalbmedical.org/classesandevents/. . . /Diabetes.
13 "The Center for Outpatient Diabetes Education," http://www.dekalbmedical.org/ProgramServices/DiabetesServicesEducation….
14 "Diabetes," DeKalb Medical – Intranet, http://intranet.drhs.org/dept/…id=9026.
15 "DeKalb Medical Center's Diabetes Education Program Lauded for Multicultural Efforts," DeKalb Medical Center—News and Media, http:// www.dekalbmedicalcenter.org/shownews.asp? id=801.

Education Services

1 Mrs. Gertrude Ennis, mathematics teacher, Sylvania High School, Sylvania, Georgia, 1946.
2 Peter M. Senge, *The Fifth Discipline: The Art and Practice of the Learning Organization*, Currency Doubleday, Publishers, 1990.
3 *The General InDecatur*, November 24, 1961; The General InDecatur, January 5, 1962.
4 The General InDecatur, January 7, 1972.
5 "Orientations Scheduled" and "Medical Terminology Course," *The General InDecatur*, December 8, 1961; "Safety First," *The General InDecatur*, February 16, 1962.
6 *The General InDecatur*, January 5, 1962.
7 Mary Hollis interview, February 28, 2006.
8 Minutes, DeKalb County Hospital Authority, June 1962.
9 Barbara Lewis, RN, interview, June 6, 2008.
10 *InDecatur*, August 2003.
11 "Our Training and Education Section," *The General InDecatur*, April 11, 1975; *The General InDecatur*, January 7, 1972.
12 Lewis interview.
13 "Our Training and Education Section."
14 Minutes, DeKalb County Hospital Authority, November 1, 1971.
15 "DeKalb Medical Training Class Descriptions," DeKalb Medical – Intranet.
16 Dannie Bell and Martin Isganitis interview, June 10, 2008.
17 Anne Fears, MBA, interview, June 6, 2008.
18 *The General InDecatur*, January 5, 1973; "Advanced EMT Program Held," *InDecatur*, September 12, 1975.
19 "Training Expands Department," *InDecatur*, March 19, 1981.
20 Lewis interview.
21 *The General InDecatur*, November 11, 1982; *The General InDecatur*, February 17, 1983.
22 "Training Staff Makes Changes," *InDecatur*, January 1985.
23 "Training and Continuing Education Department Offers Alternatives for Receiving In-services," *InDecatur*, September 1990.
24 "DHS Pilots New Video Training System," *InDecatur*, January 1989.

25 Fears interview.
26 Fears interview.
27 Fears interview.
28 Fears interview.
29 "DeKalb Medical Training Class Descriptions."
30 Fears interview.
31 "DRHS Goes High-Tech With Computer-Based Learning," *InDecatur*, December 2000.
32 Fears interview.
33 Fears interview.
34 Minutes, DeKalb County Hospital Authority, March 11, 1963.
35 Marilyn Barry, "The Health Sciences Library: Selected Moments in History."
36 Minutes, DeKalb County Hospital Authority, May 12, 1969.
37 Minutes, Quarterly Medical Staff Meeting, January 1972.
38 Minutes, Medical Staff Executive Committee, January 1973; Minutes, DeKalb County Hospital Authority, February 2, 1973.
39 "Enlargement of Medical Library at DeKalb General," *The General InDecatur*, October 11, 1974; Minutes, DeKalb County Hospital Authority, April 1, 1974.
40 Minutes, DeKalb County Hospital Authority, March 4, 1974.
41 "Enlargement of Medical Library at DeKalb General;" Minutes, Quarterly Medical Staff Meeting, April 1974.
42 "Enlargement of Medical Library at DeKalb General."
43 Ernie Atkins, MD, Lecture: "The History of DeKalb Medical Center."
44 "Enlargement of Medical Library at DeKalb General."
45 Marilyn Barry interview, October 8, 2008.
46 Marilyn G. Barry curriculum vitae.
47 Marilyn Barry, "Forty Years of Wise Investment in a DMC Library," 2002.
48 Barry, "Forty Years of Wise Investment in a DMC Library."
49 Barry, "Forty Years of Wise Investment in a DMC Library."
50 Minutes, DeKalb County Hospital Authority, August 7, 1978.
51 Barry, "Forty Years of Wise Investment in a DMC Library."
52 Marilyn Barry, "The Health Sciences Library: Selected Moments in History."
53 Barry, "Forty Years of Wise Investment in a DMC Library."
54 "Knowledge Based Sources," DeKalb Medical Center Information Management Plan, March 2007.
55 "DMC's Medical Library Becomes Health Sciences Library," *InDecatur*, September 1990.
56 "New Health Information Resource Opens," *InDecatur*, June 1996.
57 Minutes, Quarterly Medical Staff Meeting, April 1967.
58 "News from Inhalation Therapy," *The General InDecatur*, October 13, 1972.
59 Minutes, Medical Staff Executive Committee, July 1970.
60 Minutes, DeKalb County Hospital Authority, July 1973.
61 Minutes, DeKalb County Hospital Authority, October 6, 1975.
62 Minutes, DeKalb County Hospital Authority, November 3, 1975.
63 *The General InDecatur*, March 1977.
64 Barry interview.
65 Barry interview.
66 Minutes, DeKalb County Hospital Authority, December 1977.
67 "First Operating Room Technician Class Graduates at DeKalb Community College," *The General InDecatur*, July 6, 1973.
68 Minutes, DeKalb County Hospital Authority, September 1976.
69 "DRHS Increases Tuition Reimbursement," *InDecatur*, August 2001.
70 "RNs Receive Bachelor's Degrees," *InDecatur*, June 25, 1981.
71 "Master Degree Program Offered Through Satellite Program," *InDecatur*, July 1991.
72 "DRHS Partners Earn MBA on Campus," *InDecatur*, May 1999.

Emergency Services

1 Minutes, DeKalb County Hospital Authority, June 5, 1972.
2 Minutes, DeKalb Medical Center, Inc. Board of Directors, April 2, 2001; "Patrick O'Neal, MD, Named State EMS Medical Director," *InDecatur*, December 2000; "J. Patrick O'Neal, MD, Retires After 29 Years of Service," *InDecatur*, January–February 2002.
3 *InDecatur*, February 17, 1983.
4 Minutes, DeKalb Medical Center, Inc. Board of Directors, February 4, 2002; *InDecatur*, April 2002.
5 Minutes, Medical Staff Executive Committee at Hillandale, September 5, 2006.
6 *InDecatur*, April 1989.
7 *InDecatur*, January 1991.
8 *InDecatur*, June 1990.
9 *InDecatur*, January 1996.
10 "O'Neal Retires After 29 Years of Service."
11 Patrick O'Neal, MD, personal communication, December 18, 2008.
12 Minutes, DeKalb Medical Center, Inc. Board of Directors, November 6, 1995.
13 Minutes, DeKalb Regional Healthcare System, Inc. Board of Directors, April 11, 2005.
14 Minutes, DeKalb Regional Healthcare System, Inc. Board of Directors, May 9, 2005.
15 Minutes, DeKalb Medical Center, Inc. Board of Directors, October 4, 1971.
16 "New Emergency Entrance Now Open," *InDecatur*, September 12, 1975.
17 Minutes, DeKalb Medical Center, Inc. Board of Directors, October 28, 1996.
18 "O'Neal Retires After 29 Years of Service."
19 "Emergency Department Project Receives Approval," *InDecatur*, February 1995.
20 "DMC Expansion To Benefit Community," Special Edition *InDecatur*, June 1996.
21 "Emergency and ADTC Providing Faster Care," *InDecatur*, November 26, 1982.
22 "New Program for Emergency Department Patients," *InDecatur*, December 1992.
23 "Emergency Department Answers Call for Change," *InDecatur*, April 1990.
24 "Emergency Department Begins Two New Programs," *InDecatur*, September 1990.
25 Minutes, DeKalb County Hospital Authority, August 3, 1987.
26 Minutes, DeKalb County Hospital Authority, February 1, 1988.
27 Minutes, DeKalb County Hospital Authority, February 8, 1965.
28 Minutes, DeKalb County Hospital Authority, June 4, 1990.
29 "DeKalb Rape Crisis Center Honors DeKalb Medical Center Physician Assistant," DeKalb Medical Center—News & Media, http://www.dekalbmedicalcenter.org/shownews.asp?id=892, March 29, 2007.
30 "DeKalb Rape Crisis Center Honors DeKalb Medical Center Physician Assistant;" "DeKalb Rape Crisis Center: Your W.H.A.T Dollars at Work," *W.H.A.T.'s Happening: Working, Healing, Achieving Together*, June–July, 2005.
31 "DeKalb Rape Crisis Center Honors DeKalb Medical Center Physician Assistant."
32 "New Chest Pain Center Opens at DMC," *InDecatur*, December 1991.
33 Minutes, DeKalb County Hospital Authority, August 5, 1991.
34 J. Patrick O'Neal, MD, "From DeKalb General Hospital's ER to DeKalb Medical Center's ED."

35 Minutes, DeKalb County Hospital Authority, March 10, 1969
36 "Office of Emergency Medical Services/Trauma Operating Report," Georgia Department of Human Resources, Division of Public Health, 2005, p. 11
37 Minutes, DeKalb County Hospital Authority, June 3, 1985
38 Minutes, DeKalb County Hospital Authority, February 2, 1987
39 Minutes, DeKalb County Hospital Authority, January 6, 1986
40 Minutes, DeKalb County Hospital Authority, April 6, 1987
41 Minutes, DeKalb County Hospital Authority, June 6, 1988
42 Minutes, DeKalb County Hospital Authority, July 6, 1987
43 Minutes, DeKalb County Hospital Authority, June 5, 1989.
44 Minutes, DeKalb County Hospital Authority, June 5, 1989.
45 Minutes, DeKalb County Hospital Authority, November 6, 1989.
46 Minutes, DeKalb County Hospital Authority, January 2, 1990.
47 "DMC Names Trauma Service Director," *InDecatur*, September, 1997.
48 "Trauma in Georgia: Analysis of Trauma System Data," Georgia Department of Human Resources, Division of Public Health, Office of Emergency Medicine/Trauma, 2003, p. 16.
49 "Trauma Service," Report to the DeKalb Medical Center, Inc. Board of Directors, by John R. Gerlach, CEO, July 7, 1997; Minutes, DeKalb Medical Center, Inc. Board of Directors, June 4, 2001; Minutes, DeKalb Regional Healthcare System, Inc. Board of Directors, November 14, 2005.
50 "DeKalb Medical Center Trauma Service Recognized," DeKalb Medical Center—News and Media, April 11, 2005; http://www.dekalbmedicalcenter.org/shownews.asp?id=828; "DMC Trauma Service Receives Recognition: Only Adult Trauma Center in DeKalb County Re-designated," *InDecatur*, February 2005.
51 Eric Norwood, CEO, memorandum, Medical Staff Executive Committee "Future Direction for DMC Central Trauma Program," June 6, 2005.
52 "DeKalb Medical Center Trauma Service Recognized."
53 Eric Norwood, CEO, memorandum, June 6, 2005
54 Minutes, DeKalb Medical Center, Inc. Board of Directors, June 1, 1998; Minutes, DeKalb Medical Center, Inc. Board of Directors, September 3, 2002; Minutes, DeKalb Medical Center, Inc. Board of Directors, March 3, 2003.
55 Minutes, Finance Committee, DeKalb Regional Healthcare System, December 5, 2005; CEO Strategic Updates, DRHS Board of Directors, Inc., June 2006.
56 Minutes, Medical Staff Executive Committee, March 16, 2006; Minutes, Medical Staff Executive Committee, June 27, 2007; CEO Strategic Updates, DRHS Board of Directors, Inc., February 2007.
57 Andy Miller and Chandler Brown, "Trauma Network Loses DeKalb Medical Center," *The Atlanta Journal Constitution*, March 22, 2007.
58 Eric Norwood, CEO, memorandum, June 6, 2005.
59 Miller and Brown
60 Eric Norwood, CEO, memorandum, June 6, 2005
61 Minutes, DeKalb Regional Healthcare System, Inc. Board of Directors, June 13, 2005; Minutes, DeKalb Regional Healthcare System, Inc. Board of Directors, December 12, 2005
62 CEO Strategic Updates, DRHS Board of Directors, Inc., April 2007

Home Health Services

1 Minutes, DeKalb County Hospital Authority, July 8, 1967.
2 Minutes, DeKalb County Hospital Authority, May 6, 1985.
3 Minutes, DeKalb County Hospital Authority, December 5, 1988.
4 Minutes, DeKalb Regional Healthcare System, Inc., April 29, 1993.
5 Minutes, DeKalb Medical Center, Inc., December 4, 1995.
6 Minutes, DeKalb Regional Healthcare System, Inc., January 5, 1998; Minutes, DeKalb Medical Center, Inc., September 2, 1997; "DMC Now Offers Home Health Services," *InDecatur*, February 1998.
7 Minutes, DeKalb Regional Healthcare System, Inc., January 5, 1998; Minutes, DeKalb Medical Center, Inc., September 2, 1997; Minutes, DeKalb Medical Center, Inc., January 8, 1998.
8 Minutes, DeKalb Regional Healthcare System, Inc., September 9, 1998; Minutes, DeKalb Regional Healthcare System, Inc., June 7, 1999.
9 Minutes, DeKalb Regional Healthcare System Finance Committee, August 28, 1997.
10 "DMC Now Offers Home Health Services."
11 Minutes, DeKalb Medical Center, Inc., October 5, 1998.
12 Minutes, DeKalb Medical Center, Inc., January 3, 2000.
13 Minutes, DeKalb Regional Healthcare System, Inc., August 7, 2000.
14 Minutes, DeKalb Regional Healthcare System, Inc., December 4, 2000.
15 "DMC Home Health Provides Care for Home-Bound Patients," *InDecatur*, April, 2002.
16 "DMC Home Health Provides Care for Home-Bound Patients," *InDecatur*, April, 2002; Joyce Osborne, RN, Director, Home Health, personal communication, June 10, 2008.
17 CEO Strategic Update to the DeKalb Regional Health Board of Directors, October 2007; Mackay Asbury, Business Development Manager, Visiting Nurse Health System of Atlanta, personal communication, March 12, 2008.
18 CEO Strategic Update, October 2007.

Information Technology

1 DeKalb County Hospital Authority Finance Committee Report of Budget Policy Investigation, Fiscal Year 1965-66.
2 Minutes, DeKalb County Hospital Authority, November 14, 1966.
3 Minutes, Medical Staff Executive Committee, November, 1966.
4 Minutes, Medical Staff Executive Committee, May 1969.
5 Minutes, DeKalb County Hospital Authority, September 8, 1967.
6 "Bill Chapman Promoted as Data Project Manager of Computer Group," *The General InDecatur*, April 16, 1971.
7 Minutes, DeKalb County Hospital Authority, June 7, 1971.
8 "Data Collection System Update," *InDecatur*, April 8, 1977.
9 Minutes, DeKalb County Hospital Authority, November 5, 1973.
10 Minutes, Special Meeting, DeKalb County Hospital Authority, December 16, 1977; "Data Collections and Communications System," *InDecatur*, August 1, 1975.
11 Minutes, Special Meeting, DeKalb County Hospital Authority, December 16, 1977; Minutes, DeKalb County Hospital Authority, July 5, 1977.
12 Minutes, Special Meeting, DeKalb County Hospital Authority, February 22, 1978.
13 Minutes, DeKalb County Hospital Authority,

May 5, 1980.
14 Minutes, DeKalb County Hospital Authority, February 22, 1978.
15 Minutes, DeKalb County Hospital Authority, July 2, 1979; "First Patient Admitted on New Data Collection and Communication System," *InDecatur*, August 9, 1979.
16 "New Computer System By June," *InDecatur*, January 11, 1979.
17 Minutes, DeKalb County Hospital Authority, August 2, 1982; "Computer System Preparing for 1990s," *Indecatur*, August 1987.
18 "Computer System Preparing for 1990s," *Indecatur*, August 1987; Minutes, DeKalb County Hospital Authority, May 5, 1986.
19 "Computer System Preparing for 1990s," *Indecatur*, August 1987.
20 "DeKalb Regional Healthcare System Implements Document Imaging System," AMS News Release, September 18, 2001, http://www3.amsinc.com/CMC/newsroom.nsf/pr/JWAY-52SJ95.
21 "Nothing But 'Net," Health Management Technology, February 2005, http:www.healthmgttech.com/archives/0205/0205nothing_but.htm.
22 Minutes, DeKalb Regional Healthcare System, Inc. Board of Directors, February 3, 2003.
23 Reynolds, "Nothing But 'Net;" "DRHS FOCUSes on Technology," *InDecatur*, April 1, 2003; "FOCUS Implementation to Improve Business Processes, *InDecatur*, January–February 2004.
24 Reynolds, "Nothing But 'Net."
25 Barbara Kleynen, RN, Critical Care Services Coordinator, letter to DeKalb Medical Center Board of Trustees and DeKalb Regional Healthcare System Board of Trustees, March 1, 2000.
26 Minutes, DeKalb Regional Healthcare System, Inc. Finance Committee, April 23, 2002.
27 Minutes, DeKalb Regional Healthcare System, Inc. Finance Committee, April 23, 2002.
28 Minutes, DeKalb Regional Healthcare System, Inc. Finance Committee, April 23, 2002.
29 Reynolds, "Nothing But 'Net."
30 Reynolds, "Nothing But 'Net;" "Cynthia Adgate Joins DRHS as Chief Information Officer," *InDecatur*, August 2002.
31 Minutes, DeKalb Regional Healthcare System, Inc., November 22, 2003.
32 Reynolds, "Nothing But 'Net;" Minutes, DeKalb Regional Healthcare System, Inc. Finance Committee, April 23, 2002.
33 "DRHS Launches QUEST for Better Patient Care," *InDecatur*, May-June 2002.
34 Norman Jacobs, MD, interview August 13, 2008.
35 Jacobs interview.
36 "Sunrise Clinical Manager Rolled Out Hospital-wide in 14 Hours at DeKalb Medical Center," Eclipsys News Release, http://www.eclipsys.com/about/CaseStudies/customers_CS_DeKalb.asp.
37 "QUEST Training Begins in February," *InDecatur*, January–February 2004.
38 Eric Norwood, CEO, email to All Notes Users from "WOW What A Week!" September 28, 2007.
39 "DeKalb Medical Center Named to Prestigious National 'Most Wired' List," *Communique: A Newsletter for the Medical Staff of DeKalb Medical Center*, September–October 2005.
40 "DeKalb Medical Center Named 2006 Most Wired Hospital," *datelineDeKalb*, September–October 2006.
41 Norwood email.

Laboratory Services

1 Frank Matthews, MD, interview, December 10, 2008.
2 Minutes, DeKalb Medical Center, Inc. Board of Directors, March 3, 1997.
3 "Employee Beat," *InDecatur*, January 1996.
4 The General InDecatur, May 15, 1970.
5 Minutes, DeKalb County Hospital Authority, March 23, 1960; Matthews interview.
6 Frank Matthews, MD, "The Laboratory at DeKalb," February 9, 1997.
7 Matthews, "The Laboratory at DeKalb."
8 Matthews, "The Laboratory at DeKalb."
9 "FDA Rules Mandates Expanded Screening Criteria for Each Blood Donation," Transplant News, June 30, 2001, http://findarticles.com/p/articles/mi_m0YUG/is_12_11/ai_n18612098.
10 Matthews, "The Laboratory at DeKalb."
11 Roslyn Heath, MT, MBA, director, Laboratory Administrative Services, interview, October 2, 2008.
12 Matthews, "The Laboratory at DeKalb;" Matthews interview.
13 Matthews, "The Laboratory at DeKalb."
14 Heath interview; "Clinical Lab Announces Roll-Out of New Hematology Equipment," *dateline DeKalb* E-Digest, January 7, 2008.
15 Matthews interview.
16 Heath interview.
17 Heath interview.
18 Matthews, "The Laboratory at DeKalb."
19 Heath interview.
20 Matthews interview.
21 "Toxicology Lab Opens for Business," *InDecatur*, May 2000.
22 Matthews interview.
23 "Hiram Ragsdale Employed Longest at DeKalb General," *The General InDecatur*, May 12, 1972.
24 Matthews interview.
25 Minutes, Medical Staff Executive Committee, May 1, 2007.
26 "New Lab Debuts This Month," *InDecatur*, April 1997.
27 "Lab Computer Is Retired," *InDecatur*, February 1999.
28 Matthews, "The Laboratory at DeKalb."
29 "New Lab Debuts This Month."
30 *InDecatur*, April 2000.
31 "New Lab Debuts This Month."
32 Matthews interview; Heath interview.

Medical Records

1 "Medical Records," *The General InDecatur*, January 23, 1970.
2 "Medical Audit: A New Concept," *The General InDecatur,* January 3, 1975.
3 Ron McCranie interview February 15, 2008.
4 "Frances Black Retires After 23 Years," *InDecatur*, April 26, 1984.
5 McCranie interview.
6 "Faye Sophy Appointed Director," *InDecatur*, May 24, 1984.
7 Ginna Evans, "DMC Mourns Loss of Faye Sophy," *InDecatur*, August 2000.
8 Ginna Evans.
9 "Promotion," *The General InDecatur*, June 12, 1970
10 McCranie interview.
11 "DRHS Implements Document Imaging," *InDecatur*, August 2001.
12 McCranie interview.

Medical Staff

1 Minutes, DeKalb County Hospital Authority, July 7, 1969.
2 Minutes, DeKalb County Hospital Authority, May 3, 1971.
3 Minutes, DeKalb County Hospital Authority, October 1, 1973.
4 Ernest Atkins, MD, "The History of DeKalb Medical Center," oral presentation, February 27, 1997.
5 Floyd Sanders, MD, personal communication.
6 Greg Hinesley, RN, personal communication.
7 Minutes, DeKalb County Hospital Authority,

August 30, 1961.
8 Minutes, DeKalb County Hospital Authority, July 9, 1962.
9 Minutes, Professional Service Committee of the Authority, October 1969.
10 Minutes, DeKalb County Hospital Authority, May 11, 1964.
11 Minutes, DeKalb County Hospital Authority, January 19, 1969.
12 Minutes, DeKalb County Hospital Authority, March 10, 1969.
13 Minutes, DeKalb County Hospital Authority, June 7, 1971.
14 Minutes, DeKalb County Hospital Authority, April 2, 1973.
15 Minutes, DeKalb County Hospital Authority, July 2, 1973.
16 Minutes, DeKalb County Hospital Authority, May 6, 1974.
17 Minutes, DeKalb County Hospital Authority, August 4, 1974.
18 Minutes, DeKalb County Hospital Authority, September 25, 1974.
19 Minutes, DeKalb County Hospital Authority, June 6, 1988.
20 Minutes, DeKalb Medical Center, Inc., Board of Directors, March 4, 1996.
21 Minutes, DeKalb Medical Center, Inc., Board of Directors, November 5, 2001.
22 Minutes, DeKalb County Hospital Authority, August 12, 1968.
23 Minutes, DeKalb County Hospital Authority, August 9, 1962.
24 Minutes, DeKalb County Hospital Authority, January 11, 1965.
25 Minutes, DeKalb County Hospital Authority, March 11, 1966.
26 Minutes, DeKalb County Hospital Authority, January 11, 1972; Minutes, DeKalb County Hospital Authority, March 6, 1972.
27 Minutes, DeKalb County Hospital Authority, July 2, 1973; Minutes, DeKalb County Hospital Authority, September 4, 1973.
28 Minutes, DeKalb County Hospital Authority, September 4, 1973; Minutes, DeKalb County Hospital Authority, October 1, 1973.
29 Minutes, DeKalb County Hospital Authority, May 23, 1974.
30 Minutes, DeKalb County Hospital Authority, August 5, 1974; Minutes, DeKalb County Hospital Authority, September 25, 1974.
31 James L. Bouchard, D.P.M., Chairman, Podiatry Department, Decatur Hospital, letter to John R. Gerlach, CEO, DeKalb Medical Center, November 6, 1996.
32 Sanford Hartman, MD, Chief of Staff, memorandum to All Department Chiefs re: Podiatry, December 3, 1998.
33 Minutes, DeKalb Medical Center, Inc. Board of Directors, May 3, 1999.
34 Minutes, DeKalb Medical Center Medical Staff Executive Committee, February 29, 2000.
35 Minutes, Medical Staff Executive Committee, January 3, 2007.
36 *InDecatur*, July 1990.
37 Minutes, DeKalb Medical Center, Inc. Board of Directors, December 2, 1996; Minutes, DeKalb Medical Center, Inc. Board of Directors, February 2, 1998.
38 "DMC Adopts New Medical Staff Development Plan," *InDecatur*, April 1998; "Factors in Support of Rescinding the 1996 Board Resolution Creating the Medical Staff Development Plan," Minutes, DeKalb Medical Center, Inc. Board of Directors, June 2, 2003.
39 "Factors in Support of Rescinding the 1996 Board Resolution Creating the Medical Staff Development Plan."
40 Minutes, DeKalb Medical Center, Inc. Board of Directors, June 2, 2003.
41 "DMC Names New Physician Recruitment and Retention Director," *InDecatur*, September 10, 2005.
42 "Medical Staff Restructure Continues," *Medical Staff Communiqué*, March 4, 2004.
43 Eric Norwood, CEO, interview, August 21, 2008.

Mental (Behavioral) Health Services

1 Minutes, DeKalb County Hospital Authority, October 10, 1958.
2 *Decatur-DeKalb News*, January 8, 1959.
3 *Decatur-DeKalb News*, January 15, 1959.
4 *Decatur-DeKalb News*, January 15, 1959.
5 "DeKalb Hospital to Have Space for Mentally Ill," *Decatur-DeKalb News*, January 22, 1959.
6 Minutes, DeKalb County Hospital Authority, May 17, 1965.
7 Minutes, Medical Staff Executive Committee, January 21, 1967.
8 Minutes, DeKalb County Hospital Authority, July 7, 1967.
9 Minutes, Medical Staff Executive Committee, November 26, 1968.
10 Sam Nunn, Senator, letter from to Margaret Heckler, Secretary, the U.S. Department of Health and Human Resources, February 15, 1985.
11 Minutes, Medical Staff Executive Committee, October 27, 1969; Minutes, DeKalb County Hospital Authority, December 1, 1969.
12 Minutes, DeKalb County Hospital Authority, December 1, 1969.
13 Minutes, DeKalb County Hospital Authority Professional Service Committee, December 30, 1969.
14 Minutes, DeKalb County Hospital Authority, May 3, 1971.
15 "Inpatient Mental Health Unit Open," *The General InDecatur*, March 5, 1971; Minutes, DeKalb County Hospital Authority, April 5, 1971; Minutes, DeKalb County Hospital Authority, February 1, 1971.
16 "Inpatient Mental Health Unit Open."
17 Minutes, Special Committee on Mental Health, DeKalb County Hospital Authority, March 10, 1971.
18 Minutes, DeKalb County Hospital Authority, April 3, 1972; Minutes, Coordinating Committee for Central DeKalb County Mental Health Unit, March 14, 1972.
19 Jim Wooten, "Hospital Ripped on Mental Health," *The Atlanta Journal*, December 15, 1971.
20 Minutes, DeKalb County Hospital Authority, February 5, 1973.
21 Minutes, DeKalb County Hospital Authority, April 2, 1973; Minutes, DeKalb County Hospital Authority, May 3, 1973.
22 "Central DeKalb Mental Health Center Opens on Ground Floor," *The General InDecatur*, February 2, 1973.
23 Minutes, DeKalb County Hospital Authority, April 7, 1975.
24 "Dr. Douglas Talbott Heads Drug-Alcohol Treatment for DeKalb County," *The General InDecatur*, January 3, 1975.
25 Minutes, DeKalb County Hospital Authority, January 5, 1976.
26 Minutes, DeKalb County Hospital Authority, September 8, 1981; Minutes, DeKalb County Hospital Authority, January 4, 1982; Minutes, DeKalb County Hospital Authority, August 8, 1982.
27 Minutes, DeKalb County Hospital Authority, October 7, 1985; Minutes, DeKalb County Hospital Authority, December 2, 1985; Sam Nunn, letter.
28 Minutes, DeKalb County Hospital Authority, May 3, 1982.
29 "Mental Health Expands," *InDecatur*, August 13, 1976; *InDecatur*, February 1990.
30 "DeKalb Medical Center Expands Substance

Abuse Treatment Program," *InDecatur*, October 1989.
31 Minutes, DeKalb County Hospital Authority, January 4, 1988; Minutes, DeKalb County Hospital Authority, June 5, 1989.
32 "Mental Health Unit Offers Full Care," *InDecatur*, January 19, 1984.
33 Minutes, DeKalb County Hospital Authority, June 1, 1992; "New Med-Psych Unit Opens," *InDecatur*, November, 1992.
34 "Mental Health Services Expands," *InDecatur*, November, 1996.
35 Minutes, Finance Committee, DeKalb Regional Healthcare System, Inc., December 2, 1999.
36 Charlene L. McGinty letter to Bonnie L. Phipps, "Re: Merger of Strategic Decisions Systems, Inc. (SDS) into Behavioral Health Partners, Inc. (BHP)," April 24, 1997; Minutes, Finance Committee, DeKalb Regional Healthcare System, Inc. December 2, 1999.
37 "Behavioral Health Partners, Inc. Overview Presentation," made to PROMINA Health Plan, March 2, 1998.
38 "Behavioral Health Partners, Inc. Overview Presentation."
39 "Behavioral Health Partners, Inc. Overview Presentation."
40 Minutes, Behavioral Health Partners, Inc. Board of Directors Meeting, December 10, 1998.
41 Minutes, Behavioral Health Partners, Inc. Board of Directors Meeting, November 2, 1999.
42 Minutes, Finance Committee, DeKalb Regional Healthcare System, Inc., December 2, 1999.
43 Minutes, Finance Committee, DeKalb Regional Healthcare System, Inc., December 2, 1999; Minutes, Behavioral Health Partners, Inc. Board of Directors Meeting, November 2, 1999.
44 Netsmart Technologies, Inc., letter, to Gary Long, "Re: Netsmart Technologies, Inc. Acquisition of Connex Systems," December 6, 1999.
45 Ernst & Young LLP, "Internal Audit: Behavioral Health Partners, Inc. Review(Draft)," December 30, 1999.
46 Bill Sublett memorandum to Jack Gerlach, "BHP" from, April 21, 2000.
47 Minutes, Behavioral Health Partners, Inc. Board of Directors Meeting, April 26, 2000.
48 The Employees of Behavioral Health Partners letter to Bill Sublett and Michael Gardenier, April 28, 2000.
49 B. L. Sublett letter to Mr. M. Andrew McCollum, Regional Executive Director, MHMRS Region 12 Regional Board, Augusta, Georgia, May 3, 2000.
50 John R. Gerlach letter, "To Whom It May Concern," October 11, 2002.
51 *InDecatur*, March 2002.
52 Paul Olander interview, July 10, 2008.
53 Paul Olander interview; *InDecatur*, March 2002.
54 Paul Olander interview.
55 "Mental Health Unit Offers Full Care," *InDecatur*, January 19, 1984.
56 Paul Olander interview.

Nursing Home (Skilled Nursing Facility)

1 Minutes, DeKalb County Hospital Authority, February 24, 1958, Dr. Ross McCain reporting on an opinion rendered by DeKalb County attorney, Robin Harris.
2 Minutes, DeKalb County Hospital Authority, April 26, 1960, reporting on a meeting between Mr. Thrasher and Dr. Joe Beasley, Dr. Oscar Vinson, Rep. James Mackay, and Mr. William Uzzell.
3 Minutes, DeKalb County Hospital Authority, September 28, 1960.
4 Minutes, DeKalb County Hospital Authority, October 19, 1960.
5 Minutes, DeKalb County Hospital Authority, November 23, 1960.
6 Minutes, DeKalb County Hospital Authority, January 25, 1961.
7 "Development Plan of DeKalb General Hospital, DeKalb County, Georgia," Bothwell and Nash, Architects, Decatur, Georgia, Evan L. Marbut, Site Planner, Decatur, Georgia, December, 1962.
8 Minutes, DeKalb County Hospital Authority, May 9, 1963.
9 Minutes, DeKalb County Hospital Authority, March 11, 1968.
10 Minutes, DeKalb County Hospital Authority, September 9, 1963.
11 Minutes, DeKalb County Hospital Authority, May 9, 1963.
12 Minutes, DeKalb County Hospital Authority, September 9, 1963; Minutes, DeKalb County Hospital Authority, May 11, 1964.
13 Minutes, DeKalb County Hospital Authority, June 10, 1964.
14 Minutes, DeKalb County Hospital Authority, April 12, 1965.
15 Minutes, DeKalb County Hospital Authority, November 8, 1965; Minutes, DeKalb County Hospital Authority, April 11, 1966.
16 Minutes, DeKalb County Hospital Authority, April 8, 1968.
17 Minutes, DeKalb County Hospital Authority, March 11, 1968; "Federal, State and Local Participation, DeKalb General Hospital Additions," Exhibit IV, June 6, 1968; Minutes, Special Meeting, DeKalb County Hospital Authority, December 12, 1967; William H. Thrasher, Administrator, memorandum to Members of the DeKalb County Hospital Authority, "Financial Information Regarding Expansion," May 16, 1968.
18 Minutes, DeKalb County Hospital Authority, April 6, 1970.
19 Minutes, DeKalb County Hospital Authority, June 1, 1970; Minutes, DeKalb County Hospital Authority, February 7, 1972.
20 Minutes, DeKalb County Hospital Authority, June 5, 1972; Minutes, DeKalb County Hospital Authority, July 10, 1972; Minutes, DeKalb County Hospital Authority, October 11, 1972; Minutes, DeKalb County Hospital Authority, December 4, 1972; Minutes, DeKalb County Hospital Authority, March 15, 1973; Minutes, DeKalb County Hospital Authority, May 7, 1973.
21 Minutes, DeKalb County Hospital Authority, November 3, 1975.
22 Minutes, DeKalb County Hospital Authority, January 5, 1976.
23 *InDecatur*, March 1998, *InDecatur*, February 1998, *InDecatur*, January 1999, *InDecatur*, January 2001, #43.
24 "Skilled Nursing Unit Opens," *InDecatur*, November 7, 1975; "The New Day," *InDecatur*, December 5, 1975; "Granny's Parlor Heals Hair Woes of Patients and Nursing Home Residents," *InDecatur*, July 1988.
25 *InDecatur*, November 1986.
26 *InDecatur*, December 1986.
27 *InDecatur*, April 1987.
28 Minutes, DeKalb County Hospital Authority, February 2, 1976; Minutes, DeKalb County Hospital Authority, June 6, 1977.
29 "DeKalb Medical Center Closes Skilled Nursing Facility," *InDecatur*, March 2003.
30 "DeKalb Medical Center Closes Skilled Nursing Facility," *InDecatur*, March 2003.
31 Minutes, DeKalb Medical Center, Inc. Board of Directors, February 3, 2003; Minutes, DeKalb Medical Center, Inc. Board of Directors, March 3, 2003.

Nursing Services

1 Opal Hopkins Fyffe, RN, interview, March 3, 2006.
2 Kalisch, Phillip A. and Kalisch, Beatrice J.,

American Nursing: A History. Fourth Edition. Philadelphia: Lippincott Williams & Wilkins, 2004, p. 402.
3 Fyffe interview.
4 Minutes, DeKalb County Hospital Authority, August 30, 1961.
5 Fyffe interview .
6 Cathleen Conway Johnson, "The Troubles with Angels of Mercy: The Mass Resignation of Registered Nurses at DeKalb General Hospital, Decatur, Georgia, January 22, 1969." A thesis submitted to the Faculty of the Graduate School of Emory University in partial fulfillment of the requirements for the degree of Doctor of Philosophy, The Graduate Institute of Liberal Arts, 1994.
7 Johnson.
8 Naomi Harman, RN, interviews, April 22, 2008, and May 17, 2008.
9 Harman interviews.
10 Mary Hollis, RN, interview, February 28, 2006.
11 Johnson, p. 39.
12 Johnson, p. 40.
13 Harman interviews; "60 Seconds with Naomi Harman," *InDecatur*, March 1990.
14 Harman interviews.
15 Harman interviews.
16 Kalisch and Kalisch, p. 383.
17 Kalisch and Kalisch, p. 332.
18 "Refresher Course In Progress," *InDecatur*, September 18, 1980.
19 "DRHS Partners Earn MBA On Campus," *InDecatur*, May 1999.
20 Harman interviews.
21 "Nursing Division Reorganizes," *InDecatur*, January 19, 1984.
22 Harman interviews; Hollis interview; Mary Chambers interview, January 24, 2006; *The General InDecatur*, March 3, 1972.
23 *InDecatur*, October 8, 1976
24 "Clinical Ladder Program Implemented for Nurses," *InDecatur*, January 1991
25 "DMC Nurses Advance Through Clinical Ladders Program," *InDecatur*, March 1993.
26 Nursing group interview with Patricia Horton, Ellen Hargett, Beth Singleton, Gay Newton, Carol Campbell, Mary Kay Flake, Nancy Curdy, Cathy Booker, and Cathleen Wheatley, June 13, 2008.
27 "Intermediate Intensive Care Unit Opens," *InDecatur*, March 8, 1979.
28 Nursing group interview.
29 Nursing group interview.
30 Nursing group interview.
31 *InDecatur*, March 1993.
32 Ninfa Saunders curriculum vitae.
33 "DRHS Partners Earn MBA On Campus," *InDecatur*, May 1999.
34 "IV Therapy Completes Transition," *InDecatur*, October 1996.
35 Anne Fears, Director of Education Services, interview, June 6, 2008.
36 "Patient Care Services Restructures Position," *InDecatur*, August 2002.
37 "DMC Designs New Model of Patient Care," *InDecatur*, October 1999.
38 Becky Beagle, RN, "Milestones in the 90s," July 2008.
39 Nursing group interview.
40 Helen Ebaugh, RN, interview, June 10, 2008.
41 Nursing group interview.
42 "Brent Robinson Appointed Assistant VP of Patient Care Services," *InDecatur*, November 2004.
43 "Changed Give DMC Nurses More Visibility, Impact," *InDecatur*, April 2005.
44 "Growing Our Own: Center for Frontline Nursing Leadership," *InDecatur*, September–October 2005.
45 Minutes, Medical Staff Executive Committee, March 6, 2007.

Nutrition Services

1 Robert Prescott letter to William Thrasher, November 21, 1961.
2 "Mattie L. Meadows, Director of Dietary Retires," *InDecatur*, October 10, 1975.
3 Helen Scherer, RD, interview, April 17, 2008.
4 "Mattie L. Meadows, Director of Dietary Retires;" *The General InDecatur*, February 16, 1962.
5 "Mattie L. Meadows, Director of Dietary Retires."
6 "Mattie L. Meadows, Director of Dietary Retires."
7 Nancy Ward, RD, and Gail Shackelford, RD, interview, March 13, 2008.
8 Jim Wooten, "They Serve 5 Meals, Go Home Early," *The Atlanta Journal-Constitution*, October 21, 1971.
9 "Mattie L. Meadows, Director of Dietary Retires;" Minutes, Medical Staff Executive Committee, March 1968.
10 *The General InDecatur*, November 9, 1962.
11 "Maxi Meals From A Mini-Kitchen," *The General InDecatur*, March 20, 1970.
12 Wooten.
13 Scherer interview.
14 Minutes, Medical Staff Quarterly Conference, January 1967.
15 Minutes, Medical Staff Quarterly Conference.
16 Ward and Shackelford interview.
17 Ward and Shackelford interview.
18 Nancy Ward, RD, personal communication, November 20, 2008.
19 "Dennis Ryan Director of Food Services," *InDecatur*, November 7, 1975.
20 "Food Service Reorganization," *InDecatur*, November 5, 1976.
21 "Dietary Department Gives Food for Thought," *InDecatur*, September 1984.
22 Ward and Shackelford interview.
23 Ward and Shackelford interview.
24 Ward personal communication.
25 Ward and Shackelford interview.
26 "Have You Eaten With Ford Lately?" *InDecatur*, August 1986.
27 Ward and Shackelford interview.
28 "DMC's Dietary Department Dishes Up Healthier Food," *InDecatur*, September 1990.
29 "Cafeteria Gets a New Look," *InDecatur*, December 1988.
30 Ward and Shackelford interview.
31 Ward personal communication.
32 Ward personal communication.
33 "Cafeteria Completes Serving Area Renovation," *InDecatur*, September–October 1998.
34 Minutes, DeKalb Medical Center, Inc., Board of Directors, August 8, 2002.
35 "New Chef Brings Extra Spice to DMC Food Service," *InDecatur*, February 1999.
36 Ward and Shackelford interview.
37 Minutes, Medical Staff Executive Committee, September 4, 2007; "Bon Appetite! DeKalb Medical and Sodexho will Treat Your Taste Buds!" *datelineDeKalb*, October–November 2007.

Occupational Health and Infection Control

1 Sally Williams, RN, interview, July 7, 2008.
2 *The General InDecatur*, December 8, 1961.
3 *The General InDecatur*, June 26, 1970.
4 *The General InDecatur*, August 9, 1971.
5 *The General InDecatur*, November 10, 1972.
6 Williams interview.
7 *The General InDecatur*, August 9, 1971.
8 Helen Ebaugh, RN, interview, June 10, 2008.
9 *The General InDecatur*, October 12, 1962.
10 *The General InDecatur*, November 12, 1971.
11 *The General InDecatur*, January 1972.

12 *The General InDecatur*, November 10, 1972.
13 Williams interview.
14 "Your Health Nurse," *InDecatur*, October 10, 1975.
15 *The General InDecatur*, January 3, 1975.
16 Ebaugh interview.
17 *InDecatur*, March 1997; Cathy Boyles, RN, interview, June 12, 2008.
18 *InDecatur*, September 2002.
19 *InDecatur*, August 2003.
20 "Occupational Health," DeKalb Medical Interactive Directory, November 5, 2008.
21 *The General InDecatur*, January 19, 1962.
22 *The General InDecatur*, October 12, 1962.
23 "New Modified Work Program Eases Injured Employees Back Into the Work Place," *InDecatur*, July 1989.
24 Boyles interview.
25 DeKalb Medical Interactive Directory.
26 Williams interview.
27 Williams interview.
28 Williams interview.
29 Williams interview; "DeKalb General Hospital Infection Control Committee," *The General InDecatur*, March 1, 1974.
30 "Sally Williams Receives Certification," *InDecatur*, February 16, 1984; "GICN Honors Williams," *InDecatur*, November 1984.
31 Ebaugh interview.
32 Williams interview.
33 Norman Jacobs, MD, interview, August 3, 2008.
34 Betsy McCaughey, "Hospital Infections: Preventable and Unacceptable," *The Wall Street Journal*, August 14, 2008, p. A11.
35 McCaughey.
36 Virginia Brown, RN, "Staph," *The General InDecatur*, September 14, 1962.
37 Jacobs interview.
38 Marti Jaynes, RN, interviews, June 6, 2008 and November 5, 2008.
39 Jacobs interview; "MRSA Threatens Community," DeKalb Medical news release, November 6, 2007.
40 Jacobs interview.
41 Jaynes interview.
42 Jaynes interview.
43 Jaynes interview.
44 Jacobs interview.

Pastoral Services

1 J. Ross McCain, Chairman of the Committee on Personnel, letter to William Thrasher, candidate for the position of hospital administrator, February 13, 1958.
2 J. Ross McCain remarks at the DeKalb General Hospital groundbreaking ceremony, May 15, 1959.
3 Program: Dedication Ceremony, DeKalb General Hospital, April 21, 1961.
4 "DeKalb General Hospital to Lay Cornerstone Sunday," DeKalb General Hospital press release, July 11, 1960.
5 "New Addition Nearly Ready: Hospital Work Nearly Done," *DeKalb New Era*, July 9, 1970.
6 Minutes, DeKalb County Hospital Authority, May 25, 1960 and July 27, 1960.
7 Minutes, DeKalb County Hospital Authority, May 9, 1963.
8 Minutes, DeKalb County Hospital Authority, July 8, 1963.
9 Minutes, DeKalb County Hospital Authority, July 10, 1972.
10 Minutes, DeKalb County Hospital Authority, October 11, 1972.
11 Minutes, DeKalb County Hospital Authority, September 7, 1976.
12 Minutes, DeKalb County Hospital Authority, May 2, 1977.
13 Minutes, DeKalb County Hospital Authority, June 3, 1977.
14 Minutes, DeKalb County Hospital Authority, October 2, 1978; "Hospital Chaplain Named," *InDecatur*, December 14, 1978.
15 "Associate Chaplain Named," *InDecatur*, May 1987.
16 "DeKalb Medical Center Welcomes New Chaplain," *InDecatur*, September 1996.
17 Betty Castellani, DMin, interview, August 26, 2008.
18 "Chapel Dedicated at DeKalb Medical Center," *DeKalb Neighbor*, December 19, 2001.
19 Castellani interview.

Pharmaceutical Services

1 Ernie Atkins, MD, Lecture: "The History of DeKalb Medical Center."
2 Minutes, DeKalb County Hospital Authority, June 11, 1962.
3 Minutes, DeKalb County Hospital Authority, May 17, 1965.
4 Minutes, Medical Staff Executive Committee, July 1965.
5 Minutes, Medical Staff Executive Committee, May 1967.
6 Minutes, DeKalb County Hospital Authority, September 18, 1967.
7 Minutes, Medical Staff Executive Committee, May 26,1969.
8 "Pharmacy Leadership Undergoes Change," *InDecatur*, April 1, 2005.
9 Minutes, DeKalb County Hospital Authority, November 11, 1968.
10 *The General InDecatur*, March 1972.
11 Minutes, DeKalb County Hospital Authority, November 2, 1970.
12 "Briscoe Named Hospital Pharmacist of the Year," *The General InDecatur*, November 10, 1972.
13 Minutes, DeKalb County Hospital Authority, March 10, 1969.
14 Minutes, DeKalb County Hospital Authority, March 1, 1971; Minutes, DeKalb County Hospital Authority, April 5, 1971.
15 Minutes, DeKalb County Hospital Authority, October 4, 1971.
16 Minutes, DeKalb County Hospital Authority, January 3, 1972.
17 Minutes, DeKalb County Hospital Authority, February 7, 1972.
18 Minutes, DeKalb County Hospital Authority, April 3, 1972.
19 Minutes, DeKalb County Hospital Authority, July 10, 1972; Minutes, DeKalb County Hospital Authority, August 7, 1972.
20 Minutes, DeKalb County Hospital Authority, October 11, 1972.
21 "Staff Recognized I.V. Nurse Day," *InDecatur*, February 1985; "Pharmaceutical Services Dispenses More Than Just Drugs," *InDecatur*, October–November 1990.
22 "Staff Recognized I.V. Nurse Day."
23 "IV Team Sticks Together," *InDecatur*, May 1989.
24 Minutes, DeKalb Medical Center, Inc. Board of Directors, May 3, 1993.
25 "IV Therapy Completes Transition," *InDecatur*, October 1996.
26 Minutes, Medical Staff Executive Committee, March 7, 2006.
27 "Walter J. 'Jack' Linn Named Director of Pharmacy," *The General InDecatur*, May 11, 1973.
28 Minutes, DeKalb County Hospital Authority, July 10, 1974; Minutes, DeKalb County Hospital Authority, November 11, 1974.
29 *InDecatur*, September 1989.
30 "Pharmacy Leadership Undergoes Change."
31 "Pharmaceutical Services Dispenses More Than Just Drugs."
32 Scott McAuley, RPh, interview October 9, 2008.
33 McAuley interview.
34 "Pharmaceutical Services Dispenses More Than

Just Drugs."
35 McAuley interview.
36 "Pharmacy Leadership Undergoes Change."
37 "Pharmaceutical Services Dispenses More Than Just Drugs."
38 McAuley interview.
39 McAuley interview.
40 McAuley interview.
41 "DeKalb Medical Center Pharmacy Acquires Robot," *InDecatur*, March 1999.
42 McAuley interview.
43 McAuley interview.
44 "Pharmacy Operations Engagement Helps DeKalb Medical Center Identify Staffing, Technological Efficiencies," VHA Delivering Results, October 2005.
45 McAuley interview; "Pharmacy Operations Engagement. . ."
46 "Pharmacy System Undergoes Change," The *Communique: Medical Staff Newsletter*, March-April 2004.
47 McAuley interview.
48 "Pharmacy Leadership Undergoes Change."
49 McAuley interview.
50 McAuley interview.
51 McAuley interview.
52 McAuley interview

Quality

1 "Hospital Opens Monday, Medical, Administrative Staff Told," *The DeKalb New Era*, April 26, 1961.
2 "Hospital Objectives for 1971–1972," The *InDecatur*, June 1971.
3 "Mission Statement," DeKalb Medical Center Strategic Plan, 1991–1995.
4 DeKalb Medical Center Organization-Wide Performance Improvement Plan, 2001-2002.
5 "Hospital Plan of Care," Minutes, DeKalb Medical Center, Inc. Board of Directors, January 5, 2004.
6 *The General InDecatur*, January 19, 1962.
7 *The General InDecatur*, November 9, 1962.
8 Minutes, DeKalb County Hospital Authority, April 6, 1970.
9 *The General InDecatur*, November 9, 1962.
10 Minutes, DeKalb County Hospital Authority, August 30, 1961.
11 *The General InDecatur*, December 1973.
12 Minutes, DeKalb County Hospital Authority, December 3, 1973; Minutes, DeKalb County Hospital Authority, December 6, 1976.
13 "People Who Have Made Contributions to the Field of Quality Management," *The Quality Gurus*, http://www.dhutton.com/tqm/gurus.html, 1/28/08; "Deming Cycle (PDSA)," *12 Manage Management Communities*, http://www.12manage.com/methods_demingcycle.html, 1/28/08; "The Original Quality Gurus," *Department of Trade and Industry*, www.dti.gov.uk/quality/gurus, 1/28/08.
14 "Hospital Quality Initiative Overview: Centers for Medicare and Medicaid Services, December 2005," U.S. Department of Health and Human Services, http://www.cms.hhs.gov/QualityInitiativesGenInfo, 1/28/08.
15 "Quality Assurance Program Begun," *InDecatur*, December 24, 1981; Minutes, DeKalb County Hospital Authority, February 2, 1981.
16 "JCAHO Quality Assurance Guidelines," *The Accreditation Manual for Hospitals, Joint Commission on Accreditation of Healthcare Organizations*, Oak Brook, Illinois, 1991, http://www.ncbi.nih.gov/books/bv. fcgi?rid=hstat5.table.40607.
17 John R. Gerlach, CEO, and Michael Hartman, MD, chief of staff, memorandum to DeKalb Medical Center Board of Directors: "Proposal for the Establishment of a Multi-Disciplinary Quality Council for DeKalb Medical Center," May 28, 1997.
18 Gerlach and Hartman memorandum.
19 Minutes, DeKalb Medical Center, Inc. Board of Directors, October 6, 1997.
20 Minutes, DeKalb Medical Center, Inc. Board of Directors, September 2, 1997.
21 "DeKalb Medical Center Announces New Departmental Leadership," *InDecatur*, March 2003.
22 *InDecatur*, June-July 2005.
23 "DeKalb Regional Healthcare System (DRHS) Organizational Annual Report, Performance Improvement, FY 2004," Minutes, DeKalb Regional Healthcare System, Inc. Board of Directors, September 9, 2004.
24 "Service Excellence Team Forms to Focus on Customer Service, Patient Care," *InDecatur*, February 2005.
25 "Team EXCEL Introduces New Tools, Management Model," *InDecatur*, June-July 2005.
26 John Gerlach, CEO, "Current Issues," *InDecatur*, March 2003.
27 *Atlanta Business Chronicle*, May 19-25, 2006, p. 5A
28 Eric Norwood memorandum to DPHO Board Members, DRHS Board Members "Clinical Integration," May 25, 2004.
29 "DMC Develops Quality Institute, Meurer Named Director," *InDecatur*, October 2004.
30 Norwood memorandum.
31 Norwood memorandum.
32 Cathleen Wheatley, MS, RN, interview, June 24, 2008.
33 "DeKalb Medical Strengthens Management Team," DeKalb Medical press release, October 22, 2007.
34 Wheatley interview.
35 "DeKalb Regional Health System: The Quality Committee."

Radiology (Imaging) Services

1 Minutes, DeKalb County Hospital Authority, November 19, 1959.
2 Minutes, DeKalb County Hospital Authority, May 27, 1959.
3 Minutes, DeKalb County Hospital Authority, June 24, 1959.
4 Minutes, DeKalb County Hospital Authority, August 19, 1959.
5 Contract between DeKalb County Hospital Authority and Frank E. Morgan, Jr., M.D., signed January 27, 1960.
6 Jo Ann Morgan personal communication, September 29, 2008.
7 Jo Ann Morgan; Minutes, DeKalb County Hospital Authority, February 5, 1973.
8 "Mrs. Della Johnson Named Technical Director of Radiology," *The General InDecatur*, April 17, 1973.
9 "Employee Celebrates 43 Years at DeKalb Medical," DeKalb Medical news release, December 11, 2007.
10 Minutes, DeKalb County Hospital Authority, January 27, 1980.
11 Minutes, DeKalb County Hospital Authority, December 7, 1981.
12 "Radiology Expands Capabilities," *The General InDecatur*, November 9, 1973.
13 Minutes, DeKalb County Hospital Authority, October 11, 1965.
14 Minutes, Medical Staff Executive Committee, May 21, 1968.
15 Minutes, DeKalb County Hospital Authority, May 8, 1967.
16 Minutes, Medical Staff Executive Committee, May 21, 1968.
17 "Graduation: School of Radiologic Technology," *InDecatur*, July 1, 1977.
18 Minutes, DeKalb County Hospital Authority, May 5, 1973.
19 Minutes, DeKalb County Hospital Authority, September 4, 1973.

20 Minutes, DeKalb County Hospital Authority, January 6, 1975.
21 Minutes, DeKalb County Hospital Authority, March 1, 1976.
22 Minutes, DeKalb County Hospital Authority, February 7, 1977.
23 Minutes, DeKalb County Hospital Authority, July 5, 1977.
24 Minutes, DeKalb County Hospital Authority, November 7, 1977.
25 Minutes, Medical Staff Executive Committee, January, 1967.
26 Minutes, Medical Staff Executive Committee, February, 1967.
27 Minutes, DeKalb County Hospital Authority, February 3, 1975.
28 Minutes, DeKalb County Hospital Authority, February 2, 1970.
29 Minutes, DeKalb County Hospital Authority, April 7, 1975.
30 "Radiology Responds to Community's Needs: Mammography Center to Open in Mid-1984," *InDecatur*, February 16, 1984.
31 "Diagnostic Breast Center Expands Services," *InDecatur*, October 2002.
32 Jay Coffsky, MD, interview, September 24, 2008.
33 "Diagnostic Breast Center Expands Services."
34 "DMC Offers New Osteoporosis Service," *InDecatur*, June–July 2000.
35 "Computed Tomography," Wikipedia, http://en.wikipedia.org/wiki/Computerized_axial_tomography, January 24, 2008.
36 Minutes, DeKalb County Hospital Authority, February 4, 1974.
37 "Computed Tomography."
38 Minutes, DeKalb County Hospital Authority, May 6, 1974.
39 Minutes, DeKalb County Hospital Authority, March 3, 1975.
40 Minutes, DeKalb County Hospital Authority, April 7, 1975; Minutes, DeKalb County Hospital Authority, July 6, 1975.
41 Minutes, DeKalb County Hospital Authority, January 4, 1982.
42 "Radiology Expands Capabilities."
43 Minutes, DeKalb County Hospital Authority, November 2, 1970; Minutes, DeKalb County Hospital Authority, October 11, 1972.
44 "Magnetic Resonance Imaging," Wikipedia, http://en.wikipedia.org/wiki/Magnetic_resonance_imaging, January 24, 2008.
45 "Magnetic Resonance Imaging."
46 Minutes, DeKalb County Hospital Authority, March 3, 1984.
47 Minutes, DeKalb County Hospital Authority, May 5, 1986; Minutes, DeKalb County Hospital Authority, August 4, 1986; Minutes, DeKalb County. Hospital Authority, July 6, 1987.
48 Minutes, DeKalb County Hospital Authority, July 6, 1999.
49 "Open MRI Comes to Diagnostic Imaging Center," *InDecatur*, March 1999.
50 "New MRI Added at Central Campus," *InDecatur*, November 2005.
51 "PET Scanning Now Available at DeKalb Medical Center," *InDecatur*, September–October 2001.
52 "PET Scanning Now Available at DeKalb Medical Center."
53 "PET/CT Certificate of Need Approved by the State: Centerpiece of 3-Year Foundation Capital Campaign," Minutes, DeKalb Medical Center, Inc., Board of Directors, September 2, 2003.
54 "Positron Emission Tomography," Wikipedia, http://en.wikipedia.org/wiki/Pet_scans, January 24, 2008.
55 Minutes, DeKalb Regional Healthcare System, Inc. Board of Directors, December 13, 2004; "DeKalb Medical Rolls Out New System to Detect Diseases," *Health and Fitness*, November 15, 2004.
56 "Radiology Expands Capabilities."
57 "Pneumoencephalography," Wikipedia, the Free Encyclopedia, http://en.wikipedia.org/wiki/Pneumoencephalogram, January 24, 2008.
58 "Radiology Responds to Community's Needs: Mammography Center to Open in Mid-1984," *InDecatur*, February 16, 1984; "DeKalb Medical Rolls Out New System to Detect Diseases," *Health and Fitness*, November 15, 2004.
59 "Millennium Technology: Medical Milestones Improve Patient Care," *Health Lines*, Winter, 2000.
60 "Physician at DeKalb Medical Reaches Milestone," *The Champion*, August 31, 2007.
61 "Physician at DeKalb Medical Reaches Milestone."
62 "Radiology Department Unveils PACS," *InDecatur*, March 2002.
63 "DMC at Decatur Radiology Goes Digital," *InDecatur*, November 2004.

Rehabilitation Services

1 "Rehab Services Chooses New Name," *InDecatur*, March 1995.
2 Minutes, Medical Staff Executive Committee, January 9, 1967.
3 Medical Staff Executive Committee, February 10, 1967.
4 Minutes, DeKalb County Hospital Authority, March 13, 1967.
5 Minutes, DeKalb County Hospital Authority, May 8, 1967.
6 Minutes, DeKalb County Hospital Authority, June 7, 1971.
7 "Physical Therapy Department to Open," *The General InDecatur*, March 3, 1972.
8 "Physical Therapy at DeKalb General," *The General InDecatur*, July 7, 1972.
9 Mary Booth Thomas, "Therapy Unit Is Success Story," *The Atlanta Journal*, March 4, 1974.
10 "Physical Therapy Grows: Offers Evening Hours," *InDecatur*, October 5, 1978.
11 "Physical Therapy Grows: Offers Evening Hours."
12 Medical Staff Executive Committee, May 10, 1972; "Occupational Therapy at DGH," *The General InDecatur*, August 4, 1972.
13 "Occupational Therapy at DGH."
14 "Occupational Therapy," *InDecatur*, April 1985.
15 "Speech Therapy Available to Patients," *The General InDecatur*, July 5, 1974.
16 "Rehabilitative Services Center Opens," *InDecatur*, August 20, 1981.
17 Minutes, DeKalb County Hospital Authority, July 10, 1974.
18 Kevin McMullen, director of Rehabilitation Services interview, October 17, 2008.
19 "Enable the Disabled," *InDecatur*, April 1986.
20 McMullen interview.
21 Minutes, DeKalb County Hospital Authority, February 4, 1991.
22 "WorksWell Opens New Facility," *InDecatur*, February–March 1991.
23 Minutes, DeKalb Medical Center, Inc. Board of Directors, July 6, 1992.
24 McMullen interview.
25 "DGH To Offer Specialized ArthritisCare," *InDecatur*, January 1989; "ArthritisCare Opens Outpatient Clinic," *InDecatur*, February 1990.
26 "Conquering the Pain of Arthritis," *Healthy Living*, Spring 1996.
27 "DGH To Offer Specialized ArthritisCare."
28 McMullen interview.
29 "Inpatient Rehabilitation Program Debuts at DeKalb Medical Center," *InDecatur*, September 1989.
30 Minutes, DeKalb County Hospital Authority, May 1, 1989.
31 "Inpatient Rehab Unit Receives Accreditation," *InDecatur*, March 1994; "Inpatient Rehabilitation Continues To Be Successful After

10 Years of Service," *InDecatur*, May 2000; "DMC Schedules Opening of New Rehabilitation Center," *The Decatur-DeKalb News/Era Legal Review*, February 15, 1990.
32 Minutes, DeKalb County Hospital Authority, July 2, 1990.
33 McMullen interview.
34 "IRF Classification Criteria," Center for Medicare and Medicaid Services, HHS.gov.
35 McMullen interview.
36 "DMC Schedules Opening of New Rehabilitation Center."
37 McMullen interview.
38 "DMC Offers New MS Program," *InDecatur*, September 1993.
39 McMullen interview.
40 "Rehabilitation Services Develops Day Treatment Program," *InDecatur*, January 1999.
41 McMullen interview.

Respiratory Care Services

1 "Inhalation Therapy," *The General InDecatur*, August 21, 1970.
2 "Of Interest from Respiratory Therapy," *The General InDecatur*, December 7, 1973.
3 "Inhalation Therapy."
4 "News form Inhalation Therapy," *The General InDecatur*, October 13, 1972.
5 Minutes, DeKalb County Hospital Authority, December 4, 1972.
6 Minutes, DeKalb County Hospital Authority, April 4, 1974.
7 Minutes, DeKalb County Hospital Authority, May 3, 1976; Minutes, DeKalb County Hospital Authority, June 7, 1976; "New Services: Pulmonary Function," *InDecatur*, March 11, 1977.
8 Minutes, DeKalb County Hospital Authority, August 2, 1982.
9 Minutes, DeKalb Medical Center, Inc. Board of Directors, December 4, 1995.
10 *InDecatur*, January 1996.
11 *InDecatur*, April 2000.
12 "Townsend Named New Respiratory Care Director," *InDecatur*, February 2003.
13 "Townsend Named New Respiratory Care Director."
14 Interview with William Townsend, RRT, February 8, 2008.
15 "Sleep Lab Contract," Minutes, Professional Service Committee, DeKalb Medical Center, Inc., May 15, 2001.
16 Minutes, DeKalb Medical Center, Inc. Board of Directors, September 8, 1992.
17 "Sleep Lab Contract."
18 "Sleep Lab Contract."
19 "Sleep Disorders Center, DeKalb Medical Center," SleepCenters.Org, http://www.sleepcenters.org/ CentersInfo.aspx?Center_ID=175604, 1/18/08.

Social Services and Care Management

1 Minutes, Executive Committee of the Medical Staff, June 28, 1971.
2 John R. Gerlach memorandum to Mr. William H. Thrasher: "Establishment of Social Service Department," January 3, 1972.
3 "Social Services Department Established," *The General InDecatur,* January 7, 1972.
4 "DeKalb General Hospital: A Dream From the Early 1950s Became Reality," *The South DeKalb News/Sun*, July 22, 1981; "Fiscal Department Reorganization," *The General InDecatur*, June 11, 1971.
5 "Social Services," *InDecatur*, March 11, 1977.
6 "Patient Representatives Liaison Between DMC and Patients," *InDecatur*, April, 1991.
7 "Social Services."
8 "Patient Representatives Liaison Between DMC and Patients."
9 "DeKalb Stroke Club Observes 5th Anniversary," *InDecatur*, December 24, 1981; Mike Tu, "Survivor: A Story of Hope," DeKalb Medical Center—News & Media, http://www.dekalbmedicalcenter.org/shownews.asp?id =912.
10 "Stroke Club Donates Equipment," *InDecatur*, April 26, 1984; "DGH Stroke Club Donates Equipment," *InDecatur*, January 1987.
11 Mike Tu.
12 "New Benefit: Employee Assistance," *InDecatur*, June 26, 1980; "About Your Employee Assistance Program (E.A.P.): A Program of Georgia Behavioral Care, Inc.," Abou-EAP.doc, November 29, 2005, http://intranet2.drhs.drhs.org/index.cfm?p=msp&pg_8597; "Employee Assistance Program Offers Confidential Counseling," *InDecatur*, January 21, 1982.
13 Paula Simon Eissner interview, April 27, 2007.
14 "Medical Management Refocuses Patient Care," *InDecatur*, July 1997.
15 "Medical Management is Not Case Management," *InDecatur*, October 2003.
16 "Today Marks the Name Change — CASE Management Is Now CARE Management," *DatelineDeKalb E-Digest*, January 21, 2008.
17 *InDecatur*, May 1997.
18 *InDecatur*, January 1999.
19 *InDecatur*, August 2000.
20 "Medical Management is Not Case Management."
21 "A Call to Service," news story, http://dekalbmedical.org/NewsMedia/ViewAllNewsStories/tabid/74/Default.aspx?aid-430; Paul Olander interview July 10, 2008.
22 "About Care Management," DeKalb Medical – Intranet, http://intranet.drhs.org/dept/insex.cfm?p= dept_page&dept_id=187.
23 Olander interview.
24 Olander interview.
25 Olander interview.
26 Olander interview.
27 Olander interview.
28 Olander interview.

Surgical Services

1 Atkins, Earnest C., MD, lecture "The History of DeKalb Medical Center."
2 Minutes, Professional Services Committee, DeKalb County Hospital Authority, April 12, 1971.
3 *The General InDecatur*, December 8, 1961.
4 Duane Blair, MD, interview, December 9, 2008.
5 *The General InDecatur*, May 15, 1970.
6 *InDecatur*, September 1990.
7 "Health," *DeKalb Extra*, May 20, 1982.
8 "ASC Offers Quality Care, Convenience and Lower Cost," *InDecatur*, May 24, 1984.
9 "Authority Approves Surgery Center Project," *InDecatur*, December 1990.
10 "DMC Wins Approval to Build New Surgical and Obstetrical Center," *InDecatur*, February 1992.
11 "New Women's and Surgery Center Tower at DMC Central Opens for Patients," *Communiqué: A Newsletter for the Medical Staff of DeKalb Medical Center*, April 2007, p. 1.
12 "New Procedure," *InDecatur*, May 26, 1983; "DeKalb General to Offer Laser Lithotripsy," DeKalb General Hospital press release, 1988.
13 "DeKalb General to Offer Laser Lithotripsy;" "Hospital Acquires New Surgical Laser," *InDecatur*, January 1990.
14 "Laser," Wikipedia, the free encyclopedia, http://en.eikipedia.org/wiki/Laser, October 16, 2008.
15 "Hospital Acquires New Surgical Laser."
16 "Urology: Cutting Edge Technique Freezes, Kills Cancer Cells," *DeKalb Medical Center Health Lines*, Summer 2004, p. 2.
17 "Neurosurgery: Kyphoplasty Heals Cracked

Vertebrae," *DeKalb Medical Center Health Lines*, Summer 2004, p. 2.

18 "Laser;" "Eye Surgery Innovations," *DeKalb Medical Center Health Lines*, Winter 2005, p. 14.

19 "DMC Designated as 'Center of Excellence' Hospital Recognized for Weight Loss Surgery," DeKalb Medical Center — News & Media, May 2, 2007, http://www.dekalbmedicalcenter.org/shownews.asp?id=955.

20 Sood, Jayashree; Jayaraman, Lakshmi; and Kumra, V. P., "Endoscopic Surgery—Anaesthetic Challenges—a Historical Review," *Indian Journal of Anaesthesia*, Vol. 50 (3), June 2006, pp. 178-182.

21 Jayashree et al.

22 Lamaro, Vincent P., "Gynaecological Endoscopic Surgery—Past, Present and Future," *St. Vincent's Clinic Proceedings*, Vol. 12 (1), September 2004, pp. 23-29.

23 Jayashree et al.

24 Ballantyne, Garth H., "Minimally Invasive Surgery for Diseases of the Colon and Rectum: the Legacy of an Ancient Tradition," *The History of Laparoscopic Colectomy*, Churchill & Livingstone, New York, 1995, pp. 13-23, http://www.lapsurgery.com/history.htm, June 29, 2007.

25 Jayashree et al; Ballantyne; Daniel J. Riskin, Michael T. Longaker, Michael Gertner, and Thomas M. Kummel, "Innovations in Surgery: A Historical Perspective," *Annals of Surgery*, Vol. 244 (5), November 2006, pp. 686-693.

26 Ballantyne.

27 Wolfgang Wayand, "The History of Minimally Invasive Surgery," Business Briefing: Global Surgery, 2004, pp.37-38.

28 Doug Isenberg, "DeKalb Medical A Cut Above," Business Atlanta, January 1993, pp. 32 ff.

29 "DeKalb Medical Center Uses Laser Technology to Remove Gallbladders," *InDecatur*, March 1990.

30 "Not Your Mother's Hysterectomy: New Procedure Shortens Recovery and Reduces Patients' Pain," DeKalb Medical news release, January 23, 2007.

31 "New Lease On Life," DeKalb Medical press release, May 14, 2008.

32 Bill Hendrick, "State-of-the-Art Surgery: Delicate procedures done by remote control with da Vinci machine," *The Atlanta Journal-Constitution*, August 27, 2008.

33 Susan Bales Harris interview, June 30, 2008.

34 Harris interview.

35 Harris interview.

36 Harris interview; "Alert: More Details About the NICU, 2200 and 2300 Areas," *dateline DeKalb E-Digest*, June 16, 2008, DeKalb Medical Intranet, http://intranet.drhs.drhs.org.

Wellness Center

1 "DeKalb General First in Southeast With Women's Center," *InDecatur*, October 1985.

2 "New Wellness Center Urges Women to Take Time to Take Care," *Women's Wellness Center At DeKalb General*.

3 "DeKalb General First In Southeast With Women's Center," *InDecatur*, October 1985.

4 "A Wellness Center for Women," *Health In General*, Winter, 1986, p. 1.

5 "A Wellness Center for Women."

6 "New Wellness Center Builds on Healthy Tradition," *Health Lines*, Spring 1996, p. 6; "Step Up To A Better Workout Experience," *Health Lines*, Winter 2005, p. 6.

7 Holly Wolfe, "History and Overview of the Wellness Center," prepared for Dr. Earnest Atkins; "DeKalb General First in Southeast With Women's Center."

8 "A Wellness Center for Women."

9 "DeKalb General Opens Women's Wellness Center," *InDecatur*, February 1985.

10 Holly Wolfe.

11 :Employee Wellness Program Announced," *InDecatur*, July 1988.

12 "New Wellness Center Builds on Healthy Tradition."

13 "New Wellness Center Builds on Healthy Tradition;" "DeKalb General First in Southeast With Women's Center."

14 "Integrating Mind, Body and Spirit," Health Lines, Winter 2000, p.6; "Your Guide to Health and Well-being With Help From DeKalb Medical Center," *Healthy Living*, Fall 2007.

15 "DMC Wellness Center Recognized as Top Fitness Center," Press Release, February 26, 2007, http://www.dekalbmedicalcenter.org/shownews.asp?id=932.

16 "DMC Kicks Off Fitness Challenge," *InDecatur*, August 2005; "It's a Way of Life: Fitness Challenge 2005-2006," DeKalb Medical Center Intranet, http://intranet2.drhs.drhs.org/dept/index. . .8533.

17 "DMC Fitness Challenge Makes Strides for Better Employee Health," *InDecatur*, July 2004.

18 "Winston Named Director of Health Promotion," *InDecatur*, November-December 2003.

Women's and Infants' Services

1 "Gifts Welcome First Baby At Hospital," *The DeKalb New Era*, May 8, 1961.

2 Mary Chambers, RN, interview, January 24, 2006.

3 DeKalb General Hospital note associated with picture of Stacy Stull and parents, May 8, 1961.

4 Minutes, DeKalb Medical Center, Inc. Board of Directors, December 3, 2001.

5 Jimmy and Rosalyn Carter letter to John R. Gerlach, August 3, 1999; "DMC Welcomes Carter Grandson," *InDecatur*, September 1999.

6 "Parents of First Twins Born at DMC Visit Hospital," *InDecatur*, September 2004.

7 "Triplets Born at DeKalb General," *The General InDecatur*, June 3, 1975.

8 "Quadruplets Born at DGH," *InDecatur*, November 1985.

9 "DMC Delivers Miracle Baby," *InDecatur*, March 2000; "DeKalb Medical Center Has Become a Regional Referral Center for High-Risk Mothers," DeKalb Medical Center Health Lines, Summer 2004, p. 8.

10 Gary Hendricks, "Woman in Coma Delivers Baby," *The Atlanta Journal-Constitution*, March 31, 2003; Paula Eissner, memorandum, May 5, 2007.

11 Andria Simmons, "Families Chafe at Physicians' Power to Give Up Life Support: Courts Left to Decide Who Holds Patient's Fate," *The Atlanta Journal-Constitution*, February 10, 2008.

12 Virginia Anderson, "Love's Triumph," *The Atlanta Journal-Constitution*, November 25, 2004.

13 Andria Simmons.

14 Andria Simmons.

15 "OB/Delivery Holds Open House," *InDecatur*, April 17, 1983.

16 "DeKalb General's OB/GYN Services," *InDecatur*, September 29, 1983.

17 "Infant Hearing Testing at DeKalb General," *The General InDecatur*, October 11, 1974.

18 "Three DGH Nurseries Meet Special Needs," *InDecatur*, October 27, 1983.

19 Minutes, DeKalb County Hospital Authority, October 3, 1977; Minutes, DeKalb County Hospital Authority, April 3, 1978; "Neonatology Services Are Available Here," *InDecatur*, September 7, 1978.

20 "DeKalb Medical Center Acquires Second Neonatologist," *InDecatur*, May 1989.

21 Minutes, DeKalb Medical Center, Inc., Board of Directors, July 7, 1997.

22 Margie Hunter, RN, interview, June 30, 2008.

23 "Maternity Services," DeKalb Medical Center - Maternity, http://www.dekalbmedicalcenter.

org/maternity/maternity_services.asp; "Sneak a Peek in the New NICU," *datelineDeKalb–Digest*, August 4, 2008.

24 "DeKalb General's OB/GYN Services," *InDecatur*, September 29, 1983.

25 Mary Chambers interview; "We're In the Movies," *InDecatur*, July 1987.

26 "Preconceptual Counseling Is DMC First," *InDecatur*, June 1991; "Healthy Living," Summer 2007.

27 "Vorce Elected President of the Southeastern Lactation Consultants Association," *InDecatur*, August 1992.

28 Margie Hunter interview.

29 *InDecatur*, March 2003.

30 "Perinatal Bereavement Performance Improvement," *InDecatur*, November–December 2003.

31 Minutes, DeKalb County Hospital Authority, November 15, 1990.

32 "New Programs and Services Deliver High-Quality Care," *InDecatur*, May 1992; "DMC's Perinatology Services Expanded," *InDecatur*, April 1993.

33 "DMC's Perinatology Services Expanded."

34 Minutes, DeKalb Medical Center, Inc. Board of Directors, February 1, 1993.

35 Dottie W. Roach, Director, State Health Planning Agency, letter to Charles B. Eberhart, Administrator, February 20, 1992; "DMC Wins Approval to Build New Surgical and Obstetrical Center," *InDecatur*, February 1992.

36 "Maternity Center Renovation Underway," *InDecatur*, August 2003; "Maternity Center Renovation Complete," *InDecatur*, January–February 2004; "Maternity Program Enjoys Rebirth of Services, Facilities," *InDecatur*, May 1999.

37 Margie Hunter interview.

38 Paul C. Brown, MD, letter to the Board of Directors, DeKalb Regional Health Care System, December 2, 2002; Minutes, DeKalb Medical Center, Inc. Board of Directors, December 3, 2001; Minutes, DeKalb Regional Healthcare System, Inc. Board of Directors, August 7, 2000.

39 Minutes, DeKalb Regional Healthcare System, Inc. Board of Directors, July 7, 2003; Minutes, DeKalb County Hospital Authority, November 8, 2005; Minutes, DeKalb County Hospital Authority, October 26, 2004; Minutes, DeKalb County Hospital Authority, April 26, 2005.

40 "Patient Tower Comes to Life at DMC Central," dateline DeKalb, January 2006; "The Women's Center at DeKalb Medical Center (North Decatur Campus), DeKalb Medical Center—Maternity, http://www.dekalbmedicalcenter.org/maternity/facilities.asp, April 24, 1007.

Index

C

D

E

F

G

H

I

J

K

L

M

N

O

P

Q

R

S

X

Y

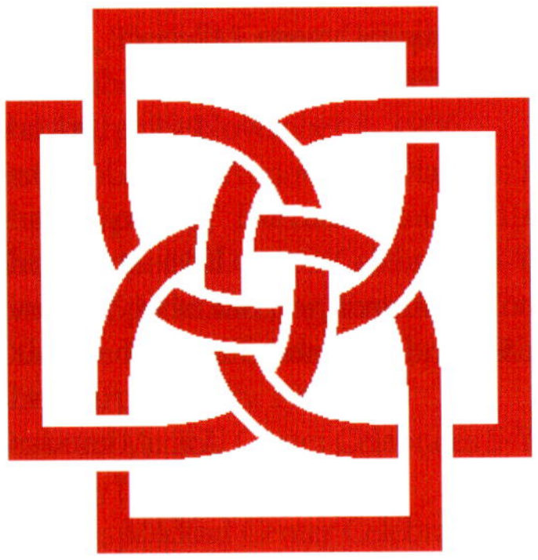

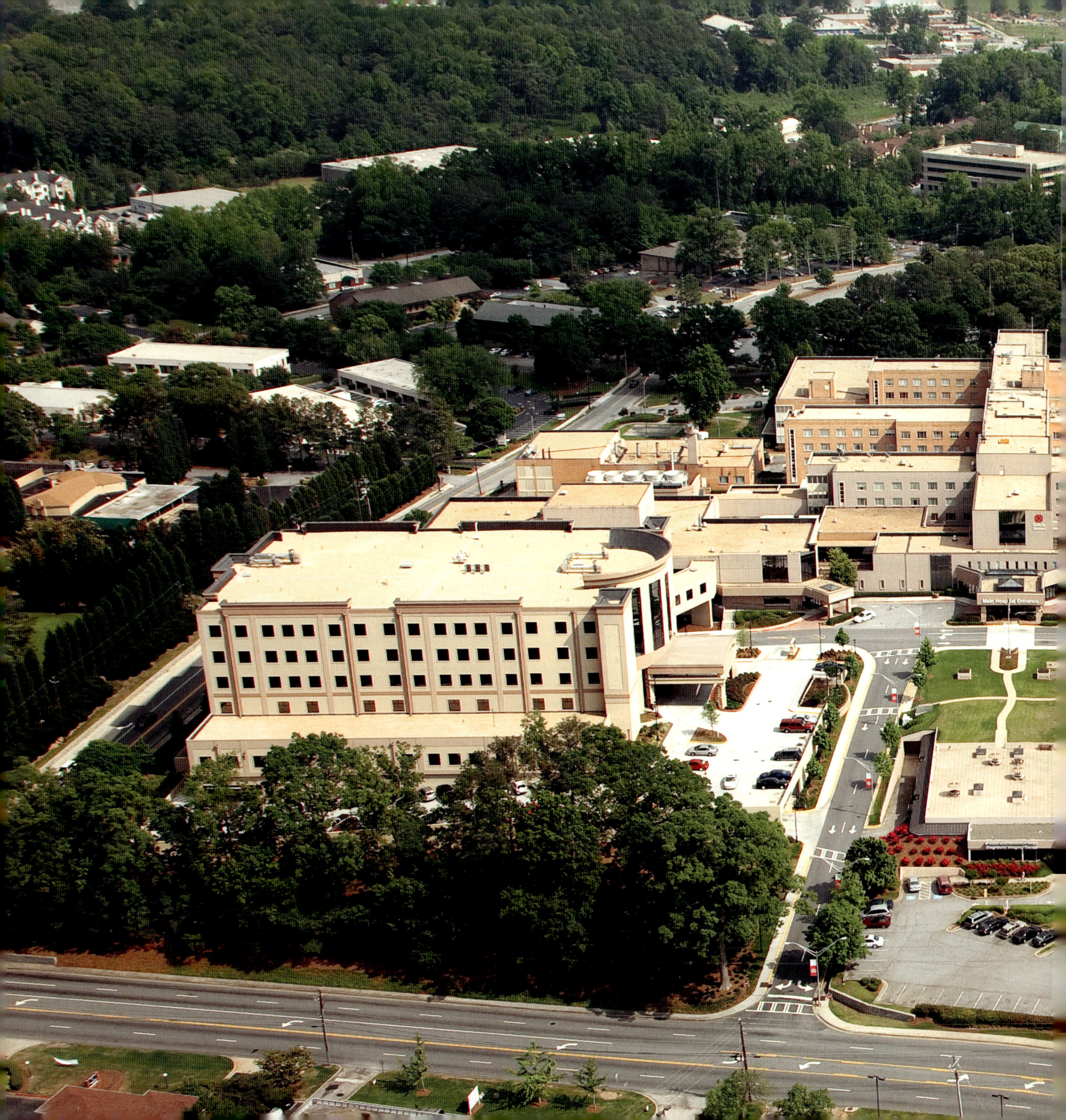
Main Hospital Entrance